D1408625

VITAMIN ANALYSIS
for the HEALTH and
FOOD SCIENCES

VITAMIN ANALYSIS
for the HEALTH and
FOOD SCIENCES

Ronald R. Eitenmiller
W.O. Landen, Jr.

Department of Food Science and Technology
University of Georgia

CRC Press
Boca Raton London New York Washington, D.C.

Library of Congress Cataloging-in-Publication Data

Eitenmiller, Ronald R. (Ronald Ray), 1944–
    Vitamin analysis for the health and food sciences / Ronald R.
Eitenmiller and W.O. Landen, Jr. ; illustrations by Toni Kathryn
White.
        p. cm.
    Includes bibliographical references and index.
    ISBN 0-8493-2668-0 (alk. paper)
    1. Vitamins--Analysis. I. Landen, W. O. II. Title.
QP771.E37 1998
612.3′99—dc21   98-21970
                                                                                              CIP

© 1999 by CRC Press LLC
Illustrated By: Kathy White and Gene Wright

No claim to original U.S. Government works
International Standard Book Number 0-8493-2668-0
Library of Congress Card Number 98-21970
Printed in the United States of America 1 2 3 4 5 6 7 8 9 0
Printed on acid-free paper

Preface

During our careers at the University of Georgia and with the U.S. Food and Drug Administration, we have been privileged to experience and participate in the rapid advance of vitamin assay methodology. From the early 1970s, our field progressed from reliance on techniques developed decades earlier to a degree of sophistication that few of us foresaw. Indeed, we clearly remember the effort required to obtain valid data on the vitamin content of the food supply using microbiological, thin-layer and open-column chromatographic, and spectrophotometric assays. We know that scientists investigating the vitamins in clinical samples had similar experiences. A great deal of discipline was required on the part of experienced analysts and graduate students to produce analytical values which, for the most part, have withstood the test of time when compared to values obtained with current, much improved, procedures.

Challenges we firmly appreciate are training of students and analysts in the proper application of the best vitamin assay methods, and the frequently required efforts to improve, develop, or adapt existing methods to meet specific analytical needs. This book was written as a source for these activities.

Our discussion on each vitamin includes a review section aimed at providing individuals who have not studied the vitamins in-depth an appreciation of the uniqueness of the vitamin and how it participates in metabolism. This section has purposefully been kept brief. However, the references provided can be highly useful for those seeking additional information.

We strongly feel that individuals involved in the analysis of any analyte must have a basic understanding of the chemistry of the compound. Therefore, chemistry and nomenclature of each vitamin is discussed. The information might be considered inadequate by the research biochemist or analytical chemist involved in basic studies on a specific vitamin; however, our goal was to produce a usable source for analysts at the bench and not to write a multi-volume treatise. Extensive information is given in tabular form on spectral properties. Such data is routinely required on a day-to-day basis at the bench. Additionally, stability properties of the vitamins are discussed. Stability considerations can be easily disregarded or forgotten during routine analysis or during method development if the chemist is not thoroughly aware of the specific properties of the vitamin that affect stability. If this happens, extensive efforts can be negated when the oversight is recognized.

In the method section of each chapter, our purpose was two-fold. First, we felt that attention needed to be given to commonly used and available handbook, compendium, and regulatory methods. These accepted procedures are in use world-wide and, from a regulatory standpoint, maintain significant status. A summary table is provided covering many of these sources. Additionally, several of the AOAC International Methods are discussed in detail. Secondly, our primary objective was to give an interpretive review of the development of advanced methods of vitamin analysis in sufficient detail to be valuable as a methodology guide.

When analysis programs are being initiated, much effort can be saved in making correct decisions about analytical approach if the analyst has a thorough grasp of research leading to available methods. For the vitamins for which high-performance liquid chromatography (HPLC) is the best approach, detailed tables are presented describing historically significant method development advances that led the way to current methods as well as significant publications which appeared in the 1990s. References used for tabular information are provided separately from text references to ease the reader's ability to quickly find the cited bibliographic information. It is evident for each vitamin that the efforts of a few research groups have driven the field to its current capability to accurately assay the vitamin. We hope that our discussion has given the credit where it is due. At the same time, the literature is voluminous and expanding extremely rapidly. It was impossible to cite all efforts playing a role in vitamin assay. If this book can lead those endeavoring to initiate a vitamin analysis program to the right groups of investigators producing the current advances, then, we have accomplished our purpose to provide a usable source for today's vitamin chemist.

Ronald R. Eitenmiller
W. O. Landen, Jr.

Authors

Dr. Ronald R. Eitenmiller is Professor of Food Biochemistry, Department of Food Science and Technology, University of Georgia. He has published widely on food composition, methods of vitamin analysis, and improvement of nutritional quality. Dr. Eitenmiller is a Fellow of the Institute of Food Technologists. He is Science Advisor to the U.S. Food and Drug Administration at the Southeastern Regional Laboratory, Atlanta Center for Nutrient Analysis. He has consulted in numerous countries on fortification, nutritional quality, and methods of vitamin analysis. Dr. Eitenmiller currently serves as Chair of the Expert Panel on Food Safety and Nutrition, Institute of Food Technologists. He is a member of the FANSA Task Force on Vitamin E.

W. O. Landen, Jr., is a research scientist at the Department of Food Science and Technology, Food Process Research and Development Laboratory, University of Georgia, Athens, Georgia. Current research centers on the improvement of methods for fat- and water-soluble vitamins in foods. He has published widely throughout his career. Mr. Landen retired from the U.S. Food and Drug Administration in 1995 after 33 years service to the FDA. He was a Research Supervisory Chemist with the Atlanta Center for Nutrient Analysis. His work with FDA was recognized by ten outstanding or special performance awards. He currently serves on the AOAC International Methods Committee on Food and Nutrition. Past service to AOAC International included membership on the AOAC-NLEA Task Force on Nutrient Analysis Methods.

Contents

Abbreviations

Acetic acid—HAC
Acetone—A
Acetonitrile—MeCN
Acyl—Carrier protein—ACP
Ammonium acetate—NH_4OAC
Angstrom—Å
Aquocobalamin—H_2OCbl
Association of Official
  Analytical Chemists—AOAC
Ascorbic acid—AA
Atlanta Center for Nutrient Analysis—ACNA

Benzenesulfonyl chloride—BSC
Butylated hydroxyanisole—BHA
Butylated hydroxytoluene—BHT
tert-Butylammonium hydroxide—TBAH
tert-Butyl methyl ether—TBME

Capillary electrophorosis—CE
Centimeter—cm
Cholecalciferol—Vitamin D_2
Chloroform—$CHCl_3$
Coefficient of variation—CV
Competitive protein bending assays—CPBA
Cyanocobalamin—Cbl

Dehydroascorbic Acid—DHAA
5′—Deoxyadenosyl cobalamin—AdoCbl
Detection limit—DL
2,6-Dichloroindophenol—DCIP
Dichloromethane—CH_2Cl_2
Diethyl ether—ET_2O
Diisopropylether—DIPE
Dimethylformamide—DMF
Dimethylsulfoxide—DMSO
2,4-Dinitrophenylhydrazine—DNPH
Dithiothreitol—DTT
Dodecyltrimethyl ammonium chloride—
  DTMAC

Electrochemical—EC
Electron impact—EI
Emission—Em
Enzyme-linked immunosorbent assay—ELISA
Enzyme protein binding assay—EPBA
Ergocalciferol—Vitamin D_2

Ethyl Acetate—EtOAC
Ethyl Alcohol—EtOH
Evaporative light scattering detector—ELSD
Excitation—Ex

Flame ionization detection—FID
Flavin adenine dinucleotide—FAD
Flavin mononucleotide—FMN
Fluorescein isothiocyanate—FITC
Formiminoglutamic acid—FIGLU

Gas liquid chromatography—GLC
Gram—g

Heptane—HEP
Hexadecyl trimethylammonium bromide—
  HDTMAB
Hexane—HEX
High performance-Gel permeation
Chromatography—HP-GPC
High performance liquid chromatography—
  HPLC
Hours—h
Hydrochloric acid—HCI
Hydroxycobalamin—OHCbl

Internal Standard—IS
International Unit—IU
Isoascorbic acid—IAA
Isooctane—iOCT
Isopropyl alcohol—IPA

Kilogram—kg

Liter—L
Liquid chromatography—LC

Mass spectrometry—MS
Menadione dimethyl pyrimidinol bisulfate—
  MPB
Menadione sodium bisulfate—MSB
Menadione sodium bisulfate complex—MSBC
Metaphosphoric acid—MPA
Methanol—MeOH
Methylcobalamin—MeCbl
Methyl-*tert*-butyl ether—MTBE

Microliter—μL

Micrograms—μg

Micrometer—μm

Milliliter—mL

Millimeter—mm

Millimole—mmol

Millimolar—m*M*

Millivolt—mV

Molar—*M*

Molar Absorptivity—ϵ

Nanometer—nm

Nanomole—nmol

National Institute of Standards and
Technology—NIST

Niacin equivalent—NE

Nicotinamide adenine dinucleotide—NAD

Nicotinamide adenine dinucleotide
Phosphate—NADP

Nitrocobalamin—NO_2Cbl

N-Methylnicotinamide—NMN

Normal—N

Normal Phase—NP

Nutritional Labeling and Education Act of
1990—NLEA

Octyldecylsilica—ODS

Orthophenyldiamine—OPD

P-Aminobenzoyl-glutamic acid—PABG

Parts per billion—PPB

Photodiode array—PDA

Picogram—pg

Platinum—Pt

2,2,5,7,8—Pentamethyl-6-hydroxy
chroman—PMC

Petroleum ether—PE

O-Phenylenediamine—OPD

Polyunsaturated fatty acid—PUFA

Prothrombin time—PT

Pyridoxamine—PM

Pyridoxamine-5′-Phosphate—PMP

Pyridoxal—PL

Pyridoxal-5′-phosphate—PLP

Pyridoxine (pyridoxol)—PN

Pyridoxine HC1—PN-HC1

Pyridoxine-5′-phosphate—PNP

Pyridoxine-glucoside—PN-glucoside

4-Pyridoxic acid—4-PA

Quantitation limit—QL

Racmic—RAC

Radial compression module—RCM

Radioimmunoassay—RIA

Radioreceptor assay—RRA

Recommended Dietary Allowance—RDA

Reference Daily Intake—RDI

Relative standard deviation—RSD

Retinol equivalent—RE

Reversed-phase—RP

Sodium acetate—NaOAC

Solid-phrase extraction—SPE

Specific extinction coefficient—$E_{1\ cm}^{1\%}$

Sulfitocobalamin—SO_3Cbl

Sulfosalicylic acid—SSA

Tetrabutylammonium phosphate—TBAP

Tetrabutylammonium hydrogen sulfate—
TBAHS

Tetrabutylammonium bromide—TBAB

Tetrahydrofuran—THF

Tetraoctylammonium bromide—TOAB

Thiachrome monophosphate—ThcMP

Thiachrome pyrophosphate—ThcPP

Thiachrome triphosphate—ThcTP

Thiamin monophosphate—TMP

Thiamin pyrophosphate—TPP

Thiamin triphosphate—TTP

Thin layer chromatography—TLC

Thymidylate—dTMP

α-Tocopherol—α-T

α-Tocotrienol—α-T3

β-Tocopherol—β-T

β-Tocotrienol—β-T3

γ-Tocopherol—γ-T

γ-Tocotrienol—γ-T3

δ-Tocopherol—δ-T

δ-Tocotrienol—δ-T3

Toluene—T

Tricarboxylic acid cycle—TCA cycle

Trichloroacetic acid—TCA

Triethylamine—TEA

Trimethyl-silyl—TMS

Ultraviolet—UV

United States Pharmacopeial Convention—
USP

Volts—V

Wavelength—λ

Fat-Soluble Vitamins

1 Vitamin A and Carotenoids

1.1 REVIEW

The relationship of night blindness to a dietary deficiency was recognized as early as 1500 B.C.[1] In 1913, McCollum and Davis reported the presence of a lipid-like substance in butter and egg yolk necessary for growth in rats. In 1916, the substance was named fat-soluble A. McCollum related fat-soluble A deficiency to xerophthalmia in children in the following year, providing the first indication of the diverse functionality of the vitamin. The name, vitamin A, was first used in 1920 to signify the early discovery of the growth factor and to differentiate it from water-soluble vitamins, collectively called vitamin B at that time. The structure of vitamin A was determined in 1931. The vitamin A activity of β-carotene was demonstrated in 1929. The term "provitamin A" is accepted to differentiate carotenoid precursors of vitamin A from carotenoids without vitamin A activity. Plant carotenoids are, therefore, the precursor of vitamin A found in the animal kingdom. Dietary vitamin A is designated preformed vitamin A when consumed as a dietary constituent of animal products.

Vitamin A deficiency is characterized by changes in the tissue of the eye that ultimately result in irreversible blindness. Clinical symptoms are collectively referred to as xerophthalmia[2] and include the following:

1. Night blindness—the inability to see in dim light
2. Conjunctival and corneal xerosis
3. Keratomalacia—ulceration and scarring of the cornea that leads to loss of vision

Other symptoms include skin lesions, loss of appetite, epithelial keratinization, lack of growth and increased susceptibility to infections.[2,3,4] Human status assessment methods include dietary assessment, content of liver, plasma and breast milk, and functional assessment by dark adaptation and conjunctival impression cytology.[4] Biochemical tests include the relative dose response test (RDR) and the modified relative dose response test (MRDR) that estimate liver stores of vitamin A. Such tests are useful to assess marginal vitamin A deficiency.[5] Toxicity can occur due to high intake from either foods high in vitamin A or high potency supplements.

Dietary sources of vitamin A include organ meats (the liver contains the highest amount), fish oils, butter, eggs, whole milk and fortified low fat milk, other dairy products, and fish (particularly fish with higher fat content like tuna and sardines). Margarine, fluid milk, and dry milk are typically fortified with retinyl palmitate in many countries. These products play a dramatic role in preventing vitamin A deficiency in countries where fortification is mandatory. In the United States, milk is fortified with not less than 2000 IU of vitamin A (retinyl palmitate). Margarine is fortified with not less than 15,000 IU per pound (retinyl palmitate and β-carotene).[6]

Provitamin A carotenoids are found throughout the plant kingdom. Food sources include carrots, dark-green leafy vegetables, and various fruits. Because of the complexity of the carotenoid profiles of fruits and vegetables, color cannot be used to predict the vitamin A activity of the food. Lycopene is frequently used to demonstrate this point. The red color of ripe tomatoes is primarily due to this carotenoid which possesses no vitamin A activity. Thus, most tomato cultivators are quite low in vitamin A activity. Approximately 75% of the vitamin A in the United States diet is derived from retinol and 25% from provitamin A carotenoids.[7] A USDA-NCI database containing compositional information on α-carotene, β-carotene, β-cryptoxanthin, lutein plus zeaxanthin, and lycopene has been compiled for over 2400 fruits, vegetables, and foods containing fruits and vegetables.[8,9,10] This database provides a valuable tool for determining dietary intake of the carotenoids.[11]

The biological activity of vitamin A is quantified by conversion of the vitamin A active components to retinol equivalents (RE). One RE is defined as 1 µg of retinol. For calculation of RE values in foods, 100% efficiency of absorption of retinol is assumed. Incomplete absorption and conversion of β-carotene is taken into account by the relationship of 1 RE = 6 µg of β-carotene. Other provitamin A active carotenoids have approximately 50% of the biological activity of β-carotene. The conversion factor is, therefore, 1 RE = 12 µg of other provitamin A carotenoids.[2] The Recommended Dietary Allowance (RDA) is 1000 RE for adult men and 800 RE for adult women. No increase in intake is recommended during pregnancy; however, the RDA is increased by 500 RE during the first six months of lactation and by 400 RE during the second six months of lactation.[2]

International units (IU) are defined by the relationship of 1 IU = 0.3 µg of all-*trans*-retinol or 0.6 µg of β-carotene. Therefore, 1 RE is equal to 3.33 IU based on retinol. RE and IU designations are both used to define vitamin A activity; however, usage of RE is preferred. Original studies that estimated the vitamin A activity of various carotenoids and defined IUs did not account for absorption and bioavailability differences compared to all-*trans* retinol.[2] International Units are commonly used for labeling of pharmaceuticals and foods. The Reference Daily Intake (RDI) set by the Nutritional Labeling and Education Act of 1990 (NLEA) is 5000 IU.[12]

Functional roles of vitamin A continue to be identified as knowledge of its participation in cell growth and differentiation expands. Well-known functions include the visual cycle, effects on immune response, and embryonic development. Steps in the visual cycle include isomerization to 11-*cis* retinol, transport by the interphotoreceptor-binding protein to the rod outer segment, enzymatic conversion to 11-*cis* retinal, and formation of rhodopsin from opsin and 11-*cis* retinal.[7] Specific sites of vitamin A action in immune response include action of T-helper and natural killer cells.

Identification of two families of nuclear receptors, RAR and RXR, led to a clearer understanding of the role of vitamin A in cell differentiation. RAR receptors bind with all-*trans* or 9-*cis* retinoic acid, and the RAX receptors bind only with 9-*cis* retinoic acid, functioning in gene expression. Pleiotrophic effects are highly varied and include the following:

1. Development of pancreatic α and β cells[13]
2. Up regulation of insulin production[14]
3. Up regulation of the genes for vitamin A transport proteins[15]
4. Down regulation of ornithine decarboxylase gene expression[16]
5. Increased insulin stimulated glucose transport and GLUT 4 mRNA in L6 muscle cells[17]

With the expanding knowledge of the diverse functions of vitamin A, its role in child health and well being becomes even more critical. Vitamin A deficiency continues to be the primary cause of blindness and chronic disease in young children in areas where dietary supply is insufficient. Fortification programs provide adequate vitamin A in supplementary form to large segments of the world's population. However, such programs need to be developed to counteract the significant public health impacts where nutritional deficiency still exists. The role of the food industry and public health organizations in this regard can still dramatically improve nutrition worldwide.

1.2 PROPERTIES

1.2.1 CHEMISTRY

1.2.1.1 General Properties

1.2.1.1.1 Vitamin A

The structure of all-*trans* retinol (vitamin A) is given in Figure 1-1. Vitamin A refers to all isoprenoid compounds from animal products that possess the biological activity of all-*trans* retinol. The retinol

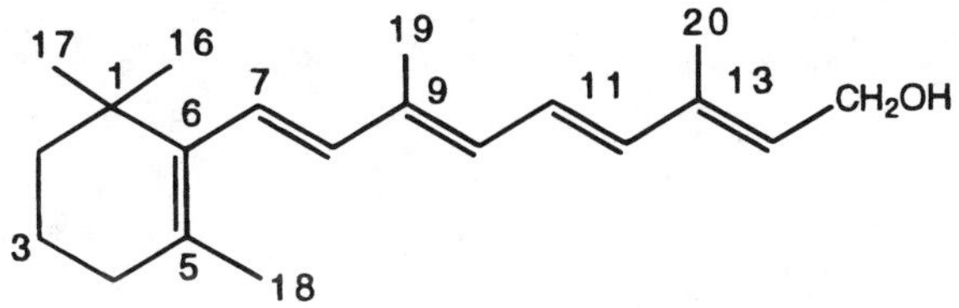

All-*trans*-retinol
vitamin A

FIGURE 1.1   Structure of all-*trans* retinol.

parent structure to most retinoids contains a substituted β-ionone ring (4-{2,6,6-trimethyl-2-cyclo-hexen-1-yl}-3-buten-2-one) with a side chain of three isoprenoid units linked at the 6-position of the β-ionone ring. The conjugated double-bond system includes the 5,6-β-ionone ring carbons and the isoprenoid side chain. Retinoids include all substances with vitamin A activity, some of which differ structurally from all-*trans*-retinol. Synthetic retinoids are increasingly being used for treatment of skin disorders such as acne and psoriasis. Effects of retinoids on cell differentiation will undoubtedly lead to many accepted therapeutic treatments that are now in the experimental stages. Such treatments include potential actions against various leukemias, malignancies, immunological abnormalities, and inflammatory conditions.

Important metabolites of all-*trans* retinol are shown in Figure 1-2. Oxidation of the alcohol moiety of all-*trans* retinol yields all-*trans* retinal. Further oxidation produces all-*trans* retinoic acid. In the visual cycle, all-*trans* retinol is isomerized to 11-*cis* retinol which is either converted to a retinyl ester or transported to the outer rod segment and oxidized to 11-*cis* retinal prior to combination with opsin to form rhodopsin.[18] Acetate and palmitate esters of all-*trans* retinol are the primary commercial forms of vitamin A available to the pharmaceutical and food industry. Esterification greatly stabilizes the vitamin toward oxidation. The USP standard for vitamin A is retinyl acetate. This standard reference material is stable and supplied in ampules to allow quick turn-over of the standard.

Physical properties of all-*trans* retinol and closely related retinoids are provided in Table 1.1. Vitamin A is water-insoluble and soluble in fats and oils, and most organic solvents.

1.2.1.1.2   Carotenoids

Over 600 carotenoids have been characterized. Nomenclature for the carotenoids specified by the International Union of Pure and Applied Chemistry (IUPAC) and the International Union of Biochemistry (IUB) was recently reviewed by Weedon and Moss.[19] The reader is urged to read this source for an easy-to-follow description of the nomenclature rules.

The structures are formed by the head-to-tail linkages of eight isoprene units to provide a C_{40} skeleton. Lycopene (Figure 1-3) shows the acyclic hydrocarbon backbone chain. This compound is regarded as the prototype of the family.[19] Structural modifications of lycopene lead to the diverse nature of the carotenoids present in the plant kingdom. β-carotene (Figure 1-3) is the most significant of the provitamin A carotenoids, characterized by the cyclicized β-ionone rings on both ends of the hydrocarbon chain. Structures of common carotenoids are shown in Figure 1-4. Addition of oxygenated functions to the molecule yields the xanthophylls. Oxygen functions include hydroxylation at the 3- or 4-position (lutein and β-cryptoxanthin) and ketolation (canthaxanthin) as well as formation of aldehydes, epoxy, carboxy, methoxy, and other oxygenated forms. Hydrocarbon carotenoids (lycopene, phytoene, and phytofluene), carotenal esters, and carotenol fatty acid esters are frequently found in plant materials.

Provitamin A active carotenoids include β-carotene, α-carotene, γ-carotene, and β-cryptoxanthin. *Cis*-isomers are less active than the all-*trans* naturally occurring carotenoids. Biological

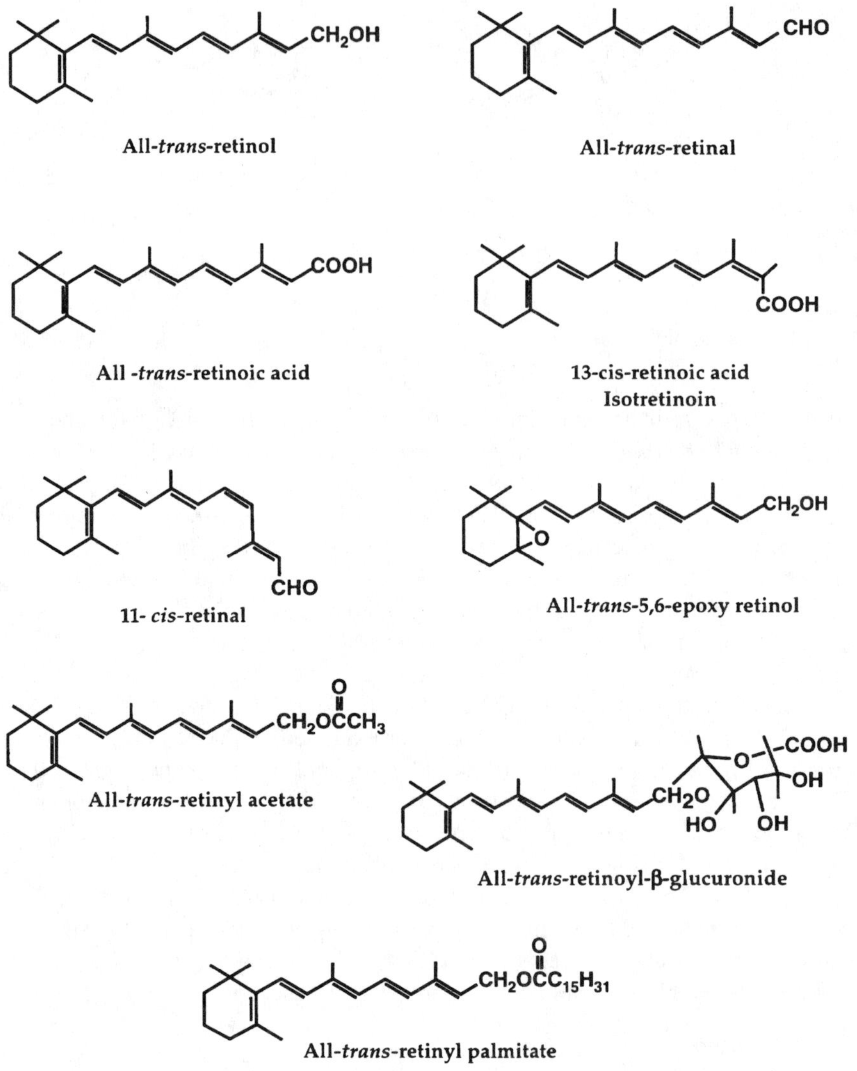

CH2OH
All-*trans*-retinol
CHO
All-*trans*-retinal
COOH
All -*trans*-retinoic acid
COOH
13-cis-retinoic acid
Isotretinoin
CHO
11- *cis*-retinal
CH2OH
O
All-*trans*-5,6-epoxy retinol
O
CH2OCCH3
All-*trans*-retinyl acetate
COOH
O
OH
CH2O
HO
OH
All-*trans*-retinoyl-β-glucuronide
O
CH2OCC15H31
All-*trans*-retinyl palmitate

FIGURE 1.2 Structures of vitamin A metabolites and esters.

activity depends on the presence of one, non-hydroxylated β-ionone ring in the provitamin A carotenoid structure. Thus, acyclic hydrocarbon carotenoids such as lycopene do not possess vitamin A activity. Compounds that have one hydroxylated ring (β-cryptoxanthin) have approximately 50% of the biological activity of β-carotene. Hydroxylation of both β-ionone rings (lutein) leads to complete inactivity from a vitamin A functional standpoint. Conversion of provitamin A carotenoids to retinol is believed to occur through central and eccentric cleavage. Oxidative central cleavage at the 15,15′ double bond yields two moles of retinol per mole of β-carotene. Eccentric or random cleavage provides only one to two moles of retinol per mole of β-carotene, depending on the cleavage sites.[20] Bioavailability is influenced greatly by absorption properties of the carotenoids, vitamin A status, metabolic digestive disorders, the food matrix, and level of fat in the meal. Certain dietary components including fiber may interfere with absorption.[21] A comparison of relative biological activities for various retinoids and carotenoids is shown in Table 1.2.

Physical properties of several carotenoids are given in Table 1.3. β-carotene and β-apo-8′-carotenal are important pigments added to margarine, salad dressings, and many other products to

TABLE 1.1
Physical Properties of Retinol and Other Retinoids

Substance[a]	Molar Mass	Formula	Solubility	Melting Point °C	Crystal Form	UV Absorption[b]			Fluorescence[c]	
						λ max nm	$E_{1cm}^{1\%}$	$\varepsilon \times 10^{-3}$	Ex nm	Em nm
all-*trans*-retinol CAS No. 68-26-8 **10150**	286.46	$C_{20}H_{30}O$	Soluble in absolute alcohol, methanol, chloroform, ether, fats, oils	**62–64**	Yellow prisms	325 **325**	1845 **1810**	**[52.8]** **[51.8]**	**325**	470
13-*cis*-retinol 11-*cis*-retinol	286.46 286.46	$C_{20}H_{30}O$ $C_{20}H_{30}O$		58–60		328 319 **318**	1689 1220 **1200**	[48.3] [34.9] **[34.3]**		
all-*trans*-retinyl acetate CAS No. 127-47-9 **10150**	328.50	$C_{22}H_{32}O_2$		57–58	Pale yellow prismatic	325 **325**	1560 **1590**	[51.2] **[52.2]**	325	470
all-*trans*-retinyl palmitate CAS No. 79-81-2 **10150**	524.88	$C_{36}H_{60}O_2$		28–29	Amorphous or crystalline	325	940	[49.3]	325	470
all-*trans*-retinal CAS No. 116-31-4 **8331**	284.44	$C_{20}H_{28}O$	Soluble in ethanol, chloroform, cyclo-hexane, petroleum ether, oils	61–64 (*trans*) 63.5–64.4 (11-*cis*)	Orange crystals	383 **368**	1510 **1690**	[42.9] **[48.0]**		
13-*cis*-retinal	284.44	$C_{20}H_{28}O$				375 **363**	1250 **1365**	[35.5] **[38.8]**		
11-*cis*-retinal	284.44	$C_{20}H_{28}O$		63.5–64.4	Orange prisms	380 **365**	878 **928**	[24.9] **[26.4]**		

TABLE 1.1 Continued

Substance[a]	Molar Mass	Formula	Solubility	Melting Point °C	Crystal Form	UV Absorption[b]			Fluorescence[c]	
						λ max nm	$E_{1cm}^{1\%}$	$\varepsilon \times 10^{-3}$	Ex nm	Em nm
all-*trans*-retinoic acid CAS No. 302-79-4 **8333**	300.44	$C_{20}H_{28}O_2$		180–182	Crystals	350	[1510]	45.3		
13-*cis*-retinoic acid CAS No. 4759-48-2 **8333**	300.44	$C_{20}H_{28}O_2$		174–175	Reddish-orange plates	354	[1325]	39.8		

[a] Common or generic name; CAS No.—Chemical Abstract Service number, bold print designates the Merck Index monograph number.
[b] In ethanol; bold values in hexane; values in brackets are calculated from corresponding ε or $E_{1cm}^{1\%}$ values.
[c] In isopropanol.

Budavari, S., *The Merck Index*.[1]
Furr, H. C. et al., *Modern Chromatographic Analysis of Vitamins*.[2]
Furr, H. C. et al., *The Retinoids, Biology, Chemistry and Medicine*.[3]
Olson, J. A., *Handbook of Vitamins*.[4]

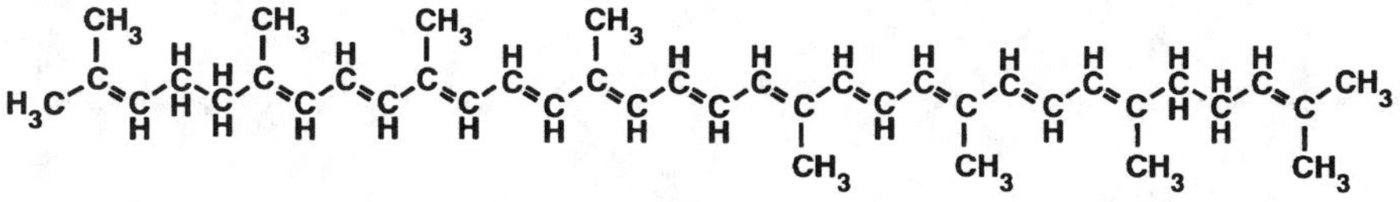

Lycopene

Acyclic $C_{40}H_{56}$ Hydrocarbon

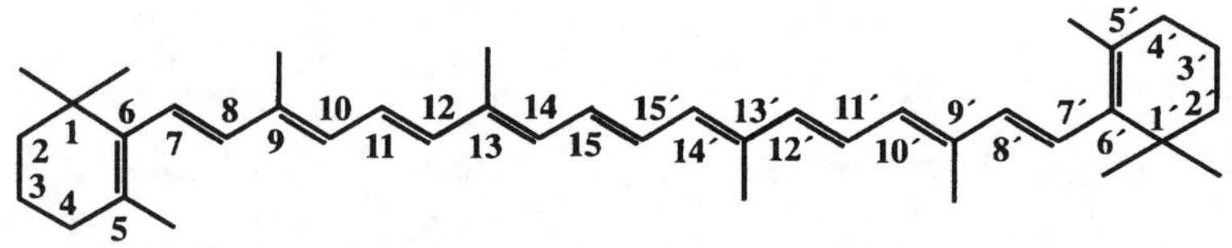

β,β-carotene

β-carotene

FIGURE 1.3   Structures of β-carotene and lycopene.

enhance color. When used in this respect, the provitamin A carotenoids can provide significant vitamin A activity to the food. In the poultry industry, xanthophyll concentrates derived from various natural products including the marigold are widely used feed ingredients that enhance yellow to red pigmentation in poultry skin and egg yolks. Vitamin A activity of the products is not affected since the xanthophylls in such concentrates lack vitamin A activity.

TABLE 1.2
Relative Biological Activity of Retinoids and Carotenoids

Compound	Relative Activity (%)
all-*trans*-retinol	100
all-*trans* retinal	100
cis-retinol isomers	23–75
Retinyl esters	10–100
β-carotene	50
α-carotene	26
γ-carotene	21
β-cryptoxanthin	28
Zeaxanthin	0
Lycopene	0
β-apo-8′-carotenal	18–36

Source: Reference 22

1.2.1.2   Spectral Properties

Retinoids possess strong UV absorption properties owing to the conjugated double bond system. UV absorption maxima vary as structural variations are introduced to the parent all-*trans* retinol. Structural variations in the large number of synthetic retinoids and effects on UV absorption were

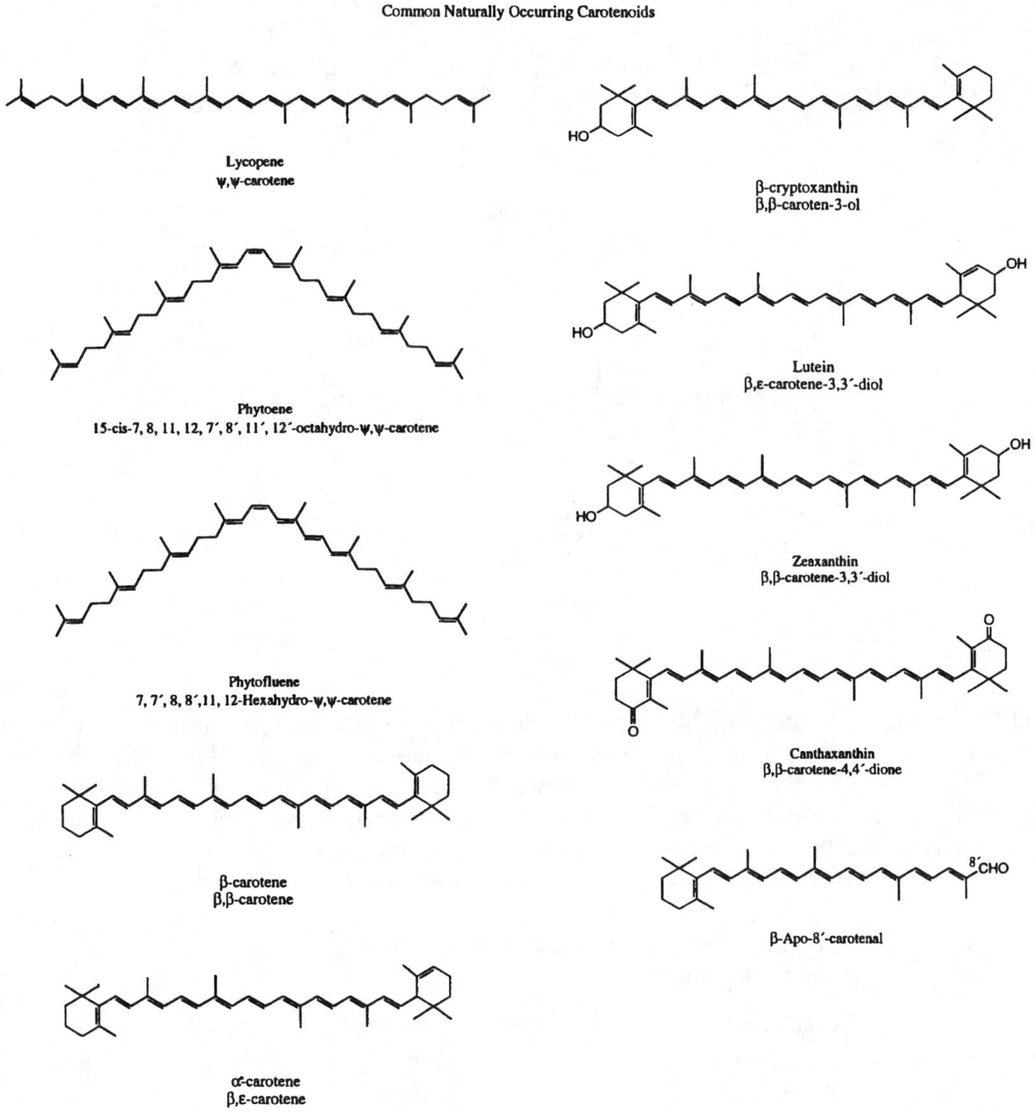

Common Naturally Occurring Carotenoids

Lycopene
ψ,ψ-carotene

β-cryptoxanthin
β,β-caroten-3-ol

Phytoene
15-cis-7, 8, 11, 12, 7′, 8′, 11′, 12′-octahydro-ψ,ψ-carotene

Lutein
β,ε-carotene-3,3′-diol

Zeaxanthin
β,β-carotene-3,3′-diol

Phytofluene
7, 7′, 8, 8′,11, 12-Hexahydro-ψ,ψ-carotene

Canthaxanthin
β,β-carotene-4,4′-dione

β-carotene
β,β-carotene

β-Apo-8′-carotenal

α-carotene
β,ε-carotene

FIGURE 1.4 Structures of commonly occurring carotenoids.

discussed by De Leenheer et al.[23] Maximal absorption occurs from 318 to greater than 360 nm
(Table 1.1). Absorption maxima vary depending on the solvent and the presence of *cis*-isomers (Z-).
Isomerization to the *cis*-form lowers the absorption maxima and $E_{1 \, cm}^{1\%}$ values relative to all-*trans*
retinol (Table 1.1).[24] The most common wavelength used for detection of all-*trans* retinol after
HPLC resolution is 325 nm. The UV spectra of all-*trans* retinol and its *cis*-isomers are provided in
Figure 1-5.[25]

Fluorescence provides an alternative to UV absorption as a detection mode for specific retinoids.
All-*trans* retinol and retinyl esters possess excellent fluorescence properties at Ex λ from 325 to 330
nm and Em λ of 470 to 490 nm.[26] Fluorescence intensity is greater in non-polar solvents, and normal phase systems with hexane based mobile phases offer ideal detector response conditions for use
of fluorescence compared to UV detection.[24] Most other retinoids other than retinol and its esters do
not fluoresce and oxidation of the alcohol results in loss of fluorescence; therefore, UV detection is
used for quantitation of many synthetic retinoids and retinoic acid.[23]

TABLE 1.3
Physical Properties of Selected Carotenoids

Substance[a]	Molar Mass	Formula	Solubility	Melting Point °C	Crystal Form	λ max	$E^{1\%}_{1\,cm}$	Absorbance[b] ε × 10⁻³	Solvent
Provitamin A Carotenoids									
β-carotene CAS NO. 7235-40-7 1902	536.88	$C_{40}H_{56}$	Soluble in CS_2, benzene, chloroform	183	Red rhombic square leaflets	425 453 479 452	— 2592 — 2505	— 139 — 134	Petroleum ether Cyclohexane Petroleum ether
α-carotene CAS No. 7488-99-5 1901	536.88	$C_{40}H_{56}$	Freely soluble in CS_2, chloroform; soluble in ether, benzene	187.5	deep purple prisms	422 444 474	— 2800 —	— 150 —	Petroleum ether
β-cryptoxanthin 2676	552.88	$C_{40}H_{56}O$	Freely soluble in chloroform, benzene, pyridine, CS_2	158–159 (racemic) 169 (natural)	Red plates with metallic luster	425 452 479 450	— 2386 — 2460	— 132 — 136	Petroleum ether Hexane
γ-carotene CAS No. 472-93-5 1903	536.88	$C_{40}H_{56}$	Somewhat less soluble than β-carotene	152–153.5 (synthetic) 177.5 (natural)	Red plates (synthetic) Deep-red prisms (natural)	437 462 494	2055 3100 2720	110 166 146	Petroleum ether
β-Apo-8'-carotenal CAS No. 1107-26-2	416.65	$C_{30}H_{40}O$	Freely soluble in chloroform; sparingly soluble in acetone	136–142 (decomp)	Powder with dark metallic sheen	457	2640	110	Petroleum ether

TABLE 1.3 Continued

Substance[a]	Molar Mass	Formula	Solubility	Melting Point °C	Crystal Form	Absorbance[b] λ max	$E_{1\ cm}^{1\%}$	$\varepsilon \times 10^{-3}$	Solvent
Other carotenoids									
Phytoene	544.95					275	—	—	Petroleum ether
						285	1250	68.1	
						296	—	—	
Phytofluene CAS No. 540-05-6 **7544**	542.93	$C_{40}H_{68}$	Freely soluble in petroleum ether, benzene; practically insoluble in H_2O, methanol, ethanol	B.P. 140–185	Pale orange viscous oil	286	915	49.8	Hexane
						331	—	—	Petroleum ether
						348	1350	73.3	
						367	—	—	
Lycopene CAS No. 502-65-8 **5650**	536.88	$C_{40}H_{56}$	Soluble in chloroform, benzene; insoluble in methanol, ethanol	172–173	Deep red needles	444	—	—	Petroleum ether
						472	3450	185	
						502	—	—	
Lutein CAS No. 127-40-2 **10197**	568.88	$C_{40}H_{56}O_2$	Soluble in fats and fat solvents	190	Yellow prisms with metallic luster	421	—	—	Petroleum ether
						445	2550	145	
						475	—	—	

Compound	Formula	MW	Solubility	MP (°C)	Appearance	λ			Solvent
Zeaxanthin CAS No. 144-68-3 **10248**	$C_{40}H_{56}O_2$	568.88	Slightly soluble in petroleum ether, ether, methanol; soluble in CS_2, benzene, chloroform, pyridine, ethyl acetate	215.5	Yellow rhombic plates with steel-blue metallic luster	426 452 479 450	— 2348 — 2540	— 133 — 144	Petroleum ether
Canthaxanthin	$C_{40}H_{52}O_2$	564.85	Soluble in chloroform, oil; very slightly soluble in acetone	207–217 (decomp)	Violet	466	2200	124	Petroleum ether
Violaxanthin CAS No. 126-29-4	$C_{40}H_{56}O_4$	600.88	Soluble in alcohol, methanol, ether; almost insoluble in petroleum ether	200	Orange prisms	420 443 470 440	— 2550 — 2550	— 153 — 153	Ethanol Hexane
Neoxanthin		600.88				416 439 467 438	— 2243 — 2470	— 135 — 148	Ethanol Hexane

TABLE 1.3 Continued

Substance[a]	Molar Mass	Formula	Solubility	Melting Point °C	Crystal Form	Absorbance[b]			Solvent
						λ max	$E_{1\,cm}^{1\%}$	$\varepsilon \times 10^{-3}$	
Astaxanthin CAS No. 472-61-7 **890**	596.85	$C_{40}H_{52}O_4$		182–183	Needles	472	2135	124	Petroleum ether

[a] Common or generic name; CAS No—Chemical Abstract Service number; bold print designates the Merck Index monograph number.

Bauernfeind, J.C., *Carotenoids as Colorants and Vitamin A Precursors, Technological and Nutritional Applications.*[1]
Budavari, S., *The Merck Index.*[2]
Britton, G. et al., *Carotenoids, Spectroscopy.*[3]
Committee on Food Chemicals Codex, *Food Chemicals Codex.*[4]
Friedrich, W., *Vitamins.*[5]
Furr, H.C. et al., *Modern Chromatographic Analysis of Vitamins.*[6]

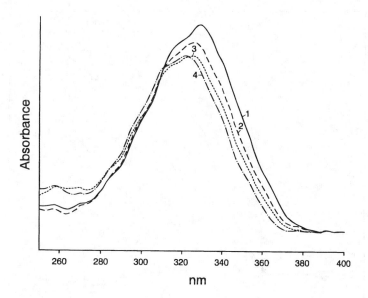

FIGURE 1.5 Spectra of retinol isomers. 1 = 13-*cis*-retinol, 2 = all-*trans* retinol, 3 5 9,13-di-*cis*-retinol, 4 = 9-*cis*-retinol. Reproduced with permission from Reference 25.

The varied and bright pigmentation of the carotenoids results from the strong primary absorption in the visible region resulting from the long conjugated double bond system. A characteristic UV absorption peak occurs in *cis*-isomers approximately 142 nm below the longest-wavelength absorption maxima of the all-*trans* carotenoid.[27] The characteristic strong absorption between 400 to 500 nm is universally used for detection after HPLC resolution. Published absorbance parameters for common carotenoids are given in Table 1.3. Spectra commonly show two to three maxima in the visible range. The UV maximum in *cis*-isomers typically occurs between 330 to 340 nm with a downward wavelength shift of the entire spectra.[23,27] Characteristic spectra of β-carotene are shown in Figure 1-6.[27]

Absorption intensity is affected by the solvent or mobile phase composition carrying the carotenoid.[28,29] Recently published absorption maxima and the solvent and/or mobile phase are given in Table 1.4 and Table 1.5.

1.2.2 STABILITY

Several excellent reviews exist on the stability of all-*trans* retinol and the carotenoids. Particularly useful reviews to the analyst include those by Ball[26] and Schiedt and Liaaen-Jensen.[31] Similar chemical properties of the vitamin A retinoids and provitamin A carotenoids contribute to common problems encountered during analytical determination. These include instability when isolated from the biological matrix, susceptibility to isomerization to *cis*-isomers with lower biological activity, and different absorption properties, and susceptibility to oxidation. Owing to the general lack of stability, artifacts formed during sample storage, extraction, and analysis can make analytical results difficult to interpret and even meaningless.

Schiedt and Liaaen-Jensen[31] provided the following general precautions necessary to minimize carotenoid changes throughout the analysis:

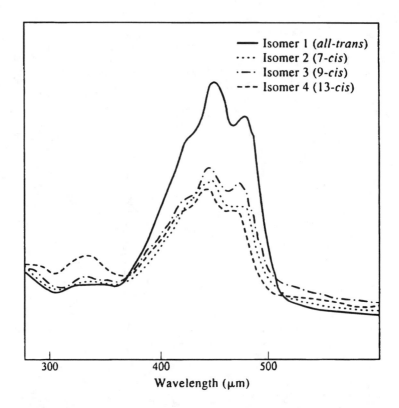

FIGURE 1.6   Spectra of β-carotene isomers. 1 = all-*trans*-β-carotene, 2 = 7-*cis*-β-carotene, 3 = 9-*cis*-β-carotene, 4 = 13-*cis*-β-carotene. Reproduced with permission from Reference 28.

1. Exclude oxygen; air should be replaced by vacuum or inert gas.
2. Addition of antioxidants such as butylated hydroxytoluene (BHT), pyrogallol, or ascorbyl palmitate are necessary prior to saponification. Low levels of antioxidants in extracting solutions and mobile phases are often added to protect the retinoids and carotenoids from oxidation.
3. *Trans*-to-*cis*-isomerization (E/Z) is promoted at higher temperatures. Therefore, use of the lowest practical temperature is recommended, and use of solvents with low boiling points are preferred. For rotary evaporation, 40°C should not be exceeded. Solutions should be stored at −20°C and preferably at lower temperature.
4. All sunlight should be avoided. Analytical steps should be completed in dim light, diffused sunlight, or under gold fluorescent light. Solutions should be stored in low actinic glassware whenever possible. Isomerization rapidly occurs through light activation and is a common source of *cis*-isomer formation in biological sample extracts.
5. Acid must be avoided. All solvents must be acid free. Addition of triethylamine (TEA) at 0.001% is useful to neutralize low acid levels occurring in some solvents.
6. Alkaline conditions can lead to base-catalyzed isomerization.

E/Z isomerization is difficult to completely avoid during sample handling and determinative analysis. Additionally, 5,6-epoxides readily rearrange to the 5,8-epoxide in the presence of acids.[31] Conversion of all-*trans* retinol to *cis*-isomers is higher in chlorinated solvents compared to nonchlorinated solvents.[32] Iron and copper supplementation of foods can increase the rate of isomerization.[32] Studies by Landers and Olson[33] showed that retinol and retinyl palmitate were isomerized much less extensively in hexane solution compared to chloroform or methylene chloride when

TABLE 1.4
Comparison of λ Maxima for Carotenoids Showing Solvent Effects

Carotenoid	λ max (nm)	
	MTBE in Methanol[a]	Petroleum Ether[b]
β-carotene		
all-trans	450	453
9-cis	444	—
13-cis	443	—
α-carotene		
all-trans	444	444
9-cis	441	—
13-cis	438	—
zeaxanthin		
all-trans	450	450
9-cis	446	—
13-cis	443	—
lutein		
all-trans	442	445
9-cis	438	—
13-cis	435	—
β-cryptoxanthin		
all-trans	449	452
9-cis	444	—
13-cis	442	—

[a] Mobile phase consisted of 5 to 38% methyl-tert-butyl ether (MTBE) in methanol. Adapted from Reference 29.

[b] See Table 1.3.

exposed to white light. Isomers included 13-cis, 11-cis, 9-cis, and 7-cis in order of decreasing amounts. Gold light exposure did not produce isomerization. Gold lighting by the Sylvania F40/GO gold fluorescent light or equivalent is considered essential for laboratories routinely involved in vitamin A or carotenoid assay.

Peng et al.[34] studied the stability of all-trans retinol in plasma. Their data showed that blood could be stored on ice in the dark for at least 24 h prior to separation of the plasma. Plasma could be stored up to 1 year at −20°C or lower without loss of vitamin A activity. Scita[35] showed β-carotene to be fairly stable over 24 h when micellar solutions in aqueous medium were held at 37°C in the dark in a 5% CO_2 and air atmosphere. Exposure to UV light and fluorescent light was highly degradative. The addition of BHT or α-tocopherol at 1 mM concentrations significantly reduced the loss of β-carotene. α-Tocopherol was approximately three times as effective as BHT in slowing oxidation. BHT (0.025%) did not prevent slow β-carotene loss under storage at −20°C in the dark under nitrogen. Rates of loss were 1.5% per month and 1.1% per month in the absence or presence of the antioxidant.

TABLE 1.5
Absorption Maxima of α-Carotene Isomers in Pure Organic Solvents[a]

Isomer	Absorption Maxima[b]	
	Hexane	*Petroleum ether*
all-*trans*	267, nd, 421, (445), 474	267, 328, 420, (443), 472
13-*cis*	267, 331, 415, (438), 465	271, 329, 413, (436), 463
13'-*cis*	270, 330, 415, (437), 465	268, 330, 413, (435), 463
9-*cis*	258, 330, 417, (440), 469	255, 328, 416, (439), 467
9'-*cis*	258, 328, 418, (441), 469	258, 328, 415, (439), 467
	MTBE	*Ethanol*
all-*trans*	268, nd, nd, (445), 474	267, nd, nd, (447), 474
13-*cis*	270, 331, nd, (438), 466	267, 331, nd, (439), 466
13'-*cis*	269, 331, nd, (438), 465	269, 331, nd, (438), 465
9-*cis*	259, 329, 420, (442), 470	258, 331, 420, (442), 470
9'-*cis*	266, 329, 420, (442), 470	259, 328, nd, (442), 470
	Dichloromethane	*Acetone[c]*
all-*trans*	271, nd, 432, (456), 484	330, nd, (448), 476
13-*cis*	273, 337, 428, (449), 476	332, nd, (440), 468
13'-*cis*	272, 337, 424, (448), 475	332, nd, (440), 467
9-*cis*	261, 339, 428, (450), 479	332, nd, (443), 471
9'-*cis*	262, 336, 429, (452), 480	332, nd, (444), 472

[a] Table adapted from Reference 30.

[b] Units are nm. Values in parentheses are the primary λ max. The nd designation indicates that no maximum was detected.

[c] Absorbance at ≤ 330 nm interfered with the detection of the overtone (~265 mn).

Many studies exist in the literature on the stability of all-*trans* retinol and β-carotene in foods during processing and storage. Conversely, little information exists on the stability of other carotenoids such as lycopene. This is largely the result of difficulties that still exist in most laboratories to accurately assess carotenoid profiles and changes in all-*trans*-isomers to multiple *cis*-isomeric forms. One of the best reviews on all-*trans* retinol and β-carotene stability in foods was presented by Ball,[26] and the reader is urged to access this reference for specific literature references. Of significance, the following observations are evident in the published studies on the stability of all-*trans* retinol, provitamin A active carotenoids, and other carotenoids in food:

1. Conversion of all-*trans* isomers to *cis*-isomers occurs easily. Light, acids, metals, lipoxygenase, and heat processing, acting independently or sometimes synergistically, can produce rapid isomerization.
2. All-*trans* retinol and the carotenoids are oxidatively unstable. The presence of autoxidizing lipid systems can lead to rapid loss of vitamin A activity. Some carotenoids are active singlet oxygen quenchers. This ability is directly related to the number of double bonds in the conjugated double bond system. β-carotene, lutein, and other carotenoids preferentially react with singlet oxygen with conversion to triplet state forms.[36] The excited triplet state carotenoid thermally disperses the excess excited state energy through a chemical reaction that destroys the carotenoid.[37] Degradation products include various cleavage products.

In addition to singlet oxygen quenching, carotenoids scavenge free radicals at low oxygen pressures of less than 155 mmHg and act as primary chain-breaking antioxidants. In this capacity, the primary mode of β-carotene is through trapping of peroxyl radicals. Mechanisms include addition of the radical at the 5,6-double bond of the carotenoid with formation of epoxides.[37]

3. All-*trans* retinol and the carotenoids become more unstable as the food matrix is disrupted or the compounds are removed from the matrix by extractions prior to analytic quantitation. Destruction of the sample matrix can liberate lipoxygenases that catalyze isomerization.

4. Blanching of plant products prior to freezing inactivates lipoxygenase and removes oxygen from the tissue. Thus, carotenoids are protected from oxidative degradation during freezer storage.

5. Air drying or freeze drying can lead to large losses in all-*trans* retinol or the carotenoids. Storage of freeze-dried material, because of the open, porous nature of the product, requires removal of oxygen with inert gas flushing or vacuum to stabilize the vitamin A activity. Losses can be considerable during the drying process. The analyst should avoid dehydration of the sample, if possible. Low temperature freezing of samples in evacuated, light protected containers is preferable.

6. All-*trans* retinol and the carotenoids are relatively stable at alkaline pH. Therefore, saponification can be used for sample extraction if the saponification vessel is evacuated and protected from light. Ambient temperature saponification is often used to slow isomerization reactions that are more predominant at elevated temperatures.

7. All-*trans* retinyl palmitate and all-*trans* retinyl acetate are the common commercial forms of vitamin A used for food fortification and by the pharmaceutical industry. The ester forms are more stable to oxidation. However, isomerization can readily occur. Most HPLC procedures will resolve the all-*trans* from the *cis*-isomers which is essential to accurately assess biological activity. Encapsulation of commercial preparations inhibits oxidation and isomerization. Antioxidants including tocopherols and other free radical interceptors are usually added to vitamin A concentrates to inhibit oxidation.

1.3 METHODS

Methodology for analysis of vitamin A and the carotenoids includes colorimetric, spectrophotometric, fluorometric, paper, open-column and thin-layer chromatography, HPLC, and capillary electrophoresis. NMR and mass spectrometry are often coupled with HPLC purification for characterization and identification studies. Because of the large number of investigators involved in retinoid and carotenoid research, many excellent method reviews exist. Selected reviews on retinoid assay were written by Wyss,[38,39] Bhat and Sundaresan,[40] De Leenheer et al.[23] and Furr et al.[41] Methodology reviews on the retinoids and carotenoids include Parrish et al.,[42] Lambert et al.,[43] Thompson,[44] Ball,[26] Tee and Lim,[45] Furr et al.,[24] and Eitenmiller and Landen.[46] Those specific for carotenoid analysis include Rodriguez-Amaya,[47,48] Craft,[49] De Leenheer et al.,[50] Tsukida,[51] Khachik et al.,[52] and O'Neil and Schartz[53] Table 1.6 summarizes various compendium and handbook methods. Methods specific for retinol or its esters are often based on spectrophotometry. Erroneous results are common unless material under analysis is a relatively concentrated source of all-*trans* retinol or its esters. Carotenoids from fruits and vegetables or from mixed foods should be assayed by liquid chromatography (LC) methodology. Other methods for food analysis are often subject to overestimation of the vitamin A activity because biologically inactive carotenoids are difficult to completely remove from the provitamin A carotenoids by open-column chromatography employed in the colorimetric or spectrophotometric methods.

TABLE 1.6
Compendium, Regulatory, and Handbook Methods for Analysis of Vitamin A and Carotenoids

Source	Form	Methods and Application	Approach	Most Current Cross-Reference
U.S. Pharmacopeia National Formulary, 1995 USP 23/NF 18, Nutritional Supplements Official Monograph[1]				
1. pages 2138, 2140	Retinol Retinyl acetate Retinyl palmitate β-carotene	Vitamin A in oil-soluble vitamin Capsules/tablets	HPLC, retinol 325 nm Spectrophotometric, β-Carotene 452 nm	None
2. pages 2142, 2143, 2146, 2150	Retinol Retinyl acetate Retinyl palmitate β-carotene	Vitamin A in oil- and water-soluble Vitamin capsules/tablets with/without Minerals	HPLC, retinol 325 nm Spectrophotometric, β-carotene 452 nm	None
3. pages 185–186	β-carotene	β-carotene capsules	Spectrophotometric 452 nm	None
4. pages 1630–1631	Retinol Retinyl acetate Retinyl palmitate	Vitamin A (NLT 95.0% of label claim)	Spectrophotometric 325 nm	None
5. page 1631	Retinol Retinyl acetate Retinyl palmitate	Vitamin A capsules	Spectrophotometric 325 nm	None
British Pharmacopoeia, 15th ed., 1993[2]				
1. pages 702–703	Natural retinyl esters	Vitamin A ester (natural)	Spectrophotometric 326 nm	None
2. pages 703–704	Retinol acetate Retinyl palmitate Retinyl propionate	Synthetic Vitamin A concentrate (oily form)	Spectrophotometric 325 nm	None
3. page 704	Retinol acetate Retinyl palmitate Retinyl propionate	Synthetic vitamin A concentrate (powder form)	Spectrophotometric 326 nm	None

	Analyte	Sample/Method	Technique	Reference
4. page 704	Retinol acetate Retinyl palmitate Retinyl propionate	Synthetic vitamin A concentrate (water dispersible form)	Spectrophotometric 326 nm	None

AOAC Official Methods of Analysis, 16th ed.,[3] 1995

	Analyte	Sample/Method	Technique	Reference
1. 45.1.01	Retinol	AOAC Official Method 960.45 Vitamin A in margarine (surplus 1980)	Spectrophotometric	
2. 50.1.02	Retinol	AOAC Official Method 985.30 Vitamin A in milk-based infant formula	HPLC 340 nm	J. AOAC Int., 76, 398, 1993[4]
3. 50.1.03	Retinol	AOAC Official Method 992.04 Vitamin A in milk-based infant formula	HPLC 325 nm	
4. 45.1.02	Retinol β-Carotene	AOAC Official Method 974.29 Vitamin A in mixed feed, premixes and feeds Carr-Price	Colorimetric 620 nm-Retinol 440 nm-β-carotene	
5. 45.1.03	β-Carotene	AOAC Official Method 941.15 Carotene in fresh plant materials and silage (Not applicable to samples containing α-carotene, γ-carotene, zea-carotene, cryptoxanthin, and xanthophyll)	Spectrophotometric 436 nm	J. Assoc. Off. Anal. Chem., 53, 181, 1970[5]
6. 45.1.04	Carotene Xanthophylls	AOAC Official Method 970.64 Carotene and xanthophylls in dried plant materials and mixed feeds	Spectrophotometric 436 nm	J. Assoc. Off. Anal. Chem., 57, 511, 1974[6]

American Feed Ingredients Association, Laboratory Methods Compendium, vol. 1, 1991[7]

	Analyte	Sample/Method	Technique	Reference
1. pages 117–120	Retinol	Vitamin A in feeds, premixes, and vitamin concentrates (>1000 IU/kg)	HPLC 326 nm or Fluorescence Ex λ = 325 Em λ = 480	Hoffmann-LaRoche, Analytical Methods for Analysis of Vitamins and Carotenoids in Feed, 1988, 5[8]
2. pages 121–124	Retinol	Vitamin A in dry feeds (<10,000 IU/lb)	Colorimetric 610 nm	None
3. pages 125–126	Retinol	Vitamin A in feeds	Colorimetric 620 nm	None
4. pages 127–129	Retinol	Vitamin A in feeds, supplements, premixes (>1000 IU/kg)	HPLC 326 nm	None

TABLE 1.6 Continued

Source	Form	Methods and Application	Approach	Most Current Cross-Reference
5. pages 131–134	Retinol	Vitamin A in feeds, premixes, and concentrates (10,000–500,000 IU/lb)	Colorimetric 610 nm	None
6. pages 135–137	Retinol	Vitamin A in premixes (250–5000 IU/g)	HPLC 325 nm	None
7. pages 139–141	Retinol	Vitamin A in premixes and vitamin mineral compounds (200–250,000 IU/g)	Spectrophotometric 325 nm	None
American Association of Cereal Chemists, *Approved Methods*, vol. 2, 1996[9]				
1. AACC 86-01 A	Retinol	Vitamin A in dry vitamin mixes, beadlets, oils and emulsions (>10,000 IU/g)	Spectrophotometric 325 nm	None
2. AACC 86-02	Retinol	Vitamin A in nonfat and instantized dry milks	Colorimetric 620 nm	None
3. AACC 83-03	Retinol	Vitamin A in enriched flour (free of carotenes)	Colorimetric 620 nm	None
4. AACC 86-05	Retinol Carotene	Vitamin A and carotene in enriched cereals and mixed feeds	Colorimetric 620 nm (retinol) Spectrophotometric 440 nm (carotene)	*J. Assoc. Off. Anal. Chem.,* 41, 593, 1958[10]
Hoffmann-LaRoche, *Analytical Methods for Vitamins and Carotenoids in Feed*, 1988[8]				
1. pages 5–7	Retinyl esters as retinol	Determination of vitamin A in complete feeds, premixes, and vitamin concentrates (>1000 IU/kg)	HPLC, 326 nm or fluorescence Ex λ = 325 Em λ = 480	None
2. pages 53–55	Ethyl 8′apo-β-caroten-8′oate	Determination of Stabilized, added apocarotenoic ester in complete feeds and Premixes with HPLC (>1 mg/kg)	HPLC 443 nm	None
3. pages 56–58	Ethyl 8′apo β-caroten-8′oate, β-carotene	Determination of added apocarotenoic Ester and β-carotene in complete feeds and various carotenoid blends by open-column chromatography on aluminum oxide (>5 mg/kg)	Spectrophotometric 456 nm (β-carotene) 446 nm (ethyl 8′-apo-β-caroten-8′-oate)	*Z. Lebensm. Unters.-Forsch.,* 163, 21, 1977[11]

4. pages 59–62	Astaxanthin	Determination of stabilized, added astaxanthin in fish feeds and premixes with HPLC (>1 mg/kg)	HPLC 470 nm	None
5. pages 62–64	Astaxanthin	Determination of stabilized astaxanthin in fish feeds by open-column chromatography on silica gel (20–200 mg/kg)	Spectrophotometric 472 nm	None
6. pages 65–67	Canthaxanthin	Determination of stabilized, added Canthaxanthin in complete feeds and Premixes with HPLC (>1 mg/kg)	HPLC 466 nm	None
7. pages 68–71	Canthaxanthin	Determination of added canthaxanthin in complete feeds and premixes by manual procedures (>1 mg/kg)	Spectrophotometric 470 nm	Z. Lebensm. Unters.-Forsch. 163, 21, 1977[11]
8. pages 72–74	β-Carotene	Determination of stabilized, added β-carotene in complete feeds and premixes with HPLC (>1 mg/kg)	HPLC 450 nm	None
9. pages 75–76	α-, β-, γ-Carotene calculated as β-Carotene	Determination of natural carotene in complete feeds and raw materials by open-column chromatography or aluminum oxide (1–200 mg/kg)	Spectrophotometric 456 nm	None
10. pages 77–78	β-Carotene	Determination of added, stabilized β-carotene in premixes by spectrophotometry (1000–2000 mg/kg)	Spectrophotometric 454 nm	None
11. pages 79–82	Paprika pigments	Determination of paprika pigments in complete feeds and various xanthophyll blends (>1 mg/kg)	Spectrophotometric 450 nm or HPLC 450 nm	Acta Aliment. 11, 309, 1982[12]
12. pages 83–85	Xanthophylls Lutein Zeaxanthin	Determination of xanthophylls, lutein and zeaxanthin in complete feeds and xanthophyll blends with HPLC (>1 mg/kg)	HPLC 450 nm	None
13. pages 86–89	Xanthophylls Lutein Zeaxanthin	Determination of total xanthophylls, lutein and zeaxanthin in complete feeds and various xanthophyll blends by manual procedures (> 1 mg/kg)	Spectrophotometric 450 nm	Z. Lebensm. Unters.-Forsch. 163, 21, 1977[11]

TABLE 1.6 Continued

Source	Form	Methods and Application	Approach	Most Current Cross-Reference
Food Chemicals Codex, 4th ed., 1996[13]				
1. page 90	β-carotene	1. β-carotene (NLT 96.0%, NMT 101.0%)	Spectrophotometric 455 nm	None
2. pages 429–430	Retinol Retinyl acetate Retinyl palmitate	Vitamin A (NLT 95.0%, NMT 100.5% of the declared vitamin A activity)	HPLC 325 nm	None
Methods for the Determination of Vitamin in Foods, COST 91, 1985[14]				
1. page 23	Retinol	Vitamin A in food saponification	HPLC 325 nm	*J. Assoc. Off. Anal. Chem.*, 66, 746, 1983[15]
2. page 33	Total carotenes	Complex foods, fruits and vegetables, beverages, saponification, aluminum oxide clean up	Spectrophotometric 450 nm	*Z. Lebensm. Unters.- Forsch.*, 163, 21, 1977[11]

1.3.1 THE CARR-PRICE COLORIMETRIC METHOD

The most widely used assay for vitamin A until the advent of LC analysis in the 1970s was the Carr-Price colorimetric procedure. Methodology is given in AOAC Official Method 974.29 (45.1.02) "Vitamin A in Mixed Feeds, Premixes, and Foods, Colorimetric Method."[54] The chemistry is based on the formation of a blue complex between antimony trichloride or trifluoroacetic acid with retinol in chloroform which is measured at 620 nm. The method is still used throughout the world, but should be replaced by LC methods in all situations unless instrumentation is not available to change to LC analysis. Often-mentioned deficiencies of the Carr-Price method include lack of specificity, unstable color that requires rapid and time-consistent measurement, and the use of corrosive and carcinogenic reagents. Procedural steps must be carefully controlled throughout the assay. Problems with the Carr-Price method were recently discussed in detail by Thiex et al.[55] Because of the practicality of their treatment detailing sources of errors in the assay, and their applicability to vitamin A assays in general, the Thiex et al.[55] summary is provided.

Systematic Errors Producing a Positive Bias

1. Presence of high levels of carotenoids or other interfering substances such as phenothiazine, ethoxyquin, or Rabon
2. Solids remaining after hydrolysis that affect dilution volume
3. Less than complete recovery of standard at the partitioning step
4. Excessive standing of the standard solution in hexane after partitioning and before partitioning
5. Failure to remove standard from the evaporator immediately after hexane removal
6. Moisture in cuvettes
7. Cloudy solutions in cuvette
8. Use of degraded standard

Systematic Errors Producing a Negative Bias

1. Sample abuse including undue storage before analysis and exposure to heat, light, and oxidants
2. Grinding of mineral mix samples
3. Failure to completely solubilize vitamin during saponification
4. Failure to add antioxidant or stabilizer during hydrolysis
5. Failure to keep sample dispersed during hydrolysis
6. Use of old potassium hydroxide solution for saponification
7. Failure to use low actinic glassware and/or subdued lighting
8. Incomplete partitioning of retinol from the hydrolyzate
9. Inclusion of sodium sulfate or other particulates from digest when removing aliquotes
10. Poor-quality hexane
11. Failure to remove sample residue from the evaporator immediately after hexane evaporation
12. Moisture in pipettes or cuvettes
13. Standard concentration actually higher than the value used in calculation

Random Errors Producing Poor Precision

1. Lack of sample homogeneity
2. Failure to properly reduce samples
3. Too small sample size
4. Use of a single standard reading from a single day to make calculations
5. Use of an unstable spectrophotometer or detector

AOAC Method 974.29 permits use of trifluoroacetic acid in place of antimony trichloride. Thiex et al.[55] report that trifluoroacetic acid is easier to use, less corrosive, and provides a more stable color compared to antimony trichloride.

1.3.2   High Performance Liquid Chromatography

For routine assessment of vitamin A activity and for characterization of retinoids and carotenoids in biological samples, LC resolution is clearly the analyst's best analytical technique. Obvious advantages of LC over older approaches are the abilities to resolve *cis*-isomers from all-*trans* retinol and all-*trans* carotenoids, to resolve provitamin A carotenoids from complex carotenoid mixtures, and to use LC resolution as a preparatory step for characterization studies. Many of the reviews cited in Section 1.3 provide excellent overviews of LC applications, and Tables 1.7 and 1.8 provide details of analysis of different biological matrices. It is important to note that these references were selected from many excellent sources published over the last decade. Because of its accepted role as the primary analytical tool for retinoid and carotenoid analysis, the remainder of this chapter concentrates on LC analysis.

1.3.2.1   Extraction Procedures for the Analysis of Retinoids and Carotenoids by Liquid Chromatography

Saponification and direct solvent extraction are commonly used to extract retinoids and carotenoids from biological samples. When applicable, direct solvent extraction is preferable to saponification because of time, lower solvent costs, and a better ability to avoid formation of artifacts in the extract. Artifact formation from the relatively unstable analytes (Section 1.2.2) can lead to underestimation of vitamin A activity, poor chromatographic resolution, and greater possibility of peak misidentification. It should always be kept in mind that all-*trans* retinol and all-*trans*-carotenoids are more subject to degradation by isomerization and oxidation as the sample matrix is destroyed and the retinoids and carotenoids are extracted into the partitioning solvent.

1.3.2.1.1   Saponification

Saponification is routinely used to extract retinol from tissues and animal based foods and carotenoids from fruits, vegetables, and prepared foods. These matrices are often difficult to extract efficiently by direct solvent extraction owing to the inability of the solvent system to effectively penetrate the sample matrix, or the need to use excessive solvent volumes to achieve satisfactory recovery of the analytes. Saponification parameters are discussed in detail for vitamin E analysis (Chapter 3). Issues relevant to the use of saponification for extraction of vitamin E apply to the extraction of retinol and the carotenoids. Details of several applications of saponification for retinol and carotenoid extraction are given in Table 1.9.

Saponification destroys lipids, chlorophyll, and other materials in the sample that potentially would interfere with chromatographic separations. Partitioning of the analytes into the organic phase can be problematic and the behavior of various partitioning solvents can be difficult to predict with complex sample digests. Following hydrolysis, the digest is diluted with water or salt solution to inhibit emulsion formation, and organic solvent is added to extract the non-saponifiable fraction. Solvents used include hexane, diethyl ether, 1:1 mixtures of hexane and diethyl ether, and hexane containing up to 15% acetonitrile. Hexane can be used as the extracting solvent, which decreases soap extraction that occurs with diethyl ether.[44] The effect of soaps on the partitioning of the saponified analytes from the aqueous phase to the organic phase must be controlled.

Thompson[44] relates use of hexane to low vitamin recoveries. In the digest, the ethanol-water-soap mixture tends to behave similarly to a hydrocarbon solvent, decreasing the affinity of the fat-soluble vitamins to the organic phase. High ingoing fat levels with increased soap formation can increase the effect with low analyte recoveries resulting. Thompson[44] stressed that the efficiency of

TABLE 1.7
HPLC Methods for the Analysis of Retinol and its Metabolites in Food, Feeds, Pharmaceuticals, and Biologicals

		Sample Preparation	HPLC Parameters				
	Analyte	Sample Extraction	Column	Mobile Phase	Detection	Quality Assurance Parameters	References
Food							
1. Dried skim milk	Retinol	Saponify, reflux 30 min; Extract with PE; Dilute with PE after addition of BHT; Evaporate aliquot to dryness; Dissolve residue in MeOH	C_8 or C_{18} 10 μm 25 cm × 4.6 mm	Isocratic MeOH : water (90 : 10) 2 mL/min	325 nm	—	*Int. Dairy Fed.* 285, 53, 1993[1]
2. Infant formula	Retinol	Saponify, ambient, 18 h; Extract with Hex : Et_2O (85 : 15); Centrifuge, reextract; Add hexadecane to extract; Evaporate aliquot; Dissolve residue in heptane	Apex silica 3 μm 15 cm × 4.5 mm	Isocratic Heptane : IPA Variable IPA (1–5%) 1–2 mL/min	324.5 nm	$S_r = 98.8$ $S_R = 265.4$ $RSD_r = 3.62$ $RSD_R = 9.72$	*J. Assoc. Off. Anal. Chem.* 76, 399, 1993[2]
3. Cheese	Retinol	Homogenize in water : EtOH : Hex (8 : 20 : 20) containing 2% BHT; Add water, centrifuge; Remove Hex layer; Dilute with Hex	LiChrosorb Si60 25 cm × 4.0 mm	Isocratic Hex : IPA (99.8 : 0.2) 2 mL/min	325 nm	% CV 2.6–8.8	*Die Nah.* 38, 527, 1994[3]
4. Milk	Retinol	Saponify, 70°C, 20 min; Extract with heptane : DIPE (3 : 1), reextract; inject extract	HS-5-Silica 12.5 cm × 4.0 mm	Isocratic Heptane : IPA (60 : 1) 1 mL/min	Fluorescence Ex λ = 344 Em λ = 472	QL <0.04 mg/L; % Recovery 98.5; % CV 3.6	*J. Dairy Res.* 61, 233, 1994[4]
5–6. Liver, liver products, infant foods	Retinol 7-cis-, 9-cis- 9,13-di-cis-	*Low fat samples* Homogenize liver and infant foods; Digest with pancreatin at pH 9.0	Spherisorb SW 3 mm 10 cm × 2.0 mm	Isocratic iOct : IPA (98.75 : 1.25)	Retinol 325 nm 13-cis-retinol	—	*Z. Lebensm. Unters-Forsch.*, 199, 206, 1994[5]

TABLE 1.7 Continued

Analyte	Sample Preparation — Sample Extraction	HPLC Parameters — Column	HPLC Parameters — Mobile Phase	HPLC Parameters — Detection	HPLC Parameters — Quality Assurance Parameters	References
13-*cis*-, 11,13-	Saponify, ambient, 16 h		0.4 mL/min	329 nm		*J. Chromatogr. A*, 693, 271, 1995[6]
di-*cis*-, 11-*cis*-	*High fat samples* Homogenize liver sausage with water : EtOH (1 : 1) Saponify, ambient, 16 h Dilute digest with water and EtOH to give 1 : 1 ratio Pass aliquot through Kieselguhr column Elute with PE Evaporate Dissolve residue in iOct					
Biologicals						
1. Blood Retinol Retinoic acid Retinoyl-β-glucuronide	Add EtOH and EtOAC Centrifuge, wash pellet with EtOAC Add water to supernatant to separate phases Add HAC to aqueous phase, reextract with EtOAC Wash pooled EtOAC extract Dry over Na$_2$SO$_4$ Evaporate under argon Dissolve residue in MeOH	Resolve C$_{18}$ 5 μm 15 cm × 3.9 mm	Isocratic MeOH : water (7 : 3) containing 10 mM NH4OAC 1.5 mL/min	355 nm	—	*Am. J. Clin. Nutr.*, 43, 481, 1986[1]

Sample	Analytes	Sample preparation	Column	Conditions	Detection	Recovery	Reference
2–3. Plasma, amniotic fluid, embryo	Retinol, retinoic acid, 13-cis-retinoic acid, 4-oxo-metabolites	Add IPA, freeze overnight in liquid N₂, centrifuge Inject directly	*Precolumn* LiChrosorb RP18 10 μm 20 cm × 4.6 mm *Analytical column* Spherisorb 3 ODS II 3 μm 4.6 mm	Column switching Gradient *Pump A*—40 mM NH₄OAC 2 mL/min *Pump B*—MeOH 2 mL/min *Pump C*—40 mM NH₄OAC at pH 7.3 : MeOH (50 : 50) *Pump D*—MeOH Preenrichment on LiChrosorb RP18	354 nm	% Recovery 90–100	*J. Liq. Chromatogr.,* 11, 2051, 1988[2] *Reprod. Toxicol.* 7, 11, 1993[3] 12.5 cm ×
4–6. Biological fluids	Retinoic acid, 13-cis-retinoic acid, 4-oxo-metabolites	Add Ro 11-6738(3) or etretin (IS) in water : MeCN (8 : 2) Centrifuge On-line solid phase extraction	*Precolumn* μBondapak C18 Corasil 37–53 μm *Analytical column* Two Spherisorb ODS 1, 5 μm, in series	Column switching Mobile Phase 10% NH₄OAC:water : MeCN (9 : 81 : 10) *Mobile phase* A. 10% NH₄OAC : water : MeCN : HAC (4 : 396 : 600 : 30) B. NH₄OAC : water : MeCN : HAC (4 : 146 : 8 50 : 10) Inject onto precolumn Switch to analytical column	360 nm	% Recovery <90 % CV <4	*J. Chromatogr.,* 424, 303, 1988; 593, 55, 1992[4,6] *Meth. Enzymol.,* 189, 146, 1990[5]
7. Plasma	Retinol Retinoic acid 13-cis-retinoic acid	Add arotinoid ethyl sulfonic acid (Ro15-1570) (IS) in EtOH Vortex, add water and Hex Acidify with 2 m HCl Centrifuge Evaporate organic layer Dissolve residue in mobile phase	Spherisorb S5W silica 5 μm 15 cm × 4.6 mm	Isocratic Hex : IPA : HAC (200 : 0.7 : 0.135) 0.9 mL/min	350 nm	% Recovery >83	*Clin. Chem.,* 40, 48, 1994[7]

TABLE 1.7 Continued

Analyte	Sample Preparation — Sample Extraction	HPLC Parameters — Column	Mobile Phase	Detection	Quality Assurance Parameters	References
8. Serum — Retinoic acid, cis-retinoic acid	Dilute serum with 10 × volume of MeCN : 100 mM NH4 OAC (1 : 3), pH 5.5; Extract with Hex; Concentrate organic phase; Evaporate under N_2; Dissolve residue in MeOH : MeCN (1 : 2); Centrifuge	Chemcosorb 5-ODS-H, 5 μm, 15 cm × 4.6 mm	Isocratic, MeCN : MeOH (2 : 1) : 100 mM NH4OAC, pH 7.0, 1 mL/min	340 nm	% Recovery 79–89, RSD 3.7–14.2	J. Chromatogr. B, 657, 53, 1994[8]; Centrifuge
9. Serum — Retinoic acid, 13-cis-retinoic acid, 4-oxo-metabolites	Add RO 13-6307 (IS) and 1 M HAC; Transfer to Bakerbond SPE octadecyl column equilibrated with MeOH and HAC; Wash with A : 1 M HAC (1 : 1); Dry under vacuum; Elute with MeCN; Evaporate; Dissolve residue in mobile phase	Lichrocast Si60, 5 μm	Isocratic, CH2Cl2 : 1,4-dioxane (180 : 40) containing 1% HAC, 0.8 mL/min	360 nm	% CV 7.2–12.4	J. Chromatogr. B, 666, 55, 1995[9]
10. Human liver — Retinol, Retinyl esters	Homogenize in EtOH containing 1% pyrogallol; Shake 30 min, 4°C; Add water; Extract 2 × with Hex; Centrifuge; Evaporate; Dissolve residue in MeOH spiked with retinyl acetate; Saponify, 30 min, 60°C, to determine total retinol	Supelcosil LC-8, 5 μm, 25 cm × 4.6 mm	Isocratic, MeOH : water (94 : 6), 1.5 mL/min	PDA 325 nm	% Recovery 80–100, % CV <11	J. Chromatogr. B, 668, 233, 1995[10]

	Matrix	Analytes	Sample preparation	Column	Mobile phase	Detection	Performance	Reference
11.	Bovine serum	Retinol Retinaldehyde Retinoic acid 13-*cis*-retinoic acid	Add MeCN and AA (0.02 M) Centrifuge Add water to make MeCN : water (4 : 6)	ODS-AQ YMC 3 μm Two columns in series 150 μm × 50 μm and 360 μm × 180 μm	Isocratic MeCN : water : MeOH (65 : 32.5 : 2.5) containing 1% TBAP, pH 5.0 4 μL/min	EC Ag/AgCl + 0.9 V	DL on-column 0.27–2.7 fmol	*J. Chromatogr. B,* 677, 225, 1996[11]
12.	Mouse plasma, embryo	Retinoic acid 4-oxo-, 5,6-epoxy-, 9-*cis*-, 13-*cis*-	Add 4-(5,6,7,8-tetrahydro-5,5,8,8-tetramethyl-2-anthracenyl) benzoic acid (IS) in MeOH Add MeCN Shake, centrifuge Evaporate to dryness Dissolve residue in mobile phase	Spherisorb ODS-2 5 μm 25 cm × 4.6 mm	Isocratic MeCN : water : MeOH : n-butyl alcohol (56 : 37 : 4 : 3) containing 10 mM NH_4OAC and 70 mM HAC 1 mL/min	325 nm	% CV 3–9	*J. Chromatogr. B,* 681, 153, 1996[12]
13.	Plasma	Retinoic acid 13-*cis*-retinoic acid	Add acitretin (IS) in MeCN containing 0.01 M BHT Add IPA containing 0.01 M BHT Vortex, centrifuge Add 1% NH_4OAC to supernatant Apply to Methyl-C_1 phase Accubond SPE cartridge Elute retinoids with MeCN (0.01 M BHT) Derivatize to pentafluorobenzyl esters Dry Dissolve in MeCN (0.01 M BHT)	Two Nova-Pak C_{18} columns in series 15 cm × 3.9 mm and 7.5 cm × 3.9 mm	Gradient A—MeCN B—0.1 M NH_4OAC, pH 5.0 0 min 80% A/20% B At 10 min initiate gradient to 90% A/10% B	PDA 369 nm MS 299 mZ	DL on-column 0.25 ng	*J. Pharmaceut. Sci.,* 85, 287, 1996[13]

TABLE 1.7 Continued

| | Sample Preparation | HPLC Parameters | | | | |
| | Sample Extraction | Column | Mobile Phase | Detection | Quality Assurance Parameters | References |
Analyte						
14. Standards						
Retinol		C_{30}, YMC 25 cm × 4.6 mm	Gradient	PDA with electro-spray—MS	DL on-column 0.5 ng–23 pg	*FASEB*, 10, 1098, 1996[14]
Retinalde-hyde			A— MeOH : water : HAC (50 : 50 : 0.5)		Retinoic acid—23 pg	
Retinoic acid			B—MeOH : *t*-butyl ether:HAC (50 : 50 : 0.5)			
Retinyl acetate			*Retinol, Retinaldehyde, Retinoic acid* 95% A/5% B to 45% A/55% B to 100% B 0.6 mL/min			
			Retinoic acid MeOH : water (80 : 20) to MeOH : *t*-butyl ether (20 : 80) containing 5 m*M* NH_4OAC in 60 min.			
15–20. Plasma	Add IPA (3 × volume) containing 0.0125% BHT Vortex, centrifuge Dilute 0.4 mL with 1.2 mL 2% NH4OAC and force through AASPC2 cartridge conditioned with	Spherisorb ODS 3 μm	Gradient A—60 m*M* NH_4OAC : MeOH (1 : 1) B—MeOH : IPA (1 : 1) 0 min	UV 340 nm 356 nm	—	*Life Sci.*, 59, Pl169, 1996[15] Related References
Retinol						
Retinoic acid						
4-oxo-retinoic acid,						
13-*cis*-4-oxo-,						
13-*cis*-retinoic						

acid, 9-cis-retinoic acid	1.7 mL MeOH and 0.6 mL 2% NH$_4$OAC After sample extraction, wash cartridge with 1.5 mL 2% NH$_4$OAC Elute on-line	90% A/10% B 8 min 45% A/55% B 8.5 min 10% A/90% B 17 min 5% A/95% B 55°C or A—60 mM NH$_4$OAC, pH 5.75 B—MeOH 0 min 85% A/15% B to 90% B at 11 min to 99% B at 11.2 min 60°C	*J. Lipid Res.,* 31, 1445, 1990[16] *Arch. Toxicol.,* 66, 652, 1992[17] *Drug Metab. Disp.,* 22, 928, 1994[18] *J. Chromatogr. A,* 685, 182, 1994[19] *Biochem. Biophys. Acta,* 1301, 1, 1996[20]

TABLE 1.8
HPLC Methods for the Analysis of Carotenoids in Food, Feeds, Pharmaceuticals, and Biologicals

		Sample Preparation	HPLC Parameters				
	Analyte	Sample Extraction	Column	Mobile Phase	Detection	Quality Assurance Parameters	References

Food

1. Tomatoes	α-, β-carotene, lycopene	Extract with A Filter, add water Extract with Hex Extract Hex with water to remove A Evaporate Saponify residue, ambient, 14 h Extract with PE	Partisil PX5-5 5 μm 25 cm × 4.6 mm	Isocratic MeCN : CHCl3 (92 : 8) 2 mL/min	470 nm	DL— on-column nmoles α-carotene—0.04 β-carotene—0.03 lycopene—0.004	*J. Chromatogr.,* 176, 109, 1979[1]
2. Fruits and vegetables	α-, β-carotene	Blend with Na2SO4, MgCO3 and THF, 2 × Concentrate, rotovap, 40°C concentrated samples, partition THF extract with PE Evaporate to dryness Dissolve residue in THF	Partisil 5 ODS 5 μm 25 cm × 4.6 mm	Isocratic MeCN : THF : water (85 : 12.5 : 2.5) 2 mL/min	470 nm	% Recovery 100.5	*Can. Inst. Food Sci. Technol. J.,* 15, 165, 1982[2]
3.–4. Carrots, green vegetables	β-carotene, 15,15'-*cis*-β-carotene	Add Decapreno-β-carotene (IS) and β-apo-8'-carotenal (IS) and Na2SO4 plus MgCO3 Extract by blending with THF, reextract Evaporate, extract residue with PE, dry over Na2SO4 Evaporate Dissolve residue in Hex (see Reference 2).	Microsorb C18 5 μm 25 cm × 4.6 mm	Isocratic *β-carotene and 15,15'-cis isomer* MeOH : MeCN : (CH2Cl2 : Hex) (1 : 1) (22 : 55 : 11.5 : 11.5) 0.7 mL/min *Xanthophylls and β-apo-8'-carotenal* 0 min MeOH : MeCN : CHCl2 : Hex	PDA 446–450 nm, 500 nm	—	*J. Chromatogr.,* 346, 237, 1985[3] *J. Agric. Food Chem.,* 34, 603, 1986[4]

	Analytes	Procedure	Column	Mobile phase	Detection	Recovery	Reference
5. Fruits and vegetables	α-, β-carotene, 9-cis- and 13-cis-isomers	Puree, mix with MeOH; Filter, extract filter cake with A : Hex (1 : 1); Extract A and MeOH with water; Saponify epilayer, ambient, 30 min; Wash with H_2O to remove bias; Dry oven Na_2SO_4; Filter, inject	$Ca(OH)_2$, 115 mesh, 25 cm × 4.6 mm	(15 : 75 : 5 : 5) followed by gradient to (15 : 40 : 22.5 : 22.5) 0.5 mL/min; Isocratic A : Hex (3 : 97) 0.9 mL/min	436 nm, 340 nm	% Recovery 90–95; DL on-column 20 µg	*J. Food Sci.*, 52, 669, 1987[5]
6. Yellow/orange vegetables	α-, β-, δ-carotene, 15,15'-cis-β-carotene, cis-δ-carotene	Add non-apreno-β-carotene (IS); Extract with mobile phase with Na_2SO_4 added at 200% sample weight and $MgCO_3$ at 10% of sample weight; Extract with THF; Filter, reextract until filtrate is colorless; Rotovap to remove most of solvent; Partition into PE : water (1 : 1); Wash water layer with PE (multiple times); Dry over Na_2SO_4, evaporate; To evaluate presence of carotenol esters, ether extracts were saponified, ambient, 3 h	Brownlee RP-18, 5 µm, 22 cm × 4.6 mm	Isocratic MeOH : MeCN : CH_2Cl_2 (22 : 55 : 23) 1 mL/min	PDA lycopene, α-, β-98 carotene—475 nm; IS—402 nm	% Recovery	*J. Agric Food Chem.*, 35, 732, 1987[6]
7–8. Squash	33 analytes xantho-phylls, carotenol esters, cartenoids,	Add isozeaxanthin (IS) 6-apo-8'-carotenol; Extraction—See Reference 6.	Microsorb C_{18}, 5 µm, 25 cm × 4.6 mm	Baby food squash *Carotenoids and carotenol esters* 0 min MeOH : MeCN : CH_2Cl_2 : Hex	See Reference 6.	% Recovery >98	*J. Agric. Food Chem.*, 36, 929, 1988[7] 36, 938, 1988[8]

TABLE 1.8 Continued

Analyte	Sample Preparation Sample Extraction	HPLC Parameters Column	Mobile Phase	Detection	Quality Assurance Parameters	References
carotenol cis esters			(15 : 65 : 10 : 10) Acorn squash 0 min MeOH : MeCN : CH$_2$Cl$_2$: Hex (10 : 85 : 2.5 : 2.5) Gradient to (10 : 45 : 22.5 : 22.5) 0.7 mL/min			
9–10. Apricots, peaches, pink grapefruit, tomatoes, green vegetables	xantho- phylls, carotenoids, carotenol esters	See Reference 6	Microsorb C$_{18}$ Vydac 201 TP54 5 µm 25 cm × 4.6 mm	Microsorb C$_{18}$ 0 min–10 min MeOH : MeCN : CH$_2$Cl$_2$: Hex (10 : 85 : 2.5 : 2.5) Gradient to 10 : 45 : 22.5 : 22.5 Vydac 201TP54 Isocratic MeOH : MeCN : CH$_2$Cl$_2$: Hex (10 : 85 : 2.5 : 2.5)	PDA	—	J. Agric. Food Chem., 37, 1465, 1989[9]; 40, 390, 1992[10]
11. Vegetables, fruits, berries	α-, β-, γ-carotene, lutein, lycopene	Extract with A with addition of NASO$_4$ and MgCO$_3$ Filter, rotovap Saponify residue, ambient, overnight, with BHT added Extract with Hex : Et$_2$O (7 : 3)	Zorbax ODS 5–6 mm or Spherisorb ODS2 5 µm 25 cm × 4.6 mm	Zorbax ODS Isocratic MeCN : CH$_2$Cl$_2$: MeOH (70 : 20 : 10) 2 mL/min Spherisorb ODS2	PDA 450 nm	% Recovery 101–103	J. Agric. Food Chem., 37, 655, 1989[11]

containing 0.1% BHT

Sample	Carotenoids	Procedure	Column	Gradient	Detection	% Recovery QL	Reference
				Gradient MeCN : MeOH : CH₂Cl₂ : Hex (75 : 15 : 5 : 5) to (40 : 15 : 22.5 : 22.5) over 20 min 1 mL/min, 30°C			
12–13. Fruits, sweet potato	α-, β-carotene, β-crypto-xanthin	Saponify, ambient, overnight Filter, extract with Hex containing 0.01% BHT Wash Hex with water saturated with NaCl Filter through Na₂SO₄ Evaporate Dissolve in mobile phase	Zorbax ODS Vydac C₁₈218TP54 5 μm 25 cm × 4.6 mm	Zorbax ODS Isocratic MeCN : CH₂Cl₂ : MeOH (350 : 150 : 1) containing 0.001% TEA 1 mL/min Vydac C₁₈218TP54 Isocratic MeOH : MeCN : THF (28 : 25 : 2) 1 mL/min	PDA 436 nm	70–100 QL 1 μg/100g	J. Food Comp. Anal., 3, 119, 1990[12]; 6, 336, 1993[13]
14. Vegetables	α-, β-, γ-carotene lutein zeaxanthin β-crypto-xanthin Phytoene Phytofluene	Add retinyl palmitate (IS) Extraction–See Reference 2. System I Dissolve residue in THF System II Dissolve residue in THF : EtOH (1 : 3)	Spherisorb-S RP-18 or Spheri-ODS 22 cm × 4.6 mm	System I Isocratic MeCN : CH₂Cl₂ : MeOH (70 : 20 : 10) 1.8 mL/min System II 0–9.5 min MeCN : MeOH (85 : 15) 1.8 mL/min At 9.5 min, increase flow rate to 3.5 mL/min	Carotenoids 450 nm Phytoene 286 nm Phytofluene 370 nm	—	J. Agric. Food Chem., 40, 2135, 1992[14]

TABLE 1.8 Continued

		Sample Preparation	HPLC Parameters				
	Analyte	Sample Extraction	Column	Mobile Phase	Detection	Quality Assurance Parameters	References
15. Vegetables	α-, β-carotene β-cryptoxanthin	Add β-apo-8′-carotenal (IS) Add MgCO$_3$ Extract with Hex : A : EtOH : T (10 : 7 : 6 : 7) Saponify, ambient, 16 h, under N$_2$ Extract with Hex with Na$_2$SO$_4$ Evaporate Dissolve in EtOAC	Phenomenex Ultramax C$_{18}$ 5 μm 25 cm × 4.6 mm	Isocratic MeCN : MeOH : EtOAC (75 : 15 : 10) 1 or 2 mL/min	PDA 450 nm	—	J. Food Prot., 56, 51, 1993[15]
16. Red peppers	14 carotenoids	Add β-apo-8′-carotenal (IS) Extract with A Extract A with Et$_2$O 10% NaCl solution Dry with Na$_2$SO$_4$ Concentrate If required, saponify residue or Et$_2$O extract, ambient, 1 h	Spherisorb ODS 2 5 μm 25 cm × 4 mm	Gradient A : water (95 : 5) to 100 A 1.5 mL/min	PDA 450 nm	—	J. Agric Food Chem., 41, 1616, 1993[16]
17. Fruit, vegetables	10 carotenoids 30 esters	Add Na$_2$CO$_3$ Extract with A Evaporate, 40°C Add NaCl saturated water Extract with B : Et$_2$O (1 : 1) Dry over Na$_2$SO$_4$ Evaporate Dissolve in CH$_3$Cl and mobile phase	LiChrosorb C$_{18}$ 10 μm 25 cm × 4.6 mm	Isocratic MeCN : IPA : water (39 : 57 : 4) or MeCN : IPA : MeOH : water (39 : 52 : 6:4) 0.9–1.5 mL/min	PDA Multiple λ	—	J. Plant Physiol., 143, 520, 1994[17]

18. Human milk	α-, β-carotene Lycopene β-crypto-xanthin	Saponify, 30 min, 25°C Extract with Hex	YMC C$_{18}$	Isocratic MeOH:THF (90 : 10) containing 025 g BHT per L 1.7 mL/min	450 nm	—	*J. Nutr. Biochem.,* 5, 551, 1994[18].
19. Carrot juice	*β-carotene* all-trans- 9-*cis*- 13-*cis*- 15-*cis*- 13,15-di-*cis*- *Lutein* 9-*cis*- 13-*cis*-	Mix with Hex : A : EtOH : T (10 : 7 : 6 : 7) and 40% methanolic KOH Saponify, ambient, 16 h Extract with Hex Dilute with 10% Na$_2$SO$_4$ Allow phase separation Evaporate Hex layer Dissolve in MeOH : CH$_2$Cl$_2$ (45 : 55)	Vydec C$_{18}$ 201TP54 5 μm 25 cm × 4.6 mm	Isocratic MeOH : CH$_2$Cl$_2$ (99 : 1) 1 mL/min	PDA 450 nm	—	*J. Agric. Food Chem.,* 43, 1912, 1995[19]
20. Carrots	α-, β-carotene Lutein	Extract with A Filter Reextract 2 × Evaporate Add NaCl saturated water and B : Et$_2$O (1 : 1) Collect organic layer Wash, dry over Na$_2$SO$_4$ Evaporate Dissolve residue in CHCl$_3$ Dilute with mobile phase	LiChrosorb ODS 6 μm 25 cm × 4.6 mm	Isocratic MeCN : IPA : MeOH : water (39 : 52 : 5 : 4)	PDA Multiple λ	—	*J. Agric. Food Chem.,* 43, 589, 1995[20]
21. Tomato juice	α-, β-, γ-, δ-carotene Lutein Lycopene Lycopene-5,6-diol β-crypto-xanthin Neuro-	Add β-apo-8′-carotenal (IS) Blend with MgCO$_3$, celite, and THF Filter, reextract until colorless Reduce volume Partition with CH$_2$Cl$_2$ and NaCl saturated water Dry over Na$_2$SO$_4$ Reduce volume to 10 mL Filter	Microsorb MV C$_{18}$ 5 μm 25 cm × 4.6 mm	Isocratic MeCN : MeOH : CH$_2$Cl$_2$: Hex (40 : 20 : 20 : 20)	PDA 450 nm except Lycopene— 470 nm β-cryptoxanthin —445 nm γ-carotene— 400 nm Phytofluene—	—	*J. Agric. Food Chem.,* 43, 579, 1995[21]

TABLE 1.8 Continued

Analyte	Sample Preparation — Sample Extraction	HPLC Parameters — Column	Mobile Phase	Detection	Quality Assurance Parameters	References
sporene Phytoene Phytofluene	Dilute with CH_2Cl_2			350 nm Phytoene—290 nm		
22. Fruits, vegetables	α-, β-carotene *cis*-β-carotene Lycopene β-crypto-xanthin zeaxanthin lutein	Add β-apo-8'-carotenal (IS) or echinenone (IS) Add $MgCO_3$ Extract with THF : MeOH (1 : 1) Filter, reextract residue Partition with PE containing 0.1% BHT Evaporate Dissolve residue in CH_2Cl_2 *For peppers and fruit:* Saponify 1 h, 30°C Extract with PE containing 0.1% BHT Evaporate Dissolve in CH_2Cl_2	ODS 2 5 μm 10 cm × 4.6 mm connected to Vydac C_{18} 201TP54 5 μm 25 cm × 4.6 mm	Isocratic MeCN : MeOH : CH_2Cl_2 (75 : 20 :) containing 0.05% TEA and 0.1% BHT MeOH contains 0.05 M NH_4OAC 1.5 mL/min	PDA 450 nm	DL (μg/mL) 0.01–0.045	*Food Chem.,* 54, 101, 1995[22]
23. Milk	β-carotene	Add IPA, vortex Extract 2 × with Hex Centrifuge Evaporate Hex aliquot Saponify, 30 min, 30°C Extract with Hex Evaporate Dissolve in Hex : CH_2Cl_2 (95 : 5)	Two ChromSep ChromoSphere PAH columns in series 5 μm 10 cm × 3 mm	Isocratic MeCN : MeOH : CH_2Cl_2 (80 : 14 : 6) 0.7 mL/min	450 nm	% Recovery 100	*J. Chromatogr. A,* 721, 355, 1996[23]

Sample	Analytes	Sample preparation	Column	Mobile phase/Conditions	Detection	DL	Reference
24. Green vegetables	α-, β-carotene 13-cis-β-carotene 9-cis-β-carotene	Blend with water containing 0.5% AA Extract with A : PE (3 : 2) containing 0.5% BHT Saponify extract, ambient, 15 min Wash 3 × with 10% NaCl solution Dry over Na$_2$SO4 Evaporate Dissolve in MeOH : CH$_2$Cl$_2$ (9 : 1)	Vydac TP-201 5 mm 25 cm × 4.6 mm	Isocratic *Prepared Isomers* MeOH : CH$_2$Cl$_2$: water (79 : 15 : 6) 0.8 mL/min *Samples* MeOH : CH$_2$Cl$_2$: water (80 : 15.2 : 4.8) 1 mL/min	450 nm	—	*Food Chem.,* 55, 63, 1996[24]
25. Vegetables	16 carotenoids	Blend with A, shake with Et$_2$O and water Collect organic layer, wash with water Dry over Na$_2$SO$_4$ Reduce volume Saponify, ambient Wash mixture with water Dry over Na$_2$SO$_4$ Saponify 1 h, 30°C Extract with PE containing 0.1% BHT Evaporate Dissolve residue in CH$_3$Cl	Two NovaPak C$_{18}$ in series 5 μm	Gradient A. MeCN : MeOH : water (50 : 25 : 15) B. MeCN : MeOH (75 : 25) Pump A for 60 min To B at 180 min Maintain B for 70 min	440 nm	—	*Food Chem.,* 56, 451, 1996[25]
26. Vegetables, plasma	α-, β-carotene β-cryptoxanthin Zeaxanthin Lycopene Lutein	*Vegetables* Lyophilize, mix with MeOH Homogenize Filter Reextract solids with THF Rotovap, 30°C Partition concentrate with PE : water (1 : 1) Dry organic layer over Na$_2$SO$_4$ evaporate Dissolve residue in mobile phase Some products with saponified *Plasma* Add echinenone (IS) Dilute 1 : 1 with water Extract with Hex Evaporate Dissolve in mobile phase	Vydac 201TP54 C$_{18}$ 5 μm 25 cm × 4.6 mm	Isocratic MeOH : THF (95 : 5) 1 mL/min	PDA 200–600 nm	DL (mg/mL) 0.02–0.7	*Int. J. Vit. Nutr. Res.,* 67, 47, 1997[26]

TABLE 1.8 Continued

	Sample Preparation	HPLC Parameters				
Analyte	Sample Extraction	Column	Mobile Phase	Detection	Quality Assurance Parameters	References
27. Mango β-carotene β-crypto-xanthin all-*trans, cis-* Zeaxanthin Luteoxan-thin isomers Violaxan-thin all-*trans-cis-* Neoxanthin all-*trans,cis-*	Extract with cold A Partition with Et_2O : PE (1 : 1) Saponify, ambient, overnight Wash organic layer free of base Concentrate Add Sudan I (IS) to aliquot Evaporate Dissolve in Hex	Spherisorb Nitrile 5 µm 15 cm × 4.6 mm	Multilinear gradient A in Hex 0 A to 15% A in 10 min to 20% A in 20 min to 30% A in 10 min to 40% A in 2 min 1 mL/min	PDA 400–500 nm identification by mass spectrometry, molecular ion, fragmentation pattern	—	*J. Agric. Food Chem.,* 45, 120, 1997[27]
28. Fruits and vegetables α-, β-carotene, lutein, lycopene, β-cryptoxanthin, zeaxanthin	Add ethyl-β-apo-8'-carotenoate (IS) to 0.5–1.0 g freeze-dried sample Add 0.2 g $MgCO_3$, Extract with MeOH : THF (1:) until colorless by homogenization at 8°C Centrifuge to remove solids after each extraction Combine extracts and extract with PE until PE extracts are colorless Evaporate to dryness Dissolve residue in MeOH : THF (75 : 25) For samples containing β-cryptoxanthin, initial MeOH : THF extract must be saponified before PE partitioning	Vydac 201TP 5 µm 25 cm × 4.6 mm Peek alloyed with Teflon frits	Isocratic MeOH : THF (95 : 5) 1.0 mL/min	450 nm	DL (mg/mL) 1.0 RSD_r 1.9–4.9% % Recovery 93–107	*Food Chem.,* 59, 599, 1997[28]

Biologicals							
1. Plasma	Six carotenoids	Add echinenone (IS) in ethanol, add Hex; Vortex, centrifuge; Transfer Hex phase; Evaporate; Dissolve in mobile phase	LC$_{18}$ 5 μm 25 cm × 4.6 mm	Isocratic MeCN : CH$_2$Cl$_2$: MeOH (70 : 20 : 10) 1.7 mL/min	PDA 436 nm	% CV 1.9–7.1	J. Liq. Chromatogr., 8, 473, 1985[1]
2. Standards	Straight chain fatty acid esters of various carotenoids	—	Spheri-5-RP-18 5 μm 25 cm × 4.6 mm	Eluent A MeOH : MeCN : CH$_2$Cl$_2$/Hex (1 : 1) (10 : 85 : 5) at 0 min 10 min—gradient to (10 : 45 : 45) at 40 min 07 mL/min Eluent B MeOH : MeCN : CH$_2$Cl$_2$/Hex (1 : 1) (15 : 65 : 20) at 0 min 23 min—Gradient to (15 : 40 : 45) at 33 min 0.7 mL/min Eluent C MeOH : MeCN : CH$_2$Cl$_2$/Hex (1 : 1) (20 : 40 : 4) 0.7 mL/min	PDA 450 nm except Violaxanthin— 442 nm Auroxanthin— 400 nm	% CV —	J. Chromatogr., 449, 119, 1988[2]
3–4. Plasma	18 carotenoids	Add ethyl β-apo-8'-carotenoate (IS) and (3R)-8'-apo-β-carotene-3,8'diol (IS) and EtOH; Vortex, centrifuge; Add EtOH, shake	Microsorb C$_{18}$ 5 μm 25 cm × 4.6 mm or Silica-based	Silica based nitrile bonded Isocratic Hex : CH$_2$Cl$_2$: MeOH : N,N-diisopropyl-	PDA MS desorption chemical ionization (DCI)	% Recovery >90 % CV <5	Anal. Chem., 64, 2111, 1992[3] Meth. Enzymol., 213, 205, 1992[4]

TABLE 1.8 Continued

Analyte	Sample Preparation — Sample Extraction	HPLC Parameters — Column	Mobile Phase	Detection	Quality Assurance Parameters	References
	Centrifuge, remove solution; Reextract residue (2×); Combine ethereal layers; Dry over Na_2SO_4; Evaporate; Dissolve residue in CH_2Cl_2; Evaporate to dryness; Dissolve in eluent B to 100 mL	nitrile bonded 5 μm 25 cm × 4.6 mm	ethylamine (74.65 : 25:0.25 : 0.1) 1 mL/1min; $Microsorb\ C_{18}$ MeCN : MeOH : CH_2Cl_2/Hex (1 : 1) 0 min (85 : 10 : 5) 10 min—Gradient to (45 : 10 : 45) at 40 min 0.7 mL/min	or electron capture negative ionization (ECNI)		
5. Plasma — α-, β-carotene β-cryptoxanthin Lycopene Lutein	Add n-butyl-β-apo-8'-carotenoate (IS) and BHT in EtOH; Extract 6 × with Hex, centrifuge following each extraction; Combine Hex fractions; Evaporate; Store at −20°C; Dissolve residue in mobile phase	Adsorbsphere C_{18} 5 μm 10 cm × 4.6 mm	Isocratic MeOH : CH_2Cl_2 : MeCN (65 : 25 : 10) containing 0.025% BHT containing 0.5 M BTP (2 mL/L) 1.5 mL/min	PDA 450 nm	% CV 2.9–4.3	J. Chromatogr., 614, 43, 1993[5]
6. Plasma — α-, β-carotene Lycopene	Add echinenone (IS) in EtOH; Vortex; Add Hex, centrifuge; Remove 100 μL Hex; Evaporate; Dissolve residue in mobile phase; Evaporate	Ultrasphere ODS- 5 μm 25 cm × 4.6 mm	Isocratic MeCN : CH_2Cl_2 : MeOH (80 : 10 : 10) 1.7 mL/min	464 nm	—	Am. J. Clin. Nutr., 59, 896, 1994[6]

Sample	Analytes	Sample Preparation	Column	Conditions	Detection	% Recovery	References

7–8. Serum	β-carotene 9-cis-, 13-cis-β-carotene	Add EtOH, vortex
		Add Hex, vortex
		Centrifuge
		Remove Hex layer, reextract
		Dry Hex over Na_2SO_4
		Fractionate on Sep-Pak alumina
		Collect 10% A in Hex fraction
		Evaporate
			$Ca(OH)_2$
			25 cm × 4.6 mm
				Isocratic
				P-methylanisole: A : Hex (1 : 1 : 98)
				Flow Gradient
				min mL/min
				0 0.6
				12.5 0.6
				13.0 0.9
					410 nm	>90	Clin. Chem., 36, 1986, 1990[7]; J. Agric. Food Chem., 42, 2746, 1994[8]

9. Plasma, blood cells	β-carotene 9-cis-β-carotene	Add EtOH containing 0.015% BHT, shake under N_2 Add 0.9% NaCl Extract with Hex Evaporate Dissolve residue in EtOH	Vydac C_{18} 201TP54 5 μm 25 cm × 4.6 mm	Isocratic MeOH : MeCN (95 : 5) containing 50 mM $NaClO_4$ 1 mL/min	450 nm	—	Lipids, 30, 493, 1995[9]
10–15. Serum	α-, β-carotene Lutein Zeaxanthin β-cryptoxanthin cis-isomers	Add β-apo-10′-carotenal (IS) in EtOH containing 30 μg/mL BHT Vortex Add Hex, vortex Centrifuge, reextract Evaporate Dissolve residue in EtOH containing 30 μg/mL BHT	*Column 1* C_{18} Narrow-bore polymeric 5 μm 25 cm × 4.6 mm *Column 2* C30 3 μm Polymeric	Gradient *Column 1* A—MeCN B—MeOH with 0.05 M NH_4OAC C—EtOAC 98% A/2% B to 75%A/18% B/7% C in 10 min to 68% A/25% B/ 7% C in 5 min *Column 2* A—water : MeOH 0.05 M NH_4OAC and 0.05% TEA B—MTBE 83% A/17% B to 59% A/4% B in 29 min To 30% A/70% B in 5 min Hold 4 min	PDA 250 nm–50 nm 450 nm	—	J. Chromatogr. B, 678, 187, 1996[10] Related References: J. Chromatogr., 619, 37, 1993[11]; 707, 205, 1995[13]; 719, 333, 1996[15] Anal. Chem., 66, 1667, 1994[12] Fres. J. Anal. Chem., 356, 1, 1996[14]

TABLE 1.8 Continued

		Sample Preparation	HPLC Parameters				
	Analyte	Sample Extraction	Column	Mobile Phase	Detection	Quality Assurance Parameters	References
16. Serum, human milk	34 carotenoids including 13 geometric isomers and 8 metabolites	*Serum* Add ethyl-β-apo-8'-carotenate (IS) for recovery studies Add equal volume of ETOH containing 0.1% BHT Centrifuge Extract 2 × with Hex Evaporate to dryness Dissolve residue in Eluent B *Human Milk* To 100 mL milk add IS for recovery studies Add 0.6 g of bile salts containing 50% Na cholate and 50% Na deoxycholate Add 1.0 g $MgCO_3$ Vortex, shake at 37°C, 15 min Add 2 mL of 50 mg/mL Pronase E and HmL 50 mg/mL lipase B in saline Incubate, 37°C, 1 h Add 100 mL ETOH (0.1% BHT) Vortex Extract 2 × with 50 mL Hex Dry Hex over Na_2SO_4, evaporate Dissolve residue in CH_2Cl_2 Filter (0.45 μm) Evaporate under N_2 Add eluent B to 30 μL	Reversed-phase Microsorb C_{18} 5 μm 25 cm × 4.6 mm Normal-phase Sillica-based nitrile 5 μm 25 cm × 4.6 mm	Reversed-phase Eluent A—Isocratic MeCN : MeOH : CH_2Cl_2 : Hex (85 : 10 : 2.5 : 2.5) followed by a linear gradient at 10 min to 40 min; ending at $M3CN$: CH_2Cl_2 : Hex : MeOH (45 : 22.5 : 22.5 : 10) 0.7 mL/min Normal-phase Eluent B—Isocratic Hex : CH_2Cl_2 : MeOH : N,N-diisopropylethyl amine (74.65 : 25 : 0.25 : 0.1) 0.7 mL/min	PDA Eluent A 470, 445, 400, 350, 325, 290, and 276 nm Eluent B 445, 340, 325, and 276 nm HPLC-MS interface Divide eluents 1 : 3, lesser amount into particle beam interface Desolvation at 45°C Electron capture negative ionization at 0.85 Torr and 250°C Collect spectra at m/z 100 to 700, 1.5z scan cycle	% Recovery >95	*Anal. Chem.*, 69, 1873, 1997[16]

| 17. Plasma, foods | lycopene, 5-cis, 9-cis, 15-cis | *Food* Add 10 g MgSO4 and 30 mL A to 1–2 g sample Homogenize, filter through sintered glass Reextract at least 2 × with A, until extract is colorless. If color cannot be removed, grind residue in mortar with sea sand, extract with Hex containing 1% A Combine filtrater, evaporate Add EtOH, reevaporate Dissolve residue in Hex and treat by aluminum oxide open-column chromatography *Plasma* To 200 μL clarified plasma, add 200 μL water and 400 μL EtOH Vortex, add 800 μL Hex, shake 10 min, centrifuge Evaporate 500 μL Hex layer Add 10 mL CH_2Cl_2, and dilute with 250 μL Hex | Nucleosil 300-S Three columns in series 25 cm × 4.6 mm | Isocratic Hex containing 0.15% *m*-ethyladi-isopropylamine 1 mL/min | PDA 470 nm | Food 90–94 Plasma 95–102 | Food Chem., 59, 459, 1997[17] |

TABLE 1.9
Saponification Parameters for Retinol and Carotenoids

Matrix	Sample Size	Hydrolysis Conditions	Antioxidant	Extractant	Internal Standard or % Recovery	Quantitation Level	Reference
Retinol							
Fish oil	1.0 g	Ethanolic KOH Ambient, overnight	Ascorbic acid Nitrogen flush	Diethyl ether	Retinol—89% 3-dehydroretinal— 89%	—	*J. Chromatogr.* 312, 423, 1984
Dried skim milk	20 g	Ethanolic KOH Reflux, 30 min	Sodium ascorbate	Petroleum ether	None	—	*Dairy Fed.,* Bulletin 285, 1993
Milk	200–1000 mg	Ethanolic KOH 70°C, 20 min	Ascorbic acid	Heptane : diisopropyl ether (3:1)	99%	0.5 µg/g	*J. Dairy Res.,* 61, 233, 1994
Liver, liver products	1–5 g	Ethanolic KOH Ambient, overnight	Ascorbic acid Nitrogen flush	Dilute to water : alcohol ratio of 1:1 Pass through Kieselguhr column Elute retinol with petroleum ether	None	—	*Z. Lebensm. Unters.Forsch.,* 199, 206, 1994
Foods Milk Liver	1–10 g	Ethanolic KOH Ambient, 16 h	BHT Ascorbic acid Nitrogen flush	Dilute to water : ethanol ratio of 1 : 1 Pass through Kieselguhr column Elute with petroleum ether	None	4.2 mg/100 g	*J. Chromatogr., A.,* 693, 271, 1995

Carotenoids

Sample	Amount	Saponification/Extraction	Antioxidant/Atmosphere	Solvent	Analyte/Recovery	Detection limit	Reference
Fruits and Vegetables	1.0 g	Ethanolic KOH Ambient overnight	Ascorbic acid Nitrogen flush	Diethyl ether	—	—	J. Chromatogr., 288, 217, 1982
Berries, fruits, vegetables	5–10 g	Extract with acetone Ethanolic KOH Ambient, overnight	Ascorbic acid	Hexane : diethyl ether (70 : 30)	β-carotene—101% lycopene—103% lutein—103%	4.0 µg/100 g	J. Agric. Food Chem., 37, 655, 1989
Fruit	50 g	Ethanolic KOH Ambient, overnight	Ascorbic acid Nitrogen flush	Hexane (0.01% BHT)	α-carotene-82% β-carotene-87% $n = 52$	2.0 µg/100 g	J. Food Comp. Anal., 3, 119, 1990
Vegetables	10 g	Solvent extraction Methanolic KOH Ambient, 16 h	Nitrogen flush	Hexane	β-apo-8′-carotenal	0.6 µg/g	J. Food Prot., 56, 51, 1993
Sweet potato	5–15 g	Blanch potato Ethanolic KOH Ambient, overnight	Ascorbic acid Nitrogen flush	Hexane (0.01% BHT)	α-, β-carotene— 90–100% $n = 28$	1.1 µg/g	J. Food Comp. Anal., 6, 336, 1993
Human milk	4.0 mL	Ethanolic KOH Ambient, 5 h		Hexane			J. Nutr. Biochem., 5, 551, 1994 Lipids, 25, 159, 1990

Fruit Vegetables	10 g	Extract with THF:MeOH (1:1) with magnesium carbonate Partition with petroleum ether Evaporate Redissolve in CH_2Cl_2 Saponify with methanolic KOH Ambient, 1 h	BHT	Petroleum ether	β-apo-8′-carotenal or echiemone	6 µg/100 g	*Food Chem.*, 54, 101, 1995
Dark green vegetables	25 g	Blanch vegetables Extract with acetone : petroleum ether : (0.5% BHT) (3 : 2) Saponify with ethanolic KOH Ambient, 15 min	BHT	Water wash to remove acetone	β-carotene 96–104%	—	*Food Chem.*, 55, 63, 1996

extraction with hexane is dependent on the concentrations of fatty acids in the digest. Control is achieved by limiting the amount of fat in the sample (sample weight), by optimizing the amount of water added before extraction, and by repeated extractions with small volumes of hexane. Examination of the methods in Table 1.9 shows that hexane, petroleum ether, diethyl ether, and hexane : diethyl ether mixtures are common extracting solvents. Extended, ambient temperature saponification decreases heat induced isomerization. Digests must include antioxidants such as ascorbic acid, pyrogallol, and/or BHT. Flushing the vessel with inert gas, usually nitrogen, provides additional protection from oxidation, and protection from light and metal contamination must be assured during all stages of the sample extraction process. To further inhibit oxidation, an antioxidant such as BHT which is soluble in the organic phase should be included in the extracting solvent.

1.3.2.1.2   Direct Solvent Extraction

Many organic solvents and solvent mixtures efficiently extract retinoids and carotenoids directly from the sample matrix. Solvent systems must be capable of penetrating tissues and breaking lipoprotein bonds to free the analytes.[26] Under most circumstances, complete lipid extraction must be assured to accomplish efficient removal of retinoids and carotenoids from the sample matrix. Most physiological fluids are extracted with simple direct solvent extraction procedures. These protocols follow the sequence of:

1. Denaturing proteins with a volume of ethanol, methanol, or acetonitrile equal to the sample volume
2. Addition of buffer or water to improve the extraction efficiency of the solvent
3. Addition of organic phase to extract the retinoids and carotenoids
4. Centrifugation to facilitate phase separation
5. Solvent evaporation.

Examination of the methods provided in Tables 1.7 and 1.8 shows that hexane is commonly used as the extracting solvent. Other solvents include diethyl ether, ethyl acetate, acetonitrile, and various solvent mixtures. Further extract cleanup by SPE can be completed but is usually not necessary for assay of retinol and its metabolites from physiological fluids. Retinoic acid and the retinoid glucuronides require acidification or addition of buffer salts to the solvent for efficient extraction. Acetonitrile is an excellent solvent for extraction of retinoic acid.[24] All-*trans* retinoic acid and its *cis*-isomers were extracted from plasma in more recent work by a combined solvent-SPE extraction.[56] Isopropyl alcohol was used to denature the protein, following addition of acetonitrile containing 0.01 M BHT. After centrifugation, 1% ammonium acetate solution was added to reduce the solvent concentration and ensure SPE retention of the lipophilic retinoic acids onto the SPE column (Methyl-C1, Accubond). Retinoids were eluted with acetonitrile/0.01 M BHT.

Under certain conditions, carotenoids can be efficiently extracted from fruit and vegetables by direct solvent extraction. Khachik and co-workers[57,58,59] used the following procedure to extract carotenol esters for characterization from squash and various fruits:

1. Add tetrahydrofuran, sodium sulfate (200% of the sample weight), and magnesium sulfate (10% of the sample weight)
2. Blend for 5 min with a blender
3. Filter and re-extract the residue until the filtrate is colorless
4. Evaporate with rotary evaporator to near dryness at 30°C
5. Partition the concentrated extract between petroleum ether and water (salt can be added to break emulsions)
6. Wash the aqueous layer with petroleum ether containing 15% methanol several times until colorless

7. Combine organic layers and dry over sodium sulfate
8. Evaporate, dissolve residue in hexane

Isozeaxanthin dipelargonate and β-apo-8'-carotenol served as internal standards. The internal standards were added prior to blending of the sample.

1.3.2.2 Chromatography Parameters

1.3.2.2.1 Supports and Mobile Phases

Most recent LC methods for resolution of retinoids and carotenoids used reversed-phase C_{18} or ODS supports (Tables 1.7 and 1.8). Advantages of reversed-phase systems compared to normal-phase chromatography include the following:

1. Less sensitive to changes in retention time due to the presence of water
2. More easily cleaned of contaminants
3. More stable to small changes in mobile phase composition
4. More quickly equilibrated to mobile phase composition changes, permitting use of gradients
5. Capable of resolving compounds with a wide range of polarities[23,24,38,39,43]

Both isocratic and gradient mobile phase systems are provided in the methods summarized in Tables 1.7 and 1.8. For retinol analysis by reversed-phase chromatography, simple, isocratic, methanol-water, acetonitrile-water, or gradients based on these solvents provide excellent resolution. When more polar metabolites (retinoic acid) or synthetic retinoids are under study, acetonitrile or methanol based mobile phases are modified by the addition of 1% or 0.1 M ammonium acetate or acetic acid. Acid addition results in ion suppression of the carboxylic acids but does not affect resolution of retinol or retinyl esters. Ammonium acetate improves resolution and decreases broadening of the retinoic acid peak.[24,39]

Normal-phase or absorption chromatography is advised when critical resolution of retinol isomers is required. Hexane or heptane mobile phases modified with isopropanol, 1,4-dioxane, or t-butyl methyl ether resolve retinol isomers more efficiently than reversed-phase systems. Retinoic acid chromatography on silica support requires acidification of the mobile phase, usually with acetic acid, to decrease the affinity of the polar analyte for the support. Wyss[39] reviewed mobile phase composition and applications of various chromatography systems to retinoid resolution.

Nöll[60] and Nöll and Kalinowski[61] recently demonstrated that identification of retinol isomers can be easily misidentified and that some identifications in the literature are inconsistent or wrong. Using Zorbax SIL and LiChrospher Si60 supports with n-hexane : 5-butyl methyl ether (97 : 3) mobile phase, retinol and retinal isomers were detected at 325 nm and 371 nm, respectively. A characteristic chromatogram is shown in Figure 1.7. Nöll[60] stressed that elution time and pressure of the system are dependent on the columns used. Factors such as specific inner surface area of the support can affect resolution time and order of elution of the various isomers. Nöll and Kalinowski[61] compared many previous chromatographic systems (51 papers) and showed that inconsistencies exist in identification of eluted peaks. They again stressed that the HPLC mode, support material, mobile phases, ratio of eluents, flow rate, pressure, detection wavelength, and column temperature are all important factors controlling retention time and order of elution of complex retinoid isomeric mixtures.

Major advances occurred over the past decade in methods for the separation of cis- and trans-isomers of the carotenoids. O'Neil and Schwartz[53] reviewed the chromatography of cis- and trans-carotenoid isomers through 1992. For β-carotene isomers, most procedures used $Ca(OH)_2$ or Vydac C_{18} supports. Vydac supports are produced using trichlorosilanes in a polymeric synthesis of C_{18} as opposed to monomeric synthesis with monochlorosilanes. The polymeric C_{18} has greater shape

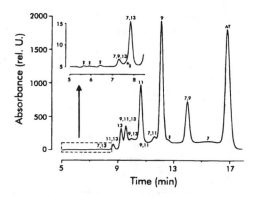

FIGURE 1.7 Chromatograms of retinal isomers on Zorbax SIL. Mobile phase was hexane : *t*-butyl methyl ether (97 : 3), 2 mL/min. Reproduced with permission from Reference 60.

selectivity towards geometric isomers compared to monomeric supports.[29] Normal-phase chromatography on $Ca(OH)_2$ provides excellent *cis*-resolution from *trans*-isomers; however, the support is not commercially available and in-house packing is irreproducible.[29,53] Therefore, polymeric C_{18} supports have routinely been used for studies on *cis*- and *trans*-carotenoids. Monomeric C_{18} supports provide resolution of some of the xanthophylls.[53] As shown in Table 1.8, a variety of solvents mixtures including methanol, acetonitrile, dichloromethane, and tetrahydrofuran are useful for carotenoid resolution by reversed-phase chromatography.

A C_{30} stationary phase was designed at the National Institute of Standards and Technology (NIST) to provide high absolute retention, enhanced shape recognition of carotenoid isomers, and moderate silanol activity.[62] The support was produced by triacontyl (C30) polymeric surface modification of a moderate pore size (~20 nm), moderate surface area (~200 m^2/g) silica, without end-capping. Superior resolution was obtained compared to monomeric and polymeric C_{18} supports. Figure 1.8 compares resolution of carotenoids and *cis*- and *trans*-isomers on the monomeric, polymeric C_{18}, and C_{30} carotenoid column.[62] The C_{30} column has improved resolution of *cis/trans* carotenoid isomers in several studies.[29,30,63,64]

In more recent work, NIST synthesized and characterized a new long-chain (C_{34}) alkyl-bonded support for carotenoid resolution.[65] This stationary phase was synthesized by polymeric and surface-polymerization synthesis. The C_{34} column slightly improved carotenoid isomer separation compared to the C_{30} stationary phase. The improvement was associated with the ability of large carotenoid molecules to more fully interact with the thicker C_{34} support. The ability to engineer "designer" supports like the C_{30} and C_{34} polymeric supports that incorporate shape selectivity or other properties of a specific analyte or class of analytes add a significant dimension to LC capabilities.

A recently published study completed in Europe gives important data about the capability of several different supports and mobile phases used to determine β-carotene in commercial foods.[66] The interlaboratory study involved fourteen different laboratories assaying four products with saponification and direct solvent extraction. LC conditions were the laboratories' normal operating systems. All methods resolved lycopene, α-carotene, and β-carotene. Repeatability (RSD_r) for total β-carotene was quite good (2.9 to 5.6%). Reproducibility (RSD_R) ranged from 6.5 to 15%. Values for all-*cis*-β-carotene were 3.3 to 5.1% (RSD_r) and 8.4 to 14% (RSD_R). Major conclusions drawn from the study were

1. Exclusion of *cis*-isomers of β-carotene can underestimate the effective β-carotene content.

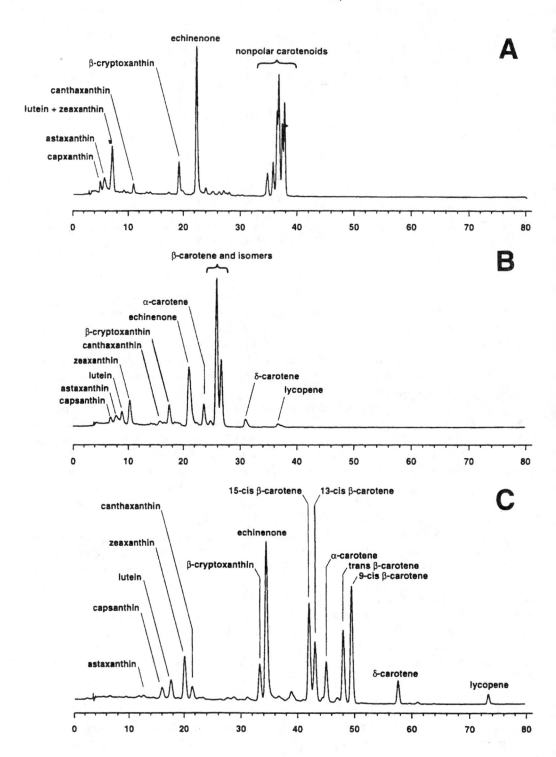

FIGURE 1.8 Separation of carotenoid standards on commercial (A) monomeric and (B) polymeric C_{18} columns, as well as the engineered C_{30} "carotenoid column." Separation conditions were as follows: 81 : 15 : 4 to 6 : 90 : 4 methanol/methyl-*tert*-butyl ether/water over 90 min; 1 mL/min; 20°C. Reproduced with permission from Reference 62.

2. Direct solvent extraction can be used for most samples if the method verifies the absence of interfering compounds by saponifying the sample after direct extraction and comparing the chromatograms. Because of the extent of the information provided by the study, the supports and mobile phases and their capabilities are reproduced from the paper in Table 1.10. However, if accurate determination of vitamin A activity is an objective of the assay, resolution of *cis*- from all *trans*-β-carotene is required.

1.3.2.2.2 Detection

1.3.2.2.2.1 Retinoids—The conjugated double-bond system present in natural and some synthetic retinoids gives quite specific and strong UV absorbance properties (Section 1.2.1.2). Most LC procedures use UV absorbance and quantitation limits can be less than 1 ng/mL. λ max are usually between 320 and 380 nm (Table 1.1). Fluorescence can be used for retinol and retinyl esters (Ex λ = 325, Em λ = 470); however, oxidation of the alcohol essentially destroys the fluorescence, and retinoic acid and many synthetic retinoids can not be detected by fluorescence. Retinol, bound to the retinol-binding proteins, fluoresces at Ex λ 333, Em λ 470.[23] Electrochemical detection has been used in a few studies. Hagen et al.[67] applied capillary LC and amperometric detection to improve detection limits three orders of magnitude compared to UV detection. Detection limits were between 0.267 and 2.73 fmol for the retinoids included in the study. The methodology was developed for assay of extremely limited quantities of embryonic tissue. Although the use of electrochemical detection is advantageous in cases where sample amounts are highly limited, most routine assays do not require such low detection limits, and UV detection is more than sufficient. PDA detectors with increased sensitivity, compared to detectors introduced throughout the 1980s, are used extensively for multiple vitamin assays. Such methods are covered in Chapter 5.

1.3.2.2.2.2 Carotenoids—The carotenoids show strong absorption bands in the visible region due to the long conjugated double-bond system.[27] Maximum absorbance is usually between 400 and 500 nm, but the λ max of individual carotenoids can vary. The strong, characteristic, visible absorption provides an ideal detection mode; however, 450 nm, a wavelength near the λ max of β-carotene, is not best for detection of many other carotenoids (Table 1.3). Variable wavelength, programmable UV/visible and PDA detectors are powerful research tools for study of complex, natural carotenoid mixtures. A multichannel PDA detector is essential for carotenoid research. Peak identification and validation of homogeneity are simplified by capabilities of the modern PDA detector. Further, multichannel capability allows detection of carotenoids with absorption maxima in the low visible to UV range (phytoene, λ max 285; phytofluene, λ max 347;[24] γ-carotene, λ max 437; and lutein, λ max 421).

1.3.2.2.3 Internal Standards

Availability of synthetic retinoids simplified the search for useful internal standards for retinol, retinoic acid, and their metabolites. Etretin,[39,68,69] RO11-6738,[39,68,69] RO13-6307,[70] acitretin,[39,71] and 11-*cis*-acitretin[39,71] have been used as internal standards in the assay of retinoic acid and its metabolites. 13-*cis*-retinoic acid is a good internal standard in the assay of synthetic retinoids.[68] If saponification is not used in extraction, retinyl esters not present in the sample can serve as the internal standard for retinol and retinyl esters.[72] Lanvers et al.[73] used arotinoid ethyl sulfone as the internal standard for assay of all-*trans*-retinol and all-*trans*-retinoic acid, various *cis*-retinoic acid isomers, and their 4-oxo metabolites.

β-apo-8′-carotenal is the most common internal standard for carotenoid assay.[57,58,74,75,76,77,78] Other carotenoid internal standards include *trans*-β-apo-10′-carotenal oxime,[63,64,79,80] decapreno-β-carotene,[81] monoapreno-β-carotene,[82] and echinenone.[78,83] Internal standards for multivitamin assays are provided in Chapter 5.

1.3.2.2.4 Method Applications

1.3.2.2.4.1 Vitamin A—AOAC International[54] Official Methods for vitamin A assay by LC are available for milk and milk-based infant formula. The Carr-Price method (Method 974.2) is

TABLE 1.10
LC Conditions Used by Participants in European Interlaboratory Study on Carotenoid Analysis

Laboratory	Precolumn	Stationary Phase	Mobile Phase	Flow mL/min	Column Temp, °C	Detection Wavelength, nm	Retention Times, min			
							Lycopene	α-Carotene	(all-E)-β-Carotene	(Z)-β-Carotene
1	None	Spherisorb ODS-2; 5 μm; 250 × 4.0 nm	CH_3CN-0.05 M $AcONH_4$,1 in CH_3OH-CH_2Cl_2 (75 + 20 + 5) CH_3CN-CH_3OH-CH_2Cl_2 (75 + 20 + 5)	1.0	RT_b	450	10.5	17.9	18.8	19.8
2	Spherisorb ODS-2, 10 × 4.6 mm + 100 × 4.6 mm	Vydac 201 TD, 5 mm, 250 × 4.6 mm	CH_3OH-CH_2Cl_2 (75 + 20 + 5)	1.5	22.5	450	16.0	20.4	22.8	2.2
3	None	Nucoeosil 100-10 C_{18}; 10 μm, 250 × 4.0 mm	CH_3OH-CH_3CN-2-propanol-0.2% $AcONH_4$ in H_2O-N-ethyldiisopropylamine (500 + 455 + 20 + 25 + 0.2) + 50 ppm BHT^c	1.0	30	445	18.6	25.7	28.0	29–32.1
4	Suplex pKb-100; 5 μm; 30 × 4.6 mm	Suplex pKb-100; 5 μm; 250 × 4.6 mm	CH_3OH-CH_3CN-2-propanol-0.2% $AcONH_4$ in H_2O-N-ethyldiisopropylamine (500 + 455 + 25 + 0.2) + 50 ppm BHT	1.0	30	445	16.0	21.3	22.9	24.4–27.5
5	RP18; 10 × 4.6 mm	Brownlee Sphen-5 ODS; 5 μm	CH_3CN-CH_3OH-THF (55 + 35 + 15)	0.8	RT	445	12.3	17.9	19.9	20.7
6	Suplex pKb-100; 5 μm; 30 × 4.6 mm	Suplex pKb-100; 5 μm; 250 × 4.6 mm	CH_3OH-CH_3CN-2-propanol-0.2% $AcONH_4$ in H_2O-N-ethyldiisopropylamine (500 + 455 + 25 + 0.2) + 50 ppm BHT	1.0	21	445	17.8	24.1	26.2	—
7	Lichrospher 100 RP18; 5 μm; 4 × 4.0 mm	Lichrospher 100 RP18; 5 μm; 250 × 4.0 mm	CH_3OH-CH_3CN-2-propanol-0.2% $AcONH_4$ in H_2O (500 + 455 + 25 + 0.2) + 50 ppm BHT	2.2	25	453	31.7	45.5	50.2	53.2
8	None	Nucleosil-100 C_{18}AB; 5 μm; 250 × 4.0 mm	CH_3OH-CH_2Cl_2-CH_3CN-2-propanol-0.2% $AcONH_4$ in H_2O (500 + 455 + 25 + 0.2) + 50 ppm BHT	1.5	25	455	14	15	17	18–19
9	None	Lichrospher 100 RP18; 5 μm; 250 × 4.0 mm	CH_3CN-CH_3OH-THF (40 + 55 + 5)	2.0	30	450	9.2	13.1	14.1	14.6–15.2

10	Lichrospher 100 RP18; 5 μm; 4 × 4.0 mm	YMC, C_{30} polymeric non-endcapped; 5 μm; 250 × 4.6 mm	CH_3OH-MTBE[d] gradient (30–80% MTBE) +0.1% BHT	1.0	22	452	18.4	11.3	12.4	10.8; 13.4
11	None	Vydac 201 TP54 protein & peptide C_{18}; 5 μm, 250 × 4 mm	CH_3CH-0.05 M $AcONH_4$ in CH_3OH-CH_2Cl_2 (75 + 20 + 5)	1.0	15	445	20.3	19.6	22.3	24–28
12	None	Vydac 201 TP54 protein & peptide C_{18}; 5 μm, 250 × 4.6 mm	CH_3OH-THF[e] (99 + 1)	0.6	RT	450	22.8	17.2	19.6	21.5–23.5
13	None	Ultrasphere ODS; 5 μm, 250 × 4.6 mm	CH_3OH-THF (95 + 5)	3.0	RT	450	12	13.6	14.6	—
14	Vydac 201 TP54; 10 × 4.6 mm	Vydac 201 TP54; 10 μm; 250 × 4.6 mm	CH_3OH-THF (95 + 5) + 0.1% BHT	1.0	20	445	24.8	13.5	15.6	17.6

[a] $AcONH_4$, ammonium acetate

[b] RT, room temperature

[c] BHT, butylated hydroxytoluene

[d] MTBE, methyl tert-butyl ether

[e] THF, tetrahydrofuran

Reproduced with permission from Reference 66.

discussed in Section 1.3.1. Method 992.04 (50.1.02) "Vitamin A (Retinol Isomers) in Milk and Milk-Based Infant Formula, Liquid Chromatographic Method" and Method 992.06 (50.1.03) "Vitamin A (Retinol) in Milk-Based Infant Formula Liquid Chromatographic Method" were collaborated in 1993.[84] Method 992.04 quantitates all-*trans* retinol and 13-*cis* retinol after sample digestion at ambient temperature for 15 h in ethanolic KOH and extraction of the digest with diethyl ether : hexane (15 : 85). Normal-phase chromatography on silica (Apex, 3 mm) is completed with heptane : isopropanol at concentrations that elute 13-*cis* retinol at 4.5 min and all-*trans* retinol at 5.5 min. Detection is at 340 nm.

Method 992.06 is specific for milk-based infant formula containing 500 IU or more of vitamin A per reconstituted quart. This method incorporates saponification at 70°C for 25 min as opposed to the 18 h digestion at ambient temperature for Method 992.04. Normal-phase chromatography uses a silica-based cyano stationary support (Sepralyte CN, 5 μm) and hexane : isopropyl alcohol (100 + 0.25 V/V). Detection is at 336 nm. Use of 336 nm assumes that the relative molar absorptivities of both isomers are virtually equal at 336 nm. International Units (IU) are corrected for the lower biological activity of 13-*cis* vitamin A palmitate in the sample by a correction factor of 0.75 for the *cis*-isomer. The assumption is made that the *cis*-isomer measured as 13-*cis* retinol after saponification is not an artifact of the digestion and extraction. A deficiency of the method is failure to adequately follow hydrolysis of all-*trans* retinyl palmitate and extraction efficiency from the sample digest. Retinyl palmitate standards are saponified with water in place of sample. Recoveries from the standard digest may well vary due to matrix effects from the sample digest.

Method 992.06 makes no provisions for use of spike recoveries or for incorporation of internal standard methodology. Methods 992.04 and 992.06 provide poor directions for saponification. Digestions are completed in a volumetric flask (992.04) or capped tubes (992.06) without evacuation or inert gas flush. The methods would be improved by use of an air condenser (Chapter 3) or air removal.

The International Dairy Federation (IDF) provides a method for the LC determination of vitamin A in dried skim milk.[85] The IDF procedure is based on saponification and extraction with light petroleum with reversed-phase resolution on C_8 or C_{18}. The saponification procedure is detailed to provide control of vitamin A degradation during the extraction phase of the method; however, like AOAC International methods, no allowance is made for use of spiked recoveries or internal standards to ensure method conformance for extraction of the retinyl ester used for the standard, retinyl ester, all-*trans* retinol, or *cis*-retinol isomers in the sample. A detailed summary of the IDF method is provided in Section 1.4.

Comprehensive reviews cited in Section 1.3 are available for methods for all-*trans* retinol, its esters and isomers, and other retinoids. Several recently published methods are summarized in Table 1.7.

1.3.2.2.4.2 Carotenoids—LC is necessary to resolve complex mixtures of carotenoids from plant materials. Additionally, a PDA detector is essential for peak identity and homogeneity confirmation.[46] Nevertheless, many laboratories around the world do not have this quite sophisticated instrumentation capability and must rely on older procedures, particularly to quantitate provitamin A activity of foods and diets. Because of this, much interest exists in the application and improvement of such methods.

Provitamin A methods were reviewed by Rodriguez-Amaya[47,48] with emphasis on the associated problems of relevant methods. Evaluated methods included:

1. AOAC International methods of which Method 941.14 (45.1.03) "Carotene in Fresh Plant Materials" is most pertinent to provitamin A estimation in foods
2. European Cooperation in Scientific and Technological Research in methods (COST)
3. Published open column methods
4. HPLC methods

AOAC[54] and COST[86] (Table 1.6, References 3 and 14) provide excellent procedural guides; however, these procedures are adequate only if β-carotene is the sole contributor of vitamin A activity.[47] In AOAC Official Method 941.14, the carotene fraction is extracted with acetone and hexane and isolated by MgO (activated) : Hyflo Super Cel (diatomaceous earth) open column chromatography. The carotenes pass through the column in visible bands with elution with acetone : hexane (1 : 9). The entire column eluate is collected, diluted to 100 mL, and absorbance read at 436 nm. Xanthophylls, carotene oxidation products, and chlorophylls remain on the column. Results are reported as mg β-carotene or IU of vitamin A activity. Overestimation of vitamin A activity is common if less active provitamin A carotenoids, other than β-carotene, are present in the sample. Method 941.14 was modified to isolate specific carotenoid fractions for improved accuracy, but such modifications add to the tediousness of the assay.[87]

COST procedures[86] apply to complex foods, total carotenes in fruit, vegetables, unaltered plant materials, and beverages. For assay of complex foods, the sample is saponified (30 min, 60°C) with methanolic KOH. Carotenes are partitioned into diethyl ether, evaporated, and redissolved in hexane. Other matrices are treated with slight modification. For each procedure, water is removed from the hexane fraction by adding ethanol and reevaporating the solvent. Residues are dissolved in hexane and passed through a deactivated alumina column. Carotenes are eluted with hexane, and absorbance is measured at 450 nm. β-carotene is calculated using a $E_{1\ cm}^{1\%}$ value of 2590 (hexane). The methods assume that contributions of α-carotene, β-cryptoxanthin, and other more uncommon provitamin A carotenoids are negligible. Rodriguez-Amaya[47] provides a complete review of open-column methods and their problems for vitamin A activity measurement of complex matrices.

Characteristics of HPLC procedures suitable for measurement of provitamin A measurement include:

1. Capability to efficiently remove interfering compounds prior to LC through proper extraction techniques
2. Capability to resolve each carotenoid in the sample extract with provitamin A activity
3. Capability to resolve cis- from trans-isomers
4. Capability to prove peak identity and homogeneity[46]

Early work on resolution of cis- and trans-isomers showed that Ca(OH)$_2$ was an effective support when acetone : hexane gradients were applied. However, owing to lack of a commercial source and problems with column to column repeatability, Ca(OH)$_2$ was never widely applied to carotenoid research.[53] More recent development of the C_{30} polymeric LC columns as discussed in Section 1.3.2.2.1 enhances capability of LC methodology to accurately measure provitamin A activity.

Excellent studies exist in which HPLC methods were used to quantitate primary provitamin A carotenoids in fruits and vegetables. Some of the later papers are Chen et al.[75] (Taiwanese vegetables), Homnava et al.[88,89] (fruits), Dokkum et al.[90] (Netherlands diets), Heinonen et al.[91] (Finnish foods), Granado et al.[92] (Spanish vegetables), Simonne et al.[93] (Sweet potatoes), Biacs and Daood[94] (fruits and vegetables), Minguez-Mosquera and Hornero-Méndez[76] (red peppers) Tonucci et al.[77] (processed tomato products), Chen et al.[95] (carrots), Nyambaka and Ryley[28] (dark green vegetables), Granelli and Helmersson[96] (milk), Hart and Scott[78] (fruits and vegetables), Wills and Rangga[97] (Chinese vegetables), Mercadante et al.[98] (mango), Riso and Porrini[83] (vegetables), and Konings and Roomans[99] (fruits and vegetables). The Konings and Roomans procedure[99] provides an easy to follow protocol and good method performance validation parameters. The procedure is presented in Section 1.4.

Concentrated efforts have extensively characterized the carotenoid profiles of specific fruits and vegetables. Khachik and co-workers at the USDA, Beltsville, Nutrient Composition Laboratory developed HPLC procedures for resolution of up to 30 components in fruit and vegetable extracts.[52,57,58,59,74,81,82,100,101] Components identified included xanthophylls, chlorophylls, hydrocarbon carotenoids, β-carotene *cis*-isomers, and carotenol fatty acid esters. Carotenoids were resolved by several different LC systems, and the isolated carotenoids were identified and characterized by thin layer chromatography, NMR, mass spectrometry, and diode array UV/visible spectroscopy. The study is described in detail in Reference 52.

Recently, Mercadente et al.[98] characterized the carotenoids in mango. Principle carotenoids identified by mass spectrometry after LC purification were all-*trans* violaxanthin, all-*trans*-β-carotene, and a *cis*-violaxanthin.

Interest in the antioxidant capability of common dietary carotenoids led to extensive research on profiling plasma and tissue carotenoid levels in order to define diet-health relationships. Definitive studies were not completed until the early 1990s. However, earlier work by Nelis and De Leenheer[102] provided the basis for carotenoid assay of serum. This work identified lutein, zeaxanthin, β-cryptoxanthin, lycopene, α-carotene, and β-carotene as the primary constituents of human serum. Subsequent work by Bieri et al.[103] identified an additional, unidentified peak in normal plasma. These authors essentially used the Nelis and De Leenheer method, substituting a C_{18} Supelco column for the Zorbax ODS support used by Nelis and De Leenheer. Comprehensive characterization studies have been completed by research led by Khachik and Beecher at the USDA Nutrient Composition Laboratory that provides extensive information on carotenoids in plasma, human milk, and other physiological samples. Initial studies published in 1991[104] identified α-cryptoxanthin as the unknown carotenoid found by Bieri et al.[103] in earlier work.

Subsequent work identified 18 carotenoids in extracts of human plasma.[105,106] Methods available for plasma analysis up to 1992 were reviewed by Khachik et al.[106] More recently, Khachik et al.[107] identified 34 carotenoids in breast milk and human serum. Identifications included 13 geometric isomers and 8 metabolites. The procedure included resolution by reversed-phase and normal-phase chromatography, PDA detection, and HPLC-MS interfaced identification by electron capture negative ionization. Because of the significance of this work, the carotenoids identified in this comprehensive study are listed in Table 1.11 along with absorption maxima and molecular mass information. Methodology is summarized in Table 1.8 (Biologicals, Reference 16). Improved methods led to recent studies that increased our understanding about diet-health relationships concerning carotenoids.[108–112]

Accurate quantitation and identification of carotenoids continues to be problematic. While HPLC coupled with PDA detection and, often, interfaced with MS is a powerful analytical research tool, such instrument sophistication is not available in the majority of analytical laboratories worldwide. Additionally, advantages of LC resolution are often negated by stability problems with the analytes that can cause the inexperienced analyst a great deal of difficulty. Scott[113] discussed specific problems associated with carotenoid analysis that all analysts should be aware of before initiating LC analysis. These include:

1. Variation in results owing to inconsistencies in retention times, peak identification, and inconsistencies in peak homogeneity because of variations in mobile-phase composition and stationary supports.
2. On-column loss owing to degradation by interaction with stainless steel frits: Frits made of Peek Alloyed with Teflon (PAT) eliminates the problem.
3. Reaction of carotenoids with injection solvents and mobile phase: Failure to include an antioxidant such as BHT in the mobile phase and extraction solvent will intensify this problem. Also, low acid levels in solvents used for reversed-phase chromatography (e.g., methylene chloride) can be easily neutralized by addition of 0.001% triethylamine.[114]
4. Potential loss of labile carotenoids during solvent evaporation: inclusion of antioxidant in the extraction solvent tends to decrease degradation. Also, some methods call for the inclusion of a saturated hydrocarbon like decanoate in the solvent to protect labile analytes from oxidation during solvent evaporation. This can be particularly helpful if rotary evaporation is

TABLE 1.11

HPLC Peak Identification of Carotenoids in Human Serum and Milk Extracts from Their Wavelengths of Absorption Maxima and Mass Spectral Data Determined by HPLC Photodiode Array Detection Mass Spectrometry in the Order of Elution with Eluents B and A

Peak No.	Serum/Milk Carotenoids[a]	Absorption Maxima (nm)[c]	Molecular Mass (m/z)[d]
	Eluent B		
1[a]	ε,ε-carotene-3,3′-dione	420, 442, 472	564
2[a]	3′-hydroxy-ε,ε-caroten-3-one	422, 442, 472	566, 548 (M-H_2O)
3[a]	2,6-cyclolycopene-1,5-diol I	434, 458, 492	570
4[a]	3-hydroxy-β-ε-caroten-3′-one	(424), 448, 476	566, 548 (M-H_2O)
5[a]	(Z)-3-hydroxy-β-ε-caroten-3′-one	(420), 442, 470	566, 548 (M-H_2O)
6	(3S,6S,3′S,6′S)-ε,ε-carotene-3,3′-diol (lactucaxanthin)	416, 442, 470	566, 550 (M-H_2O)
7	(13Z,13′Z,3R,3′R,6′R)-β-ε-carotene-3,3′-diol[(13Z,13′Z,3R,3′R,6′R)-lutein]	274, 336, 410, 432, 460	568, 550 (M-H_2O)
8	(all-E,3R,3′R,6′R),β-ε-carotene,3,3′diol [(all-E,3R,3′R,6′R)-lutein]	(424), 448, 476	568, 550 (M-H_2O)
9[a]	2,6-cyclolycopene-1,5 diol II	432, 458, 490	570
10	(all-E,3R,3′R),β-β-carotene,3,3′-diol [(all-E,3R,3′R)-zeaxanthin]	(428), 454, 482	568
11[a]	(all-E,3R,3′S,6′R),β-ε-carotene,3,3′-diol [(all-E)-3′-epilutein]	(424), 448, 476	568, 550 (M-H_2O)
12	(9Z,3R,3′R,6′R)-lutein	334, (420), 442, 470	568, 550 (M-H_2O)
13	(9′Z,3R,3′R,6′R)-lutein	334, (420), 444, 472	568, 550 (M-H_2O)
14	(13Z)-lutein + (13′Z)-lutein	334, (418), 440, 468	568, 550 (M-H_2O)
15	(9Z)-zeaxanthin	340, (424), 450, 474	568
16	(13Z)-zeaxanthin	338, (419), 446, 472	568
17	(15Z)-zeaxanthin	338, (426), 450, 478	568
	Eluent A		
18[a]	(3R,6′R)-3-hydroxy-3′,4′-didehydro-β-γ-carotene	334, (424), 446, 476	550
19[a]	(3R,6′R)-3-hydroxy-2′,3′-didehydro-β-ε-carotene (2′,3′-anhydrolutein)	336, (424), 448, 476	550
20	β-ε-caroten-3-ol (α-cryptoxanthin)	(424), 446, 476	552
21	3-hydroxy-β-carotene (β-cryptoxanthin)	(428), 454, 480	552
22	(Z)-3-hydroxy-β-carotene [(Z)-β-cryptoxanthin]	(424), 450, 476	552
23	ψ,ψ-carotene (lycopene)	446, 474, 502	536
24	(Z)-ψ,ψ-carotene [(Z)-lycopene]	348, 362, 438, 466, 494	536
25	7,8-dihydro-ψ,ψ-carotene (neurosporene)	418, 442, 470	538
26	β,ψ-carotene (γ-carotene)	(440), 462, 492	536

TABLE 1.11 Continued

Peak No.	Serum/Milk Carotenoids[a]	Absorption Maxima (nm)[c]	Molecular Mass (m/z)[d]
27	7,8,7′,8′-tetrahydro-ψ,ψ-carotene (ζ-carotene)	378, 400–402, 426	540
28	β-ε-carotene (α-carotene)	(428), 446–448, 474	536
29	(all-E)- β,β-carotene [(all-E)-β-carotene]	(430), 454, 478	536
30	(9Z)-β,β-carotene [(9Z)-β-carotene]	340, (426), 450, 474	536
31	(13Z)-β,β-carotene [(13Z)-β-carotene]	340, (424), 448, 472	536
32	(all-E)-or (Z)-7,8,11,12,7′,8′-hexahydro-φ,φ-carotene [(all E)-or (Z)-phytofluene]	334, 350, 368	e
33	[(Z)- or (all-E)-phytofluene]	344, 350, 368	e
34	7,8,11,12,7′,8′,11′,12′-octahydro-ψ,ψ-carotene (phytoene)	(276), 286, (295)	e

[a] Refers to carotenoid metabolites.

[b] Common names for certain carotenoids are shown in parentheses.

[c] Values in parentheses represent points of inflection.

[d] The molecular ions appeared as the base peak (100% intensity). In some cases, the ion due to the loss of H_2O from the molecular parent ion (M) could also be observed.

[e] Due to the coelution of cholestryl esters with this compound, its molecular parent ion was not observed by HPLC-MS.

Reproduced with permission from Reference 107. Chromatography parameters given in Table 8, Reference 16, Biologicals.

used. The hydrocarbon can form a thin film oxygen barrier on the rotary flask, protecting the carotenoids from low levels of oxygen that are potentially present in the evaporation system.

5. Potential for degradation during saponification (see Section 1.3.2.1.1).

Carotenoid identification from complex mixtures is still hampered by lack of reliable standards. Commercial, pure standards are limited. Craft et al.[115] evaluated all-*trans*-β-carotene sources by reversed-phase chromatography and found that impurities and *cis*-isomers accounted for 16 to 75% of the absorbance at 450 nm. Analytical purity ranged from 7.1 to 82.9%. Probably, use of impure standards, failure to document purity of commercially available standards, and use of degraded standards will continue to be an impediment to reliable carotenoid data collection for the foreseeable future. We often learn the "hard" way about stability of the carotenoids and associated assay problems.

Improved sensitivity of PDA detectors, use of multiple detection modes, and improved resolution systems have led to the rapid employment of methods for the simultaneous determination of multiple fat-soluble vitamins and their metabolites. These methods are discussed in Chapter 5.

Other approaches for retinoid and carotenoid analysis include gas chromatography, supercritical fluid chromatography, and capillary electrophoresis (CE). Wyss[39] reviewed application of these techniques to retinoid research. Of these approaches, CE shows excellent promise, and several recent papers document the usefulness of CE, particularly for retinoid quantitation. The reader is referred to the following publications for information regarding CE: Bampong et al.,[116] Ma et al.,[117] Shi et al.,[118] and Hsieh and Kuo.[119]

1.4   METHOD PROTOCOLS

Dried Skimmed Milk—Determination of Vitamin A—Colorimetric and Liquid Chromatographic Methods

Method B—High Performance Liquid Chromatographic Method

Liquid Chromatographic Method

Principle
- Dried skimmed milk is saponified and extracted with light petroleum.
- Retinol is quantitated by reversed-phase LC with detection at 325 nm.

Chemicals
- Ethanol, 95%
- Sodium ascorbate solution, 200 g/L
- Potassium hydroxide, 50% in water wt/wt
- Potassium hydroxide, ethanolic; dissolve 3 g in water, add 10 mL ethanol, and dilute to 100 mL with water
- Light petroleum, boiling range 40 to 60°C or 60 to 80°C
- Methanol
- USP vitamin A—all-*trans* retinyl acetate
- BHT

Apparatus
- Liquid chromatograph
- UV detector
- Saponification vessel fitted with reflux condenser
- Steam bath, boiling water bath, or electric heating mantle
- Water bath operating at a temperature up to 40°C

Procedure

Saponification
- Weigh 20 g sample (nearest 0.001 g) into beaker or conical flask, dissolve in 50 mL hot water (60 to 80°C). Cool to ambient temperature. Transfer to 100 mL volumetric and dilute with water.
- Transfer 25 mL of the solution to a saponification flask.
- Add 20 mL potassium hydroxide aqueous solution, 10 mL sodium ascorbate solution and 50 mL ethanol, mix.
- Reflux 30 min on steam bath, water bath, or heating mantle.
- Swirl occasionally, cool immediately.

Extraction
- Transfer to separatory funnel with two 30 mL portions of water, two 10 mL portions of ethanol and two 40mL portions of light petroleum.
- Shake vigorously for 30 s, allow phase separation.
- Transfer aqueous phase to second separatory funnel, shake with a mixture of 10 mL ethanol and 40 mL light petroleum
- Allow phase to separate, repeat extraction for a third time, add washings to the first separatory funnel.
- Shake the aqueous phase with 40 mL light petroleum and 10 mL ethanol, add the petroleum phase to the first separatory funnel.
- Wash the combined light petroleum extracts three times with 40 mL portions of ethanolic potassium hydroxide.
- Wash with 40 mL portions of water until washing is neutral.
- Dry extract by adding two sheets of 9 cm filter paper cut into strips.
- Transfer extract to 200 mL volumetric, add 10 to 20 mg BHT, dilute to volume with light petroleum.

Chromatography

Column	25 cm × 4.6 mm
Stationary phase	C_8 or C_{18}, 10 mm
Mobile phase	Methanol : water (90 : 10 or ratio to accomplish resolution)
Flow	2 mL/min
Column temperature	Ambient
Injection	20 ml
Detection	325 nm
Calculation	Peak area, linear regression

Note: Even though the extraction procedure is based upon multiple solvent extractions, the method has unacceptable repeatability and reproducibility characteristics. Stated limits were 14% for one analyst based on two observations (repeatability), and 42% for two analysts working in different laboratories (reproducibility).

Evaluation of an LC Method for the Analysis of Carotenoids in Vegetables and Fruit

Principle
- Carotenoids were extracted with methanol/THF (1 : 1) by homogenization. Following centrifugation, supernatants were, in some cases, saponified. After centrifugation or saponification, NaCl was added and carotenoids partitioned with petroleum ether. Organic layers were evaporated and the residue dissolved in methanol/THF (75 : 25). Carotenoids were resolved by reversed-phase chromatography with PDA detection.

Chemicals
- α-carotene, β-carotene,
- β-cryptoxanthin, lutein, lycopene, zeaxanthin (standards)
- Ethyl-β-apo-8′-carotenate (IS)
- Potassium hydroxide
- Ethanol, absolute
- Methanol
- THF
- Hexane
- Acetone
- Petroleum ether
- BHT
- Sodium chloride
- Magnesium carbonate

Apparatus
- Liquid chromatograph fitted with PAT column frits
- UV detector
- Homogenizer
- Centrifuge
- Rotary evaporator
- Sonicator

Procedure

Extraction
- Add 0.2 g $MgCO_3$ to 0.5 to1.0 g freeze-dried sample.
- Add ethyl-β-apo-8′-carotenoate (IS), amount approximately equal to carotenoids in sample.
- Homogenize with methanol/THF (1 : 1) until extract is colorless. Use 100 mL of extracting solution followed by 50 mL for subsequent extractions.
- Centrifuge to collect supernatants.
- If β-cryptoxanthin is present, extract was saponified at ambient temperature for 2 h with equal volume of 10% KOH.
- Add 50 mL 10% NaCl to extract (saponified or non-saponified).
- Extract with 50 mL portions of petroleum ether until the petroleum ether is colorless.
- For saponified extract, wash petroleum ether with 100 mL portions of water until washes are neutral.
- Evaporate petroleum ether to dryness.
- Dissolve residue in methanol : THF (75 : 25) with sonication.

Chromatography

Column	25 cm $\times$ 4.6 mm
Stationary phase	Vydac 201 TP, 5 mm
Mobile phase	Methanol : THF (95 : 5)
Flow	1 mL/min
Column temperature	Ambient
Detection	PDA, 450 nm
Calculation	Peak area, linear regression, internal standard

Notes: RSD_r ranged from 1.9 to 4.9%; recovery ranged from 93 to 107%.

Lycopene recovery is adversely affected by stainless steel frits in the pump. Replace with Peek Alloyed with Teflon (PAT).

All solvents contain 0.1% BHT (w/v).

Food Chem., 59, 599, 1997

1.5 REFERENCES

Text

1. Friedrich, W., Vitamin A and its provitamins, in *Vitamins,* Walter de Gruyter, Berlin, 1988, chap. 2.
2. National Research Council, *Recommended Dietary Allowances,* 10th ed., National Academy Press, Washington, D. C., 1989, chap. 7.
3. Machlin, L. J. and Hüni, J. E. S., *Vitamins Basics,* Hoffmann-LaRoche, Basel, 1994, 3.
4. van den Berg, H., Vitamin A intake and status, *Eur. J. Clin. Nutr.,* 50, 57, 1996.
5. Gibson, R. S., *Principles of Nutritional Assessment,* Oxford University Press, New York, 1990, chap. 18.
6. *21 CFR, 131, Milk and Cream and 166, Margarine.*
7. Olson, J. A., Vitamin A, in *Present Knowledge in Nutrition,* 7th ed., Ziegler, E. E. and Filer, L. J., Jr., Eds., ILSI Press, Washington, D.C., 1996, chap. 11.
8. Margels, A. R., Holden, J. M., Beecher, G. R., Forman, M. R., and Lanza, E., Carotenoid content of fruits and vegetables: an evaluation of analytic data, *J. Am. Diet. Assoc.,* 93, 284, 1993.
9. Chug-Ahuja, J. K., Holden, J. M., Forman, M. R., Mangels, A. R., Beecher, G. R., and Lanza, E., The development and application of a carotenoid database for fruits, vegetables, and selected multicomponent foods, *J. Am. Diet. Assoc.,* 93, 318, 1993.
10. USDA, NCI, *Carotenoid food composition database version I,* 1993.
11. Yong, L. C., Forman, M. R., Beecher, G. R., Graubard, B. I., Campbell, W. S., Reichman, M. E., Taylor, P. R., Lanza, E., Holden, J. M., and Judd, J. T., Relationship between dietary intake and plasma concentrations of carotenoids in premenopausal women: application of the USDA-NCI carotenoid food-composition database, *J. Am. Clin. Nutr.,* 60, 223, 1994.
12. Nutritional Labeling and Education Act of 1990, *Fed. Reg.,* 58, 2070, 1993.
13. Chertow, B. S., Driscoll, H. K., Blaner, W. S., Meda, P., Cordle, M. B., and Matthews, K. A., Effects of vitamin A deficiency and repletion on rat glucagon secretion, *Pancreas,* 9, 475, 1994.
14. Clark, A. R., Wilson, M. E., London, N. J. M., James, R. F. L., Docherty, K., Identification and characterization of a functional retinoic acid/thyroid hormone response element upstream of the human insulin gene enhancer, *Biochem. J.,* 309, 863, 1995.
15. Levin, M. S. and Davis, A. E., Retinoic acid increases cellular retinol binding protein II mRNA and retinol uptake in the human intestinal Caco-2 cell line, *J. Nutr.,* 127, 13, 1997.
16. Mao, Y., Gurr, J. A., and Hickok, N. J., Retinoic acid regulates ornithine decarboxylase gene expression at the transcriptional level, *Biochem J.,* 295, 641, 1993.
17. Sleeman, M. W., Zhou, H., Rogers, S., Ng, K., and Best, J. D., Retinoic acid stimulates glucose transporter expression in L6 muscle cells, *Mol. Cell. Endocrinol.,* 108, 161, 1995.
18. Olson, J.A., Vitamin A, in *Handbook of Vitamins,* Machlin, L. J., Ed., Marcel Dekker, New York, 1991, chap. 1.

19. Weedon, B. C. L. and Moss, G. P., Structure and nomenclature, in *Carotenoids,* Vol. 1A, *Isolation and Analysis,* Britton, G., Liaan-Jensen, S., and Pfander, H., Eds., Birkhaüser Verlag, Basel, 1995, chap. 3.

20. Parker, R. S., Bioavailability of carotenoids, *Eur. J. Clin. Nutr.,* 51, 586, 1997.

21. Erdman, J. W., Jr., Bierer, T. L., and Gugger, E. T., Absorption and transport of carotenoids, *Ann. NY Acad. Sci.,* 691, 76, 1993.

22. Combs, G. F., Jr., Characteristics of the vitamins, in *The Vitamins,* Academic Press, Harcourt Brace Jovanovich, New York, 1992, chap. 3.

23. De Leenheer, A. P., Lambert, W. E., and Meyer, E., Chromatography of retinoids, in *Retinoids, Progress in Research and Clinical Applications,* Livnea, M. A. and Packer, L., Eds., Marcel Dekker, New York, 1993, chap. 37.

24. Furr, H., Barua, A., and Olson, J., Retinoids and carotenoids, in *Modern Chromatographic Analysis of the Vitamins,* De Leenheer, A. P., Lambert, W. E., and Nelis, H. J., Eds., Marcel Dekker, New York, 1992, chap. 1.

25. Brinkmann, E., Dehne, L., Oei, H. B., Tiebach, R., and Baltes, W., Separation of geometrical retinol isomers in food samples by using narrow-bore high performance liquid chromatography, *J. Chromatogr. A,* 693, 271, 1995.

26. Ball, G. F. M., Chemical and biological nature of the fat-soluble vitamins, *Fat-Soluble Vitamin Assays in Chap. 2 Food Analysis—A Comprehensive Review,* Elsevier Applied Science Publishers, London, 1988, chap. 2.

27. Britton, G., UV/Visible spectroscopy, in *Carotenoids,* Vol. 1B: *Spectroscopy,* Britton, B., Liaaen-Jensen, S., and Pfander, H., Eds., Birkhäuser Verlag, Basel, 1995, chap. 2.

28. Nyambaka, H. and Ryley, J., An isocratic reversed-phase HPLC separation of the stereoisomers of the provitamin A carotenoids (α- and β-carotene) in dark green vegetables, *Food Chem.,* 55, 63, 1996.

29. Emenhiser, C., Sander, L. C., and Schwartz, S. J., Capability of a polymeric C_{30} stationary phase to resolve *cis-trans* carotenoid isomers in reversed-phase liquid chromatography, *J. Chromatogr. A,* 707, 205, 1995.

30. Emenhiser, C., Englert, G., Sander, L. C., Ludwig, B., and Schwartz, S. J., Isolation and structural elucidation of the predominant geometrical isomers of α-carotene, *J. Chromatogr. A,* 719, 333, 1996.

31. Schiedt, K. and Liaaen-Jensen, S., Isolation and analysis, in *Carotenoids,* Vol. 1A, *Isolation and Analysis,* Britton, G., Liaaen-Jensen, S., and Pfaner, H., Eds., Birkhäuser Verlag, Basel, 1995, chap. 5.

32. Manan, F., Guevara, L. V., and Ryley, J., The stability of all-*trans* retinol and reactivity towards transition metals, *Food Chem.,* 40, 43, 1991.

33. Landers, G. M. and Olson, J. A., Absence of isomerization of retinyl palmitate, retinol, and retinal in chlorinated and nonchlorinated solvents under gold light, *J. Assoc. Off. Anal. Chem.,* 69, 50, 1986.

34. Peng, Y. M., Xu, M. J., and Alberts, D. S., Analysis and stability of retinol in plasma, *JNCI,* 78, 95, 1987.

35. Scita, G., The stability of β-carotene under different laboratory conditions, *J. Nutr. Biochem.,* 3, 124, 1992.

36. Reische, D. W., Lillard, D. A., and Eitenmiller, R. R., Antioxidants, in *Food Lipids,* Akoh, C. and Min, D., Eds., Marcel Dekker, New York, 1998, chap. 16.

37. Liebler, D. C., Antioxidant reactions of carotenoids, *Ann. NY Acad. Sci.,* 69, 20, 1993.

38. Wyss, R., Chromatography of retinoids, *J. Chromatogr.,* 531, 481, 1990.

39. Wyss, R., Chromatographic and electrophoretic analysis of biomedically important retinoids, *J. Chromatogr. B,* 671, 381, 1995.

40. Bhat, P. V. and Sundaresan, P. R., High-performance liquid chromatography of vitamin A compounds, *CRC Crit. Rev. Anal. Chem.,* 20, 197, 1988.

41. Furr, H. C., Barua, A. B., and Olson, J. A., Analytical methods, in *The Retinoids, Biology, Chemistry and Medicine,* Sporn, M. B., Roberts, A. B., and Goodman, D. S., Eds., Raven Press, New York, 1994, Chap. 3.

42. Parrish, D., Moffitt, R., Noci, R., and Thompson, J., Vitamin A, in *Methods of Vitamin Analysis,* Augustin, J., Klein, B. P., Becker, D. A., and Venugopal, Eds., John Wiley & Sons, New York, 1984, 153.

43. Lambert, W. E., Nelis, H. J., De Ruyter, M. G. M., and De Leenheer, A. P., Vitamin A: retinol, carotenoids and related compounds, in *Modern Chromatographic Analysis of the Vitamins,* De Leenheer, A. P., Lambert, W. E., and De Ruyter, M. G. M., Eds., Marcel Dekker, New York, 1985, 1.

44. Thompson, J. N., Review: Official methods for measurement of vitamin A. Problems of official methods and new techniques for analysis of foods and feeds for vitamin A, *J. Assoc. Off. Anal. Chem.,* 69, 727, 1986.

45. Tee, E. S. and Lim, C. L., The analysis of carotenoids and retinoids: a review, *Food Chem.,* 41, 147, 1991.

46. Eitenmiller, R. R. and Landen, W. O., Jr., Vitamins, in *Analyzing Food for Nutrition Labeling and Hazardous Contaminants,* Jeon, I. J. and Ikins, W. G., Eds., Marcel Dekker, 1995, chap. 9.

47. Rodriguez-Amaya, D., Critical review of provitamin A determination in plant foods, *J. Micronutr. Anal.,* 5, 191, 1989.

48. Rodriguez-Amaya, D., Provitamin A determination—problems and possible solutions, *Food Lab. News,* 19, 35, 1990.

49. Craft, N., Carotenoid reversed-phase high-performance liquid chromatography methods: reference compendium, *Meth. Enzymol.,* 213, 185, 1992.

50. De Leenheer, A. P. and Nelis, H. J., Profiling and quantitation of carotenoids by high performance liquid chromatography and photodiode array detection, *Meth. Enzymol.,* 213, 251, 1992.

51. Tsukida, K., Separation of *cis*-β-carotenes, *Meth. Enzymol.,* 213, 291, 1992.

52. Khachik, F., Beecher, G., Goli, M., and Lusby, W., Separation and quantitation of carotenoids in foods, *Meth. Enzymol.,* 213, 205, 1992.

53. O'Neil, C. A. and Schwartz, S. J., Chromatographic analysis of *cis/trans* carotenoid isomers, *J. Chromatogr.,* 624, 235, 1992.

54. AOAC International, *Official Methods of Analysis,* 16th ed., AOAC International, Arlington, VA, 1995.

55. Thiex, N., Smallidge, R., and Beine, R., Sources of error in vitamin A analysis, *J. AOAC Int.,* 79, 1269, 1996.

56. Lehman, P. A. and Franz, T. J., A sensitive high-pressure liquid chromatography/particle beam/mass spectrometry assay for the determination of all-*trans*-retinoic acid and 13-*cis*-retinoic acid in human plasma, *J. Pharm. Sci.,* 85, 287, 1996.

57. Khachik, F. and Beecher, G. R., Separation and identification of carotenoids and carotenol fatty acid esters in some squash products by liquid chromatography. 1. Quantification of carotenoids and related esters by HPLC, *J. Agric. Food Chem.,* 36, 929, 1988.

58. Khachik, F., Beecher, G. R., and Lusby, W. R., Separation and identification of carotenoids and carotenol fatty acid esters in some squash products by liquid chromatography. 2. Isolation and characterization of carotenoids and related esters, *J. Agric. Food Chem.,* 36, 938, 1988.

59. Khachik, F., Beecher, G. R., and Lusby, W. R., Separation, identification, and quantification of the major carotenoids in extracts of apricots, peaches, cantaloupe, and pink grapefruit by liquid chromatography, *J. Agric. Food Chem.,* 37, 1465, 1989.

60. Nöll, G. N., High-performance liquid chromatographic analysis of retinal and retinol isomers, *J. Chromatogr. A,* 721, 247, 1996.

61. Nöll, G. N. and Kalinowski, H. O., Identification of retinolisomers by high performance liquid chromatography not unequivocal up to now, *Vision Res.,* 36, 1887, 1996.

62. Sander, L. C., Sharpless, K. E., Craft, N. E., and Wise, S. A., Development of engineered stationary phases for the separation of carotenoid isomers, *Anal. Chem.,* 66, 1667, 1994.

63. Brown Thomas, J., Kline, M. C., Schiller, S. B., Ellerbe, P. M., Sniegoski, L. T., Duewer, D. L., and Sharpless, K. E., Certification of fat-soluble vitamers, carotenoids, and cholesterol in human serum: Standard Reference Material 968b, *Fres. J. Anal. Chem.,* 356, 1, 1996.

64. Sharpless, K. E., Brown Thomas, J., Sander, L. C., and Wise, S. J., Liquid chromatographic determination of carotenoids in human serum using an engineered C_{30} and a C_{18} stationary phase, *J. Chromatogr. B,* 678, 187, 1996.

65. Bell, C. M., Sander, L. C., Fetzer, J. C., and Wise, S. A., Synthesis and characterization of extended length alkyl stationary phases for liquid chromatography with application to the separation of carotenoid isomers, *J. Chromatogr. A,* 753, 37, 1996.

66. Schüep, W. and Schierle, J., Determination of β-carotene in commercial foods, Interlaboratory study, *J. AOAC Int.,* 80, 1057, 1997.

67. Hagen, J. J., Washco, K. A., and Monnig, C. A., Determination of retinoids by reverse-phase capillary liquid chromatography with amperometric electrochemical detection, *J. Chromatogr. B,* 677, 225, 1996.

68. Wyss, R., Determination of retinoids in plasma by high performance liquid chromatography and automated column switching, *Meth. Enzymol.,* 189, 146, 1990.

69. Wyss, R. and Buchreli, F., Use of direct injection precolumn techniques for the high performance liquid chromatographic determination of the retinoids acitretin and 13-*cis*-acitretin in plasma, *J. Chromatogr.,* 593, 55, 1992.

70. LeFebvre, P., Agadin, A., Cornic, M., Gourmel, B., Hue, B., Dreux, C., Degos, L., and Chomienne, C., Simultaneous determination of all-*trans* and 13-*cis* retinoic acids and their 4-oxo metabolites by adsorption liquid chromatography after solid-phase extraction, *J. Chromatogr. B,* 666, 55, 1995.

71. Lehman, P. A. and Franz, T. J., A sensitive high pressure liquid chromatography/particle beam/mass spectrometry assay for the determination of all-*trans*-retinoic acid and 13-*cis*-retinoic acid in human plasma, *J. Pharm. Sci.,* 85, 3, 1996.

72. Got, L., Gausson, T., and Delacoux, E., Simultaneous determination of retinyl esters and retinol in human livers by reversed-phase high performance liquid chromatography, *J. Chromatogr. B,* 668, 233, 1995.

73. Lanvers, C., Hempel, G., Blaschke, G., and Boos, J., Simultaneous determination of all-*trans*-, 13-*cis*- and 9-*cis*-retinoic acid, their 4-oxo metabolites and all-*trans*-retinol in human plasma by high-performance liquid chromatography, *J. Chromatogr. B,* 685, 233, 1996.

74. Khachik, F., Beecher, G. R., and Whittaker, N. F., Separation, identification, and quantification of the major carotenoids and chlorophyll in extracts of several green vegetables by liquid chromatography, *J. Agric. Food Chem.,* 34, 603, 1986.

75. Chen, B. H., Chuang, J. R., Lin, J. H., and Chiu, C. P., Quantification of provitamin A compounds in Chinese vegetables by high-performance liquid chromatography, *J. Food Prot.,* 56, 51, 1993.

76. Minguez-Mosquera, M. I. and Hornero-Méndez, D., Separation and quantification of the carotenoid pigments in red peppers (*Capsicum annum* L.), paprika, and oleoresin by reversed-phase HPLC, *J. Agric. Food Chem.,* 41, 1616, 1993.

77. Tonucci, L. H., Holden, J. M., Beecher, G. R., Khachik, F., Davis, C. F., and Mulokzi, G., Carotenoid content of thermally processed tomato-based food products, *J. Agric. Food Chem.,* 43, 579, 1995.

78. Hart, D. J. and Scott, J., Development and evaluation of an HPLC method for the analysis of carotenoids in foods, and the measurement of the carotenoid content of vegetables and fruits commonly consumed in the UK, *Food Chem.,* 54, 101, 1995.

79. Handelman, G. J., Shen, B., and Krinsky, N.I., High resolution analysis of carotenoids in human plasma by high performance liquid chromatography, *Meth. Enzymol.,* 213, 336, 1992.

80. Groenendijk, G. W. T., De Grip, W. J., and Daeman, F. J. M., Quantitative determination of retinals with complete retention of their geometric configuration, *Biochim. Biophys. Acta,* 617, 430, 1980.

81. Khachik, F. and Beecher, G. R., Decapreno-β-carotene as an internal standard for the quantification of the hydrocarbon carotenoids by high performance liquid chromatography, *J. Chromatogr.,* 346, 237, 1985.

82. Khachik, F. and Beecher, G. R., Application of C-45-β-carotene as an internal standard for the quantification of carotenoids in yellow/orange vegetables by liquid chromatography, *J. Agric. Food Chem.,* 35, 732, 1987.

83. Riso, P, and Porrini, M., Determination of carotenoids in vegetable foods and plasma, In. *J. Vit. Nutr. Res.,* 67, 47, 1997.

84. Tanner, J. T., Barnett, S. A., and Mountford, M. K., Analysis of milk-based infant formula. Phase V. Vitamins A, and E, folic acid, and pantothenic acid: Food and Drug Administration—Infant Formula Council: collaborative study, *J. AOAC Int.,* 76, 399, 1993.

85. de Vries, E. J., Olling, Ch.C. J., Manz, U., and Tagliaferri, E., Dried skim milk—Determination of vitamin A—colorimetric and liquid chromatographic methods, *Bull. IDF,* 285, 1993, p. 53.

86. Brubacher, G., Müller-Mulot, W., and Southgate, D. A. T., *Methods for the Determination of Vitamins in Foods Recommended by COST 91,* Elsevier Applied Science Publishers, London, 1985.

87. Gebhardt, S., Elkins, E., and Humphrey, J., Comparison of two methods for determining the vitamin A value of clingstone peaches, *J. Agric. Food Chem.,* 25, 629, 1977.

88. Homnova, A., Rogers, W., and Eitenmiller, R. R., Provitamin A activity of specialty fruit marketed in the United States, *J. Food Compos. Anal.,* 3, 119, 1990.

89. Homnova, A., Payne, J., Koehler, P. E., and Eitenmiller, R. R., Provitamin A (α-carotene, β-carotene, and β-cryptoxanthin) and ascorbic acid content of Japanese and American persimmons, *J. Food. Anal.,* 13, 85, 1990.

90. Van Dokkum, W., De Vos, R., and Schrijver, J., Retinol, total carotenoids, β-carotene, and tocopherols in total diets of male adolescents in the Netherlands, *J. Agric. Food Chem.,* 38, 211, 1990.

91. Heinonen, M. I., Ollilainen, V., Linkola, E. K., Varo, P. T., and Koivistoinen, P. E., Carotenoids in Finnish foods: vegetables, fruits, and berries, *J. Agric. Food Chem.,* 37, 655, 1989.

92. Granado, F., Olmedilla, B., Blanco, I., and Rojas-Hidalgo, E., Carotenoid composition in raw and cooked Spanish vegetables, *J. Agric. Food Chem.,* 40, 2135, 1992.

93. Simonne, A. H., Kays, S. J., Koehler, P. E., and Eitenmiller, R. R., Assessment of β-carotene in sweet potato breeding lines in relation to dietary requirements, *J. Food Comp. Anal.,* 6, 336, 1993.

94. Biacs, P. A. and Daood, H. G., High performance liquid chromatography with photodiode array detection of carotenoid and carotenoid esters in fruits and vegetables, *J. Plant Physiol.,* 143, 520, 1994.

95. Chen, B. H., Peng, H. Y., and Chen, H. E., Changes of carotenoids, color, and vitamin A contents during processing of carrot juice, *J. Agric. Food Chem.,* 43, 1912, 1995.

96. Granelli, K. and Helmersson, S., Rapid high-performance liquid chromatographic method for determination of β-carotene in milk, *J. Chromatogr. A,* 721, 355, 1966.

97. Wills, R. B. H. and Rangga, A., Determination of carotenoids in Chinese vegetables, *Food Chem.,* 56, 451, 1996.

98. Mercadante, A. Z., Rodriguez-Amaya, D. B., and Britton, G., HPLC and mass spectrometric analysis of carotenoids from mango, *J. Agric. Food Chem.,* 45, 120, 1997.

99. Konings, E. J. M and Roomans, H. H. S., Evaluation and validation of an LC method for the analysis of carotenoids in vegetables and fruit, *Food Chem.,* 59, 599, 1997.

100. Khachik, F. and Beecher, G., Separation of carotenol fatty acid esters by high performance liquid chromatography, *J. Chromatogr.,* 449, 119, 1988.

101. Khachik, F., Goli, M., Beecher, G., Holden, J., Lusby, W., Tenorio, M., and Barrera, M., Effect of food preparation on qualitative and quantitative distribution of major carotenoid constituents of tomatoes and several green vegetables, *J. Agric. Food Chem.,* 40, 390, 1992.

102. Nelis, H. J. and De Leenheer, A. P., Isocratic nonaqueous reversed-phase liquid chromatography of carotenoids, *Anal. Chem.,* 55, 270, 1983.

103. Bieri, J. G., Brown, E. D., and Smith, J. C., Jr., Determination of individual carotenoids in human plasma by high performance liquid chromatography, *J. Liq. Chromatogr.,* 8, 473, 1985.

104. Khachik, F., Beecher, G. R., Goli, M., and Lusby, W. R., Separation, identification, and quantification of carotenoids in fruits, vegetables and human plasma by high performance liquid chromatography, *Pure Appl. Chem.,* 63, 71, 1991.

105. Khachik, F., Beecher, G. R., Goli, M.B., Lusby, W. R., and Smith, J. C., Jr., Separation and identification of carotenoids and their oxidation products in extracts of human plasma, *Anal. Chem.,* 64, 2111, 1992.

106. Khachik, F., Beecher, G. R., Goli, M. B., and Daitch, C. E., Separation and quantitation of carotenoids in human plasma, *Meth. Enzymol.,* 213, 205, 1992.

107. Khachik, F., Spangler, C. J., Smith, J. C., Jr., Canfield, L. M., Steck, A., and Pfander, H., Identification, quantification, and relative concentrations of carotenoids and their metabolites in human milk and serum, *Anal. Chem.,* 69, 1873, 1997.

108. Yong, L., Forman, M., Graubard, B., Reichman, M., Judd, J., Khachik, F., Beecher, G., Campbell, W., and Taylor, P., Diet-plasma carotenoid asociation: application of the U.S. Department of Agriculture—National Cancer Institute Carotenoid Food Composition Data Base, *Am. J. Epidemiol.,* 138, 638, 1993.

109. Khachik, F., Englert, G., Beecher, G. R., and Smith, J. C., Jr., Isolation, structural elucidation, and partial synthesis of lutein dehydration products in extracts from human plasma, *J. Chromatogr. B,* 670, 219, 1995.

110. LeMarchand, L., Hankin, J. H., Bach, F., Kolonel, L. N., Wilkens, L. R., Stacewicz-Sapuntzakis, M., Bowen, P. E., Beecher, G. R., Laudon, F., Baqué, P., Daniel, R., Seruvatu, L., and Henderson, B. E., An ecological study of diet and lung cancer in the South Pacific, *Int. J. Cancer,* 63, 18, 1995.

111. Forman, M. R., Beecher, G. R., Muesing, R., Lanza, E., Olson, B., Campbell, W.S., McAdam, P., Ramond, E., Schulman, J. D., and Graubard, B. I., The fluctuation of plasma carotenoid concentrations by phase of the menstrual cycle: a controlled diet study, *Am. J. Clin. Nutr.,* 64, 559, 1996.

112. Schierle, J., Bretzel, W., Bühler, I., Faccin, N., Hess, D., Steiner, K., and Schüep, W., Content and isomeric ratio of lycopene in food and human blood plasma, *Food Chem.,* 59, 459, 1997.

113. Scott, K., Observations on some of the problems associated with analysis of carotenoids in foods by HPLC, *Food Chem.,* 45, 357, 1992.
114. Landen, W. O., Jr. and Eitenmiller, R. R., Application of gel permeation chromatography and non-aqueous reverse phase chromatography to high pressure liquid chromatographic determination of retinyl palmitate and β-carotene in oil and margarine, *J. Assoc. Off. Anal. Chem.,* 62, 283, 1979.
115. Craft, N., Sander, L., and Pierson, H., Separation and relative distribution of all-*trans*-β-carotene and its *cis*-isomers in *b*-carotene preparations, *J. Micronutr. Anal.,* 8, 209, 1990.
116. Bampong, D. K., Honigberg, I. L., and Meltzer, N. M., Separation of 13-*cis* and all-*trans*-retinoic acid and their photodegradation products using capillary zone electrophoresis and micellar electrokinetic chromatography (MEC), *J. Pharmaceut. Biomed. Anal.,* 11, 829, 1993.
117. Ma, Y., Wu, Z., Furr, H. C., Lammi-Keefe, C., and Craft, N. E., Fast microassay of serum retinoid (vitamin A) by capillary zone eletrophoresis with laser-excited fluorescence detection, *J. Chromatogr.,* 616, 31, 1993.
118. Shi, H., Ma, Y, Humphrey, J. H., and Craft, N. E., Determination of vitamin A in dried human blood spots by high-performance capillary electrophoresis with laser-excited fluorescence detection, *J. Chromatogr. B,* 665, 89, 1995.
119. Hsieh, Y. Z. and Kuo, K. L., Separation of retinoids by micellar electrokinetic capillary chromatography, *J. Chromatogr. A,* 761, 307, 1997.

Table 1 Physical Properties of Retinol and Other Retinoids

1. Budavari, S., *The Merck Index,* 12th ed., Merck and Company, Whitehouse Station, New Jersey, 1996, 1403, 1404, 1709.
2. Furr, H. C., Barua, A. B., and Olson, J. A., Retinoids and carotenoids, in *Modern Chromatographic Analysis of Vitamins,* 2nd ed., De Leenheer, A. P., Lambert, W. E., and Nelis, H. J., Eds., Marcel Dekker, New York, 1992, chap. 1.
3. Furr, H. C., Barua, A. B., and Olson, J. A., Analytical methods, in *The Retinoids, Biology, Chemistry and Medicine,* 2nd ed., Sporn, M. B., Roberts, A. B., and Goodman, D. S., Eds., Raven Press, New York, 1994, chap. 3.
4. Olson, J. A., Vitamin A, in *Handbook of Vitamins,* 2nd ed., Machlin, L.J., Ed., Marcel Dekker, New York, 1991, chap. 1.

Table 3 Physical Properties of Selected Carotenoids

1. Bauernfeind, J. C., *Carotenoids as Colorants and Vitamin A Precursors, Technological and Nutritional Applications,* Academic Press, New York, 1981, Appendix.
2. Budavari, S., *The Merck Index,* 12th ed., Merck and Company, Whitehouse Station, NJ, 1996, 145, 303, 304, 442, 961, 1271, 1719, 1731.
3. Britton, G., Liaaen-Jensen, S., and Pfander, H., *Carotenoids, Spectroscopy,* Vol. 1B, Birkhäuser Verlag, Boston, 1995, chap. 2.
4. Committee on Food Chemicals Codex, *Food Chemicals Codex,* 4th ed., National Academy of Sciences, Washington, D.C., 1996, 32.
5. Friedrich, W., Vitamin A and its provitamins, in *Vitamins,* Walter de Gruyter, Hawthorne, NY, 1988, chap. 2.
6. Furr, H. C., Barua, A. B., and Olson, J. A., Retinoids and carotenoids, in *Modern Chromatographic Analysis of Vitamins,* 2nd ed., De Leenheer, A. P., Lambert, W.E., and Nelis, H. J., Eds., Marcel Dekker, New York, 1992, chap. 1.

Table 6 Compendium, Regulatory and Handbook Methods for Analysis of Vitamin A and Carotenoids

1. United States Pharmacopeial Convention, *U.S. Pharmacopeia National Formulary,* USP 23 N/F 18, Nutritional Supplements, Official Monographs, United States Pharmacopeial Convention, Rockville, MD, 1995.
2. Scottish Home and Health Department, *British Pharmacopoeia,* 15th ed., British Pharmacopoeic Commission, United Kingdom, 1993.

3. AOAC International, *Official Methods of Analysis,* 16th ed., AOAC International, Arlington, VA, 1995.
4. Tanner, J. T., Barnett, S. A., and Mountford, M. K., Analyis of milk-based infant formula. Phase V. Vitamins A and E, folic acid, and pantothenic acid: Food and Drug Administration—Infant Formula Council: collaborative study, *J. AOAC Int.,* 76, 399, 1993.
5. Quackenbush, F. W., Dyer, M. A., and Smallidge, R. L., Analysis for carotenes and xanthophylls in dried plant materials, *J. Assoc. Off. Anal. Chem.,* 53, 181, 1970.
6. Quackenbush, F. W., Extraction and analysis of carotenoids in fresh plant materials, *J. Assoc. Off. Anal. Chem.,* 57, 511, 1974.
7. American Feed Ingredients Association, *Laboratory Methods Compendium* Vol. I: *Vitamins and Minerals,* American Feed Ingredients Association, West Des Moines, IA, 1991, 117.
8. Keller, H. E., *Analytical Methods for Vitamins and Carotenoids,* Hoffmann-LaRoche, Basel, 1988, 5.
9. American Association of Cereal Chemists, *AACC Approved Methods,* 9th ed. Vol. 2, American Association of Cereral Chemists, St. Paul, MN, 1996.
10. Parrish, D. B., Report on vitamin A in mixed feeds, *J. Assoc. Off. Anal. Chem.,* 41, 593, 1958.
11. Manz, U. and Vuilleumier, J. P., Bestimmung der pigmentierenden carotinoids in futtermittelm und konzentraten für Eierproduletion und geflügelmast, *Z. Lebensm. Unters. Forsch.,* 163, 21, 1977.
12. Baranyai, M., Matus, Z., and Szaboles, J., Determination by HPLC of carotenoids in paprika products, *Acta Aliment.,* 11, 309, 1982.
13. Committee on Food Chemicals Codex, *Food Chemicals Codex,* 4th ed., National Academy Press, Washington, D.C., 1996, 90, 429.
14. Brubacher, G., Müller-Mulot, W., and Southgate, D. A. T., *Methods for the Determination of Vitamins in Foods, Recommended by COST 91,* Elsevier, New York, 1985, 23.
15. Mulry, M. C., Schmidt, R. H., and Kirk, J. R., Isomerization of retinyl palmitate using conventional lipid extraction solvents, *J. Assoc. Off. Anal.Chem.,* 66, 746, 1983.

Table 7. HPLC Methods for the Analysis of Retinol and Its Metabolites in Food, Feeds, Pharmaceuticals, and Biologicals

Food

1. deVries, E. J., Olling, Ch. C. J., Manz, U., and Tagliaferri, E., Dried skimmed milk—determination of vitamin A—colorimetric and liquid chromatographic methods, *Int. Dairy Fed.,* 285, 53, 1993.
2. Tanner, J. T., Barnett, S. A., and Mountford, M. K., Analysis of milk-based infant formula: phase V. Vitamins A and E, folic acid, and pantothenic acid: Food and Drug Administration—Infant Formula Council: collaborative study, *J. Assoc. Off. Anal. Chem.,* 76, 399, 1993.
3. Marsh, R., Kajda, P., and Ryley, J., The effect of light on the vitamin B$_2$ and the vitamin A content of cheese, *Die Nahr.,* 38, 527, 1994.
4. Jensen, S. K., Retinol determination in milk by HPLC and fluorescence detection, *J. Dairy Res.,* 61, 233, 1994.
5. Brinkmann, E., Mehlitz, I., Oei, H. B., Tiebach, R., and Baltes, W., Determination of vitamin A in liver and liver-containing products using narrow-bore normal- phase HPLC, *Z. Lebensm. Unters. Forsch.,* 199, 206, 1994.
6. Brinkmann, E., Dehne, L., Oei, H. B., Tiebach, R., and Balters, W., Separation of geometrical retinol isomers in food samples by using narrow bore-high-performance liquid chromatography, *J. Chromatogr. A,* 693, 271, 1995.

Biologicals

1. Barua, A. B., and Olson, J. A., Retinoyl β-glucuronide: an endogenous compound of human blood, *Am. J. Clin. Nutr.,* 43, 481, 1986.
2. Kraft, J. C., Echoff, C., Kuhnz, W., Löfberg, B., and Nau, H., Automated determination of β-*cis*- and all-*trans*-retinoic and their 4-oxo metabolites and retinol in plasma, amniotic fluid and embryo by reversed-phase high-performance liquid chromatography with a precolumn switching technique, *J. Liq. Chromatogr.,* 11, 2051, 1988.
3. Kraft, J. C., Shepard, T., and Juchau, M. R., Tissue levels of retinoids in human embryos/fetuses, *Reprod. Toxicol.,* 7, 11, 1993.

4. Wyss, R. and Bucheli, F., Quantitative analysis of retinoids in biological fluids by high-performance liquid chromatography using column switching, *J. Chromatogr.,* 424, 303, 1988.

5. Wyss, R., Determination of retinoids in plasma by high-performance liquid chromatography and automated column switching, *Meth. Enzymol.,* 189, 146, 1990.

6. Wyss, R. and Bucheli, F., Use of direct injection precolumn techniques for the high-performance liquid chromatographic determination of the retinoids acitretin and β-*cis*-acitretin in plasma, *J. Chromatogr.,* 593, 55, 1992.

7. Meyer, E., Lambert, W. E., and De Leenheer, A. P., Simultaneous determination of endogenous retinoic acid isomers and retinol in human plasma by isocratic normal-phase HPLC with ultraviolet detection, *Clin. Chem.,* 40, 48, 1994.

8. Takeda, N. and Yamamoto, A., Simultaneous determination of β-*cis*- and all-*trans*-retinoic acids and retinol in human serum by high-performance liquid chromatography, *J. Chromatogr. B,* 657, 53, 1994.

9. LeFebvre, P., Agadir, A., Cornic, M., Gourmel, B., Hue, B., Dreux, C., Degos, L., and Chomienne, C., Simultaneous determination of all-*trans* and β-*cis* retinoic acids and their 4-oxo-metabolites by adsorption liquid chromatography after solid-phase extraction, *J. Chromatogr. B,* 666, 55, 1995.

10. Got, L., Gousson, T., and Delacoux, E., Simultaneous determination of retinyl esters and retinol in human livers by reversed-phase high-performance liquid chromatography, *J. Chromatogr. B,* 668, 233, 1995.

11. Hagen, J. J., Washco, K. A., and Monnig, C. A., Determination of retinoids by reversed-phase capillary liquid chromatography with amperometric electrochemical detection, *J. Chromatogr. B,* 677, 225, 1996.

12. Dimitrova, B., Poyre, M., Guiso, G., Badiali, A., and Caccia, S., Isocratic reversed-phase liquid chromatography of all-*trans*-retinoic acid and its major metabolites in new potential supplementary test systems for developmental toxicology, *J. Chromatogr. B,* 681, 153, 1996.

13. Lehman, P. A. and Franz, T. J., A sensitive high-pressure liquid chromatography/particle beam/mass spectrometry assay for the determination of all-*trans*-retinoic acid and β-*cis*-retinoic acid in human plasma, *J. Pharm. Sci.,* 85, 287, 1996.

14. Van Breeman, R. B. and Huang, C.-R., High-performance liquid chromatography-electrospray mass spectrometry of retinoids, *FASEB,* 10, 1098, 1996.

15. Arnhold, T., Tzimas, G., Wittfoht, W., Plonait, S., and Nau, H., Identification of 9-*cis*-retinoic acid, 9,13-di-*cis*-retinoic acid, and 14-hydroxy-4, 14-retro-retinol in human plasma after liver consumption, *Life Sci.,* 59, PL169, 1996.

16. Eckhoff, C. and Nau, H., Identification and quantitation of all-*trans*- and β-*cis*-retinoic acid and β-*cis*-4-oxoretinoic acid in human plasma, *J. Lipid Res.,* 31, 1445, 1990.

17. Collins, M. D., Eckhoff, C., Chahoud, I., Bochert, G., and Nau, H., 4-methylpyrazole partially ameliorated the teratogenicity of retinol and reduced the metabolic formation of all-*trans*-retinoic aid in the mouse, *Arch. Toxicol.,* 66, 652, 1992.

18. Tzimas, G., Sass, J. O., Wittfoht, W., Elmazar, M. M. A., Ehlers, K., and Nau, H., Identification of 9,13-di-*cis*-retinoic acid as a major plasma metabolite of 9-cis-retinoic acid and limited transfer of 9-cis-retinoic acid and 9,13-di-*cis*-retinoic acid to the mouse and rat embryos, *Drug Metab. Disp.,* 22, 928, 1994.

19. Sass, J. O. and Nau, H., Single-run analysis of isomers of retinoyl-β-D-glucuronide and retinoic acid by reversed-phase high-performance liquid chromatography, *J. Chromatogr. A,* 685, 182, 1994.

20. Tzimas, G., Collins, M. D., and Nau, H., Identification of 14-hydroxy-4,14-retro-retinol as an *in vivo* metabolite of vitamin A, *Biochem. Biophys. Acta,* 1301, 1, 1996.

Table 8. HPLC Methods for the Analysis of Carotenoids in Food and Plasma

Food

1. Zakaria, M., Simpson, K., Brown, P. R., and Krstulovic, A., Use of reversed-phase high-performance liquid chromatographic analysis for the determination of provitamin A carotenes in tomatoes, *J. Chromatogr.,* 176, 109, 1979.

2. Bushway, R. J. and Wilson, A. M., Determination of α- and β-carotene in fruit and vegetables by high-performance liquid chromatography, *Can. Inst. Food Technol. J.,* 15, 165, 1982.

3. Khachik, F. and Beecher, G. R., Decapreno-β-carotene as an internal standard for the quantification of the hydrocarbon carotenoids by high-performance liquid chromatography, *J. Chromatogr.,* 346, 237, 1985.

4. Khachik, F., Beecher, G. R., and Whittaker, N. F., Separation, identification and quantification of the major carotenoids and chlorphyll constituents in extracts of several green vegetables by liquid chromatography, *J. Agric. Food Chem.,* 34, 603, 1986.

5. Chandler, L. A. and Schwartz, S. J., HPLC separation of *cis-trans* carotene in fresh and processed fruits and vegetables, *J. Food Sci.,* 52, 669, 1987.

6. Khachik, F. and Beecher, G. R., Application of a C-45-β-carotene as an internal standard for the quantification of carotenoids in yellow/orange vegetables by liquid chromatography, *J. Agric. Food Chem.,* 35, 732, 1987.

7. Khachik, F. and Beecher, G. R., Separation and identification of carotenoids and carotenol fatty acid esters in some squash products by liquid chromatography. 1. Quantification of carotenoids and related esters by HPLC, J. Agric. Food Chem., 36, 929, 1988.

8. Khachik, F., Beecher, G. R., and Lusby, W. R., Separation and identification of carotenoids and carotenol fatty acid esters in some squash products by liquid chromatography. 2. Isolation and characterization of carotenoids and related esters, *J. Agric. Food Chem.,* 36, 938, 1988.

9. Khachik, F., Beecher, G. R., and Lusby, W. R., Separation, identification, and quantification of the major carotenoids in extracts of apricots, peaches, cantaloupe, and pink grapefruit by liquid chromatography, *J. Agric. Food Chem.,* 37, 1465, 1989.

10. Khachik, F., Goli, M. B., Beecher, G. R., Holden, J., Lusby, W. R., Tenoria, M. D., and Barrera, M. R., Effect of food preparation on qualitative and quantitative distribution of major carotenoid constituents of tomatoes and several green vegetables, *J. Agric. Food Chem.,* 40, 390, 1992.

11. Heinonen, M. I., Ollilainen, V., Linkola, E. K., Varo, P. T., and Koivistoinen, P. E., Carotenoids in Finnish foods: Vegetables, fruits, and berries, *J. Agric. Food Chem.,* 37, 655, 1989.

12. Homnava, A., Rogers, W., and Eitenmiller, R. R., Provitamin A activity of specialty fruit marketed in the United States, *J. Food Comp. Anal.,* 3, 119, 1990.

13. Simonne, A. H., Kays, S. J., Koehler, P. E., and Eitenmiller, R. R., Assessment of β-carotene content in sweet potato breeding lines in relation to dietary requirements, *J. Food Comp. Anal.,* 6, 336, 1993.

14. Granado, F., Olmedilla, B., Blanco, I., and Rojas-Hidalgo, E., Carotenoid composition in raw and cooked Spanish vegetables, *J. Agric. Food Chem.,* 40, 2135, 1992.

15. Chen, B. H., Chuang, J. R., Lin, J. H., and Chiu, C. P., Quantification of provitamin A compounds in Chinese vegetables by high-performance liquid chromatography, *J. Food Prot.,* 56, 51, 1993.

16. Mínguez-Mosquera, M. I., and Hornero-Méndez, D., Separation and quantification of the carotenoid pigments in red peppers (*capsicum annum* L.), paprika, and oleoresin by reversed-phase HPLC, *J. Agric. Food Chem.,* 41, 1616, 1993.

17. Biacs, P. A. and Daood, H. G., High-performance liquid chromatography with photodiode-array detection of carotenoids and carotenoid esters in fruits and vegetables, *J. Plant Physiol.,* 143, 520, 1994.

18. Giuliano, A. R., Neilson, E. M., Yap, H. H., Baier, M., and Canfield, L. M., Quantitation of and inter-intra-individual variability in major carotenoids of mature human milk, *J. Nutr. Biochem.,* 5, 551, 1994.

19. Chen, B. H., Peng, H. Y., and Chen, H. E., Changes of carotenoids, color, and vitamin A contents during processing of carrot juice, *J. Agric. Food Chem.,* 43, 1912, 1995.

20. Biacs, P. A., Daood, H. G., and Kádár, I., Effect of Mo, Se, Zn, and Cr treatments on the yield, element concentration, and carotenoid content of carrot, *J. Agric. Food Chem.,* 43, 589, 1995.

21. Tonucci, L. H., Holden, J. M., Beecher, G. R., Khachik, F., Davis, C. S., and Mulokzi, G., Carotenoid content of thermally processed tomato-based food products, *J. Agric. Food Chem.,* 43, 579, 1995.

22. Hart, D. J. and Scott, K. J., Development and evaluation of an HPLC method for the analysis of carotenoids in foods, and the measurement of the carotenoid content of vegetables and fruits commonly consumed in the UK, *Food Chem.,* 54, 101, 1995.

23. Granelli, K. and Helmersson, S., Rapid high-performance liquid chromatographic method for the determination of β-carotene in milk, *J. Chromatogr. A,* 721, 355, 1996.

24. Nyambaka, H. and Ryley, J., An isocratic reversed-phase HPLC separation of the stereoisomers of the provitamin A carotenoids (α- and β-carotene) in dark green vegetables, *Food Chem.,* 55, 63, 1996.

25. Wills, R. B. H. and Rangga, A., Determination of carotenoids in Chinese vegetables, *Food Chem.,* 56, 451, 1996.

26. Riso, P. and Porrini, M., Determination of carotenoids in vegetable foods and plasma, *Int. J. Vit. Nutr. Res.,* 67, 47, 1997.

27. Mercadante, A. Z., Rodriguez-Amaya, D.B., and Britton, G., HPLC and mass spectrometric analysis of carotenoids from mango, *J. Agric. Food Chem.,* 45, 120, 1997.

28. Konings, E. J. M. and Roomans, H. H. S., Evaluation and validation of an LC method for the analysis of carotenoids in vegetables and fruits, *Food Chem.,* 59, 599, 1997.

Biologicals

1. Bieri, J. G., Brown, E. D., and Smith, J. C., Jr., Determination of individual carotenoids in human plasma by high performance liquid chromatography, *J. Liq. Chromatogr.,* 8, 473, 1985.

2. Khachik, F. and Beecher, G. R., Separation of carotenol fatty acid esters by high-performance liquid chromatography, *J. Chromatogr.,* 449, 119, 1988.

3. Khachik, F., Beecher, G. R., Goli, M. B., Lusby, W.R., and Smith, J.C., Jr., Separation and identification of carotenoids and their oxidation products in the extracts of human plasma, *Anal. Chem.,* 64, 2111, 1992.

4. Khachik, F., Beecher, G. R., Goli, M. B., Lusby, W. R., and Daitch, C. E., Separation and quantification of carotenoids in human plasma, *Meth. Enzymol.,* 213, 205, 1992.

5. Franke, A. A., Custer, L. J., and Cooney, R. V., Synthetic carotenoids as internal standards for plasma micronutrient analyses by high-performance liquid chromatography, *J. Chromatogr.,* 614, 43, 1993.

6. Carughi, A. and Hooper, F. G., Plasma carotenoid concentrations before and after supplementation with a carotenoid mixture, *Am. J. Clin. Nutr.,* 59, 896, 1994.

7. Rushin, W. G., Catignani, G.L., and Schwartz, S.J., Determination of β-carotene and its *cis*-isomers in serum, *Clin. Chem.,* 36, 1986, 1990.

8. Schmitz, H. H., Schwartz, S. J., and Catignani, G. L., Resolution and quantitation of the predominant geometric β-carotene isomers present in human serum using normal-phase HPLC, *J. Agric. Food Chem.,* 42, 2746, 1994.

9. Tamai, H., Marinobu, T., Murata, T., Manago, M., and Mino, M., 9-*cis*-β-carotene in human plasma and blood cells after ingestion of β-carotene, *Lipids,* 30, 493, 1995.

10. Sharpless, K. E., Brown, Thomas, J., Sander, L. C., and Wise, S. A., Liquid chromatographic determination of carotenoids in human serum using an engineered C_{30} and a C_{18} stationary phase, *J. Chromatogr. B,* 678, 187, 1996.

11. Epler, K. S., Ziegler, R. G., and Craft, N. E., Liquid chromatographic method for the determination of carotenoids, retinoids, and tocopherols in human serum and in food, *J. Chromatogr.,* 619, 37, 1993.

12. Sander, L. C., Sharpless, K., Epler, K. S., Craft, N.E., and Wise, S. A., Development of engineered stationary phases for the separation of carotenoid isomers, *Anal. Chem.,* 66, 1667, 1994.

13. Emenhiser, C., Sander, L. C., and Schwartz, S. J., Capability of a polymeric C_{30} stationary phase to resolve *cis-trans* carotenoid isomers in reversed-phase liquid chromatography, *J. Chromatogr. A,* 707, 205, 1995.

14. Brown Thomas, J., Kline, M. C., Schiller, S. B., McEllerge, P. M., Smiegoski, L. T., Duewer, D. L., and Sharpless, K. E., Certification of fat-soluble vitamins, carotenoids and cholesterol in human serum: standard reference materials, *Fres. J. Anal. Chem.,* 356, 1, 1996.

15. Emenhiser, C., Englert, G., Sander, L.C., Ludwig, B., and Schwartz, S. J., Isolation and structural elucidation of the predominant geometrical isomers of α-carotene, *J. Chromatogr. A,* 719, 333, 1996.

16. Khachik, F., Spangler, C. J., and Smith, J. C., Jr., Identification, quantification and relative concentrations of carotenoids and their metabolites in human milk, *Anal. Chem.,* 69, 1873, 1997.

17. Schierle, J., Bretzel, W., Bühler, I., Faccin, N., Hess, D., Steiner, K., and Schüep, W., Content and isomeric ratio of lycopene in food and human blood plasma, *Food Chem.,* 59, 459, 1997.

2 Vitamin D

2.1 REVIEW

Rickets was first described in 1645. It was not until 1919 that rickets was experimentally induced in dogs by feeding fat-free diets and, then, cured by feeding cod liver oil.[1] Thus, rickets was recognized as a dietary deficiency of a fat-soluble factor. The antirachitic factor was named vitamin D by McCollum's research group in 1925 and, later that same year, the vitamin was proven to be produced in the skin by ultraviolet irradiation.[2] Vitamin D was isolated as Vitamin D_2 (ergocalciferol) from irradiated ergosterol from yeast in 1931, and its structure was identified in 1932. Vitamin D_3 (cholecalciferol) was structurally characterized in 1936 and was shown to be the antirachitic factor in cod liver oil.[1] The intermediary metabolism of the vitamin was more fully understood in the 1970s with the identification of the hydroxylated metabolites, 25-hydroxyvitamin D_3 ($25(OH)D_3$) and $1\alpha,25$-dihydroxyvitamin D_3 ($1\alpha,25(OH)_2(D_3)$). Biologically, $1\alpha,25(OH)_2D_3$ is the primary metabolically active form known as calcitrol. $1\alpha,25(OH)_2D_3$ and other hydroxylated, metabolically active forms such as $24R,25(OH)_2D_3$ are produced in the kidney by the action of $25(OH)D_3$-1-hydroxylase and $25(OH)D_3$-24-hydroxylase, and in the liver by D_3-25-hydroxylase.[3] Vitamin D metabolism is complex, and over 40 metabolites have been characterized from clinical samples.[4]

The metabolic functions of vitamin D are accepted as that of a steroid hormone. Vitamin D_3 must be converted to the biologically active hydroxylated forms. $25(OH)D_3$ is formed in the liver and further hydroxylated to the dihydroxy forms and transported to target organs where receptor binding occurs. The overall biological system is described as the vitamin D endocrine system. Biological responses include mobilization and accretion of calcium and phosphorous (bone), calcium absorption (intestine), and reabsorption of calcium and phosphorous (kidney). Other accepted roles for vitamin D related to the vitamin D endocrine system include osteoblast formation, fetus development, pancreatic function, neural function, immunity, and $1\alpha,25(OH)_2D_3$ mediated cellular growth and differentiation effects. The vitamin D endocrine system is described by Norman,[3] and the reader is encouraged to refer to this review.

Vitamin D deficiency is rickets in infants and children and osteomalacia in adults. Deficiency due to inadequate intake or lack of exposure to sunlight responds to vitamin D therapy; however, vitamin D-resistant rickets does not. Vitamin D-resistant rickets results through genetic disorders and includes loss of the renal resorption system for phosphate, absence of 12-hydroxylase in the kidney, and through mutations in the vitamin D receptor gene.[5] Some types of vitamin D-resistant rickets can be treated with high doses of calcitrol.

Levels of vitamin D metabolites in serum and tissue are accepted status indicators for the human. Older indices include indirect measures of calcium and phosphorous levels in the serum and alkaline phosphatase activity. These measurements are considered non-specific.[6] Concentration of $25(OH)D_3$ in the serum is an accepted index of vitamin D status in humans; however, the level correlated with clinical signs of deficiency needs further clarification. Circulatory levels below 3 ng/mL are associated with frank deficiency or rickets in children and osteomalacia in adults.[6] Liquid chromatography (LC) methods for the measurement of serum vitamin D are discussed in Section 2.3.

Food sources of vitamin D are limited. Provitamin D compounds, however, are abundant in plant and animal tissue that can be converted to previtamin D compounds by UV irradiation. 7-Dehydrocholesterol (provitamin D_3) in animals is converted to previtamin D_3 by exposure of the skin to sunlight. Previtamin D_3 then undergoes isomerization to cholecalciferol (vitamin D_3). Vitamin D_3 concentration in animal tissue is dependent on dietary intake and exposure of the animal to sunlight. Formation through sunlight exposure provides humans with most of their vitamin D requirement.[7] Ergosterol (provitamin D_2) in plant tissue is converted to previtamin D_2 by irradiation. Previtamin D_2 isomerizes to ergocalciferol (vitamin D_2). The vitamin is limited in nature but is easily and cheaply synthesized. It is the primary synthetic form of vitamin D used for pharmaceuticals. The biological activities of vitamins D_2 and D_3 are approximately equal for humans. An International Unit (IU) of vitamin D is defined as the activity of 0.025 μg of cholecalciferol (vitamin D_3) measured by the rat or chick bioassay. The USP reference standard for vitamin D is ergocalciferol (D_2) and/or cholecalciferol (D_3).

Sources of vitamin D include the vitamin D_3 synthesized in the body and food sources. Fortified fluid milk containing 10 μg (400 IU) per quart is a concentrated source of vitamin D_3. Although permitted in the United States, margarine fortification is not the rule as most margarines are not fortified. If added to margarine, the product must contain at least 1500 IU per pound (21 CFR 166).[8] Fortified breakfast cereals, eggs, butter, and some fish oils (cod liver oil) are sources of vitamin D. The Recommended Dietary Allowance (RDA) ranges from 5 μg for the 21 to 51+ year-old male or female to 10 μg per day for children and younger adults and pregnant and lactating women.[9] The Reference Daily Intake (RDI) is 10 μg or 400 IU.[10]

Vitamin D at excessive intake levels is toxic with the greatest threat to young children.[9] Consumption of as little as 45 μg of vitamin D_3 per day can lead to hypervitaminosis D in young children, an intake level that is nearly 5 times the RDA.[9] The toxic dose for adults is approximately 2.5 mg (100,000 IU) per day for one to two months.[2] Excessive intake by the adult is likely to be associated with misuse of supplements. Symptoms of excessive intake include hypercalcemia, hypercalciuria, and irreversible renal and cardiovascular damage.[9] Incidents of overfortification of fluid milk and infant formula have occurred and problems of variability of vitamin D addition to the fluid milk supply have been documented.[11,12]

2.2   PROPERTIES

2.2.1   CHEMISTRY

2.2.1.1   General Properties

Vitamin D is the inclusive term for steroids that are antirachitic. Structures of cholecalciferol (vitamin D_3) and the steroid nucleus are given in Figure 2.1. IUPAC-IUB nomenclature rules for steroid structure are used to characterize the ring system. The A, B, C, and D rings are derived from the cyclopentanoperhydrophenanthrene steroid structure with cholesterol serving as the parent compound.[13] Formation of previtamin D forms from the provitamins (7-dehydrocholesterol and ergosterol) requires opening of the B ring at the 9,10 bond. The vitamin D structures with the open ring are secosteroids. Accepted IUPAC-IUB systematic names are 9,10-seco(5Z,7E)-5,7,10(19) cholestatriene-3β-ol for vitamin D_3 and 9,10-seco(5Z,7E)-5,7,10(19),22 ergostate-traene-3β-ol for vitamin D_2. Conversions of the provitamins by irradiation to vitamin D_2 and vitamin D_3 along with the structures of the hydroxylated metabolites, 25(OH)D_3 and 1α-25(OH)$_2$$D_3$, are shown in Figure 2.2. Vitamin D_2 and vitamin D_3 differ structurally by only a double bond and an additional methyl group in the side chain of vitamin $D^{2.4}$ Due to the close structural similarity, their chemical and physical properties are similar (Table 2.1).

2.2.1.2   Spectral Properties

All vitamin D forms show a characteristic broad UV spectrum with maximum absorption near 264 nm and a minimum near 228 nm.[1] A characteristic UV absorption spectrum of vitamin D is shown in Figure 2.3.[14] Vitamin D does not fluoresce.

2.2.2   STABILITY

Vitamin D is stable in the absence of water, light, acidity, and at low temperatures. Isomerization to the 5,6-*trans*-isomer and isotachysterol[14] results under acid conditions or light exposure. The

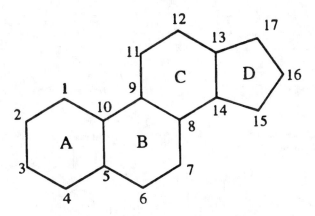

Steroid Nucleus
Cyclopentanoperhydrophenanthrene

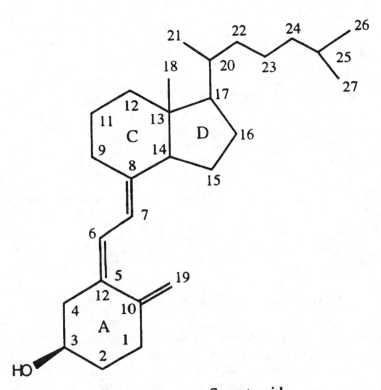

Secosteroid
Vitamin D₃
Cholecalciferol
9, 10 seco (5Z,7E)-5, 7, 10, (19) cholestatriene-3β-ol

FIGURE 2.1   Structures of the steroid nucleus and vitamin D₃.

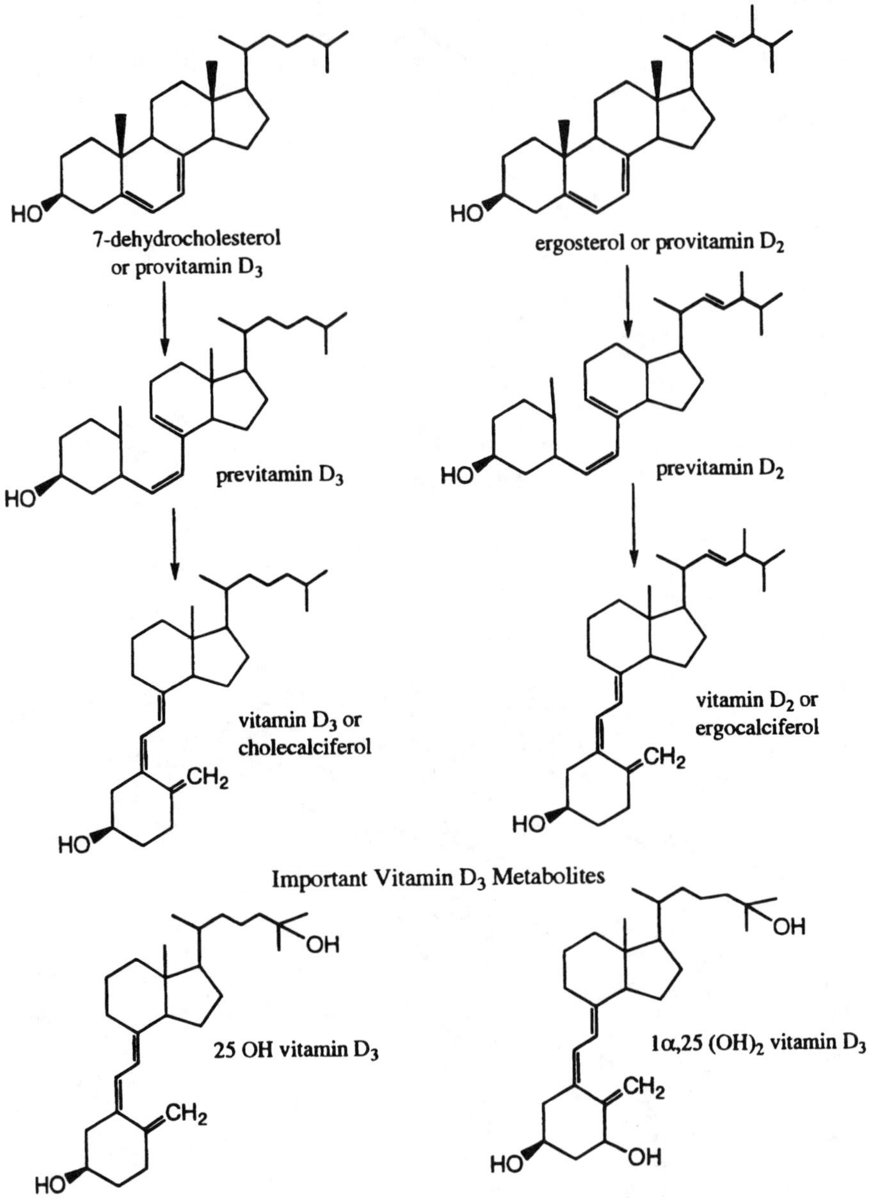

FIGURE 2.2   Structures of vitamin D, its precursors and metabolites.

vitamin withstands alkalinity, and saponification is often used as the initial sample treatment for extraction of complex matrices. Oxidation can be a predominant route for decomposition at the conjugated double bonds at the 5,6 and 7,8 positions of the secosteroid structure; however, vitamin D is less susceptible to oxidative losses than vitamin E, β-carotene, and retinol.

Various environmental conditions can cause isomerization of vitamin D_2 and vitamin D_3 to the previtamin D forms. Thermal interconversion is difficult to avoid completely during sample handling, and commercial concentrates and even standards can contain appreciable amounts of previtamin D. This fact requires that analytical methods account for all biologically active forms, including the previtamins, to accurately assess vitamin D activity.

TABLE 2.1
Physical Properties of Vitamin D and Hydroxylated Forms

Substance[a]	Molar Mass	Formula	Solubility	Melting Point °C	Crystal Form	Spectral Properties		
						λ max nm	$E^{1\%b}_{1\ cm}$	ε × 10^{-3}
D$_3$ CAS No. 67-97-0 **10157**	384.65	C$_{27}$H$_{44}$O	Soluble in most organic solvents Insoluble in water	84–85	Fine needles Yellow to white	264	485	18.3
D$_2$ CAS No. 50-14-6 **10156**	396.66	C$_{28}$H$_{44}$O	Soluble in most organic solvents Insoluble in water	115–118	Prisms Yellow to white	264	462	19.4
25(OH)D$_3$ **1677**	400.65	C$_{27}$H$_{44}$O$_2$	Soluble in most organic solvents Insoluble in water	82–83		265	[449]	18.0
1α,25(OH)$_2$D$_3$ **1681**	416.64	C$_{27}$H$_{44}$O$_3$	Slightly soluble in methanol, ethanol and ethylacetate Insoluble in water	111–115	White crystalline powder	264	[418]	19.0

a Common or generic name; CAS No.—Chemical Abstract Service number, bold print designates the Merck Index monograph number.
b Values in brackets are calculated from corresponding ε value, in ethanol.

Budavari, S. *The Merck Index*, 12th ed., 1996.[1]
Freidrich, W., *Vitamins*, 1988.[2]
DeLuca, H.F., *The Fat-Soluble Vitamins*, 1978.[3]

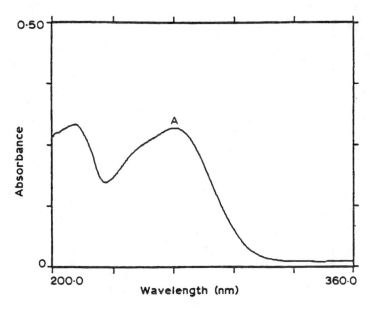

FIGURE 2.3 UV absorption spectrum of vitamin D_2 in ethanol, 2 max (peak A) = 265 nm.
Reproduced with permission from Reference 14.

From a food processing standpoint, vitamin D is quite stable. Because of the significance of fortified fluid milk and nonfat dry milk as vehicles for the delivery of vitamin D, its stability in these products has been documented. Renken and Warthesen[15] showed that light exposure caused only slight loss of vitamin D_3 in fortified milk. Air exposure did not affect the added vitamin. Recently, Indyk et al.[16] followed the processing steps for production of spray-dried, fortified whole milk. Thermal processing included preheating and direct steam injection to 95°C, five-stage evaporation, and spray-drying at 149°C. The process did not produce statistically significant losses of vitamin D_3.

2.3 METHODS

2.3.1 GENERAL APPROACH AND CURRENT SITUATION

Methods for assay of vitamin D in foods, clinical samples, vitamin premixes, concentrates, and pharmaceuticals are varied in the chemical or biological approach depending on the matrix and concentration level. Available procedures are colorimetric, spectrophotometric, chromatographic, immunological, ligand binding, or biological in approach.

Excellent methods based on competitive protein binding assays (CPBA) and radioreceptor assay (RRA) using [^{3}H] metabolites have been available for the past two decades for the analysis of serum.[17] These methods rely upon extensive prepurification of extracts by LC or solid-phase chromatography. Methodology is shown in Figure 2.4 that incorporates LC for vitamin D_2, vitamin D_3, 25(OH)D_2 and -D_3, CPBA for 24,25(OH)$_2D_2$ and -D_3, and RRA for 1,25(OH)$_2D_2$ and -D_3.[18] This approach combines currently accepted assay methods for serum analysis.

CPBA and RRA are specific and sensitive enough to measure 1,25(OH)$_2$D at circulating levels less than 100 pg/mL. However, the extensive extract purification and use of [^{3}H]-labeled compounds has been an impediment to general clinical use.[19] This situation led to the recent improvement of radioimmunoassays (RIA) using ^{125}I-labeled metabolites, and the elimination of the extensive cleanup and concentration steps. Recently published methods for 25(OH)D and 1,25(OH)$_2$D require little sample preparation and use serum calibrators that allow direct quantitation without the need for recovery determinations for each sample.[19,20] RIA analysis of serum includes the following steps:

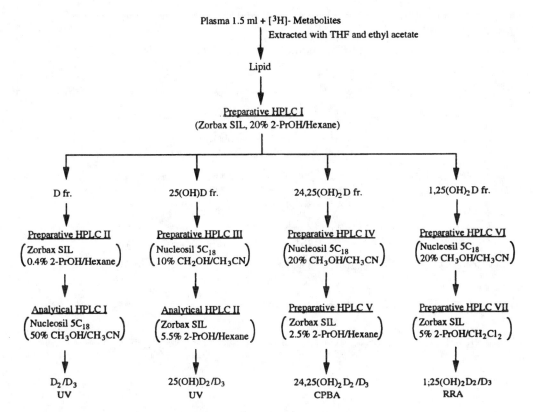

FIGURE 2.4   Procedure for determination of vitamin D_2, vitamin D_3, and hydroxylated metabolites in serum. Reproduced with permission from Reference 18.

1. Preparation of assay calibrators by stripping $1,25(OH)_2D$ with activated charcoal and addition of crystalline $1,25(OH)_2D_3$ at concentrations of 0, 5, 10, 20, 50, 100, and 200 ng/L.
2. Extraction of serum with acetonitrile.
3. Pretreatment of the extract with sodium periodate to convert $24,25(OH)_2D_3$ and $25,26(OH)_2D_3$ into aldehydes and ketones to facilitate their removal by subsequent solid phase chromatography.
4. Isolation of $1,25(OH)_2D$ by two successive C_{18}-OH silica cartridge chromatography passes.
5. Radioimmunoassay.

The assay can be completed within 5 h with a detection limit of 2.4 ng/L. Results compare with accepted RRA techniques.[20] Incorporation of the RIA procedures will dramatically change the operation of clinical laboratories for assay of 25(OH)D and $1,25(OH)_2D$.

Older methods not based on LC, CPBA, RRA, or RIA were reviewed by Singh.[21] Reviews on the use of LC for food and clinical sample analysis include Porteous et al.,[22] Norman et al.,[23] De Leenheer et al.,[24] Rizzolo and Polesollo,[25] Ball,[14] Jones et al.,[26] and Eitenmiller and Landen.[4] Various handbook, regulatory, and compendium methods for the analysis of vitamin D are summarized in Table 2.2. However, as is the case for many vitamin assay methods, these procedures have not kept abreast of available methodology.

Of significance, AOAC International Official Method 936.14 (45.3.02) "Vitamin D in Milk, Vitamin Preparations, and Feed Concentrates, Rat Bioassay" is the often quoted and still commonly

TABLE 2.2

Compendium, Regulatory and Handbook Methods for the Analysis of Vitamin D

Source	Form	Methods and Application	Approach	Most Current Cross-Reference
U.S. Pharmacopeia National Formulary, 1995 USP23/NF18 Nutritional Supplements Official Monographs[1]				
1. pages 2138, 2140	Ergocalciferol Cholecalciferol	Vitamin D in oil-soluble vitamin capsules/tablets	HPLC 265 nm	None
2. pages 2142, 2144, 2147, 2150	Ergocalciferol Cholecalciferol	Vitamin D in oil- and water-soluble vitamin capsules/tablets with/without minerals	HPLC 265 nm	None
3. pages 365–366	Cholecalciferol	Cholecalciferol (NLT 97.0%, NMT 103.0%)	HPLC 254 nm	None
4. pages 599–600	Ergocalciferol	Ergocalciferol (NLT 97.0%, NMT 103.0%)	HPLC 254 nm	None
5. pages 600–601	Ergocalciferol	Ergocalciferol capsules	HPLC 254 nm	None
6. pages 601–602	Ergocalciferol	Ergocalciferol oral solution	HPLC 254 nm	None
7. page 602	Ergocalciferol	Ergocalciferol tablets	colorimetric 500 nm	None
British Pharmacopoeia, 15th ed., 1993[2]				
1. Vol. 1, 248–250	Ergocalciferol	Ergocalciferol, calciferol injection, tablets, oral solution	HPLC 254 nm	None
2. Addendum, 1995, 1508–1509	Calcitriol	Calcitriol (1α,25 dihydroxycholecalciferol)	HPLC 265 nm	None
AOAC Official Methods of Analysis, 16th ed., 1995[3]				
1. 45.1.17	Ergocalciferol Cholecalciferol	AOAC Official Method 975.42 Vitamin D in Vitamin Preparations (200–20,000,000 IU/g)	colorimetric 550 nm	*J. Assoc. Off. Anal. Chem.,* 60, 151, 1977[4]
2. 45.1.18	Ergocalciferol Cholecalciferol	AOAC Official Method 979.24 Vitamin D in Vitamin Preparations (25,000–20,000,000 IU/g)	HPLC 254 nm	*J. Assoc. Off. Anal. Chem.,* 64, 58, 1981[5]
3. 45.1.19	Ergocalciferol Cholecalciferol	AOAC Official Method 980.26 Vitamin D in Multivitamin Preparations (≥ 200 IU/g)	HPLC 254 nm	*J. Assoc. Off. Anal. Chem.,* 64, 61, 1981[6]
4. 45.1.20	Ergocalciferol Cholecalciferol	AOAC Official Method 985.27 Vitamin D in Vitamin AD Concentrates (≥ 5000 IU/g)	HPLC 254 nm	*J. Assoc. Off. Anal. Chem.,* 68, 822, 1985[7]
5. 45.1.21	Ergocalciferol Cholecalciferol	AOAC Official Method 981.17 Vitamin D in Fortified Milk and Milk Powder (≥ 1 IU/g)	HPLC 254 nm	*J. Assoc. Off. Anal. Chem.,* 65, 1228, 1982[8]

Source	Form	Methods and Application	Approach	Most Current Cross-Reference
6. 45.1.22	Ergocalciferol Cholecalciferol	AOAC Official Method 982.29 Vitamin D in Mixed Feeds, Premixes and Pet Foods ($> 2 < 200$ IU/g) (< 200 IU/g)	HPLC 254 nm	*J. Assoc. Off. Anal. Chem.,* 66, 751, 1983[9]
7. 45.3.01	Ergocalciferol Cholecalciferol	AOAC Official Method 936.14 Vitamin D in Milk, Vitamin Preparations and Feed Concentrates	Rat bioassay	*Anal. Chem.,* 24, 1841, 1952;[10] *J. Assoc. Off. Anal. Chem.,* 46, 160, 1963[11]
8. 45.3.03	Cholecalciferol	AOAC Official Method 932.16 Vitamin D_3 in Poultry Feed Supplements	Chick bioassay	*J. Assoc. Off. Anal. Chem.,* 51, 591, 1968[12]
9. 50.1.05	Cholecalciferol	AOAC Official Method 992.26 Vitamin D_3 (Cholecalciferol) in Ready-to-Feed Milk-Based Infant Formula (488–533 IU/L)	HPLC 254 nm	*J. AOAC Int.,* 76, 1042, 1993[13]

American Feed Ingredients Association, *Laboratory Methods Compendium,* Vol. 1, 1991[14]

Source	Form	Methods and Application	Approach	Most Current Cross-Reference
1. pages 169–171	Cholecalciferol	Vitamin D_3 in vitamin D concentrates (100,000–500,000 IU/g)	HPLC 265 nm	None
2. pages 173–175	Cholecalciferol	Determination of vitamin D_3 in complete feeds and premixes (1.0–100 IU/g)	HPLC 264 nm	None
3. pages 177–179	Ergocalciferol Cholecalciferol	HPLC procedure for vitamin D in dry preparations and liquid dispersions ($500–40 \times 10^6$ IU/g)	HPLC 265 nm	None
4. pages 181–182	Cholecalciferol	HPLC procedure for vitamin D_3 in concentrates (2.0×10^5–1.0×10^6 IU/g)	HPLC 265 nm	None
5. pages 183–186	Cholecalciferol	HPLC procedure for low levels of vitamin D_3 in feeds (1.0×10^5–15×10^6 IU/lb)	HPLC 254 nm	None
6. pages 187–190	Cholecalciferol	Assay of vitamin D_3 in premixes and feeds ($2.0–1 \times 10^4$ IU/g)	HPLC 265 nm	None
7. pages 191–195	Cholecalciferol	HPLC procedure for vitamin D_3 in resin (20×10^6–32×10^6 IU/g)	HPLC 254 nm	None
8. pages 197–200	Cholecalciferol	Vitamin D_3 and vitamin E in concentrates and premixes (≥ 2000 IU/g)	HPLC 260 nm	None

Food Chemicals Codex, 4th ed., 1996[15]

Source	Form	Methods and Application	Approach	Most Current Cross-Reference
1. pages 432–433	Ergocalciferol	Vitamin D_2 (NLT 97.0%, NMT 103.0%)	HPLC 254 nm	None

TABLE 2.2 Continued

Source	Form	Methods and Application	Approach	Most Current Cross-Reference
2. page 434	Cholecalciferol	Vitamin D_3 (NLT 97.0%, NMT 103.0%)	HPLC 254 nm	None

Hoffmann-LaRoche, *Analytical Methods for Vitamins and Carotenoids in Feed,* 1988[16]

1. pages 8–11	Cholecalciferol	Determination of vitamin D_3 in complete feeds and premixes with HPLC (> 1000 IU/kg)	HPLC 264 nm	None
IDF Standard 177: 1996[17]	Cholecalciferol Ergocalciferol	Determination of vitamin D_2 or D_3 in dried skimmed milk	HPLC 265 nm	None

used line test.[27] Weanling rats are depleted of vitamin D over a 16 to 25-day depletion course and, after depletion, standard vitamin D doses and test samples are fed for 7 to 12 days. Recalcification of the tibia or distal end of a radius or ulna is determined by staining newly calcified areas with silver nitrate. Length and width of the calcification line determines potency of the sample. The assay is sensitive with detection limits as low as one IU of vitamin D. The assay is time-consuming and expensive, and few laboratories world-wide have maintained the capability to conduct the assay. In the United States, the Center for Food Safety and Nutrition (CFSAN), Food and Drug Administration, maintains the capability. AOAC International Method 932.16 (45.3.03) "Vitamin D^3 in Poultry Feed Supplements, Chick Bioassay" specifically is used for analysis of vitamin D_3 in supplements for poultry rations. Vitamin D_3 is 10 times more potent than vitamin D_2 for bone development in the chick.[28] Vitamin D deficient diets are fed to newly hatched chicks with standard doses of vitamin D_3. Bone ash of the tibia is assayed after 3 weeks.

Development of LC procedures for measurement of vitamin D in food and clinical samples has progressed to the point that methods are reliable and routinely applicable to most laboratory situations. Our review will concentrate on LC analysis of complex biologicals. The reader is directed to informative sources on the clinical application of CPBA, RRA, and RIA for the assay of vitamin D and its metabolites in serum.[17,19,20,22,26,29]

2.3.2 HIGH PERFORMANCE LIQUID CHROMATOGRAPHY

HPLC methods are available for the quantitation of vitamin D from most matrices. Further, it has been the primary tool for purification and concentration of hydroxylated metabolites prior to quantitation by more sensitive CPBA and RRA techniques (Section 2.3.1). Selected HPLC methodology papers are provided in Table 2.3.

2.3.2.1 Extraction Procedures for Vitamin D for HPLC

As shown in Table 2.3, saponification has been used almost exclusively as the initial extraction step for analysis of vitamin D in foods. In order to concentrate and clean the extract from the saponified digest, solid-phase extraction is the most common approach. Other less commonly applied purification procedures use gel permeation chromatography and semi-preparative LC. Because of the significance of saponification to analysis of vitamin D in food, we summarize various saponification procedures in Table 2.4. Most procedures are completed at ambient temperatures with pyrogallol or ascorbic acid added as antioxidants. Care must be taken to limit thermal isomerization of vitamin D to previtamin D. Ball[30] discusses the problem of resolution of previtamin D from coeluting

TABLE 2.3
HPLC Methods for the Analysis of Vitamin D and Its Metabolites in Foods, Feed, Pharmaceuticals and Biologicals

Sample Matrix	Analyte	Sample Preparation		HPLC Parameters				References
		Sample Extraction	Clean Up	Column	Mobile Phase	Detection Quantitation	Quality Assurance Parameters	
Food								
1. Milk	D_2, D_3	Saponification, ambient, overnight Extract with Et_2O	Hydroxy-alkoxypropyl sephadex	LiChrosorb S_i60 5 μm, 25 cm × 3.2 mm	Isocratic 0.6% IPA in Hex (50% water-saturated) 1 mL/min	265 nm	QL 0.08 μg/100 ml % Recovery >97	*J. Assoc. Off. Anal. Chem.,* 60, 998, 1977[1]
2. Nonfat dried milk	D_3	Extract with CH_2Cl_3–tribasic sodium phosphate with BHT	a. Sep-Pak silica b. 10 μm Partisil—10 PAC	LiChrosorb NH2 10 μm, 25 cm × 4 mm	Isocratic CH_2Cl_2 : Hex : IPA (50 : 50 : 0.2) 1 mL/min	264 nm	DL (ng) On–column 5 % Recovery 97.7	*J. Assoc. Off. Anal. Chem.,* 63, 1163, 1980[2]
3. Fortified milk, margarine, infant formula	D_2, D_3	Saponification, ambient, overnight Extract with Hex	a. Milk, infant formula, silica b. Margarine, alumina	Spherisorb ODS, 10 μm, 25 cm × 4.6 mm	Isocratic MeOH : MeCN (1 : 9) 1 mL/min	265 nm	—	*J. Assoc. Off. Anal. Chem.,* 65, 624, 1982[3]
4. Whole milk powder	D_2, D_3	Saponification ambient, overnight Extract with PE : Et_2O (90 : 10)		Two RCM100 units with Rad-PAK C_{18} 5 μm, 8 mm/ID	Isocratic MeOH (100%) or MeOH : THF (99 : 1)	Dual wavelength 250 nm 280 nm	QL 30 IU/100 g % Recovery 95	*New Zealand J. Dairy Sci. Tech.,* 19, 19, 1984[4]
5. Fortified milk infant formula	D_2, D_3	Homogenize with IPA-CH_2Cl_2 with $MgSO_4$ to remove water Evaporate, dissolve in CH_2Cl_2	a. Gel permeation chromatography Four μ styragel (100 Å) in series b. μ Bondapak/ NH2	Zorbax ODS 6 μm, 25 cm × 4.6 mm	Isocratic MeCN : CH_2Cl_2 : MeOH (700 : 300 : 2) 1 mL/min	Dual wavelength 280 nm 254 nm	% Recovery 89.6 % CV 7.5	*J. Assoc. Off. Anal. Chem.,* 68, 183, 1985[5]

TABLE 2.3 continued

Sample Matrix	Analyte	Sample Extraction	Clean Up	Column	Mobile Phase	Detection Quantitation	Quality Assurance Parameters	References
6.–7. Milk, infant formula	D_2, D_3	Saponification 75°C, 30 min Extract with Et_2O Evaporate Redissolve in Hex	Partisil—5 PAC 25 cm × 4.6 mm	Apex silica 3 µm, 15 cm × 4.5 mm	Isocratic Hex : amyl alcohol (100 : 0.15) 3 mL/min	254 nm	QL 100 IU/L RSD 7.7%	*J. Assoc. Off. Anal. Chem.*, 68, 177, 1985[6]. *J. AOAC Int.*, 76, 1042, 1993[7]
8. Milk powder, infant formula	D_2, D_3	Saponification Add ^3H-D_3 and $^3[H]$-25(OH)D_3 for recovery Steam bath, 45 min Evaporate Dissolve in MeOH containing 1.5% digitonin Extract with Hex	1. Aluminum oxide 2. Polygosil S, 60-5 25 cm × 4.6 mm Isocratic 0.5% IPA in Hex			CBPA	QL 0.1 IU/g % Recovery 90–110	*J. Agric. Food Chem.*, 34, 264, 1986[8]
9. Fortified milk, infant formula, porridge, gruel	D_3	Saponification Boiling water bath, 60 min Extract with B	Polygosil Si 60-5 30 cm × 8.0 mm Monitor at 254 nm	Two Shandon ODS columns in series, 5 µm, 25 cm × 4.6 mm	Isocratic MeOH	265 nm	QL 5 µg/L % Recovery 95	*Int. J. Vit. Nutr. Res.* 57, 357, 1987[9]
10. Human milk, infant formula	D_3	Add $^3[H]$-D_3 for recovery Deproteinize with NH_4OH and ethanol Extract with EtOH and PE Evaporate to dryness and saponify, 50°C, 15 min Extract with PE	1. Sep-Pak silica 2. LC cleanup µBondapak C_{18}, 10 µm, 36 cm × 3.9 mm Collect vitamin D fraction Isocratic MeOH : water (90 : 10) 1.3 mL/min	—	—	CPBA	QL 2 µg/L % Recovery 65–75	*Clin. Chem.*, 33, 796, 1987[10]

Sample	Vitamers	Sample preparation	Cleanup	Column	Mobile phase	Detection	Performance	Reference
11. Fortified milk, milk powder, infant formula	D_2, D_3	Saponification ambient, overnight extract with 1-chlorobutane Evaporate Redissolve in 2,2,4-trimethylpentane	Polygosil 60-5 CN 12.5 cm x 4 mm	Polygosil 60-5 NH$_2$ CN 12.5 cm × 4 mm	Isocratic 0.35% 1-pentanol in Hex 1 mL/min	254 nm 265 nm 280 nm	% Recovery 94.8	Neth. Milk. Dairy J., 42, 423, 1988[11]
12.–13. Infant formula, enteral nutritionals	D_2, D_3	Add D_2 (IS) Saponification 60°C, 30 min Extract with Hex Evaporate	SPE B & J Silica 9054 Evaporate, redissolve in MeCN	Vydac 201TP54 5 um, 25 cm × 4.6 mm (not endcapped)	Gradient MeCN MeOH EtoAC 0.7–2.5 mL/min	265 nm	QL 8 IU/quart % Recovery 99 RSD$_R$ = 13.48	J. AOAC Int., 75, 566, 1992[12] J. AOAC Int., 79, 73, 1996[13]
14. Milk	D_3	Saponification Ambient, overnight, Extract with PE : Et$_2$O (90 : 10) Evaporate Redissolve in Hex	SPE bond elute silica Evaporate Redissolve in MeCN	Vydac C$_{18}$ 5 μm, 25 cm × 4.6 mm	Isocratic MeCN : MeOH (90 : 10) 1.5 mL/min	254 nm	% Recovery 93	J. Food Sci., 58, 552, 1993[14]
15. Milk	D_2, D_3	Add D_2 (IS) Saponification 60°C, 30 min Extract with Hex Evaporate Redissolve in Hex	SPE Florisil Sep-Pak Evaporate Redissolve in MeCN	Vydac C$_{18}$ 5 μm, 25 cm × 4.6 mm	Isocratic MeCN : MeOH (97 : 3) 1 mL/min	265 nm	QL 1.6 μg/L % Recovery 81–96	J. AOAC Int., 77, 1047, 1994[15]
16.–17. Milk	D_2, D_3	Add D_2 (IS) Saponification Ambient, overnight, Extract with Hex : Et$_2$O (9 : 1) Evaporate Redissolve in Hex	a. SPE b. Semi-Prep LC Resolve silica, 5 μm, 8 × 10 RCM	Rad-Pak Resolve C$_{18}$ 5 μm, 8 × 10 RCM at 30°C	Isocratic MeOH : THF : water (93 : 2 : 5) 1 mL/min	280 nm 265 nm DAD	QL 0.06 IU/g fat RSD$_R$ = 2.7 % Recovery >80	Food Chem., 50, 75, 1994[16] 57, 283, 1996[17]

TABLE 2.3 continued

Sample Matrix	Analyte	Sample Preparation		HPLC Parameters				References
		Sample Extraction	Clean Up	Column	Mobile Phase	Detection Quantitation	Quality Assurance Parameters	
18. Fish	D_3	Extract fat (Bligh and Dyer) Saponification of fat ambient, overnight Extract with Hex Evaporate Redissolve in MeOH	—	JASCOSil SS-10-ODS-B	Isocratic MeCN : MeOH (80 : 20) 1 mL/min	265 nm	QL 1.4 µg/100 g	*J. Agric. Food Chem.*, 36, 803, 1988[18]
19. Fish	D_3, 25(OH)D_3 7-dehydro cholesterol (7-DHC)	Add ^{3}[H]-D_3 and 25-OH^3[H]-D_3 for recovery determination Saponification Extract with B Evaporate Redissolve in MeOH : Hex : CHCl$_3$ (2 : 23 : 75)	Sephadex LH-20	a. RP-HPLC Zorbax ODS 5 µm, 15 cm × 4.6 mm b. ND-HPLC Zorbax-SIL 5 µm, 15 cm × 4.6 mm	Isocratic a. RP-HPLC MeOH : MeCN (50 : 50) 2 ml/min b. NP-HPLC Hex : IPA (99.6 : 0.4) for D_3, 7-DHC and Hex : IPA (97.5 : 2.5) for 25(OH)D_3 2 mL/min	265 nm	% Recovery 95–98	*Comp. Biochem. Physiol.*, 111A, 191, 1995[19]
20. Fish, fish products	D_3, 25(OH)D_3	Add D_2 and 25(OH)D_2 (IS) Saponification Extract with PE : Et$_2$O (1 : 1) Evaporate Redissolve in Hex	Semiprep HPLC Gradient elution from µ-Parisil Collect 25(OH)D_2 and 25(OH)D_3 fraction and D_2 and D_3 fraction	Vydac 201TP54 25 cm × 4.6 mm	Isocratic a. For 25(OH)D_2 and D_3 MeOH : Water (83 : 17) b. For D_2 and D_3 MeOH : Water (93 : 7)	264 nm % Recovery 17–25(OH)D_3	DL (ng) On-column D_2, D_3 — 1.5 25(OH)D_2, 25(OH)D_3 — 0.5 76–100 CV% 3-D_3	*J. Food Comp. Anal.*, 8, 232, 1995[20]

	Compounds	Sample preparation	Cleanup	HPLC column	Mobile phase	Detection	Performance	Reference
21. Baby foods	D_2, D_3	Add D_2 or D_3 (IS) Saponification 70°C, 30 min Extract with Et_2O : PE (1 : 9) Evaporate Redissolve in iOct	Semi-Prep LC Polygosil-60 ~5 μm, 25 cm × 8 mm	Two Shandon ODS-5 columns in series 5 μm, 25 cm × 4.6 mm	Isocratic MeOH (100%) 1 mL/min	265 nm	QL 350–420 IU/Kg % Recovery 84 DL (ng) On-column 2	Neth. Milk Dairy J., 48, 31, 1994[21]
22. Egg yolk	D_2, D_3	Add D_2 (IS) Saponification ambient, overnight Extract with Hex Evaporate Redissolve in Hex	a. SPE Mega Bond Elut Silica b. HPLC μPorasil, 10 μm 30 cm × 3.9 mm	Vydac 201TP54 5 μm, 25 cm × 4.6 mm	Isocratic MeOH : water (94 : 6) 1 mL/min	264 nm	QL 0.4 μg/100g % Recovery 94 CV% = 3.6	J. Food Comp. Anal., 5, 281, 1992[22]
23. Egg yolk	25(OH)D_3	Add 25(OH)D_2 (IS) Saponification Ambient, overnight Extract with Hex	SPE Mega Bond Elut Silica	Vydac 201TP54 5 μm, 25 cm × 4.6 mm	Isocratic MeOH : water (83 : 17) 1 mL/min	264 nm	DL (ng) On-column 2-8 % Recovery 98	J. Food Comp. Anal., 6, 250, 1993[23]
24. Meat, animal fat	D_3, 25(OH)D_3	Saponification Extract with Hex : CH_2Cl_2 (85 : 15) Evaporate Redissolve in Hex No IS	a. Alumina, open-column b. HPLC (for D_3) Apex Silica, 3 μm 15 cm × 4.5 mm Collect D_3 fraction Evaporate Redissolve in IPA : Water (90 : 10)	RCM module Resolve 8C28, 5 μm	Isocratic MeOH, 100% 1.5 m./min	254 nm	—	Food Chem., 46, 313, 1993[24]
25. Medical nutritionals	D_2, D_3	Saponification Extract with Et_2O Add D_2 (IS) Evaporate Redissolve in Hex	Semi-prep HPLC Nucleosil 50-5, 5 μm	Hitachi Gal 3056, 5 μm, 25 cm × 4 mm	Isocratic MeCN : MeOH : 50% perchloric acid 97.0 : 30 : 1.2) Containing 0.057 M Sodium perchlorate 1.2 mL/min	Dual electrode EC redox mode Detector 1— 0.65 V Detector 2— 0.20 V H_2/H reference	DL (pg) On-column 200 % Recovery 97.5 $RSD_R = 3.6$	J. Chromatogr. 605, 215, 1992[25]

TABLE 2.3 continued

Sample Matrix	Analyte	Sample Preparation — Sample Extraction	Sample Preparation — Clean Up	HPLC Parameters — Column	HPLC Parameters — Mobile Phase	HPLC Parameters — Detection Quantitation	Quality Assurance Parameters	References
26.–27. Mushrooms	D_2, 25(OH)D_2, Pre-D_2	Add D_3 and 25(OH)D_3 (IS) Saponification Extract with PE : Et$_2$O (1 : 1) Evaporate	a. Semi-prep HPLC μ-Porisil gradient Collect 25(OH)D_2 and 25(OH)D_3 fraction and D_2 fraction and D_3 fraction and Pre-D_2 and Pre-D_3 fraction Evaporate b. Semi-prep HPLC Vydac 201TP54	a. For D_2, D_3, Pre-D_2, Pre-D_3 Vydac 201TP54 25 cm × 4.6 mm	Isocratic a. For D_2, D_3, Pre-D_2, Pre-D_3, MeOH : water (93 : 7) 1 mL/min b. For 25(OH)D_2, 25(OH)D_3, Hex : IPA (98 : 2) 1 mL/min	264 nm	DL (ng) On-column D_2 = 0.5 D_3 = 25(OH)D_2 = 0.5 25(OH)D_3 = 0.7 % Recovery 98 ± 9.2	J. Agric. Food Chem., 42, 2449, 1994[26] J. Food Chem., 57, 95, 1996[27]
Feeds								
1. Animal feeds, Premixes	D_2, D_3	Saponification ambient, overnight Extract with Hex No IS	—	SupelcoSil LC-18, 5 μm, 25 cm × 4.6 mm	Isocratic MeCN : MeOH (90 : 10) 1.8 m/min	301 nm	QL 1 IU/g	J. AOAC Int., 75, 812, 1992[1]
2. Fish meal	D_3, Pre-D_3	Saponification Extract with Et$_2$O Evaporate Redissolve in MeOH No IS	—	Two in series a. HC ODS/PAH 25 cm × 2.6 mm b. LC-18, 5 μm, 15 cm × 4.6 mm;	MeCN : MeOH : water (74 : 18 : 8) 1.5 mL/min;	255 nm	—	Animal Feed Sci. Tech., 47, 99, 1994[2]

Sample	Analyte	Sample preparation	Cleanup	Column	Mobile phase	Detection	DL/QL/Recovery	Reference
Plasma 1.	D3, 25(OH)D2, 25(OH)D3	Add ^{3}[H]-D3 and ^{3}[H]-25(OH)D3 (IS) for recovery calculation. Denature protein with MeOH:IPA (90:10). Extract with Hex	—	SupelcoSil LC-18 C18, 5 µm, 25 cm × 4.6 mm	Linear gradient MeOH:water (85:15) to MeOH:IPA:water (87.5:10:2.5) 2.3 mL/min	265 nm	DL 5 nmol/L; % Recovery 79.9; % CV 5.3–7.0	Scand. J. Clin. Invest. 52, 177, 1992[1]
2. Plasma	D2, D3, 25(OH)D2, -D3, 24R-(OH)2 D2, 1α-25-(OH)2	Add [1α,2α(n)-^{3}H]-D3, [23,24 (n)-^{3}H]-25(OH)D3, 23,24(n)-^{3}H-24, 25(OH)2D3, and [26,27-methyl-^{3}H]-1,25(OH)2D3 for recovery. Add THF and EtOAC. Centrifuge. Remove EtOAC layer. Reextract with EtOAC. Evaporate. Redissolve in IPA:Hex (20:80)	Semi-prep HPLC a. For D2, D3 Zorbax SIL b. For 25(OH)D2, D3, Nucleosil 5 C18 c. For 24,25 (OH)2-D2-D3 1. Nucleosil 5 C18 2. Zorbax SIL For 1,25(OH)2D2, D3 1. Nucleosil 5 C18 2. Zorbax SIL	a. For D2, D3, Nucleosil 5 C18 30 cm × 7.5 mm b. For 25(OH)D2, D3 Zorbax SIL 25 cm × 4.6 mm	Isocratic a. For D2, D3 MeCN:MeOH (50:50) 2 mL/min b. For 25(OH)D2, D3 Hex:IPA (97.5:2.5) 1.3 ml/min	a. For D2, D3, 25(OH)D2, 25(OH)D3 265 nm b. For 24,25 (OH)2D2, D3, CPBA c. 1,25 (OH)2 D2-D3 Radio receptor assay RRA	DL (ng) On-column D3—0.3; 25(OH)D3—.5; 24,25 (OH)2D3—12.5 pg; 1,25(OH)2D3—2 pg; CV% (intraassay) D3-9.6; 25(OH)D3—9.0; 24,25(OH)2D3—4.6; 1,25(OH)2D3—5.4	Food Chem. 45, 215, 1992[2]
3. Plasma	25(OH)D2,3S	Add 25(OH)-7-dehydrocholesterol (IS) in EtOH. Deproteinize with EtOH. Centrifuge. Dilute supernatant with 0.4 M phosphate, pH 7.5	SPE a. Bond Elut C18 b. PHP-LH 20 c. Bond Elut C18	YMC-Pack ODS-AM, 5 µm, 15 cm × 4.6 mm at 40°C	Isocratic MeCN:NaCLO4 (98:2) 1 mL/min	265 nm	QL 5 ng/ml; % Recovery 95–104; RSD 1.4–3.2%	Biomed. Chromatogr. 9, 229, 1995[3]
4. Plasma	25(OH)D3	Add ^{3}[H]-25-D3 for recovery calculation and 5Z-22-OH-24, 25,26,27-tetranor vitamin D3 (IS)	Sep-Pak silica	Zorbax SIL, 5 µm, 25 cm × 4.6 mm	Isocratic Hex:CHCl3:MeOH (100:25:2) 1.5 mL/min	265 nm	QL 19 ng/ml	J. Chromatogr. B: Biomed. Appl. 672, 63, 1995[4]

TABLE 2.3 continued

| Sample Matrix | Analyte | Sample Preparation | | HPLC Parameters | | | | |
		Sample Extraction	Clean Up	Column	Mobile Phase	Detection Quantitation	Quality Assurance Parameters	References
5. Plasma	$1,25(OH)_2D_3$	Add [^{3}H]-$1,25(OH)_2D_3$ Extract with CH_2Cl_2 : MeOH (1 : 2)	Bond Elute NH_2 LiChrosphere Si60 Pool fractions between 11 and 14 min Dry in vacuo Add DMEQ-TAD in CH_2Cl_2 Stop reaction with MeOH Dry under Ar Fluorescent products were purified by SPE on Bond Elut PSA Evaporate	YMC-Pak ODS-AM302	Gradient 55% to 100% MeOH in water for 40 min	DMEQ-TAD adducts Fluorescence Ex λ = 370 Em λ = 440	QL 12 pg/mL % Recovery 88–106	J. Chromatogr. B, 690, 15, 1997[5]

TABLE 2.4
Saponification Parameters for the Analysis of Vitamin D

Matrix	Sample Size	Hydrolysis Conditions	Antioxidant	Extractant	Internal Standard or % Recovery	Quantitation Level	Reference
Fortified milk	50 mL	KOH Ambient overnight	Ethanolic pyrogallol	Diethyl ether : Hexane (5 : 1)	D_3—98%	1.08 µg/mL	J. AOAC, 60, 998, 1977
Fish	20 g	Ethanolic KOH Ambient overnight	—	Diethyl ether : petroleum ether (1 : 1)	D_2 (IS) and 25(OH)D_2(IS)	0.2 µg/100 g	J. Food Comp. Anal., 8, 232, 1995
Baby foods	50 g	Ethanolic KOH 70°C, 30 min	Pyrogallol Nitrogen flush	Diethyl ether : petroleum ether (1 : 9)	D_2 (IS) or D_3 (IS) depending on product form	400 IU/kg	Neth. Milk Dairy J., 48, 31, 1994
Egg yolk	20 g	Ethanolic KOH Ambient overnight	Ascorbic acid	Diethyl ether : petroleum ether (1 : 1)	D_2 (IS) or 25(OH)D_2 (IS)	D_2—0.4 µg/100 g 25(OH)D_2— 0.87 µg/100 g	J. Food Comp. Anal., 5, 281, 1992; 6, 250, 1993
Mushrooms	1.0 g (dry)	Ethanolic KOH Ambient overnight	Ascorbic acid	Diethyl ether : petroleum ether (1 : 1)	D_3 (IS) or 25(OH)D_3 (IS)	2.8 µg/100 g	J. Agric. Food Chem., 42, 2449, 1994
Feeds, premixes	Feed 1.2 g Premix 0.5 g	Ethanolic KOH Ambient overnight	Pyrogallol	Hexane	92%—premix 87%—feed	1.0 IU/g	J. AOAC Int., 75, 812, 1992
Milk, margarine, infant formula	Milk—15 mL Infant formula—10 mL Margarine—5g	KOH Ambient, 18 h	Ethanolic pyrogallol	Hexane	D_2—96–99%	382 IU/100 g	J. AOAC, 65, 624, 1982

TABLE 2.4 Continued

Matrix	Sample Size	Hydrolysis Conditions	Antioxidant	Extractant	Internal Standard or % Recovery	Quantitation Level	Reference
Fortified milk powder	10 g	Ethanolic KOH Ambient overnight	Ethanolic pyrogallol Nitrogen flush	Diethyl ether : petroleum ether (10 : 90)	> 95%	30 IU/100 g	*New Zealand J. Dairy Sci.*, 19, 19, 1984
Milk Infant formula	Powder 4 g Infant formula, 30 mL	Ethanolic KOH 75°C, 30 min	Ascorbic acid	Diethyl ether : petroleum ether (1 : 1)	96–97%	348 IU/L	*J. AOAC*, 68, 177, 1985
Milk powder, Infant powder	10 g	Ethanolic KOH Reflux, 45 min	Sodium ascorbate	Benzene	[^{3}H]D$_3$	5 IU/g	*J. Agric. Food Chem.*, 34, 264, 1986
Fortified milk, Infant formula, Milk powder	Powder—20 g Liquid—12 g	Ethanolic KOH Ambient overnight	Sodium ascorbate Nitrogen flush	1-chlorobutane	D$_3$—95%	19.3 IU/100 g (powder)	*Neth. Milk Dairy J.*, 42, 423, 1988
Infant formula Enteral nutritionals	15 mL	Ethanolic KOH 60°C, 30 min	—	Hexane (IS) depending on product form	D$_2$ (IS) or D$_3$	136 IU/qt	*J. AOAC Int.*, 75, 571, 1992; 79, 73, 1996
Fortified milk	15 mL	Ethanolic KOH 60°C, 30 min	—	Hexane	D$_2$ (IS) 81–96%	1.6 μg/L	*J. AOAC Int.*, 77, 1047, 1994

interfering compounds in both normal-phase and reversed-phase LC systems. Reflux temperatures lead to previtamin D formation and, if not resolved by chromatography, calculations must correct for the percentage conversion during extraction.[30] For this reason, internal standards (Section 2.3.2.3) are routinely used for food analysis and considered essential. Recovery is often determined by addition of [^{3}H]-D_2 or -D_3 to the initial digest.[26]

Extraction of serum does not require saponification; therefore, degradative conditions can be avoided. Initial procedures rely on protein denaturation and solvent partitioning. Commonly used procedures are summarized in Table 2.3. Jones et al.[26] classified solvent extractions into the following general approaches:

1. Total lipid extraction—methanol : chloroform : water (2 : 1 : 0.8) which is the Bligh and Dyer technique or ethanol : water (9 : 1).
2. Selective lipid extraction—ether, ethyl acetate : cyclohexane (1 : 1), hexane, dichloromethane, or hexane : isopropanol (1 : 2).

Jones et al.[26] point out that the Bligh and Dyer extraction using methanol and chloroform is highly efficient for extraction of hydroxylated metabolites. Also, dichloromethane can be substituted for chloroform to avoid the use of the carcinogen. Such extractions based on lipid extraction provide the initial procedural step in methods that rely upon CPBA, RRA, or RIA for quantitation of low-level metabolites.

Solid-phase chromatographic cleanup is an indispensable approach for both food and clinical sample analysis. Use of normal-phase silica and reversed-phase C_{18} cartridges are routine (Table 2.3).

2.3.2.2   Chromatography Parameters

2.3.2.2.1   Supports and Mobile Phases

Both normal- and reversed-phase systems offer efficient resolution of vitamins D_2, D_3, the previtamins, and hydroxylated metabolites, if properly prepared extracts are available. Masuda et al.[18] (Figure 2-4) effectively demonstrated the usefulness of both chromatography modes in an integrated analytical approach to serum analysis. For vitamins D_2 and D_3, preparative LC or Zorbax SIL was followed by analytical LC on Nucleosil $5C_{18}$. 25(OH)D_2 and -D_3 and the dihydroxy metabolites were concentrated by preparative LC on Nucleosil $5C_{18}$ and analytical LC on Zorbax SIL. Vitamins D_2 and D_3, 25(OH)D_2 and -D_3 were detected by UV at 265 nm. 24,25(OH)$_2$$D_2$ and -D_3 were assayed by CPBA, and 1,25(OH)$_2$$D_2$ and -D_3 by RRA. Recovery was determined through addition of [$1\alpha,2\alpha(n)$-^{3}H]-D_3, [$23,24(n)$-^{3}H]-25(OH)D_3, [$23,24(n)$-^{3}H]-24,25(OH)$_2$$D_3$, and [26,27-methyl-^{3}H]-1,25(OH)$_2$$D_3$ in ethanol prior to lipid extraction by tetrahydrofuran and ethyl acetate.

Jones et al.[26] classified supports and mobile phase for resolution of vitamin D and various metabolites into the following groups:

1. Silica with isopropanol-hexane mixtures, methanol-methylene chloride mixtures, and methylene chloride-isopropanol. The latter mobile phase separates 25(OH)D_3-26,23-lactone and 24(R),25(OH)$_2$$D_3$. As shown in Table 2.3, these solvent systems are common in recently published papers with resolution based on normal-phase chromatography. Normal-phase chromatography on silica has been incorporated into semi-preparative cleanup and concentration steps of more recently published assays for fluid milk,[31] and spray-dried milk powder,[16] and for procedures applicable to most food matrices.[32–38]
2. C_{18} supports with methanol-water and acetonitrile-methanol-water. Jones et al.[26] discusses difficulties presented by the use of aqueous mobile phases if the determinative step is CPBA. Water is difficult to evaporate, tends to dissolve supports, and might introduce oxygen that would promote oxidation of the 5,7-diene double bond system. Aqueous

mobile phases provide excellent resolution for vitamins D_2 and D_3; however, resolution of dihydroxy metabolites is poorer compared to silica.[26] Reversed-phase systems provide excellent resolution of 25(OH)D_2 and -D_3.

3. Cyano supports for resolution of hydroxylated forms including separation of 25(OH)D_3-26,23-ketone from 24,25-(OH)$_2D_3$.

2.3.2.2.2   Detection

Detection at wavelengths near the UV maximum for vitamin D of 265 nm is sensitive enough for most matrices for the detection of vitamins D_2 and D_3 and 25(OH)D_2 and -D_3, provided proper extract purification steps are included in the sample preparation protocol (Section 2.3.2.1).[18] UV detection is not sensitive and specific enough for the quantitation of dihydroxy metabolites in serum and tissue at the normal physiological levels of less than 100 pg per mL. Requirements for the clinical assay of dihydroxy metabolites were the impetus for the development of the CPBA, RRA, and RIA procedures more than two decades ago (Section 2.3).

Since vitamin D does not fluoresce, this powerful detection mode has not been available for routine vitamin D assay. Recently, Shimizu et al.[39] reported a fluorometric method for analysis of 1,25(OH)$_2D_3$ from plasma. The method entailed the fluorescence labeling of the vitamin D metabolite with 4-[2-(6,7-dimethoxy-4-methyl-3-oxo-3,4-dihydro-quinoxalyl)ethyl]-1,2,4-triazoline-3,5-dione (DMEQ-TAD). The adducts were fluorometrically detected at Ex λ = 370 and Em λ = 440. The limit of detection for 1,25(OH)$_2D_3$ was 5 pg and CV% values were around 10%. Recoveries were low, but values corrected for recovery compared closely to RRA determined values. In its present state, the new procedure is more tedious and time consuming compared to RRA methodology. However, it is the first successful application of fluorescence detection to 1,25(OH)D_3 in plasma.

2.3.2.3   Internal Standards

Owing to the complexity of sample treatments for vitamin D analysis, internal standards are required to compensate for extraction losses. Vitamin D_2 can be used as the internal standard for vitamin D_3 procedures or vice-versa, provided the internal standard is proven to be absent from the matrix. Likewise, for 25(OH)D_2 or -D_3, the hydroxylated metabolite not present in the matrix can be conveniently used as the internal standard. Deuterated metabolites are routinely added to clinical samples for recovery calculations pertinent to the assay of low-level metabolites.

2.3.3   RECENT ADVANCES IN METHOD DEVELOPMENT FOR FOOD ANALYSIS

In general, methods for food analysis did not advance as rapidly as those used in the clinical area. AOAC International[27] methods include the line test bioassay (AOAC Official Method 936.14, 45.3.02) (Section 2.3) and an older colorimetric procedure for vitamin preparations (AOAC Official Method 975.42, 45.1.17). AOAC methods based on LC include Method 979.24 (45.1.18) and Method 980.26 (45.1.21) for fortified milk and milk powder, Method 982.29 (45.1.22) for mixed feeds, premixes and pet foods and Method 992.26 (50.1.05) for vitamin D_3 in ready-to-feed milk-based infant formula. These methods are suitable only for concentrated preparations or fortified foods.

AOAC Official Method 992.26 for milk-based infant formula was based on the work of Sertl and Molitar[40] published in 1985. The method was collaborated by AOAC International in 1993.[41] Procedural steps include saponification, extraction with ethyl ether and petroleum ether (1 : 1), LC cleanup on a Partasil-5 PAC column, and determinative LC on 3 μm Apex silica. Mobile phases for the cleanup and analytical columns were 0.8% amyl alcohol in hexane and 0.15% amyl alcohol in hexane, respectively. Cleanup provided by the Partisil-5 PAC (amino-cyano) column was insufficient to provide clean chromatograms by analytical chromatography. Vitamin D was quantitated on the slope of a large interfering peak. Of note, most cleanup procedures utilize chromatography modes of different separation chemistries compared to the analytical system. In order to maximize cleanup, reversed-phase supports are used prior to determinative chromatography on normal-phase supports or vice-versa. While the method was accepted by AOAC International as official, RSD$_r$ and RSD$_R$ values were greater than 20%, an unacceptably high degree of method performance variability.

Sliva et al.[42] presented a method for vitamin D in infant formula and enteral nutritionals that was recently collaborated by AOAC International.[43] The procedure incorporates saponification, hexane extraction, SPE on silica, and analytical chromatography on C_{18}. The procedure provides RSD$_r$ values of 13.48 and 9.44, respectively, which is a significant improvement over Method 992.26[42,43] Chromatograms showed excellent resolution of vitamin D_2 (internal standard), vitamin D_3, and pre-vitamins D_2 and -D_3. Levels of previtamins were below detection limits following the saponification at 60°C for 30 minutes, indicating excellent control during the extraction.

In 1996, the International Dairy Federation (IDF) published IDF Standard 177: 1996 "Dried Skimmed Milk, Determination of Vitamin D Content."[44] The method was chosen after results of an intercomparison study of methods by the Measurements and Testing Program of the Community Bureau of Reference (BCR) of the European Commission. The procedure is based upon saponification, exhaustive partitioning of the digest with light petroleum, semi-preparative LC on silia, and analytical LC on C_{18} or ODS. The limit of detection is 2.5 μg/100 g. Vitamin D_2 is used as the internal standard for determination of vitamin D_3. However, the absence of vitamin D_2 at detectable levels must be verified by assaying the sample with and without addition of the internal standard.

Recent procedures that offer excellent approaches for analysis of vitamin D in foods at endogenous levels include methods by Kurmann and Indyk[31] for milk and other dairy products and procedures developed by Mattila et al.[32–38] for most food matrices. Both approaches use semi-preparative LC for sample clean up and concentration. These methods are presented in detail in Section 2.4.

2.4   METHOD PROTOCOLS

Vitamin D_3 in Fluid and Spray Dried Milk

Principle
- Samples were saponified, extracted with hexane : diethyl ether (9 : 1), and fractionated by SPE silica and semi-preparative LC on Resolve silica Rad-Pak columns. The purified extracts were chromatographed on Resolve C_{18} with UV detection of vitamin D at 265 nm. Vitamin D_2 was added prior to saponification as the internal standard.

Chemicals
- Ethanol
- Potassium hydroxide
- Hexane
- Anhydrous diethyl ether
- Pyrogallol
- Methanol
- Ethyl acetate
- Tetrahydrofuran
- Isopropyl alcohol
- Anhydrous sodium sulfate
- Vitamin D_2 and -D_3 USP standards

Apparatus
- Liquid chromatograph
- UV detector
- Sep-Pak silica cartridges
- Rotary evaporator

Sample Preparation

- Add 250 mL of 30% ethanolic KOH containing 1% pyrogallol to 100 mL fluid milk, vitamin D_2 internal standard, 1 mL
- Flush with N_2, saponify 16 h at ambient temperature
- Transfer to separatory funnel with 100 mL water wash
- Extract 2 × with 500 mL hexane : diethyl ether (9 : 1)
- Wash combined organic phase with water until neutral
- Filter extract through 25 g Na_2SO_4
- Evaporate to near dryness
- Dissolve residue in 1 mL hexane

SPE Purification

- Pass 10 mL hexane through Sep-Pak silica cartridge
- Load sample extract
- Wash cartridge with 3 mL hexane : ethyl acetate (90 : 10)
- Elute vitamin fraction with 5 mL hexane : ethyl acetate (80 : 20)

Semi-Preparative HPLC Fractionation

- Inject entire vitamin D fraction on 8 × 10 Radial Compression Module containing Resolve silica Rad-Pak (5 μm) column
- Mobile phase—hexane : isopropyl alcohol (99 : 1), isocratic, 1 mL/min
- Monitor eluate at 265 nm
- Collect vitamin D fraction between 2 min before and 2 min after established peak retention time
- Evaporate to dryness under N_2
- Dissolve immediately in 100 μL methanol

Analytical Chromatography Parameters*

Column	Resolve C_{18} (5 μm) Rad-Pak 8 × 10 Radical Compression Module
Mobile phase	Methanol : THF : water (93 : 2 : 5), isocratic
Flow	1 mL/min
Temperature	Ambient
Detection	265 nm and PDA
Calculation	Internal standard, peak height

*See Figure 2.5.

Source: Food Chem., 50, 75, 1994 and 57, 283, 1996.

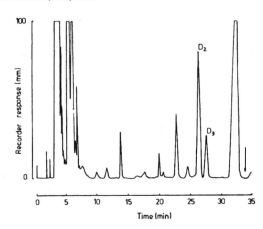

FIGURE 2.5   Chromatogram of endogenous vitamin D_3 in bovine milk by the method of Kurmann and Indyk. Reproduced with permission from Reference 31.

An Integrated Approach to Vitamin D Analysis of Foods

Principle
- Saponified samples are extacted with diethyl ether : petroleum ether (1 : 1), purified by SPE on silica and fractioned by semi-preparative LC on μPorasil or μPorsail followed by reversed-phase chromatography on Vydac 201TP54. Analytical chromatography used either normal-phase or reversed-phase systems with detection at 264 nm.

Chemicals
- Vitamin D_2, D_3, 25(OH)D_3, and 25(OH)D_2 standards
- Ethanol
- Potassium hydroxide
- Diethyl ether
- Methanol
- Hexane
- Isopropanol

Apparatus
- Liquid chromatograph
- UV detector, diode array detector
- Rotary evaporator
- Vacuum oven

Procedure

Sample Extraction
- Add internal standards—vitamin D_3 for vitamin D_2 and 25(OH)D_3 for 25(OD)D_2 or vice-versa. External spiking used if sample contains both D_2 and D_3 for recovery corrections
- Saponify oernight—ambient
- Extract with petroleum ether : diethyl ether (1 : 1)
- Wash extract with water until neutral
- Evaporate with Rotavapor
- Dissolve in 1.5 mL hexane

Sep-Pak Purification (Margarine, Egg Yolk)
- Dilute extract with 10 mL hexane and add to Mega Bond Elut silia column previously washed with 20 mL hexane
- Wash with 20 mL hexane
- Wash with 50 mL of 0.5% isopropanol in hexane
- Elute vitamin D fraction with 35 mL of 0.5% isopropanol in hexane
- Wash column with 50 mL of 0.5% isopropanol in hexane
- Elute 25(OH)D_2 and -D_3 with 40 mL of 6% isopropanol in hexane
- Evaporate 25(OH)D fraction to dryness and redissolve in 1.5 mL hexane
- Filter, 0.45 μm

Semi-Preparative HPLC Fractionation
- Inject 1 mL extract on µPorasil column
- Gradient elution

> Isocratic, 15 min, hexane : isopropanol (98.8 : 1.2)
> Linear gradient, 0.3 min to hexane : isopropanol (94.2 : 5.8)
> Isocratic, 9.7 min, hexane : isopropanol (94.2 : 5.8)
> Column purification, 10 min, hexane : isopropanol (85 : 15)
> Equilibration, 10 min, hexane : isopropanol (98.8 : 1.2)

Notes:
- Previtamin D_2 and D_3, and D_3 elute as one peak at 8 and 12 min, respectively
- 25(OH)D_2 and -D_3 resolve between 20 to 25 min
- Collection times—1.5 min before and after retention times of previtamins and D_2 and D_3; 2 min before 25(OH)D_2 and 2 min after 25(OH)D_3 elution

Analytical Protocol

See Figures 2.6 and 2.7.

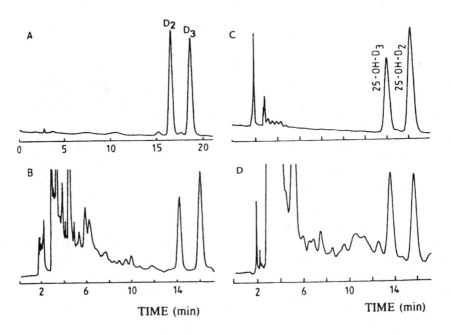

FIGURE 2.6 Chromatograms of vitamin D_2 and vitamin D_3 standards (A), vitamin D_2 (IS) and vitamin D_3 in Pike (B), 25(OH)D_2 and -D_3 standards (C), and 25(OH)D_2 (IS) and 25(OH)D_3 in whitefish. Reproduced with permission from Reference 38.

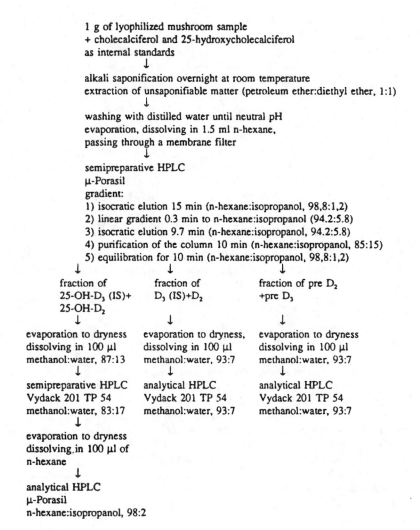

FIGURE 2.7 Analysis protocol for the analysis of vitamin D_2, $25(OH)D^2$, previtamin D_2 in mushrooms. Reproduced with permission from Reference 34.

2.5   REFERENCES

Text

1. Friedrich, W., Vitamin D, in *Vitamins,* Walter de Gruyter, Berlin, 1998, chap. 3.
2. Machlin, L. J. and Hüni, J. E. S., *Vitamin Basics,* Hoffmann-LaRoche, Basel, 1994, 12.
3. Norman, A. W., Vitamin D, in *Present Knowledge in Nutrition*, 7th ed., Ziegler, E. E. and Filer, L. J., Jr., Eds., ILSI Press, Washington, D. C., 1996, chap. 12.
4. Eitenmiller, R. and Landen, W. O., Jr., Vitamins, in *Analyzing Food for Nutrition Labeling and Hazardous Contaminants*, Jeon, I. J. and Ikins, W. G., Eds., Marcel Dekker, New York, 1995, chap. 9.
5. Olsen, R. E. and Munson, P. L., Fat-soluble vitamins, in *Principles of Pharmacology,* Munson, P. L., Mueller, R. A., and Breese, G. R., Eds., Chapman and Hall, New York, 1994, chap. 58.
6. Gibson, R. S., *Principles of Nutritional Assessment,* Oxford University Press, New York, 1990, 391.
7. Holick, M. F., McCollum Award Lecture, 1994; Vitamin D—new horizons for the 21st century, *Am. J. Clin. Nutr.,* 60, 619, 1994.
8. *21 CFR 166, Margarine.*

9. National Research Council, *Recommended Dietary Allowances,* 10th ed., National Academy Press, Washington, D. C., 1989, chap. 8.
10. *Nutritional Labeling and Education Act of 1990, Fed. Reg.,* 58, 2070, 1993.
11. Tanner, J. T., Smith, J., Defibaugh, P., Angyal, G., Villalobos, M., Bueno, M., McGarrihan, E., Wehr, H. M., Muniz, J., Hollis, B. W., Koh, Y., Reich, P., and Simpson, K., Survey of vitamin content of fortified milk, *J. Assoc. Off. Anal. Chem.,* 71, 607, 1988.
12. Holick, M. F., Shao, Q., Liu, W., and Chen, T. C., The vitamin D content of fortified milk and infant formula, *N. Engl. J. Med.,* 326, 1178, 1992.
13. IUPAC-IUB, Nomenclature of vitamin D, Recommendations 1981, *Eur. J. Biochem.,* 124, 223, 1982.
14. Ball, G. F. M., Chemical and biological nature of the fat-soluble vitamins, in *Fat-Soluble Vitamin Assays in Food Analysis: A Comprehensive Study,* Elsevier Applied Science, London, 1988, chap. 2.
15. Renken, S. A. and Warthesen, J. J., Vitamin D stability in milk, *J. Food Sci.,* 58, 552, 1993.
16. Indyk, H., Littlejohn, V., and Woollard, D. C., Stability of vitamin D_3 during spray-drying of milk, *Food Chem.,* 57, 283, 1996.
17. Holick, M. F., The use and interpretation of assays for vitamin D and its metabolites, *J. Nutr.,* 120, 1464, 1990.
18. Masuda, S., Okano, T., and Kobayashi, T., A method for the simultaneous determination of vitamins D_2, D_3 and their metabolites in plasma and its application to plasma samples obtained from normal subjects and patients, *Food Chem.,* 45, 215, 1992.
19. Hollis, B. W., Assessment of vitamin D nutritional and hormonal status: what to measure and how to do it, *Calcif. Tissue Int.,* 58, 4, 1996.
20. Hollis, B. W., Kamerud, J. Q., Kurkowski, A., Beaulieu, J., and Napoli, J. L., Quantification of circulating 1,25,dihydroxy-vitamin D by radioimmunoassay with an[125] I-labeled tracer, *Clin. Chem.,* 42, 586, 1996.
21. Singh, L., Vitamin D, in *Methods of Vitamin Assay,* 4th ed., Augustin, J., Klein, B.P., Becker, D.A., and Venugopal, P.B., Eds., John Wiley and Sons, New York, 1985, chap. 9.
22. Porteous, C. E., Coldwell, R. D., Trafford, D., and Makin, H., Recent developments in the measurement of vitamin D and its metabolites in human body fluids, *J. Steroid Biochem.,* 28, 785, 1987.
23. Norman, A. W., Bouillon, R., and Thomasset, M., *Vitamin D, a Pluripotent Steroid Hormone: Structural* Studies, *Molecular Endocrinology and Clinical Applications. Proceedings of the Ninth Workshop on Vitamin D,* Walter de Gruyter, New York, 1994.
24. De Leenheer, A. P., Nelis, H. J., Lambert, W. E., and Bauwens, R. M., Chromatography of fat-soluble vitamins in clinical chemistry, *J. Chromatogr.,* 429, 3, 1988.
25. Rizzolo, A. and Polesello, S., Chromatographic determination of vitamins in foods, *J. Chromatogr.,* 624, 103, 1992.
26. Jones, G., Trafford, D., Makin, H., and Hollis, B. W., Vitamin D: cholecalciferol, ergocalciferol, and hydroxylated metabolites, in *Modern Chromatographic Analysis of Vitamins,* 2nd ed., De Leenheer, A. P., Lambert, W. E., and Nelis, H. J., Eds., Marcel Dekker, New York, 1992, chap. 2.
27. AOAC International, *Official Methods of Analysis,* 16th ed., AOAC International, Arlington, VA, 1995.
28. Collins, E. D. and Norman, A. W., Vitamin D, in *Handbook of Vitamins,* Machlin, L. J., Ed., Marcel Dekker, New York, 1991, chap. 2.
29. van den Berg, H., Vitamin D, flair concerted action no. 10 status papers, introductory conclusions and recommendations, *Internat. J. Vit. Nutr. Res.,* 63, 247, 1993.
30. Ball, G. F. M., High-performance liquid chromatography (HPLC), in *Fat-Soluble Vitamin Assays in Food Analysis, A Comprehensive Review,* Elsevier Applied Science, London, 1988, chap. 8.
31. Kurmann, A. and Indyk, H., The endogenous vitamin D content of bovine milk: influence of season, *Food Chem.,* 50, 75, 1994.
32. Mattila, P., Piironen, V., Asunmaa, A., Bäckman, C., Uusi-Rauva, E., and Koivistoinen, P., Determination of vitamin D_3 in egg yolk by high-performance liquid chromatography with diode array detection, *J. Food Comp. Anal.,* 5, 281, 1992.
33. Mattila, P., Piironen, V., Uusi-Rauva, E., and Koivistoinen, P., Determination of 25-hyroxycholecalciferol content in egg yolk by HPLC, *J. Food Comp. Anal.,* 6, 250, 1993.
34. Mattila, P., Piironen, V., Uusi-Rauva, E., and Koivistoinen, P., Vitamin D content in edible mushrooms, *J. Agric. Food Chem.,* 42, 2449, 1994.
35. Mattila, P., Piironen, V., Lehikoinen, K., Bäckman, C., Uusi-Rauva, E., and Koivistoinen, P., Cholecalciferol contents in fortified margarine and milk, Fin. *J. Dairy Sci.,* 51, 37, 1995.

36. Mattila, P., Piironen, V., Uusi-Rauva, E., and Koivistoinen, P., Cholecalciferol and 25-hydroxychole-calciferol contents in fish and fish products, *J. Food Comp. Anal.*, 8, 232, 1995.

37. Mattila, P., Piironen, V., Uusi-Rauva, E., and Koivistoinen, P., The contents of cholecalciferol, ergo-calciferol, and their 25-hydroxylated metabolites in raw meat and milk products as determined by HPLC, *J. Agric. Food Chem.*, 43, 2394, 1995.

38. Mattila, P., Piironen, V., Uusi-Rauva, E., and Koivistoinen, P.,P New analytical aspects of vitamin D in foods, *Food Chem.*, 57, 95, 1996.

39. Shimazu, M., Wang, X., and Yamada, S., Fluorometric assay of $1\alpha,25$-dihydroxyvitamin D_3 in human plasma, *J. Chromatogr. B*, 690, 15, 1997.

40. Sertl, D. C. and Molitor, B. E., Liquid chromatographic determination of vitamin D in milk and infant formula, 68, 177, 1985.

41. Tanner, J. T., Barnett, S. A., and Mountford, M. K., Analysis of milk-based infant formula. Phase IV. Iodide, linoleic acid, and vitamins D and K: U. S. Food and Drug Administration—Infant Formula Council: Collaborative Study, *J. AOAC Int.*, 76, 1042, 1993.

42. Sliva, M. G., Green, A. E., Sanders, J. K., Euber, J. R., and Saucerman, J. R., Reversed-phase liquid chromatographic determination of vitamin D in infant formulas and enteral nutritionals, *J. AOAC Int.*, 75, 566, 1992.

43. Sliva, M. G. and Sanders, J. K., Vitamin D in infant formula and enteral products by liquid chromatography: collaborative study, *J. AOAC Int.*, 79, 73, 1996.

44. International Dairy Federation, *IDF Standard 177: 1996, Dried Skimmed Milk, Determination of Vitamin D Content*, International Dairy Federation, Brussels.

Table 2.1   Physical Properties of Vitamin D and Hydroxylated Metabolites

1. Budavari, S., *The Merck Index*, 12th ed., Merck and Company, Whitehouse Station, N J, 1996, 268, 1711.

2. Freidrich, W., Vitamin D, in *Vitamins*, Walter de Gruyter and Company, Hawthorne, NY, 1988, chap. 3.

3. DeLuca, H. F., Vitamin D, in *The Fat-Soluble Vitamins*, Plenum Press, New York, 1978, chap. 2.

Table 2.2   Compendium, Regulatory and Handbook Methods for the Analysis of Vitamin D

1. United States Pharmacopeial Convention, *U.S. Pharmacopeia National Formulary*, USP 23, NF 18, Nutritional Supplements, Official Monographs, United States Pharmacopeial Convention, Rockville, MD, 195, 1995.

2. Scottish Home and Health Department, *British Pharmacopoeia*, 15th ed., British Pharmacopoeic Commission, UK, 1993.

3. AOAC International, *Official Methods of Analysis*, 16th ed., AOAC International, Arlington, VA, 1995.

4. Mulder, F. J., De Vries, E. J., and Borsje, B., Analysis of fat-soluble vitamins, XIV. Collaborative study of the determination of vitamin D in multivitamin preparations, *J. Assoc. Off. Anal. Chem.*, 60, 151, 1977.

5. Mulder, F. J., DeVries, E. J., and Borsje, B., Analysis of fat-soluble vitamins. XXIV. High performance liquid chromatographic determination of vitamin D in vitamin D resin containing powders: collaborative study, *J. Assoc. Off. Anal. Chem.*, 64, 58, 1981.

6. DeVries, E. J., Mulder, F. J., and Borsje, B., Analysis of fat-soluble vitamins. XXV. High performance liquid chromatographic determination of vitamin D in multivitamin preparations: collaborative study, *J. Assoc. Off. Anal. Chem.*, 64, 61, 1981.

7. DeVries, E. J. and Borsje, B., Analysis of fat-soluble vitamins. XXIX. Liquid chromatographic determination of vitamin D in AD concentrates: collaborative study, *J. Assoc. Off. Anal. Chem.*, 68, 822, 1985.

8. DeVries, E. J. and Borsje, B., Analysis of fat-soluble vitamins. XXVII. High performance liquid chromatographic and gas-liquid chromatographic determination of vitamin D in fortified milk and milk powder: collaborative study, *J. Assoc. Off. Anal. Chem.*, 65, 1228, 1982.

9. DeVries, E. J., Van Bemmel, P., and Borsje, B., Analysis of fat-soluble vitamins. XXVII. High performance liquid chromatographic determination of vitamin D in pet foods and feeds: collaborative study, *J. Assoc. Off. Anal. Chem.*, 66, 751, 1983.

10. Shue, G. M., Friedman, L., and Tolle, C. D., An improvement in the vitamin D line test, *Anal. Chem.,* 24, 1841, 1952.

11. Association of Official Analytical Chemists, Nutritional adjuncts, *J. Assoc. Off. Anal. Chem.,* 46, 160, 1963.

12. Fritz, J. C. and Roberts, T., Use of toe ash as a measure of calcification in the chick, *J. Assoc. Off. Anal. Chem.,* 51, 591, 1968.

13. Tanner, J. T., Barnett, S. A., and Mountford, M. K., Analysis of milk-based infant formula. Phase IV. Iodine, linoleic acid and vitamin D and K: U. S. Food and Drug Administration—Infant Formula Council: collaborative study, *J. AOAC Int.,* 76, 1042, 1993.

14. American Feed Ingredients Association, *Laboratory Methods Compendium* Volume One: *Vitamins and Minerals,* American Feed Ingredients Association, West Des Moines, IA, 1991, 169.

15. Committee on Food Chemicals Codex, *Food Chemicals Codex,* 4th ed., National Academy Press, Washington, D.C., 1996, 432.

16. Keller, H. E., *Analytical Methods for Vitamins and Carotenoids,* Hoffmann-LaRoche, Basel, 1988, 8.

17. International Dairy Federation, *IDF Standard 177:* 1996, *Dried Skimmed Milk, Determination of Vitamin D Content,* International Dairy Federation, Brussels.

Table 2.3   HPLC Methods for the Analysis of Vitamin D and Its Metabolites in Foods, Feeds, Pharmaceuticals and Biologicals

Food

1. Thompson, J. N., Maxwell, W. B. and L'Abbé M., High pressure liquid chromatographic determination of vitamin D in fortified milk, *J. Assoc. Off. Anal. Chem.,* 60, 998, 1977.

2. Cohen, H. and Wakeford, B., High pressure liquid chromatographic determination of vitamin D_3 in instant nonfat dried milk, *J. Assoc. Off. Anal. Chem.,* 63, 1163, 1980.

3. Thompson, J. N., Hatina, G., Maxwell, W. B., and Duval, S., High performance liquid chromatographic determination of vitamin D in fortified milks, margarine and infant formulas, *J. Assoc. Off. Anal. Chem.,* 65, 624, 1982.

4. Indyk, H. and Woolard, D. C., The determination of vitamin D in milk powders by high performance liquid chromatography, *New Zealand J. Dairy Sci. Tech.,* 19, 19, 1984.

5. Landen, W. O., Jr., Liquid chromatographic determination of vitamins D_2 and D_3 in fortified milk and infant formulas, *J. Assoc. Off. Anal. Chem.,* 68, 183, 1985.

6. Sertl, D. C. and Molitor, B. E., Liquid chromatographic determination of vitamin D in milk and infant formula, *J. Assoc. Off. Anal. Chem.,* 68, 177, 1985.

7. Tanner, J. T., Barnett, S. A., and Mountford, M. K., Analysis of milk-based infant formula. Phase IV. Iodide, linoleic acid, and vitamins D and K. U. S. Food and Drug Administration—Infant Formula Council: Collaborative Study, *J.AOAC Int.,* 76, 1042, 1993.

8. van den Berg, H., Boshuis, P. G., and Schreurs, W. H. P., Determination of vitamin D in fortified and nonfortified milk powder and infant formula using a specific radioassay after purification by high performance liquid chromatography, *J. Agric. Food Chem.,* 34, 264, 1986.

9. Johnsson, H. and Hessel, H., High performance liquid chromatographic determination of cholecalciferol (Vitamin D_3) in food—a comparison with a bioassay method, *Int. J. Vit. Nutr. Res.,* 57, 357, 1987.

10. Ballester, I., Cortes, E., Moya, M., and Campello, M. J., Improved method for quantifying vitamin D in proprietary infants' formulas and in breast milk, *Clin. Chem.,* 33, 796, 1987.

11. Bakhof, J. J. and van den Bedem, J. W., Study on the determination of vitamin D in fortified milk, milk powder, and infant formula by HPLC using a column switching technique, *Neth. Milk Dairy J.,* 42, 423, 1988.

12. Sliva, M. G., Green, A. E., Sanders, J. K., Euber, J. R., and Saucerman, J. R., Reversed-phase liquid chromatographic determination of vitamin D in infant formulas and enteral nutritionals, *J. AOAC Int.,* 75, 566, 1992.

13. Sliva, M. G. and Sanders, J. K., Vitamin D in infant formula and enteral products by liquid chromatography: collaborative study, *J. AOAC Int.,* 79, 73, 1996.

14. Renken, S. A. and Warthesen, J. J., Vitamin D stability in milk, *J. Food Sci., 58,* 552, 1993.

15. Hagar, A. F., Madsen, L., Wales, L., Jr., and Bradford, H.B., Jr., Reversed-phase liquid chromatographic determination of vitamin D in milk, *J. AOAC Int.*, 77, 1047, 1994.

16. Kurmann, A. and Indyk, H., The endogenous vitamin D content of bovine milk: influence of season, *Food Chem.*, 50, 75, 1994.

17. Indyk, H., Littlejohn, V., and Woollard, D.C., Stability of vitamin D_3 during spray-drying of milk, *Food Chem.*, 57, 283, 1996.

18. Suzuki, H., Hahayawa, S., Wade, S., Okazaki, E., and Yamazawa, M., Effect of solar drying on vitamin D_3 and provitamin D_3 contents in fish meat, *J. Agric. Food Chem.*, 36, 803, 1988.

19. Rao, D. S. and Raghuramula, N., Vitamin D and its related parameters in fresh-water wild fishes, *Comp. Biochem. Physiol.*, 111A, 191, 1995.

20. Mattila, P., Piironen, V., Uusi-Rauva, E., and Koivistoinen, P., Cholecalciferol and 25-hydroxychole-calciferol contents in fish and fish products, *J. Food Comp. Anal.*, 8, 232, 1995.

21. Konings, E. J. M., Estimation of vitamin D in baby foods with liquid chromatography, *Neth. Milk and Dairy J.*, 48, 31, 1994.

22. Mattila, P., Piironen, V., Bäckman, C., Asunmaa, A., Uusi-Rauva, E., and Koivisoinen, P., Determination of vitamin D_3 in egg yolk by high-performance liquid chromatography with diode array detection, *J. Food Comp. Anal.*, 5, 281, 1992.

23. Mattila, P., Piironen, V., Uusi-Rauva, E., and Koivistoinen, P., Determination of 25-hydroxycholecalciferol content in egg yolk by HPLC, *J. Food Comp. Anal.*, 6, 250, 1993.

24. Thompson, J. N. and Plouffe, L., Determination of cholecalciferol in meat and fat from livestock fed normal and excessive quantities of vitamin D, *Food Chem.*, 46, 313, 1993.

25. Hasegawa, H., Vitamin D determination using high-performance liquid chromatography with internal standard-redox mode electrochemical detection and its application to medical nutritional products, *J. Chromatogr.*, 605, 215, 1992.

26. Mattila, P. H., Piironen, V. I., Uusi-Rauva, E. J., and Koivistoinen, P. E., Vitamin D contents in edible mushrooms, *J. Agric. Food Chem.*, 42, 2449, 1994.

27. Matilla, P. H., Piironen, V. I., Uusi-Rauva, E. J., and Koivistoinen, P. E., New analytical aspects of vitamin D in foods, *Food Chem.*, 57, 95, 1996.

Feed

1. Agarwal, V. K., Liquid chromatographic determination of vitamin D in animal feeds and premixes, *J. AOAC Int.*, 75, 812, 1992.

2. Scott, K. C. and Latshaw, J. D., The vitamin D_3 and precholecalciferol content of menhaden fish meal as affected by drying conditions, *Anim. Feed Sci. Tech.*, 47, 99, 1994.

Plasma

1. Aksnes, L., A simplified high-performance liquid chromatographic method for determination of vitamin D_3, 25-hydroxyvitamin D_2 and 25-hydroxyvitamin D_3 in human serum, *Scand. J. Clin. Lab. Invest.*, 52, 177, 1992

2. Masuda, S., Okano, T., and Kobayashi, T., A method for the simultaneous determination of vitamins D_2, D_3 and their metabolites in plasma and its application to plasma samples obtained from normal subjects and patients, *Food Chem.*, 45, 215, 1992.

3. Shimada, K., Mitamura, K., and Kitama, N., Quantitative determination of 25-hydroxy-vitamin D_3 3-sulphate in human plasma using high performance liquid chromatography, *Biomed. Chromatogr.* 9, 229, 1995.

4. Shimizu, M., Iwasaki, Y., Ishida, H., and Yamada, S., Determination of 25-hydroxy-vitamin D_3 in human plasma using a non-radioactive tetranorvitamin D analogue as an internal standard, *J. Chromatogr. B: Biomed. Appl.*, 672, 63, 1995.

5. Shimizu, M., Wang, X., and Yamada, S., Fluorimetric assay of 1α,25-dihydroxyvitamin D_3 in human plasma, *J. Chromatogr. B*, 690, 15, 1997.

3 Vitamin E
Tocopherols and Tocotrienols

3.1 REVIEW

The existence of vitamin E was first indicated through reproductive studies with animals in the early part of this century. The vitamin was characterized as a fat-soluble nutritional factor, "Factor X," necessary for reproductive functions and the prevention of fetal death by Evans and Bishop in 1922.[1] It then became known as the antisterility factor with the designation of vitamin E, since its discovery closely followed vitamin D. Vitamin E (α-tocopherol) was isolated from wheat germ oil by Evans' research group (1936). These researchers called vitamin E "tocopherol" from the Greek terms *pherein* ("carry") and *tocos* ("to birth"), owing to its essentiality for rats to bear young.[2]

Deficiency occurs infrequently in humans and is almost always due to factors other than dietary insufficiency. Vitamin E deficiency can occur through various conditions that affect absorption of fat and/or vitamin E. Malabsorption results from pancreatic and liver abnormalities that lower fat absorption, abnormalities of the intestinal cells, length of the intestine, and defects in the synthesis or assembly of the chylomicrons.[5] Genetic abnormalities in lipoprotein metabolism that produce low to non-detectable circulating chylomicrons, VLDL, and LDL levels affect both absorption and plasma transport of vitamin E.[3] Genetic defects in the α-tocopherol transfer protein gene are associated with the syndrome "ataxia with vitamin E deficiency (AVED)" characterized by neurologic abnormalities.[4]

Symptoms of vitamin E deficiency are difficult to categorize owing to varying effects among species and the fact that vitamin E deficiency in the human is primarily due to fat malabsorption syndromes or genetic abnormalities. At the cellular level, vitamin E deficiency produces increased oxidation of cellular membranes.[2] Related events might include decreased energy production by mitochondria, DNA mutation, and changes in plasma membrane transport mechanisms. Olson and Munson[5] give the following disorders associated with vitamin E deficiency: reproduction disorders, abnormalities of muscle, liver, bone marrow, brain function, and defective embryogenesis diathesis (capillary permeability disorder). Skeletal muscle dystrophy is species specific and involves cardiomyopathy which is severe in ruminants, mild in rabbits and nonexistent in primates. The variable occurrence by species of vitamin E deficiency symptoms was noted as an impediment to in-depth understanding of the vitamin function at the cellular and molecular level.[5] Primary symptoms in humans include mild hemolytic anemia characterized by increased erythrocyte hemolysis and spinocerebellar diseases, usually in children suffering from fat malabsorption syndrome.[5] Clinical status of vitamin E in the human is difficult to assess owing to extremely slow depletion of body stores. Biochemical indices include serum, erythrocyte, platelet, and tissue tocopherol levels; however, none are effective status indices.[6]

Human deficiency is generally not due to dietary insufficiency. Vitamin E is a plant product, widely distributed at good concentrations in plant oils. The contribution of vitamin E activity by oils and fats to the human diet is highly significant. This fact is apparent from data derived from U.S. consumption surveys.[7, 8] Data from the second National Health and Nutrition Examination Survey (NHANES II) showed that fats and oils accounted for over 20% of the vitamin E in the United States diet. Data collected from the Continuing Survey of Food Intakes by Individuals (CSFII, 1994) is summarized in Table 3.1.[9] Salad and cooking oils, margarine, salad dressings, mayonnaise, and

TABLE 3.1
Significant Sources of Vitamin E in the
American Diet, CSFII (1994)[a]

Product	% Vitamin E in the U.S. Diet
Salad and cooking oils	8.2
Margarines	6.8
Cereals, RTE	4.9
Salad dressings	4.4
Tomatoes and products	4.3
Mayonnaise	3.8
Shortening	3.7
Peanut butter	2.3
Potato chips, plain	2.3
Eggs	1.9
Milk, whole, 2%	1.6
Apples	1.1
Rolls and buns	1.0
Cumulative total	46.3

[a]Reprinted with permission from Reference 9.

shortening provide approximately 27% of the vitamin E in the U.S. diet. The role of low-fat margarine and spreads is not clearly indicated by this data. Increasing use of low-fat products will impact the order of available sources. Low-fat margarines are not normally fortified with vitamin E in the United States, and vitamin E content decreases as fat content decreases. Low-fat mayonnaise-type products usually contain added α-tocopheryl acetate. Since soybean oil is the primary oil used in these products in the United States, its role as a major vitamin E source is apparent. Worldwide, the contribution of palm oil to oil supplies and, therefore, as a vitamin E source is increasing.[9]

Vitamin E and other antioxidant food components have, indeed, captured the interest of the world's consumers. Antioxidant components of the diet include vitamin E, ascorbic acid, carotenoids, selenium and others such as the flavonoids.[9] Oxidative stress damage to the human includes the onset of disease states including:

1. Cancer—through initiation of carcinogenesis, promotion of tumor development mutogenesis, and stimulation of cell division.
2. Cardiovascular disease—through oxidation of blood lipoproteins and the development of atherosclerosis, and oxidative damage to tissues during heart attack and stroke
3. Cataracts—through oxidative damage to the lens of the eye.[9, 10]

Block and Langseth[10] stressed that new knowledge on disease-preventing effects of micronutrients will lead to new views on supplementation to close "the gap between the amounts of antioxidant nutrients found in typical diets and higher levels needed for optimal protection against chronic diseases."

Evidence indicates that antioxidant components of the diet have beneficial effects in prevention of various cancers, cardiovascular disease, and cataracts.[11, 12] Studies indicate difficulty in differentiating the specific effects of vitamin E from other dietary antioxidants. Strong evidence exists that the antioxidant nutrients prevent development of cardiovascular disease. Kritchevsky[13] reviewed the role of vitamin E, vitamin C, and β-carotene in decreasing the susceptibility of low-density lipoproteins to oxidation. Oxidized LDL is viewed as an initiator of atherosclerosis. Vitamin E was indicated as the most effective antioxidant in LDL, but the total antioxidant effect is a combined effect of all available antioxidants. Large epidemiological studies published as the Health Professional Studies involved 87,245 female nurses and 39,910 male health professionals and provided evidence of an association between a high intake of vitamin E and a lower risk of coronary heart disease in women and men. However, the studies could not prove cause-and-effect relationships.[14, 15]

Generally, epidemiological studies indicate that diets high in fruit and vegetables are associated with reduced risks for several cancers.[12, 16] Again, it is difficult to ascertain specific effects for vitamin E. In a large nutrient intervention trial in Linxian, China, β-carotene, vitamin E, and selenium supplementation of the adult diet reduced stomach cancer risk in the population. No significant protective effects were present for other combinations of supplements.[17]

Cataracts are theorized to develop by photochemical generation of superoxide in the intraocular chambers of the eye.[12] Several studies have shown that supplementation with antioxidant vitamins and high dietary intakes are associated with lower cataract risk.[10] Likewise, low blood levels of vitamin E and β-carotene have been linked to increased risks.[18]

Recent clinical trials reported success of all-rac-α-tocopherol supplementation as a treatment to delay onset of Alzheimer's disease.[19] These and other reported health benefits continue to increase interest in antioxidants in the diet. Without a doubt, we have just begun to understand overall relationships of diet and health. Vitamin E stands at the center of this important interface of biochemistry and nutrition.

3.2   PROPERTIES

3.2.1   CHEMISTRY

3.2.1.1   General Properties

Vitamin E is the collective term for fat-soluble 6-hydroxychroman compounds that exhibit the biological activity of α-tocopherol—the representative compound shown in Figure 3.1. Tocol (the parent compound for the vitamin E family) (Figure 3.1) is 2-methyl-2(4′,8′,12′-trimethyltridecyl)-chroman-6-ol. At present, eight naturally occurring homologs are included in the vitamin E family. The eight vitamin E forms are α-, β-, γ- and δ-tocopherol characterized by a saturated side chain consisting of three isoprenoid units, and the corresponding unsaturated tocotrienols (α-, β-, γ-, and δ-). The tocotrienols have double bonds at the 3, 7, and 11 positions of the isoprenoid sidechain. Structural interrelationships are shown in Figure 3.2. The tocopherol and tocotrienol homologs vary structurally by the number and location of methyl groups on the chromanol ring. α-Homologs contain three methyl groups, and β- and γ-homologs are dimethylated positional isomers. δ-Tocopherol and δ-tocotrienol are monomethylated. Wide differences exist in biological activity among the homologs depending on structure and stereo-chemistry (Table 3.2, Section 3.2.1.2).

The chiral centers at position two of the chroman ring and the 4′ and 8′ carbons of the side chain produce eight isomeric forms. All-rac-α-tocopherol, formerly referred to as dl-α-tocopherol, is the synthetic form of α-tocopherol and contains equal amounts of the eight stereoisomers. Only RRR-stereoisomers (2′R, 4′R, 8′R) are found in nature.

Vitamin E is fat-soluble and soluble in organic fat solvents. All forms are colorless to pale yellow, viscous oils.

In this chapter, the abbreviations α-T and α-T3 will be used for α-tocopherol and α-tocotrienol, respectively. Likewise, β-, γ-, δ-homologs and their corresponding tocotrienols will be abbreviated in a similar manner.

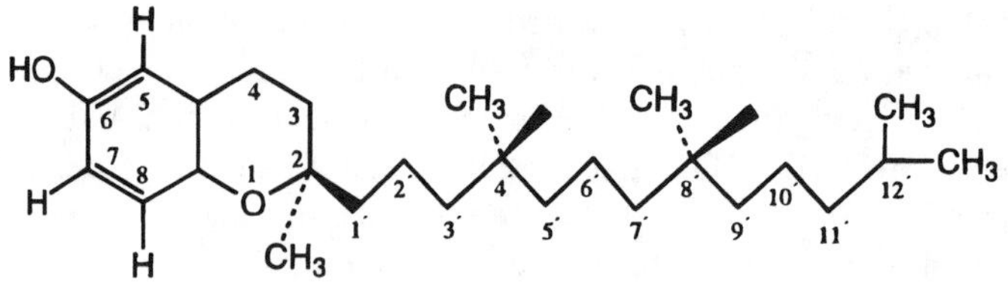

2-methyl-2-(4′, 8′, 12′,-trimethyltridecyl) chroman-6-ol

Tocol

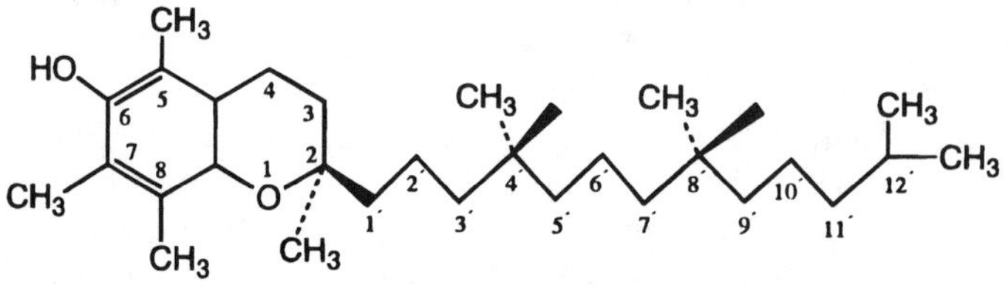

2R, 4′R, 8′R - α-tocopherol
RRR-α-tocopherol

Vitamin E

FIGURE 3.1   Structure of tocol and RRR-α-tocopherol.

3.2.1.2 Biological Activity

The National Research Council defined dietary vitamin E activity in terms of RRR-α-tocopherol equivalents (α-TEs).[20] One α-TE is the activity of 1 mg of RRR-α-T. For mixed diets containing only natural forms of vitamin E, currently accepted factors for the conversion of tocopherols and tocotrienols to α-TE units are the following:[20]

α-tocopherol—mg × 1.0
β-tocopherol—mg × 0.5
γ-tocopherol—mg × 0.1
δ-tocopherol—mg × 0.03
α-tocotrienol—mg × 0.3
β-tocotrienol—mg × 0.05
γ-tocotrienol—unknown
δ-tocotrienol—unknown
all-rac-α-T—mg × 0.74
all-rac-α-tocopheryl acetate—mg × 0.67
all-rac-α-tocopheryl succinate-mg × 0.6

The Recommended Dietary Allowance (RDA) ranges from 3 α-TE units for the infant to 12 α-TE units for breast-feeding mothers during the first 6 months of lactation.[20]

International Units (IU) define the biological activity of the vitamin E forms as measured by the rat fetal resorption test. All-rac-α-tocopheryl acetate was the reference standard with a biological

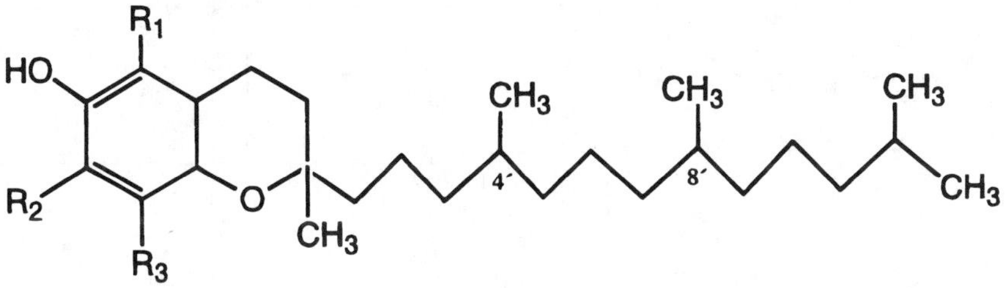

Tocopherols

Ring Position

Trivial Name	Chemical Name	Abbreviation	R_1	R_2	R_3
Tocol	-	-	H	H	H
α-Tocopherol	5,7,8-Trimethyltocol	α-T	CH_3	CH_3	CH_3
β-Tocopherol	5,8-Dimethyltocol	β-T	CH_3	H	CH_3
γ-Tocopherol	7,8-Dimethyltocol	γ-T	H	CH_3	CH_3
δ-Tocopherol	8-Methyltocol	δ-T	H	H	CH_3

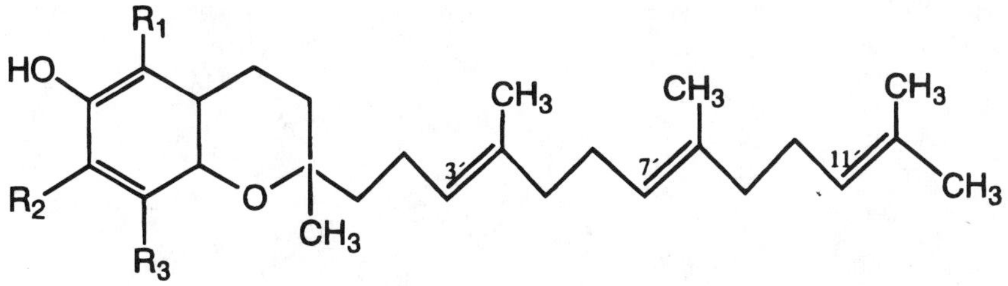

Tocotrienols

Ring Position

Trivial Name	Chemical Name	Abbreviation	R_1	R_2	R_3
Tocotrienol	-	-	H	H	H
α-Tocopherol	5,7,8-Trimethyltocotrienol	α-T3	CH_3	CH_3	CH_3
β-Tocopherol	5,8-Dimethyltocotrienol	β-T3	CH_3	H	CH_3
γ-Tocopherol	7,8-Dimethyltocotrienol	γ-T3	H	CH_3	CH_3
δ-Tocopherol	8-Methyltocotrienol	δ-T3	H	H	CH_3

FIGURE 3.2 Structural interrelationships of tocopherols and tocotrienols.

activity of 1.0 IU/mg. RRR-α-T exhibits the greatest biological activity (1.49 IU/mg) relative to all-rac-α-tocopheryl acetate. Chemically synthesized vitamin E is all-rac-α-T. The racemic mixture has a biological activity of 1.1 IU/mg. All-rac-α-tocopheryl acetate is the form commonly used for fortification. Esterification at the C-6 hydroxyl group of the chroman ring greatly stabilizes the vitamin by eliminating the ability of the vitamin to provide a hydrogen atom to free radicals through its biological role as a primary antioxidant. Therefore, addition of all-rac-α-tocopheryl acetate to foods does not provide antioxidant activity; however, biological activity is not affected for the human as the ester bond is easily hydrolyzed during digestion.[21] Table 3.2 provides the biological activity measures for the natural and synthetic forms of vitamin E.[22]

TABLE 3.2
Biological Activity of Vitamin E Forms

Vitamin E Forms	Biological Activity[a]	
	IU/mg	Compared to RRR-α-T (%)
Natural Vitamin E (RRR-)		
α-tocopherol	1.49	100
β-tocopherol	0.75	50
γ-tocopherol	0.15	10
δ-tocopherol	0.05	3
α-tocotrienol	0.75	50
β-tocotrienol	0.08	5
γ-tocotrienol	not known	not known
β-tocotrienol	not known	not known
Synthetic		
2R4'R8'R α-tocopherol	1.49	100
2S4'R8'R α-tocopherol	0.46	31
all-rac-α-tocopherol	1.10	74
2R4'R8'S α-tocopherol	1.34	90
2S4'R8'S α-tocopherol	0.55	37
2R4'S8'S α-tocopherol	1.09	73
2S4'S8'R α-tocopherol	0.31	21
2R4'S8'R α-tocopherol	0.85	57
2S4'S8'S α-tocopherol	1.10	60
RRR α-tocopheryl acetate	1.36	91
RRR-α-tocopheryl acid succinate	1.21	81
all-rac-α-tocopheryl acetate	1.00	67
all-rac-α-tocopheryl acid succinate	0.89	60

[a]Biological activity values from Reference 22.

Since natural vitamin E occurs in nature as eight different vitamers (RRR-T and T3), estimation of vitamin E activity in natural products requires quantitation of each form. Current conversion factors to convert content to α-TE units undoubtedly will change as more is learned about the biological activity of the different forms of the vitamin. Calculation of vitamin E intake in α-TEs assumes that the various homologs can substitute for α-T at efficiencies of 10% for γ-T, 50% for β-T, 30% for α-T3 and at lower efficiencies for other forms. Functionally, other forms are not equivalent to α-T,[23, 24] and a clear understanding of changes in conversion factors needed to accurately assess vitamin E from a metabolic standpoint is not yet available.

Biologically, vitamin E functions as a primary antioxidant and as a peroxyl free radical scavenger. In tissue, it prevents cell damage by preventing *in vivo* peroxidations. In cellular membranes, α-T is associated with polyunsaturated fatty acids (PUFA). This association is biologically significant and several researchers recommend quantification of vitamin E not only as total α-TE, but as a ratio of total α-TE to grams PUFA.[20,25,26,27] The vitamin E requirement in animals increases as PUFA intake increases.[28] For adult males, ten α-TE per day provides an α-TE to gram PUFA ratio of 0.4 which is thought to be adequate for the adult. Recent studies reported that tocotrienols possess antioxidant activity comparable or better than their tocopherol counterparts. γ-T3 had greater antioxidant activity than γ-T when added to dilinoleoylphosphatidyl-choline liposome solutions.[29] The homologs had similar antioxidant activity when incorporated into the liposomal membrane.

Interest in the tocotrienols from a health promoting standpoint has greatly increased in recent years. An inhibitor of cholesterol biosynthesis was isolated from barley and proven to be α-T3.[30] Qureshi et al.[31] and Tan et al.[32] conducted human studies with Palmvitee, a T3 rich fraction from palm oil. Both studies led to a reduction of LDL-cholesterol. γ-T3, δ-T3, and α-T3 are effective inhibitors of cholesterol synthesis in rat hepatocytes; whereas, α-T exhibits no inhibition.[33] Other research reported anticarcinogenic effects for the tocotrienols.[34,35,36] Isoprenoid constituents of the diet have been suggested to suppress tumor growth by depriving the cells of mevalonate-derived products.[37] The hypercholesterolemic and anticarcinogenic properties of the tocotrienols led Hendrich et al.[38] to suggest that the tocotrienols should be considered as a nutrient independent of the tocopherols. Data reported by Ong[39] indicated that palm oil is the only edible oil consumed in quantity that provides tocotrienols. Cereal oils (wheat, barley, oats, and rice bran) contain tocotrienols but their low consumption limits their significance as vitamin E sources. Cereals and legumes represent other sources of tocotrienols in the Western diet.

3.2.1.3   Spectral Properties

UV and fluorescence properties of vitamin E compounds are given in Table 3.3. UV spectra for tocopherols and the esters in ethanol show maximum absorption between 280 and 300 nm with minimum absorption between 250 and 260 nm.[1] Esterification at the C-6 hydroxyl group shifts the absorption maximum to 284 to 286 nm.[1,40] Tocotrienols have similar UV absorption properties. Tocopherols and tocotrienols possess intense native fluorescence when excited at 210 nm or 290 to 292 nm.[41] Excitation of the chroman ring at these wavelengths produces maximal emission at 320 nm or slightly higher wavelengths. The strong and specific fluorescence of the chroman ring system provides an ideal detection system for LC detection (Section 3.3.2.2.2). Older literature often states that α-tocopheryl acetate is not fluorescent. However, the ester shows weak fluorescence which is measurable by newer, highly sensitive fluorescence detectors. Several investigators utilized the fluorescence of α-tocopheryl acetate to assay all-rac-α-tocopheryl acetate in the presence of native tocopherols.[42,43,44,45] Such methods which do not use saponification for sample extraction allow more accurate quantitation of biological activity, since the biological activity of synthetic all-rac-α-tocopheryl acetate is lower than RRR-α-T (Section 3.2.1.3). Characteristic UV absorption spectra for tocopherols and tocotrienols are shown in Figure 3.3.

3.2.2   STABILITY

Since vitamin E is a natural antioxidant serving as a chain breaking peroxyl free radical scavenger in biological systems, it interacts as an antioxidant in any fat system containing unsaturated fatty acids undergoing oxidation. Oxidative losses can become substantial quite rapidly, and losses are accelerated by light, heat, alkali pH, lipoxidase reactions, various metals, primarily iron and copper, and by the presence of free radicals in the fat that can initiate autoxidation. In the absence of oxygen, tocopherols and tocotrienols are stable to heat and alkali conditions such as those used to saponify lipid containing samples. Use of edible oils for frying can lead to rapid decreases in vitamin E levels. Incorporation of air during the frying operation and the fact that edible oils are usually polyunsaturated produces an ideal environment for antioxidant action by the vitamin E components of the oil and their subsequent inactivation. Refining of edible oil results in some loss of vitamin E activity. However, plant oils after refining are more stable to oxidation since the refining process effectively removes pro-oxidants. Most vitamin E loss during refining occurs at the deodorization stage of the process.[9] Due to its instability to oxidation, all analytical procedures must be completed under conditions that ensure the absence of oxygen and pro-oxidants. The addition of synthetic antioxidants to the sample and extracts at all stages of the analysis are essential (Section 3.3.2.1.1). α-Tocopheryl acetate and α-tocopheryl succinate are stable to oxidation since the hydroxyl group at C-6 is essential to the antioxidant activity of vitamin E.

TABLE 3.3
UV and Fluorescence Properties of Vitamin E

Substance[a]	Molar Mass	Formula	λ max nm	Absorbance[b] $E_{1cm}^{1\%}$	ε	Fluorescence[c] Ex nm	Em nm
α-T CAS No. 59-02-9 **10159**	430.71	$C_{29}H_{50}O_2$	292	75.8	[3265]	295	320
β-T CAS No. 148-03-8 **9632**	416.69	$C_{28}H_{48}O_2$	296	89.4	[3725]	297	322
γ-T CAS No. 7616-22-0 **9633**	416.69	$C_{28}H_{48}O_2$	298	91.4	[3809]	297	322
δ-T CAS No. 119-13-1 **9634**	402.66	$C_{27}H_{46}O_2$	298	87.3	[3515]	297	322
α-T3 CAS No. 2265-13-4 **9636**	424.67	$C_{29}H_{44}O_2$	292	86.0	[3652]	290	323
β-T3 CAS No. 49-23-3 **9635**	410.64	$C_{28}H_{42}O_2$	296	86.2	[3540]	290	323
γ-T3 CAS No. 14101-61-2	410.64	$C_{28}H_{42}O_2$	297	91.0	[3737]	290	324
δ-T3 CAS No. 25612-59-3	396.61	$C_{27}H_{40}O_2$	297	85.8	[3403]	292	324
α-tocopheryl acetate CAS No. 52225-20-4 (dl) CAS No. 58-95-7 (l) **10160**	472.75	$C_{31}H_{52}O_3$	286	40–44	[1891–2080]	285	310
α-tocopheryl succinate CAS No. 4345-03-3 **10159**	530.79	$C_{33}H_{54}O_5$	286	38.5	[2044]	—	—

[a] Common or generic name; CAS No.—Chemical Abstract Service number, bold print designates the Merck Index monograph number.

[b] Values in brackets are calculated from corresponding $E_{1cm}^{1\%}$ values, in ethanol.

[c] In hexane.

Ball, G. F. M., *Fat-Soluble Vitamin Assays in Human Nutrition,* 1988.[1]
Budavari, S. *The Merck Index,* 12th ed., 1996.[2]
Mino, M. et al., *Vitamin E,* 1993.[3]
Machlin, L. J., *Handbook of Vitamins,* 2nd edition, 1991.[4]

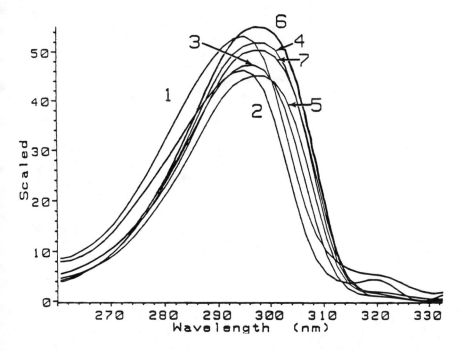

FIGURE 3.3   UV absorption spectrum of tocopherols and tocotrienols (1 = α-T, 2 = α-T3, 3 = β-T, 4 = γ-T, 5 = γ-T3, 6 = δ-T, 7 = δT3). Reproduced with permission from Reference 68.

3.3   METHODS

Comprehensive reviews are available on vitamin E quantification from food and clinical samples.[40,41,46,47,48,49,50,51] Older procedures such as colorimetric, spectrophotometric, spectrofluorometric, polarimetric, thin-layer and open-column chromatographic methods are adequately covered from a historical and applications standpoint. Compendium and handbook methods published with standard, routine protocols are summarized in Table 3.4. The AOAC International *Official Methods of Analysis*[52] provides several methods based on older, chemical approaches. These include colorimetric and polarimetric methods. AOAC Official Method 971.30 (45.1.24) "alpha-Tocopherol and alpha Tocopheryl Acetate in Foods and Feeds" and AOAC Official Method 948.26 (45.1.26), "alpha-Tocopherol Acetate (Supplemental) in Foods and Feeds" require saponification and quantitation of α-T by thin layer chromatography. If the isomeric form of α-tocopheryl acetate is unknown, AOAC Method 975.43 (45.1.25) "Identification of RRR- or all-rac-alpha-Tocopherol in Drugs and Food or Feed Supplements" must be used to determine the isomeric form of the added α-tocopheryl acetate. Method 975.43 is a polarimetric method that measures the optical rotation of the ferricyanide oxidation product of α-T present after saponification of the sample extract. Optical rotation is negligible for all-rac-α-T and positive for RRR-α-T. It is necessary to know the isomeric form of supplemental α-tocopheryl acetate to correctly calculate biological activity in IUs or α-TEs (Section 3.2.1.2). Method 975.43 is only applicable to concentrated supplements which are concentrated to ≥200 mg α-T/g before the ferricyanide oxidation step. In terms of utility, the above methods are extremely cumbersome and subject to analytical error due to their complexity. Although not available as AOAC International collaborated methods for the above matrices, HPLC methods have largely replaced the colorimetric and polarimetric procedures in the modern analytical laboratory.

TABLE 3.4
Compendium, Regulatory and Handbook Methods for Vitamin E Analysis

Source	Form	Methods and Applications	Approach	Most Current Cross-Reference
U.S. Pharmacopeia, National Formulary, 1995, USP 18/NF 18; Nutritional Supplements Official Monograph[1]				
1. pages 1631–1633	all-rac- or RRR-α-tocopherol all-rac- or RRR-α-tocopheryl acetate all-rac- or RRR-α-tocopheryl succinate	Vitamin E Vitamin E in preparations and capsules	GC flame ionization	None
2. pages 2139, 2141	all-rac- or RRR-α-tocopherol all-rac- or RRR-α-tocopheryl acetate all-rac- or RRR-α-tocopheryl succinate	Vitamine E in oil-soluble Vitamin capsules/tablets	HPLC 254 nm	None
3. pages 2142, 2144, 2147, 2151	all-rac-or RRR-α-tocopherol all-rac- or RRR-α-tocopheryl acetate all-rac- or RRR-α-tocopheryl succinate	Vitamin E in oil- and water-soluble capsules/tablets with/without minerals	HPLC	None
4. page 2315	RRR-α-tocopherol RRR-β-tocopherol RRR-γ-tocopherol RRR-δ-tocopherol	Tocopherols Excipient	GC flame ionization	None
British Pharmacopoeia, 15th ed., 1993[2]				
1. page 675, vol. I	all-rac-α-tocopherol	α-Tocopherol	GC flame ionization	None
2. pages 676–677, vol. I	all-rac-α-tocopheryl acetate	α-Tocopherol acetate	GC flame ionization	None
3. page 677, vol. I	all-rac-α-tocopheryl acetate	α-Tocopherol acetate concentrate (powder form)	GC flame ionization	None
4. page 1394, addend., 1994	RRR-α-tocopheryl succinate	α-Tocopheryl succinate	GC flame ionization	None
5. page 1464, addend., 1954	RRR-α-tocopheryl succinate	α-Tocopheryl succinate tablets	GC flame ionization	None
AOAC Official Methods of Analysis, 16th ed., 1995[3]				
1. 45.1.24	all-rac- or RRR-α-tocopherol all-rac- or RRR-α-tocopheryl acetate	AOAC Official Method 971.30 α-Tocopherol and α-Tocopheryl Acetate in Foods and Feeds Colorimetric Method	colorimetric 534 nm	*J. Assoc. Off. Anal. Chem.,* 54, 1, 1974[4]

No.	Method	Substance	Method title	Analysis	Reference
2.	45.1.25	all-rac- or RRR-α-tocopherol all-rac- or RRR-α-tocopheryl acetate	AOAC Official Method 975.43 Identification of RRR- or all-rac-α-Tocopherol in Drugs and Food or Feed Supplements (≥ 200 mg/g)	Polarimetric	J. Assoc. Off. Anal. Chem., 58, 585, 1975[5]
3.	45.1.26	all-rac- or RRR-α- tocopherol all-rac- or RRR-α-tocopheryl acetate	AOAC Official Method 948.26 α-Tocopheryl Acetate (Supplemental) in Foods and Feeds	Colorimetric 534 nm	J. Assoc. Off. Anal. Chem., 54, 1, 1971[4]
4.	45.1.27	RRR-tocopherol RRR-β-tocopherol + RRR γ-tocopherol RRR-δ-tocopherol	AOAC Official Method 988.14 Tocopherol Isomers in Mixed Tocopherols Concentrate	GC flame ionization	J. Assoc. Off. Anal. Chem., 71, 1168, 1988[6]
5.	45.1.28	all-rac-α-tocopheryl acetate	AOAC Official Method 989.09 α-Tocopheryl Acetate in Supplemental Vitamin E Concentrates	GC flame ionization	J. Assoc. Off. Anal. Chem., 61, 475, 1978[7]
6.	45.1.29	all-rac- or RRR-a-tocopherol all-rac- or RRR-α-tocopheryl acetate all-rac- or RRR-α-tocopheryl succinate	AOAC Official Method 969.40 Vitamin E in Drugs	GC flame ionization	
7.	50.1.04	all-rac-α-tocopheryl acetate as α-tocopherol	AOAC Official Method 992.03 Vitamin E Activity (All-rac-α-tocopherol) in Milk-Based Infant Formula	HPLC 280 nm	J. AOAC Int., 76, 399, 1993[8]

American Feed Ingredients Association, *Laboratory Methods Compendium*, 1991, vol. 1[9]

No.	Pages	Substance	Method title	Analysis	Reference
1.	pages 197–200	all-rac-α-tocopheryl acetate	Vitamin D₃, vitamin E in concentrates and premixes (≥ 50 IU/g)	HPLC 292 nm	None
2.	pages 201–202	all-rac-α-tocopheyl acetate as α-tocopherol	Vitamin E (coated) in powders containing no other vitamins	Colorimetric 520 nm	None
3.	pages 203–205	all-rac-α-tocopheryl acetate as tocopherol	Determination of vitamin E in feeds, supplements and premixes (> 1mg/kg)	HPLC 284 nm or fluorescence Ex λ 290, Em λ 325	None

TABLE 3.4 Continued
Compendium, Regulatory and Handbook Methods for Vitamin E Analysis

Source	Form	Methods and Applications	Approach	Most Current Cross-Reference
4. pages 207–209	α-, β-, γ-, δ-tocopherol (all-rac- or RRR-tocopherols or esters)	Method for the determination of vitamin E in feed and tissue by HPLC	HPLC fluorescence Ex λ 254, Em λ 325	*J. Agric. Food Chem.*, 31, 1330, 1983[10] Hoffmann-LaRoche, *Analytical Methods for Vitamins and Carotenoids in Feeds*, 1988[11]
5. pages 211–213	all-rac- or RRR-α-tocopherol	Determination of vitam E in premixes by HPLC (1–20 mg/g)	HPLC, 292 nm	None
Hoffman-LaRoche, Analytical Methods for Vitamins and Carotenoids, in Feeds, 1988[11]				
1. pages 12–14	RRR-α-tocopherol and added esters as α-tocopherol. Applicable to other homologs	Determination of α-tocopherol in complete feeds, premixes and vitamin concentrates with the aid of HPLC (> 1 mg/kg)	HPLC fluorescence Ex λ 293, Em λ 326	*Int. J. Vit. Nutr. Res.*, 51, 341, 1981[12]
2. pages 15–16	all-rac-α-tocopheryl acetate	Determination of α-tocopheryl acetate in feed premixes with HPLC (> 1000 mg/kg)	HPLC 280 nm	None
Food Chemicals Codex, 4th Edition, 1996[13]				
1. pages 417–418	all-rac-α-tocopherol	all-rac-α-tocopherol (NLT 96.0%, NMT 102.0%)	GC flame ionization	None
2. page 418	RRR-α-tocopherol	all-rac-α-tocopherol concentrate (concentrates from edible oil deodorizer distillate)	GC flame ionization	None

3. pages 419–420	RRR-α-tocopherol RRR-β-tocopherol RRR-γ-tocopherol RRR-δ-tocopherol	Tocopherols concentrate, mixed (concentate from edible oil deodorizer distillate)	GC flame ionization	None
4. pages 420–421	α-tocopheryl acetate (NLT 96.0%, NMT 102.0%)	RRR-α-Tocopheryl acetate (acetylization of α-tocopherol from edible oil)	GC flame ionization	None
5. pages 421–422	all-rac-α-tocopheryl acetate (NLT 96.0%, NMT 102.0%)	all-rac-α-Tocopheryl acetate	GC flame ionization	None
6. page 422	RRR-α-tocopheryl acetate	RRR-α-Tocopheryl acetate concentrate	GC flame ionization	None
7. pages 422–424	RRR-α-tocopheryl succinate	all-rac-α-tocopheryl acid succinate	GC flame ionization	None

Methods for the Determination of Vitamins in Foods, COST 91[14]

1. page 91	RRR-α-tocopherol or all-rac-α-tocopheryl acetate	foods	HPLC fluorescence Ex λ 293, Em λ 326	None
2. page 107	RRR-tocopherols RRR-tocotrienols	Fats and oils	HPLC Fluorescence Ex λ 293, Em λ 326	None

3.3.1   GAS LIQUID CHROMATOGRAPHY

Gas liquid chromatography (GLC) procedures were developed for vitamin E assay before the advent of HPLC methodology. For GLC methods applicable to vitamin E determination, Nelis et al.[47] provides an excellent literature review up to 1985. GLC can be used to quantify the 8 vitamin E homologs and their isomeric forms. The chroman derivatives can be chromatographed as the free forms or as trimethyl-silyl (TMS) derivatives with FID detection. Other useful derivatives suitable for FID detection include acetates, propionates and butyrates.[47] Electrochemical detection can be coupled with trifluoroacetate and perfluoro esters. AOAC International offers the following GLC methods:

1. AOAC Official Method 988.14 (45.1.27) "Tocopherol Isomers in Mixed Tocopherols Concentrates"
2. AOAC Official Method 989.09 (45.1.28) " *a*-Tocopheryl Acetate in Supplemental Vitamin E Concentrates"
3. AOAC Official Method 969.40 (45.1.29), "Vitamin E in Drugs"

These methods offer good precision compared to the AOAC colorimetric and polarimetric methods, but are time demanding. HPLC methods have not been collaborated for these products.

GLC resolution of β-T, γ-T, β-T3 and γ-T3 can only be efficiently accomplished as their TMS derivatives on capillary columns. GLC has been used in the analysis of vitamin E content of a wide variety of foods and biological samples.[53] One of the most recent applications of GLC successfully assayed α-T without derivatization by cold on-column injection in combination with a fused-silica capillary column coated with methylsilicone.[54] The procedure was applied to rat liver, tuna liver, wheat flour and a test diet with good results. Recovery ranged from 97 to 101% for α-T. In 1991, the effective use of heptafluorobutyryl-imidazole derivatives was demonstrated for the GLC resolution of α-T from cholesterol in foods of animal origin.[55] Appearance of GLC applications for vitamin E analysis has slowed during the 1980s and 1990s as HPLC became the preferred method.

3.3.2   HIGH PERFORMANCE LIQUID CHROMATOGRAPHY

Since the late 1970s, many HPLC methods were published for the measurement of tocopherols and tocotrienols in biological samples. Table 3.5 provides summaries of several methodology papers showing applications to a wide selection of matrices.

3.3.2.1   Extraction Procedures for Vitamin E for HPLC Analysis

A large number of diverse extraction procedures have been used for extraction and quantification of vitamin E as well as other fat soluble vitamins from biological matrices. Except for quantification of vitamin E in oils, which can be directly injected onto a normal-phase HPLC column after dilution with *n*-hexane or mobile phase, the vitamin E must be concentrated and in many cases freed from the sample matrix. Preparation of the vitamin E fraction usually requires saponification of the entire sample matrix or of an isolated lipid fraction or extraction of the total lipid from the sample with suitable solvent. The following is a brief review of currently used extraction procedures. Table 3.5 provides specific information on extraction methods used for several matrices.

3.3.2.1.1   Saponification

Saponification is a general term referring to alkaline hydrolysis. Usually, KOH is used, although NaOH is specified by some procedures. Hydrolysis results in cleavage of the ester linkages of

TABLE 3.5
HPLC Methods for the Analysis of Vitamin E in Foods, Feeds, Pharmaceuticals, and Biologicals

Sample Matrix	Analyte	Sample Preparation		HPLC Parameters				Reference
		Sample Extraction	Clean Up	Column	Mobile Phase	Detection	Quality Assurance Parameters	
Foods *Oils and Fats*								
1. Seed oils	α-, β-, γ-, δ-T3	Dilution with Hex Direct injection	—	Polygosil 60-5 5 μm 4.6 mm × 25 cm	Isocratic Hex : DIPE (90 : 10) 1.8 m/min	Fluorescence Ex λ = 296 Em λ = 320 % Recovery 93–95	QL 4 μg/g CV% 2.9–8.4	J. Food Sci., 50, 121, 1985[1]
2. Vegetable oils, cod liver oil margarine, butter, dairy spread	α-, β-, γ-, δ-T α-, β-, γ-, δ-T3	Dilution with Hex Direct injection	—	LiChrosorb Si60 5 μm 4.0 mm × 25 cm 30°C	Gradient 8 to 17% DIEP in Hex	Fluorescence Ex λ = 290 Em λ = 325	QL 0.25 mg/100 g	J. Am. Oil Chem. Soc., 63, 328, 1986[2]
3. Vegetables oils	α-, β-, γ-, δ-T	Dilution with Hex Direct injection	—	LiChrosorb Si60 5 μm 4.6 mm × 25 cm	Isocratic 3% dioxane in Hex 1 mL/min	Fluorescence Ex λ = 295 Em λ = 330	—	J. Food Comp. Anal., 1, 231, 1988[3]
4. Rice bran oil	α-, β-, γ-, δ-T α-, β-, γ-, δ-T3 γ-oryzanol	Dilution with Hex MeCN : MeOH : IPA (50 : 45 : 5) Direct injection	—	Hypersil ODS 5 μm 2.1 mm × 20 cm	Gradient a. 0–5 min MeCN : MeOH : IPA : Water (45 : 45 : 5 : 5) b. 5–10 min MeCN : MeOH : IPA (50 : 45 : 5) 1 mL/min	Fluorescence a. Vitamin E Ex λ = 290 Em λ = 320 b. Oryzanol 325 nm	—	J. Am. Oil Chem. Soc., 70, 301, 1993[4]
5. Vegetable oils	α-, β-, γ-, δ-T	Add tocol (IS) Dilute with CH₂Cl₂ GPC cleanup Collect vitamin fraction Evaporate Redissolve in mobile phase	GPC four columns in series 1. Ultrasphere 1000Å 2. Ultrasphere 500Å 3. μStyragel 100Å 4. μStyragel 100Å	Ultrasphere silica 5 μm 25 cm × 4.6 mm	Hex : IPA (99.3 : 0.7) 1 mL/min	1. Evaporative light scattering (ELSD) 2. Fluorescence Ex λ = 290 Em λ = 330	DL On-column (ng) ELSD 250 fluorescence 25	J. Am. Oil Chem. Soc., 71, 877, 1994[5]

TABLE 3.5 Continued
HPLC Methods for the Analysis of Vitamin E in Foods, Feeds, Pharmaceuticals, and Biologicals

Sample Matrix	Analyte	Sample Preparation		HPLC Parameters				Reference
		Sample Extraction	Clean Up	Column	Mobile Phase	Detection	Quality Assurance Parameters	
6. Olive oil	α-, β-, γ-, δ-T α-, β-, γ-, δ-T3	a. NP-HPLC Dilute with Hex Direct injection b. RP-HPLC Dilute with THF Dilute with MeOH Direct injection	—	a. LiChrosorb Si60 5 μm 25 cm × 4 mm b. Spherisorb ODS 5 μm 25 cm × 4.6 mm	Isocratic NP-HPLC Hex : IPA (99.7 : 0.3) 1.7 mL/min RP-HPLC 0.05 M NaClO$_4$: MeOH (10 : 90) 2.0 mL/min	NP-HPLC a. Fluorescence Ex λ = 290 Em λ = 330 b. PDA 280 nm RP-HPLC Amperometric 0.6V	QL γ-T3 1.9 mg/100 g RSDR α-T—0.5 α-T3—0.9 β-T3—6.8 γ-T3—1.5 δ-T3—5.3	*J. Am. Oil Chem. Soc.*, 72, 1505, 1995[6]
7. Rapeseed oil w/wo added antioxidants	α-, β-, γ-, δ-T	Dilute with Hex Direct injection	—	Apex Silica 5 μm 25 cm × 4.6 mm	Isocratic Hex : IPA (98.5 : 1.5) 1 mL/min	Fluorescence Ex λ = 290 Em λ = 330	—	*Food Chem.*, 52, 175, 1995[7]
Infant Formula, Milk								
8. Infant formula, milk powder	a-tocopheryl acetate	Extract with dimethysulfoxide : dimethylformamide : CHCl$_3$ (200 : 200 : 100) Partition with Hex Clarify Hex layer by centrifugation	—	Rad-Pak silica cartridge 5 μm, 8 mm, id Z-Module compression unit	Isocratic Hex : IPA (99.92 : 0.08) 2 mL/min	280 nm	QL 0.7 IU/100 g % Recovery 92–93	*J. Micronutr. Anal.*, 2, 97, 1986[8]
9. Infant formula	α-tocopheryl acetate, α-T	Extract fat by the Ross-Gottlieb procedure Saponify lipid fraction Extract with Hex Evaporate Redissolve in IPA : EtOH : Hex (1 : 0.5 : 98.5)	—	LiChrosorb Si60 12 cm × 4.6 mm	Isocratic IPA : EtOH : Hex (1 : 0.5 : 98.5) 1 mL/min	Fluorescence Ex λ = 292 Em λ = 320	% Recovery 96–108	*J. Micronut. Anal.*, 6, 35, 1989[9]

No. Food	Vitamers	Sample Preparation		Column	HPLC Conditions	Detection	QL/DL/Recovery	Reference
10. Infant formula, milk various foods	α-, β-, δ-T	Saponify Extract with light petroleum : DIEP (2 : 1) Centrifuge Inject 10 μL of upper layer	—	a. Rad-Pak silica cartridge, 5 μm RCM-100 b. Rad-Pak C$_{18}$ cartridge, 5 μm RCM-100	Isocratic a. NP-HPLC Hex : IPA (99 : 1) 1 mL/min b. RP-HPLC 100% MeOH 1 mL/min	Fluorescence Ex λ = 295 Em λ = 330	QL 0.4 mg/100 g % Recovery 93–97 CV% within run 1.9–5.7	Analyst, 113, 1217, 1988[10]
11. Infant formula	α-T	Saponify 70°C, 25 min Extract with Hex : CH$_2$Cl$_2$ (3 + 1) Evaporate Redissolve in mobile phase Hex : IP (99.92 : 0.08)	—	Hypersil silica 5 μm 25 cm × 4.6 nm	Isocratic Hex : IP (99.92 : 0.8) 1 mL/min	280 mm	—	J. AOAC Int., 76, 399, 1993[11]

Other Foods

No. Food	Vitamers	Sample Preparation		Column	HPLC Conditions	Detection	QL/DL/Recovery	Reference
12. Vegetable oils, wheat flour, barley, milk, frozen dinners, beef, spinach, infant formula	α-, β-, δ-, γ-T α-, β-, γ-, T3	Extract with boiling IPA Filter Extract with A Add water, Hex Collect Hex layer	—	LiChrosorb Si60 5 μm 25 cm ×3.2 mm	Isocratic Moist hexane : Et$_2$O (95 : 5) 2 mL/min	Fluorescence Ex λ = 290 Em λ = 330	DL On-column 4 ng	J. Liq. Chromatogr., 2, 327, 1979[12]
13. 40 food products	α-, β-, δ-T	Saponification, overnight, ambient Extract with Hex	—	Zorbax ODS 5 μm 25 cm × 4.6 mm	Isocratic MeCN : MeCl$_2$: MeOH (700 : 300 : 50) 1 mL/min	Fluorescence Ex λ = 290 Em λ = 330	QL 0.1 mg/100 g	J. Food Comp. Anal., 2, 200, 1989[13]
14–22. Finnish foods	α-, β-, γ-, δ-T α-, β-, γ-, δ-T3	a. Butter, margarine Dissolve in Hex Direct injection	—	LiChrosorb Si60 5 μm 25 cm × 4 mm	Isocratic Hex : DIEP (93 : 7) 2.1–2.5 mL/min	Fluorescence Ex λ = 290 Em λ = 325	% Recovery 80–99 CV%	Int. J. Vit. Nutr. Res., 53, 35, 1984[14] Int. J. Vit. Nutr. Res., 53, 41, 1984[15]

TABLE 3.5 Continued
HPLC Methods for the Analysis of Vitamin E in Foods, Feeds, Pharmaceuticals, and Biologicals

Sample Matrix	Analyte	Sample Preparation		HPLC Parameters				Reference
		Sample Extraction	Clean Up	Column	Mobile Phase	Detection	Quality Assurance Parameters	
b. Other foods		Saponification, overnight, ambient					3.8–7.2	J. Agric. Food Chem., 33, 1215, 1985[16] J. Am. Oil chem. Soc., 62, 1245, 1985[17] Int. J. Vit. Nutr. Res., 55, 159, 1985[18] J. Agric. Food Chem., 34, 742, 1986[19] Cereal Chem., 63, 78 1986[20] J. Food Comp. Anal., 1, 53, 1987[21] J. Food Comp. Anal., 1, 124, 1988[22]
23. Chicken muscle	α-, δ-T	Saponification, overnight, ambient, followed by 2h at 50°C Extract with Hex Evaporate Redissolve in MeOH	—	BioSil ODS-5S 25 cm × 4 mm	Isocratic MeOH : 100% 1 mL/min	Fluorescence Ex λ = 296 Em λ = 330	% Recovery 92–93	J. Food Sci., 55, 1536, 1990[23]
24–26. Pecans, Peanuts	α-, β-, γ-, δ-T	Soxhlet Hex containing 0.01% BHT, 90°C, 6 h Evaporate Redissolve in Hex containing 0.01% BHT	—	LiChrosorb Si60 5 μm 25 cm × 4 mm	Isocratic Hex : IPA (99 : 1) 1 mL/min	Fluorescence Ex λ = 290 Em λ = 330	DL (ng) On-column α-T—2 β-T—1 γ-T—2 δ-T—0.6 % Recovery 84–96	J. Food Sci., 57, 1194, 1992[24] Peanut Sci., 20, 21, 1993[25] J. Am. Oil Chem. Soc., 70, 633, 1993[26]

	Sample	Analytes	Sample Preparation	Column	Mobile Phase	Detection	QC	Reference
27.	Grain amaranths	α-, β-, γ-, δ-T; α-, β-, γ-, δ-T3	Extract with MeOH; Evaporate; Extract with Hex	Water silica 30 cm × 4.0 mm	Isocratic Hex : IPA (99.8 : 0.2) 1 mL/min	Fluorescence Ex λ = 295 Em λ = 330	— (DL)	*Lipids*, 29, 177, 1994[27]
28.	Multivitamin juices, isotonic beverages breakfast cereals, infant formula human milk	α-, β-, γ-, δ-T; α-, β-, γ-, δ-T3; α-tocopheryl acetate; plastochromanol-8	Add water, EtOH; Shake and sonicate; Add TBME, PE; Centrifuge; Repeat extraction twice; Add EtOH; Evaporate; Redissolve in Hex; For infant formula and human, add either 25% ammonia solution or 35% dipotassium oxalate prior to the first addition of EtOH	LiChrospher 100 diol 5 μm 25 cm × 4 mm	Gradient 1. a. 0–4 min Hex b. 4–5 min up to Hex : BME (97 : 30) c. 5–41 min Isocratic d. 41–42 min up to Hex : BME (95 : 5) e. 42–60 min Isocratic f. 2 min down to Hex g. 10 min Hex 2. a. 0–4 min Hex b. 4–5 min up to Hex : BME (97 : 3) c. 5–23 min Isocratic d. 2 min down to Hex e. 10 min Hex	Fluorescence Ex λ = 280 Em λ = 335 or Ex λ = 295 Em λ = 330	DL On-column (ng) α-tocopheryl acetate 2.2–4.6; % Recovery 100–103; %CV 2	*Fat Sci. Technol.*, 95, 215, 1993[28]

Animal Feeds

	Sample	Analytes	Sample Preparation	Column	Mobile Phase	Detection	QC	Reference
29.	Laboratory chow	α-, β-, γ-, δ-T	Add tocol (IS); Saponify; 70°C, 30 min; Extract with Hex or Et₂O or PE; Redissolve in MeOH	Yanapak ODS-T 25 cm × 4 mm	Isocratic MeOH containing 0.05 M NaClO₄ 1 mL/min	a. EC 0.8 V vs Ag/AgCl b. Fluorescence Ex λ = 297 Em λ = 327 a. Fluorescence	DL—On-column (ng) a. EC 0.1 b. Fluorescence 2.0 % Recovery 96–109	*J. Micronutr. Anal.*, 1, 31, 1985[29]
30.	Animal feed	α-tocopheryl acetate, α-T	Extract with dimethyl sulfoxide : dimethyl formamide : CHCl₃ (4 : 4 : 2) with 500 mg AA per L; Add water, Hex; Centrifuge; Transfer Hex aliquot to auto injection vial	Radical Pak Silicia cartridge 5 μm 8 mm, id	Isocratic Hex : IPA (99.92 : 0.08) 2 mL/min	% Recovery Ex λ = 260 Em λ = 330 b. 280 nm	88–102	*J. Micronutr. Anal.*, 2, 259, 1986[30]

TABLE 3.5 Continued
HPLC Methods for the Analysis of Vitamin E in Foods, Feeds, Pharmaceuticals, and Biologicals

		Sample Preparation		HPLC Parameters			
Sample Matrix	Analyte	Sample Extraction	Clean Up	Column	Mobile Phase	Detection	Quality Assurance Parameters	Reference
31. Pet foods	α-T	Saponify, reflux for 30 min Extract with light petroleum (BP 40–60°C) Evaporate Redissolve in Hex (NP-HPLC) or IPA (RP-HPLC)	Sep-Pak silica	a. NP-HPLC LiChrosorb Si60 5 μm 12.5 cm × 5 mm b. RD-HPLC ODS-Silica 10 μm 25 cm × 5 mm	Isocratic a. NP-HPLC Hex : 1,4-dioxane (97 : 3) b. RP-HPLC MeOH : Water (95 : 5)	a. Fluorescence Ex λ = 295 Em λ = 330 b. 295 nm	—	Analyst, 116, 421, 1991[31]
Biologicals								
1. Plasma	α-, β- + γ-, δ-T	Add δ-T in MeCN (IS) Extract with n-butanol : EtOAC : MeCN (1 : 1 : 1) Centrifuge Inject organic phase	—	LiChrocart Supersphere 100 RP-18 4 μm 25 cm × 4 mm	Isocratic EtOH : MeOH (90 : 10) at 2.5 mM $HClO_4$ and 7.5 mM $NaClO_4$ 0.6 mL/min	EC + 0.35 V	DL (pg) On-column α-T 60	J. Chromatogr., 620, 268, 1993[1]
2. Rat, blood and tissue	α-T Stereoisomers	Add PMC, NaCl, ethanolic pyrogallol Saponify 70°C, 60 min Extract with Hex : EtOAC (90 : 10) Collect Hex layer Evaporate	Acetylate Hex residue	Chiral pak OP (+) 25 cm × 4.6 mm	Isocratic MeOH : Water (96 : 4) 35°C, 0.3 mL/min	284 mm	% Recovery 91–100	J. Nutr. Sci. Vitaminol., 39, 207, 1993[2]
3. Plasma, erythrocytes	α-T	Add α-tocopheryl acetate (IS) in EtOH Extract with Hex Centrifuge Transfer Hex phase Evaporate Redissolve in MeOH : Et_2O (75 : 25)	—	Spherisorb ODS-2 5 μm 25 cm × 4.6 mm	Isocratic MeOH, 100% 1mL/min	PDA 280–400 nm λ = 280 nm	DL (mmol/L) 5.18 QL 7.56	J. Chromatogr. B, 660, 395, 1994[3]

Sample	Analyte	Sample preparation		Column	Mobile phase	Detection	DL / Recovery	Reference
4. Serum, human and rat tissue	α-T, oxidized and reduced co-enzyme Q	a. Serum: Add water, EtOH and menaquione-8 (IS), Extract with Hex, Centrifuge, Evaporate Hex, Redissolve in EtOH. b. Tissue: Homogenize in water, Add ethanol, menaquinone-8 (IS), Extract with Hex, Centrifuge, Evaporate Hex, Redissolve in EtOH	—	Capsell Pak C87, 5 μm, 15 cm × 4.6 mm	Isocratic EtOH : MeOH : water (8.2 : 0.8 : 1.0) containing 0.05 M $NaClO_4$, 0.8 mL/min	Post-column reduction of oxidized CoQ by Pt-reduction column EC + 0.6 V vs Ag/AgCl	DL (pg) On-column αT-20 CoQ homologs 70–100	Biol. Pharm. Bull., 17, 997, 1994[4]
5. Plasma	α-T, α-tocopheryl acetate	Add MeOH, Centrifuge, Filter, Direct injection	—	LiChrosorb RP-18, 10 μm, 20 cm × 4.6 mm	Isocratic MeOH, 100%, 1 mL/min	292 nm	QL (μg/mL) α-T — 0.59 α-T acetate—	J. Liq. Chromatogr., 18, 1251, 1995[5]
6. Liver tissue	α-, (γ + β), δ-T	Homogenize 0.2–0.8 g in A with 0.1–1.0 mL 50 mM AA in MeOH, Vortex, centrifuge, Filter	—	3 μm, 10 cm × 4.6 mm, Spherisorb ODS-2	Isocratic MeOH : water (95 : 5), 22°C, 1.5 mL/min	290 nm and Fluorescence Ex λ = 290 Em λ = 330	0.17 % Recovery α-T–98	Comp. Biochem. Physiol., 113B, 143, 1996[6]
7. Plasma	α-T	Add 20 mL Na tungstate : Mg Cl_2 (0.06 : 1 M) and 1 mL MeOH to 100 mL, Centrifuge	—	Kromasil C_{18}, 5 μm, 10 cm × 4.6 mm	Isocratic MeOH : MeCN : water (50 : 35 : 15), 1.5 mL/min	292 nm	% Recovery 98 CV% 2.6–5.6	J. Chromatogr. B., 690, 355, 1997[7]

TABLE 3.5 Continued
HPLC Methods for the Analysis of Vitamin E in Foods, Feeds, Pharmaceuticals, and Biologicals

		Sample Preparation		HPLC Parameters				
Sample Matrix	Analyte	Sample Extraction	Clean Up	Column	Mobile Phase	Detection	Quality Assurance Parameters	Reference
8. Tissue	α-, β-, γ-T α-, β-, γ- δ-T3	Pulverize (1 g) at dry ice temperature Add 2 mL ice-cold water Add 5 mL cold absolute EtOH Add 4 µg of a specific tocopherol as IS Sonicate, 45 s Rinse probe with 5 mL EtOH Add Hex (10 mL) Vortex Centrifuge Flash evaporate 5 mL of Hex layer Dissolve residue in 1 mL Hex	—	Supelcosil LC-Diol 5 µm	Isocratic Hex : IPA (99 : 1) 1 mL/min	Fluorescence Ex λ = 296 Em λ = 330	% Recovery 95 ± 7	Lipids, 32, 323, 1997[8]

glycerides, phospholipids and sterols, destroys pigments, and disrupts the sample matrix which facilitates vitamin extraction. Ball[40] provides a guide for the digestion mixture which includes 5 ml of 60% w/v aqueous KOH and 15 ml of ethanol per 1 g of fat. Because of the instability of vitamin E under alkaline conditions, care must be taken to avoid destruction of the vitamin E homologs during the saponification. Steps required to avoid undue loss during digestion include flushing the digestion vessel with nitrogen, addition of antioxidant (pyrogallol or ascorbic acid, and protection from light. Temperatures and times used for saponification range from ambient temperature for 12 h or longer[56,57,58] to 70°C for 30 min or less.[59,60] Saponification parameters such as sample size, volumes of alkali and ethanol, and time and temperature can be varied to optimize the digestion. Most efficient saponification and highest recovery of vitamin E is obtained when the digestion is completed under reflux conditions. Use of an air condenser greatly simplifies the saponification step in vitamin E assay (Figure 3.4).

Following the saponification, the digest is diluted with water or 1% NaCl to inhibit emulsion formation and is extracted with ether, petroleum ether, hexane or ethyl acetate in hexane, or other solvent mixtures. The unsaponifiable components including vitamin E are extracted into the solvent while the fatty acid soaps, glycerols, and many other potentially interfering substances remain in the alkaline aqueous phase.

Problems exist in getting efficient transfer of the tocopherol and tocotrienol homologs into the organic solvent phase from the aqueous phase. Ueda and Igarashi reviewed factors affecting extraction of vitamin E from the saponification medium.[59,61] Significant factors include ethanol concentration of the digest, composition of the extracting solvent, and the level of lipids used in the digest. When n-hexane is the extraction solvent, ethanol concentrations must be kept below 30% to ensure complete extraction of δ-T and tocol (an internal standard) and below 15% if 2,2,5,7,8-pentamethyl-6-hydroxy chroman (PMC) is used as the internal standard. Ethanol concentration has no effect on the extraction of α-T and only a slight effect on β-T and γ-T.[61]

n-Hexane is the most commonly used solvent for extraction of saponification digests. However, addition of ethyl acetate which is more polar than n-hexane to levels up to 10% v/v to the n-hexane can improve recoveries for β-T, γ-T and δ-T, tocol and PMC.[62] Increasing the level of ethyl acetate above 10% causes the volume of the solvent layer to decrease as the solvent becomes more miscible in the aqueous phase.

Fatty acid salts from the lipid can increase solubility of the vitamin E homologs in the aqueous phase and decrease extraction into the non-polar solvent. Ueda and Igarashi,[63] working with corn oil, showed that recovery losses of β-T, γ-T, δ-T and tocol can be significant. Recovery losses were observed with oil levels as low as 5 mg. Extraction of α-T was not affected by the lipid level in the digest. Recovery of tocol was most severely affected.

With some food matrices, extraction of the lipid prior to saponification has been advantageous. As an example, Tuan et al.[64] reported that lipid extraction from infant formula before saponification provided extracts with fewer interferences than extracts obtained by saponification of the entire formula. However, in our experience, most samples can be handled with direct saponification without prior fat extraction. Details of published saponification procedures are given in Table 3.6.

Various saponification procedures for the extraction of vitamin E from biological matrices have been designed to decrease time and solvent requirements.[60, 62] Procedures of Indyk[60] and Uega and Igarashi[62] are briefly summarized to provide methodology applicable to a wide variety of biological samples.

1. *Procedure Applicable to Dairy Products, Food and Tissues* (Indyk[60])

Sample Size:. 0.5 g whole milk powder, powdered infant formula, freeze-dried organs, fish, cereal, 5.0 g of fluid milk; 0.1 to 0.2 g butter, margarine or vegetable oil.
Procedure: Weigh sample into test tube and add 10.0 mL ethanol containing 1% pyrogallol. Add α-T standard (200 μL of known concentration (20 to 30 μg/100 mL absolute

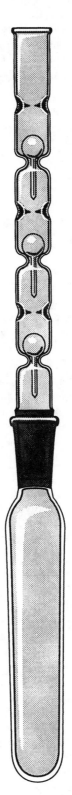

FIGURE 3.4   Saponification reflux condenser.

TABLE 3.6
Saponification Conditions Used for Extraction of Vitamin E

Matrix	Hydrolysis Sample Size	Conditions	Antioxidant	Internal Standard or % Extractant	Recovery	Reference
Feeds	0.5 g	Ethanolic KOH 70°C, 30 min	Pyrogallol	Hexane Diethyl ether Petroleum ether	Tocol—found to be not suitable for addition prior to sponification	J. Micronutr. Anal., 1, 31, 1985
Meat	10 g	Ethanolic KOH Ambient overnight	Ascorbic acid	Hexane	α-T—97% β-T—100% γ-T—97%	J. Agric. Food Chem., 33, 1215, 1985
Infant formula	1 g	Ethanolic KOH Reflux 30 min	Pyrogallol	Hexane	δ-T—68% α-T—96–109%	J. Micronutr. Anal., 6, 35, 1989
Dairy products Foods Tissues	10 g	Ethanolic KOH 70°C, 7 min	Pyrogallol	Petroleum ether : isopropyl ether (3 : 1)	α-T (IS) added to unfortified sample	Analyst, 113, 1217, 1988
40 foods	10 g	Ethanolic KOH Ambient overnight	Ascorbic acid Nitrogen flush	Hexane	>80% for α-T and γ-T in all samples	J. Food Comp. Anal., 2, 200 1989
Infant formula	10 mL	Ethanolic KOH 70°C, 25 min	Pyrogallol	Hexane : methylene chloride (3 : 1)	None	J. AOAC Int., 76, 399, 1993
Human diets	10–20 g	Ethanolic KOH Ambient, overnight	Ascorbic acid	Hexane	α-T—99% β-T—95% γ-T—99% δ-T—80%	Int., J. Vit. Nutr. Res., 53, 35, 1984
Seeds oils	1–5 g	Ethanolic KOH Reflux, 30 min	Sodium ascorbate	Diisopropyl ether	α-T—93% γ-T—94% α-T3—95%	J. Food Sci., 50, 121, 1985

ethanol) to the unfortified sample to provide a parallel assay for recovery data. Add 2 mL of 50% KOH and loosely stopper the tubes. Incubate at 70° for 7 min with periodic agitation. Cool the tubes and add 20 mL of light petroleum ether : diisopropyl ether (3 + 1). Shake mechanically for 5 min. Add 30 mL water, invert ten times, and centrifuge at 180 × g for 10 min. A 10 μL volume of the clear upper layer is injected directly into an isocratic HPLC system.

2. *Procedure Applicable to Blood and Tissues.* (Ueda and Igarashi[62])

Blood: To 200 μL plasma or 400 μL of 50% hematocrit RBC suspension in two 10 mL centrifuge tubes with teflon coated screw-caps, add 1 mL 6% ethanolic pyrogallol to each tube. Preheat the solution to 70°C for 3 min and to one tube add 1 mL of an ethanolic solution of PMC (0.3 μg) as an internal standard, to the other tube add 3 mL of an ethanolic solution containing 3.0 μg each of α-, β-, γ-, and δ-T and PMC. Add 0.2 mL of 60% KOH and saponify at 70°C for 30 minutes. Cool tubes in ice water and add 4.5 mL of 1% NaCl. The saponification mixture is extracted with 3 mL of 10% ethyl acetate in *n*-hexane. Centrifuge the saponified extracts at 3000 rpm for 5 min and pipet 2 mL of *n*-hexane layer into a 10 mL conical glass tube. Evaporate the *n*-hexane under a stream of nitrogen. Redissolve the unspiked residue in 200 μL of *n*-hexane and the residue from the spiked sample in 2.0 mL of *n*-hexane. For each, inject 10 μL into the HPLC system.

Tissues: Weigh 100 mg of tissue into a 10 mL centrifuge tube with teflon coated screw-cap. Add 100 μL of 1% NaCl, 1 mL of 6% ethanolic pyrogallol and 2.0 mL of 60% KOH. Saponify at 70°C for 60 min. Add 4.5 mL of 1% NaCl to the cooled digest and extract with 3 mL of 10% ethyl acetate in *n*-hexane. Centrifuge the saponified extracts at 3000 rpm for 5 min and pipet 2 mL of the *n*-hexane layer into a conical glass tube for concentration under a stream of nitrogen. Redissolve the residue in 200 μL of *n*-hexane and inject 10 μL into the HPLC. Recoveries can be determined by use of a parallel spike or by use of PMC internal standard.

3.3.2.1.2   Solvent Extraction

Methods normally used for total lipid extraction from biological matrices have been used for vitamin E extraction prior to quantification. Some of the earliest studies on the vitamin E content of food used hot absolute ethanol. Ball[40] stated that solvents for fat-soluble vitamin extraction must be capable of effectively penetrating tissues and breaking lipoprotein bonds while minimizing oxidative destruction of the vitamin. Some of the most commonly used solvents for vitamin E extraction include the Folch extraction with chloroform: methanol (2 : 1), acetone, diethyl ether, and Soxhlet extraction with a variety of solvents.[40] If the sample is dry, Soxhlet extraction is often the simplest and most efficient method for vitamin E extraction. Wet samples can be ground in the presence of excess anhydrous sodium sulfate to produce a dry powder suitable for Soxhlet extraction.[40] Suitable solvents include absolute ethanol, acetone, *n*-hexane, and petroleum ether. Because of the extensive time required for the extraction, an antioxidant such as BHT must be added to the extraction solvent. Protection from light is required throughout the procedure. If the sample contains polar lipids in quantity, *n*-hexane might not be sufficiently polar to efficiently extract the lipids, and the recovery of vitamin E homologs will be low.

Hakansson et al.[65] developed a Soxhlet extraction procedure for the determination of vitamin E in wheat products. The extraction used 5 to 15 g of cereal ground to pass a 1.0 mm sieve. Extraction was completed with 125 mL of *n*-hexane containing 1 mg of BHT at 90°C for 4 h. After extraction, the hexane extract was evaporated to near dryness using a rotary evaporator at 50°C. The residue was redissolved with 15 mL hexane and 15 mL of 99.5% ethanol and re-evaporated. The residue was redissolved in *n*-hexane and filtered through a 0.45 μm filter prior to HPLC quantification. The extract could be stored in amber bottles overnight if refrigerated. The Soxhlet procedure was compared to the solvent extraction procedure of Thompson and Hatina.[46] Recoveries of α-T and β-T for the Soxhlet extraction (95 to 100%) exceeded those obtained by the isopropanol/acetone solvent system developed by Thompson and Hatina.[46]

Thompson and Hatina's[46] solvent extraction procedure for tocopherols and tocotrienols has been used by many investigators for vitamin E extraction from a wide array of natural products. The procedure is based on isopropanol and acetone extraction combined with partitioning of the vitamin E fraction into *n*-hexane. A summary of the procedure follows: homogenize 10 g of sample with 100 mL of boiling isopropanol in the cup of a Virtis homogenizer. After 1 min of homogenization, add 50 mL of acetone and filter the mixture through Whatman GF/A glass fiber paper into a 500 mL separatory funnel. The residue was extracted with 50 mL of acetone, and the filter paper and its contents were homogenized with 100 mL of acetone. This extract was also filtered into the separatory funnel and the residue washed with 50 mL of acetone. Add 100 mL of hexane to the pooled extracts and swirl the funnel to mix the contents. Add 100 mL of water and swirl the funnel to mix the phases. After phase separation, the *n*-hexane epiphase was transferred to a second funnel and the aqueous hypophase was extracted two more times with 10 mL portions of *n*-hexane. The pooled *n*-hexane extracts were washed twice with 100 mL portions of water and evaporated under vacuum. The efficiency of the procedure was 97% or greater depending on the matrix being extracted.

Landen[66] used high performance gel permeation chromatography HP-GPC and reversed-phase chromatography (RP-HPLC) after extraction to simultaneously determine all-rac-α-T acetate and vitamin A palmitate in infant formulas. By avoiding saponification, this HPLC method can be used to simultaneously determine all-rac-α-T acetate and the natural vitamin E forms present in infant formulas. Landen et al.[67] successfully applied HP-GPC and RP-HPLC techniques for the determination of all-rac-α-T acetate and vitamin A palmitate levels in a large number of infant formulas, representing different batches and different matrices, with further application to medical foods and other products. The extraction method uses magnesium sulfate to dehydrate the sample and extraction with isopropanol and methylene chloride. The fat was removed from the extract by gel permeation chromatography followed by quantitation on reversed-phase LC with UV detection. The method is discussed in Chapter 5. Chase et al.[45] recently modified Landen's extraction procedure for infant formula by eliminating methylene chloride from the extraction. The extraction was completed with isopropanol and hexane : ethyl acetate (85 : 15).

3.3.2.2 Chromatography Parameters

3.3.2.2.1 Supports and Mobile Phases

Both reversed-phase and normal-phase LC are useful for resolution of vitamin E.[51] Reversed-phase systems will not resolve β- and γ-T. Studies conducted with reversed-phase methods report the combined positional isomers as (β- + γ-T). Normal-phase chromatography completely resolves the eight homologs. Tan and Brzuskiewicz[68] studied various columns and mobile phases for resolution of RRR-tocopherols and RRR-tocotrienols. Normal-phase systems showed elution of the homologs in order of increasing polarity with separation based on methyl substituents on the chromanol ring. Reversed-phase systems showed class separations based on the saturation of the phytyl side chain with the more saturated tocopherols being retained on the column longer. These authors reported optimal normal-phase chromatography on Zorbax SIL with a binary isocratic mobile phase of hexane : isopropanol (99 : 1). For normal-phase chromatography on Zorbax NH_2, the optimal solvent system was an isocratic mobile phase of hexane : isopropanol (99 : 2). Optimal reversed-phase chromatography was on Zorbax ODS with an isocratic mobile phase of acetonitrile : methanol : methylene chloride (60 : 35 : 5). Typical chromatograms for the tocopherols and tocotrienols are given in Figure 3-5. Direct injection of oils requires a normal-phase system because the triacylglycerols remain soluble in the mobile phase and do not interfere with the chromatography.

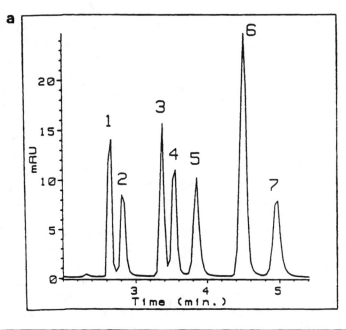

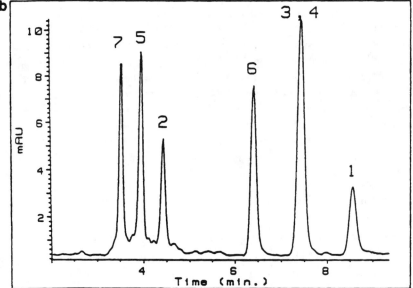

FIGURE 3.5 Chromatograms of tocopherols and tocotrienols.
a. Normal phase—Zorbax SIL with hexane : isopropanol (99 : 1).
b. Reverse phase—Zorbax ODS with acetonitrile : methanol : methylene chloride (60 : 35 : 5). α-T (1), α-T3 (2), β-T (3), γ-T (4), γ-T3 (5), δ-T (6), δ-T3 (7). Reproduced with permission from Reference 68.

Normal-phase chromatography on silica can accommodate up to 2 mg of fat per injection.[46] Examination of the current methods presented in Table 3.5 show that normal-phase chromatography is almost universally used for quantitation of vitamin E. Gradient systems are useful for better resolution of the eight homologs. Particularly, increased resolution of γ-T and γ-T3 can be obtained with gradient chromatography. Slightly elevated column temperatures can increase resolution.

Abidi and Mounts[69] showed the effects of various mobile phase conditions on the separation of β- and γ-T using aminopropyl silica or diol-silica supports. Previous work showed the molecular

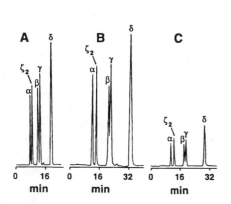

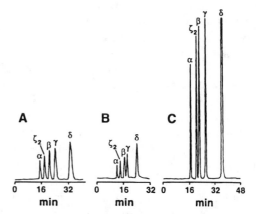

FIGURE 3.6   Vitamin E chromatography with strongly polar modifiers. A—amino-Si, hexane : dioxane (90 : 10); B—diol-Si (10 μm), hexane : dioxane (95 : 5); C—diol-Si (5 μ/m), cyclohexane-dioxane (97 : 3). Reproduced with permission from Reference 69.

FIGURE 3.7   Vitamin E chromatography with weakly polar modifiers. A—amino-Si, cyclohexane : t-butyl methyl ether (90 : 10); B—diol-Si (10 μm), hexane : t-butyl methyl ether (90 : 10); C—diol-Si (5 μm), hexane : diisopropyl ether (90 : 10). Reproduced with permission from Reference 69.

polarity and steric factors of the 5-, 7-, and 8-methyls interact with the 6-hydroxy group to significantly affect resolution. The dimethyl homologs, because of close polarity, are the most difficult vitamin E homologs to resolve by normal-phase chromatography and impossible to resolve by reversed-phase chromatography. The study showed that the ability of mobile phases containing a weakly polar modifier such as an ester (ethyl acetate) or a mono-functional ether (t-butyl methyl ether) was significantly greater compared to mobile phases containing more polar alcohol or polar ether modifiers. Chromatograms given in Figure 3.6 and Figure 3.7 show the differences in a variety of mobile phases to resolve the β- and γ-T dimethyl homologs on diol silica support.

Vitamin E mixtures were highly resolved using an amino-column and hexane : t-butyl ether (90 : 10) on a 5 μm diol column with hexane : t-butyl methyl ether (95 : 5). Mobile phases modified with mono-functional ethers were highly recommended by the authors to improve tocopherol and tocotrienol resolution.

3.3.2.2.2   Detection

Fluorescence detection provides sensitivity, specificity, and cleaner chromatograms compared to UV detection. Fluorescence detection is essential to the successful assay of vitamin E in complex food matrices. Notable studies using fluorescence detection coupled with LC include Piironen et al.,[57,70,71,72] Syväoja et al.,[56,73,74] Blott and Woollard,[42] Woollard et al.,[43] Chase et al.,[45] Speek et al.,[75] Balz et al.,[44] Rammell and Hoogenboom,[76] Deseai et al.,[77] Hogarty et al.,[58] Ang et al.,[78] Tuan et al.,[64] Hakansson et al.,[65] Rogers et al.,[79] Marero et al.,[80] Indyk,[60] Miyagawa et al.,[81] and Koprivnjak et al.[82] Again, normal-phase HPLC is the predominant method of choice. The products examined include edible oils, biological materials, human milk, corn, nuts, spices, vegetables, fruits, berries, infant formula, dairy products, cereals, fish, tomato products, chicken, and feeds. Procedural details of some of these studies are provided in Table 3.5.

UV detection can be used for concentrated supplements or fortification premixes. Cooper et al.[83] recently used UV detection at 292 nm for RRR-α-T analysis of plasma.[83]

HPLC in combination with electrochemical (EC) detection is becoming an excellent analytical procedure especially for clinical samples using very small volumes that require increased sensitivity. A 1985 review by Ueda and Igarashi[59] describes the application of LC/EC in determining tocopherols in feeds. Ueda and Igarashi[63] effectively used EC to reduce the effect of sodium salts of fatty acids on extraction losses. Because of a 20 fold increase in sensitivity using EC, the amount of fat could be reduced to an acceptable level by reducing sample size. Only δ-T in adipose tissues had a recovery of less than 75% using a reduced sample size. Ueda and Igarashi[59] also applied LC/EC to feeds and found that adding tocol as an internal standard prior to saponification was not satisfactory due to extraction losses. EC detectors also need traces of an electrolyte, therefore, EC is limited to reversed-phase chromatography.

Chou et al.[84] working with neonates measured tocopherols in microsamples of serum using a 5 μm Bio-Sil ODS-55 column and a mobile phase containing sodium acetate solution (pH-5) with δ-T as the internal standard. The α-T levels ranged from 4.3 to 9.7 mg/L and the total β- and γ-T ranged from 1.8 to 3.9 mg/L with the minimum level detectable at 0.1 mg/L. The maximum signal to noise ratio was obtained at an oxidizing potential of 1.0 mV and a pH of 5.0.

Pascoe et al.[85] determined fentamole (fmol) quantities of α-T, γ-T, δ-T and α-tocopheryl quinones (Tq) in biological tissues using a dual electrode detector. LC/EC enables the simultaneous analysis of α-T and its oxidation product of α-Tq. Because quinones do not fluoresce and are insensitive to UV, EC detection is preferred. The detection level for tocopherol was 1.0 fmol with α-Tq at 10 fmol. Murphy and Kehrer[86] further substantiated the degree of selectivity and high sensitivity offered by LC/EC by determining endogenous levels of α-T and α-Tq in tissue at 0.05 pmol levels in homogenates of chicken liver and muscle. The HPLC support was Ultrasphere-ODS 5 μm with a mobile phase of isopropanol : acetonitrile: water : triethylamine : acetic acid (60 : 20 : 19.4 : 0.5 : 0.1), pH 4.0.

A sensitive LC sequential UV and EC detection system for simultaneous determination of α-T, γ-T and δ-T, oxidized co-enzyme Q and reduced co-enzyme Q (ubiquinols) in various tissues was reported by Lang and Packer.[87] The tocopherols and ubiquinols are detected by EC detection.

Evaporative light-scattering detection offers another alternative for HPLC detection of vitamin E compounds. The evaporative light-scattering detector (ELSD) is a universal detector with the ability to detect every compound eluting off the column with or without a chromophore or fluorophore.[88] The column effluent is converted to a fine mist by passage through a nebulizer assisted by a carrier gas. The atomized droplets are carried through a temperature-controlled drift tube where vaporization occurs. The less volatile droplets pass through a laser light beam, and the droplets scatter the light. Light scatter is detected by a photodiode system. The detector response is a function of the mass of the solute particles. ELSD has seen considerable use in lipid analysis. Chase et al.[88] compared ELSD and fluorescence for the detection of tocopherols in the LC analysis of vegetable oils. Fluorescence was ten times more sensitive than ELSD. Our experiences with the ELSD detector provided no evidence of advantages of ELSD over fluorescence detection for vitamin E analysis. Carrier gas expense for the ELSD can be considerable.

3.3.2.2.3   Internal Standards

For some matrices, internal standards can simplify vitamin E analysis. For serum and plasma, δ-tocopherol is normally not detectable in the sample and can be used as an excellent internal standard for either UV or fluorescence detection. α-Tocopheryl acetate, with UV detection or a sensitive fluorescence detector, is suitable. Several studies used tocol as an internal standard; however, analytical problems are associated with its use. Ueda and Igarashi[63] determined tocol to be an unsuitable internal standard for saponification procedures owing to low recoveries in relation to the analytes. These investigators introduced 2,2,5,7, 8-pentamethyl-6-chromanol (PMC) as an internal standard for vitamin E methods requiring saponification.[62] Tocotrienols, because of their absence from most foods and biological samples, could be effectively applied as internal standards. However, the tocotrienols are generally not available commercially.

Our experience at the University of Georgia through extensive vitamin E analysis studies have shown that uneven recoveries can be a major problem. Uneven recovery refers to the variation in recoveries determined for α-, β-, γ-, and δ-T from the sample. Our solution has been to heavily rely upon spiked recoveries with the standards always added prior to saponification or solvent extraction.

3.4 METHOD PROTOCOLS

Analysis of Vitamin E in Food Products Using Liquid Chromatography

Principle

Fruit, Vegetables, Meat:

- Products were saponified with KOH for 30 min with reflux at 70°C and the unsaponifiable materials extracted with hexane (0.1% BHT). The combined organic phases were diluted to volume and 20 μL was injected onto a normal-phase HPLC column connected to a fluorescence detector (Ex λ 290, Em λ 330).

Margarine and Vegetable Oil Spreads:

- Products were dissolved in hexane and $MgSO_4$ was added to remove water. The extracts were filtered and diluted to volume in hexane (0.1% BHT) for normal-phase LC analysis with fluorescence detection (Ex λ 290, Em λ 330).

Reagents and Solvents

- 0.1% BHT in hexane for extraction
- 6% pyrogallol in ethanol for antioxidant
- Ethanol
- Potassium hydroxide
- α-tocopherol standard $E_{1\,cm}^{1\%} = 71$ at 294 nm
- γ-tocopherol standard $E_{1\,cm}^{1\%} = 92.8$ at 298 nm
- β-tocopherol standard $E_{1\,cm}^{1\%} = 86.4$ at 297 nm
- δ-tocopherol standard $E_{1\,cm}^{1\%} = 91.2$ at 298 nm
- $MgSO_4$ for margarine and vegetable oil spreads
- Sodium chloride
- Compressed nitrogen

Apparatus

- Saponification flask equipped with reflux condenser
- Bell jar filtration apparatus for margarine and vegetable oil spreads
- Liquid chromatograph
- Fluorescence detector (Ex λ 290, Em λ 330)
- Millipore filtration apparatus

Procedure

Vegetable, Fruit, and Meat Products

- Add 10 mL 6% (W/V) pyrogallol to sample weight, mix, and flush with N_2
- Heat at 70°C for 10 min with sonication
- Add 2 mL 60% KOH solution, mix and flush with N_2
- Digest for 30 min at 70°C under reflux
- Sonicate 5 min
- Cool to room temperature, add sodium chloride and water
- Extract with hexane (0.1% BHT) three times
- Add 0.5 g $MgSO_4$, mix

- Filter through Millipore filtration apparatus (0.45 μm)
- Dilute to volume with hexane
- Inject 20 μL

Margarine and Vegetable Oil Spreads

- Add 40 mL hexane (0.1% BHT) to 10 g sample and mix
- Add 3 g $MgSO_4$, mix, let stand ≥ 2 h
- Filter and dilute combined filtrate to volume with hexane (0.1% BHT)
- Inject 20 μL

Chromatography

Column	25 cm × 4.6 mm
Stationary phase	LiChrosorb Si60, 5 μm
Mobile phase	0.9% isopropanol in hexane
Column temperature	Ambient
Flow	1 mL/min
Injection	20 μL
Detector	Fluorescence, Ex λ = 290, Em λ = 330
Calculation	External standard, peak area, linear regression

Special Comments

- Determine tocopherol recovery for each food product
- Sample weight may vary between 1 to 10 g depending on oil content and vitamin level, with lipid content of the sample at less than 0.2 g
- Prior to hexane extraction add water if necessary to reduce alcohol below 30%, V/V
- For some food products such as raw shrimp, raw chicken, raw fish, it is necessary to blend with sea-sand (hexane washed) to prevent clumping and aid in KOH digestion
- For margarine and vegetable oil spreads the amount of $MgSO_4$ added varies, depending on water content, 1 g for each g water plus 1 g excess
- For vegetable oil spreads containing ≥ 50% fat, blend product at room temperature to prevent separation of water and fat prior to weighing sample

---

University of Georgia Protocol, *Peanut Sci.,* 20, 21, 1993; *Am. Oil Chem. Soc.,* 70, 633, 1993; *Nutr., Lipids, Health Dis,* chap. 37, 1995

Vitamin E Content of Margarine and Reduced Fat Products Using a Simplified Extraction Procedure and HPLC Determination

Liquid Chromatographic Method

Principle

- Tocopherol is extracted in hexane with anhydrous magnesium sulfate added to remove water. Vitamin E is quantitated by normal-phase LC with fluorescent detection (Ex λ = 290, Em λ = 330).

Reagents and Solvents

- 0.1% BHT in hexane for extraction
- Isopropanol
- $MgSO_4$

- α-, γ-, and δ-tocopherol standards
- Polyoxyethylene sorbitan monooleate (Tween 80)

Apparatus

- Bell jar filtration apparatus
- Liquid chromatograph
- Sonicator
- Fluorescence detector

Procedure

Sample Preparation and Extraction

- Weigh 5.0 g margarine or spread
- Add 40 mL hexane (0.1% BHT)
- Sonicate
- Rinse flask with 10 mL hexane (0.1% BHT)
- Add 3 drops of Tween 80
- Add 3 g MgSO$_4$
- Let stand ≥ 2 h
- Filter
- Quantitatively transfer filtrate to 100 mL volumetric flask
- Dilute to volume with hexane (0.1% BHT)
- Transfer 1.0 mL to 50 mL volumetric flask
- Dilute to volume with hexane (0.1% BHT)
- Inject extract

Chromatography

Column	25 cm × 4.6 mm
Stationary phase	LiChrosorb Si 60, 5 μm
Mobile phase	0.9% isopropanol in hexane
Column temperature	Ambient
Flow	0.9 mL/min
Injection	20 μL
Detector	Fluorescence, Ex λ = 290, Em λ = 330
Calculation	External standard, peak area, linear regression

J. Liq. Chromatogr. Rel. Technol., 21, 1227, 1998

3.5   REFERENCES

Text

1. Friedrich, W., Vitamin E, in *Vitamins,*.Walter de Gruyter, Berlin, 1988, chap. 4.
2. Sokol, R. J., Vitamin E, in *Present Knowledge in Nutrition,* 7th ed., Ziegler, E. E. and Filer, L. J., Jr., Eds., ILSI Press, Washington, D.C., 1996, chap. 13.
3. Rader, D. J. and Brewer, H. B., Abetalipoproteinemia—new insights into lipoprotein assembly and vitamin E metabolism from a rare genetic disease, *JAMA,* 270, 865, 1993.
4. Ouahchi, K., Arita, M., Kayden, H., Hentati, F., Ben Hamida, M., Sukol, R., Arai, H., Inoue, K., Mandel, J. L., and Koenig, M., Ataxia with isolated vitamin E deficiency is caused by mutations in the α-tocopherol transfer protein, *Nat. Genet.,* 9, 141, 1995.

5. Olson, R. E. and Munson, P. L., Fat-soluble vitamins, in *Principles of Pharmacology,* Munson, P. L., Mueller, R. A., and Breese, G. R., Eds., Chapman and Hall, New York, 1994, chap. 58.

6. Gibson, R. S., Assessment of the status of vitamins A, D, and E, in *Principles of Nutrition Assessment,* Oxford University Press, New York, 1990, chap. 18.

7. Murphy, S. P., Subar, A. F., and Block, G., Vitamin E intakes and sources in the United States, *Am. J. Clin. Nutr.,* 52, 361, 1990.

8. Block, G. and Langseth, L., Antioxidant vitamins and disease prevention, *Food Technol.,* 48, 80, 1994.

9. Eitenmiller, R. R., Vitamin E content of fats and oils— nutritional implications, *Food Technol.,* 51, 78, 1997.

10. Block, G., The data support a role for antioxidants in reducing cancer risk, *Nutr. Rev.,* 50, 207, 1992.

11. Packer, L. and Fuchs, J., *Vitamin E in Health and Disease,* Marcel Dekker, New York, 1993, chap. 1.

12. Diplock, A. T., Antioxidants and disease prevention, *Molec. Aspects Med.,* 15, 293, 1994.

13. Kritchevsky, D., Antioxidant vitamins in the prevention of cardiovascular disease, *Nutr. Today,* 27, 30, 1992.

14. Stampfer, M. J., Hennekens, C. H., Manson, J. E., Colditz, G. A., Rosner, B., and Willett, W. C., Vitamin E consumption and the risk of coronary heart disease in women, *N. Engl. J. Med.,* 328, 1444, 1993.

15. Rimm, E. B., Stampfer, M. J., Ascherio, A., Giovannucci, E., Colditz, G. A., and Willett, W. C., Vitamin E consumption and the risk of coronary heart disease in men, *N. Engl. J. Med.,* 328, 1450, 1993.

16. Block, G., Patterson, B., and Subar, A., Fruit, vegetable and cancer prevention: a review of the epidemiological evidence, *Nutr. Cancer,* 18, 1, 1992.

17. Blot, W. J., Li, J. Y., Taylor, P. R., Guo, W., Dawsey, S., Wang, G. Q., Yang, C. S., Zheng, S. F., Gail, M., Li, G. Y., Yu, Y., Liu, B., Tangrea, J., Sun, Y. H., Liu, R., Fraumeni, J. F., Zhang, Y. H., and Li, B., Nutrition intervention trials in Linxian, China: supplementation with specific vitamin/mineral combinations, cancer incidence and disease-specific mortality in the general population. *J. Natl. Cancer Inst.,* 1483, 1993.

18. Knekt, P., Heliovaara, M., Rissanen, A., Aromaa, A., and Aaran, R. K., Serum antioxidant vitamins and risk of cataract, *Br. Med. J.,* 305, 1392, 1992.

19. Sano, M., Ernesto, C., Thomas, R., Klauber, M., Schafer, K., Grundman, M., Woodbury, P., Growdon, J., Cotman, C., Pfeiffer, E., Schneider, L., and Thal, L., A controlled trial of selegiline, alpha-tocopherol, or both as treatment for Alzheimer's disease, *N. Engl. J. Med.,* 336, 1216, 1997.

20. National Research Council, *Recommended Dietary Allowances,* 10th ed., National Academy of Sciences, Washington, D.C., 1989, chap. 7.

21. Cheesemen, K. H., Holley, A. E., Kelley, F. J., Wasil, M., Hughes, L., and Burton, G., Biokinetics in humans of RRR-α-tocopherol: the free phenol, acetate ester, and succinate ester forms of vitamin E, *Free Rad. Biol. Med.,* 19, 591, 1995.

22. Pryor, W. A., *Vitamin E Abstracts,* VERSIS, The Vitamin E Research and Information Service, LaGrange, IL, 1995, p. VII.

23. Traber, M. G. and Kayden, H. J., Preferential incorporation of α-tocopherol vs. γ-tocopherol in human lipoproteins, *Am. J. Clin. Nutr.,* 49, 517, 1989.

24. Traber, M. G., Carpentier, Y. A., Kayden, H. J., Richelle, M., Galeano, N., and Deckelbaum, R. J., Alterations in plasma α- and γ-tocopherol concentrations in response to intravenous infusion of lipid emulsions in humans, *Metabolism,* 42, 701, 1993.

25. Bieri, J. G. and Evarts, R., Tocopherols and fatty acids in American diets, *J. Am. Diet. Assoc.,* 62, 147, 1973.

26. Horwitt, M. K., Status of human requirements for vitamin E, *Am. J. Clin. Nutr.,* 27, 1182, 1974.

27. Witting, L. A. and Lee, L., Dietary levels of vitamin E and polyunsaturated fatty acids and plasma vitamin E, *Am. J. Clin. Nutr.,* 28, 571, 1975.

28. Sokol, R. J., Vitamin E, in *Present Knowledge in Nutrition,* 7th ed., Ziegler, E. E. and Filer, J. J., Jr., Eds., ILSI Press, Washington, D.C., 1996, chap. 13.

29. Yamaoka, M., Carrillo, M. J. H., Nakahara, T., and Komiyama, K., Antioxidative activities of tocotrienols on phospholipid liposomes, *JAOCS,* 68, 2, 1991.

30. Qureshi, A. A., Burger, W. C., Peterson, D. M., and Elson, C. E., The structure of an inhibitor of cholesterol biosynthesis isolated from barley, *J. Biol. Chem.,* 261, 10544, 1986.

31. Qureshi, A. A., Qureshi, N., Wright, J. J. K., Shen, S., Kramer, G., Gabor, A., Chong, Y. H., DeWitt, G., Ong, A. S. H., Peterson, D., and Bradlow, B. A., Lowering of serum cholesterol in hypercholesterolemic humans by tocotrienols (palmvitee), *Am. J. Clin. Nutr.,* 53, 1021, 1991.

32. Tan, D. T. S., Knor, R. T., Low, W. H. S., Ali, A., and Gapor, A., The effect of palm oil vitamin E concentrate on the serum and lipoprotein lipids in humans, *Am. J. Clin. Nutr.,* 53, 1027, 1991.

33. Pearce, B. C., Parker, R. A., Deason, M. E., Qureshi, A. A., and Wright, J. J. K., Hypocholerolemic activity of synthetic and natural tocotrienols, *J. Med. Chem.,* 35, 3595, 1992.

34. Gould, M. N., Hang, J. D., Kennan, W. S., Tanner, M. A., and Elson, C. E., A comparison of tocopherol and tocotrienol for the chemo-prevention of chemically induced rat mammary tumors, *Am. J. Clin. Nutr.,* 53, 1068S, 1991.

35. Kato, A., Yamaoka, M., Tanaka, A., Komiyama, K., and Umezawa, I., Physiological effect of tocotrienol, *J. Jpn. Oil Chem. Soc.,* 34, 375, 1985.

36. Ngah, W. Z. W., Jarien, Z., San, M. M., Marzuki, A., Top, G. M., Shamaan, N. A., and Kadir, K. A., Effect of tocotrienols on hepatocarcinogenesis induced by 2-acetylaminofluorene in rats, *Am. J. Clin. Nutr.,* 53, 1076s, 1991.

37. Elson, C. E. and Yu, S. G., The chemoprevention of cancer by mevalonate-derived constituents of fruits and vegetables, *J. Nutr.,* 124, 607, 1994.

38. Hendrich, S., Lee, K. W., Xu, X., Wang, H. J., and Murphy, P. A., Defining food components as new nutrients, *J. Nutr.,* 124, 1789S, 1994.

39. Ong, A. S. H., Natural sources of tocotrienols, in *Vitamin E in Health and Disease,* Packer, L. and Fuchs, J., Eds., Marcel Dekker, New York, 1993, chap. 1.

40. Ball, G. F. M., Chemical and biological nature of the fat-soluble vitamins, in *Fat-Soluble Vitamin Assays in Food Analysis,* Elsevier, New York, 1988, chaps. 2, 8.

41. Lang, J. K., Schillaci, M., and Irvin, B., Vitamin E, in *Modern Chromatographic Analysis of Vitamins,* 2nd ed., De Leenheer, A. P., Lambert, W. E., and Nelis, H. J., Eds., Marcel Dekker, New York, 1992, chap. 3.

42. Blott, A. D., and Woollard, D. C., Rapid determination of α-tocopheryl acetate in animal feeds by high-performance liquid chromatography, *J. Micronutr. Anal.,* 2, 259, 1986.

43. Woollard, D. C., Blott, A. D., and Indyk, H., Fluorometric detection of tocopheryl acetate and its use in the analysis of infant formulae, *J. Micronutr. Anal.,* 3, 1, 1987.

44. Balz, M. K., Schulte, E., and Thier, H. P., Simultaneous determination of α-tocopheryl acetate, tocopherols, and tocotrienols by HPLC with fluorescence detection in foods, *Fat. Sci. Technol.,* 95, 215, 1993.

45. Chase, G. W., Jr., Eitenmiller, R. R., and Long, A. P., Liquid chromatographic analysis of all-rac-α-tocopheryl acetate, tocopherols, and retinyl palmitate in Infant Formula SRM 1846, *J. Liq. Chromatogr. Rel. Technol.,* 20, 2317, 1997.

46. Thompson, J. N. and Hatina, G., Determination of tocopherols and tocotrienols in foods and tissues by high performance liquid chromatography, *J. Liq. Chromatogr.,* 2, 327, 1979.

47. Nelis, H. J., DeBevere, V. O. R. C., and De Leenheer, A. P., Vitamin E: tocopherols and tocotrienols in *Modern Chromatographic Anaylsis of the Vitamins,* De Leenheer, A. P., Lambert, W. E., and DeRuyter, M. G. M., Marcel Dekker, New York, 1985, chap. 3.

48. Ball, G. F. M., Applications of HPLC to the determination of fat-soluble vitamins in foods and animal feeds, *J. Micronutr. Anal.,* 4, 255, 1988.

49. Bourgeois, C., *Determination of Vitamin E: Tocopherols and Tocotrienols,* Elsevier, New York, 1992, 21.

50. Lumley, I. D., Vitamin analysis in foods, in *The Technology of Vitamins in Foods,* Chapman and Hall, New York, 1993, chap. 8.

51. Eitenmiller, R. R. and Landen, W. O., Jr., Vitamins, in *Analyzing Food for Nutrition Labeling and Hazardous Contaminants,* Jeon, I. J. and Ikins, W. G., Eds, Marcel Dekker, New York, 1995, chap. 9.

52. AOAC International, *Official Methods of Analysis,* 16th ed., AOAC International, Arlington, VA, 1995.

53. Davidek, J. and Velisek, J., Gas-liquid chromatography of vitamins in foods: the fat-soluble vitamins, *J. Micronutr. Anal.,* 2, 81, 1986.

54. Smidt, C. R., Jones, A.D, and Clifford, A. J., Gas chromatography of retinol and α-tocopherol without derivatization, *J. Chromatogr.,* 434, 21, 1988.

55. Ulberth, F., Simultaneous determination of vitamin E isomers and cholesterol by GLC, *J. High Res. Chromatogr.,* 14, 343, 1991.

56. Syväoja, E. L., Piironen, V., Varo, P., Koivistoinen, P., and Salminen, K., Tocopherols and tocotrienols in Finnish foods: human milk and infant formulas, *Int. J. Vit. Nutr. Res.,* 55, 159, 1985.

57. Piironen, V., Syväoja, E. L., Varo, P., Salminen, K., and Koivistoinen, P., Tocopherols and tocotrienols in Finnish foods: meat and meat products, *J. Agric. Food Chem.,* 33, 1215, 1985.

58. Hogarty, C. J., Ang., C., and Eitenmiller, R. R., Tocopherol content of selected foods by HPLC/fluorescence quantitation, *J. Food Comp. Anal.,* 2, 200, 1989.

59. Ueda, T. and Igarashi, O., Evaluation of the electrochemical detector for the determination of tocopherols in feeds by high-performance liquid chromatography, *J. Micronutr. Anal.,* 1, 31, 1985.

60. Indyk, H. E., Simplified saponification procedure for the routine determination of total vitamin E in dairy products, foods and tissues by high-performance liquid chromatography, *Analyst,* 113, 1217, 1988.

61. Ueda, T. and Igarashi, O., Determination of vitamin E in biological specimens and foods by HPLC–pretreatment of samples and extraction of tocopherols, *J. Micronutr. Anal.,* 7, 79, 1990.

62. Ueda, T. and Igarashi, O., New solvent system for extraction of tocopherols from biological specimens for HPLC determination and the evaluation of 2,2,5,7,8-pentamethyl-6-chromanol as an internal standard, *J. Micronutr. Anal.,* 3, 185, 1987.

63. Ueda, T. and Igarashi, O., Effect of coexisting fat on the extraction of tocopherols from tissues after saponifiation as a pretreatment for HPLC determination, *J. Micronutr. Anal.,* 3, 15, 1987.

64. Tuan, S., Lee, T. F., Chou, C. C., and Wei, Q. K., Determination of vitamin E homologues in infant formulas by HPLC using fluorometric detection, *J. Micronutr. Anal.,* 6, 35, 1989.

65. Hakansson, B., Jägerstad, M., and Öste, R., Determination of vitamin E in wheat products by HPLC, *J. Micronutr. Anal.,* 3, 307, 1987.

66. Landen, W. O., Jr., Application of gel permeation chromatography and nonaqueous reverse phase chromatography to high performance liquid chromatographic determination of retinyl palmitate and α-tocopheryl acetate in infant formulas, *J. Assoc. Off. Anal. Chem.,* 65, 810, 1982.

67. Landen, W. O., Hines, D. M., Jr., Hamill, T. W., Martin, J. I., Young, E. R., Eitenmiller, R. R., and Soliman, A. G. M., Vitamin A and vitamin E content of infant formulas produced in the United States, *J. Assoc. Off. Anal. Chem.,* 68, 509, 1985.

68. Tan, B. and Brzuskiewicz, L., Separation of tocopherol and tocotrienol isomers using normal- and reverse-phase liquid chromatography, *Anal. Biochem.,* 180, 368, 1989.

69. Abidi, S. L. and Mounts, T. L., Normal phase high-performance liquid chromatography of tocopherols on polar phases, *J. Liq. Chromatogr. Rel. Technol.,* 19, 509, 1996.

70. Piironen, V., Varo, P., Syväoja, E. L., Salminen, K., and Koivistoinen, P., High-performance liquid chromatographic determination of tocopherols and tocotrienols and its application to diets and plasma of Finnish men, *Int. J. Vit. Nutr. Res.,* 53, 35, 1984.

71. Piironen, V., Syväoja, E. L., Varo, P., Salminen, K., and Koivistoinen, P., Tocopherols and tocotrienols in Finnish foods: vegetables, fruits, and berries, *J. Agric. Food Chem.,* 34, 742, 1986.

72. Piironen, V., Syväoja, E. L., Varo, P., Salminen, K., and Koivistoinen, P., Tocopherols and tocotrienols in cereal products from Finland, *Cereal Chem.,* 63, 78, 1986.

73. Syväoja, E. L., Salminen, K., Piironen, V., Varo, P., Kerojoki, O., and Koivistoinen, P., Tocopherols and tocotrienols in Finnish foods: fish and fish products, *JAOCS,* 62, 1245, 1985.

74. Syväoja, E. L., Piironen, V., Varo, P., Koivistoinen, P., and Salminen, K., Tocopherols and tocotrienols in Finnish foods: oils and fats, *JAOCS,.* 63, 328, 1986.

75. Speek, A. J., Schrijver, J., and Schreurs, W. H. P., Vitamin E composition of some seed oils as determined by high-performance liquid chromatography with fluorometric detection, *J. Food Sci.,* 50, 121, 1985.

76. Rammell, C. G., and Hoogenboom, J. J. L., Separation of tocols by HPLC on an amino-cyano polar phase column, *J. Liq. Chromatogr.,* 8, 707, 1985.

77. Desai, I. D., Bhgavan, H., Salkeld, R., and Dutra De Oliveira, J. E., Vitamin E content of crude and refined vegetable oils in southern Brazil, *J. Food Comp. Anal.,* 1, 231, 1988.

78. Ang, C. Y. W., Searcy, G. K., and Eitenmiller, R. R., Tocopherols in chicken breast and leg muscles determined by reverse phase liquid chromatography, *J. Food Sci.,* 55, 1536, 1990.

79. Rogers, E. J., Rice, S. M., Nicolosi, R. J., Carpenter, D. R., McClelland, C. A., and Romancyzk, L. J., Identification and quantitation of γ-oryzanol components and simultaneous assessment of tocols in rice bran oil, *JAOCS.,* 70, 301, 1993.

80. Marero, L. M., Payumo, E. M., Aquinaldo, A. R., Homma, S., and Igarashi, O., Vitamin E constituents of weaning foods from germinated cereals and legumes, *J. Food Sci.,* 56, 270, 1991.

81. Miyagawa, K., Hirai, K., Takezoe, R., Tocopherol and fluorescence levels in deep-frying oil and their measurement for oil assessment, *JAOCS,* 68, 163, 1991.

82. Koprivnjak, J. F., Lum, K. R., Sisak, M. M., and Saborowski, R., Determination of α-, γ(+ β)-, and δ-tocopherols in a variety of liver tissues by reverse-phase high pressure liquid chromatography, *Comp. Biochem. Physiol.,* 113B, 143, 1996.

83. Cooper, J., Thadwal, R., and Cooper, M., Determination of vitamin E in human plasma by high-performance liquid chromatography, *J. Chromatogr. B,* 690, 355, 1997.

84. Chou, P. P., Jaynes, P. K., and Bailey, J. L., Determination of vitamin E in microsamples of serum by liquid chromatography with electrochemical detection, *Clin. Chem.,* 31, 880, 1985.

85. Pascoe, G. A., Duda, C. T., and Reed, D. J., Determination of α-tocopherol and γ-tocopherylquinone in small biological samples by high-performance liquid chromatography with electrochemical detection, *J. Chromatogr.,* 414, 440, 1987.

86. Murphy, M. E. and Kehrer, J. P., Simultaneous measurement of tocopherols and tocopheryl quinones in tissue fractions using high-performance liquid chromatography with redox-cycling electrochemical detection, *J. Chromatogr.,* 421, 71, 1987.

87. Lang, J. K. and Packer, L., Quantitative determination of vitamin E and oxidized and reduced coenzyme Q by high-performance liquid chromatography with in-line ultraviolet and electrochemical detection, *J. Chromatogr.,* 385, 109, 1987.

88. Chase, G. W., Jr., Akoh, C. C., and Eitenmiller, R. R., Analysis of tocopherols in vegetable oils by high-pressure liquid chromatography: comparison of fluorescence and evaporative light-scattering detection, *JAOCS,* 71, 877, 1994.

Table 3.3 UV and Fluorescence Properties of Vitamin E

1. Ball, G. F. M., Chemical and biological nature of the fat-soluble vitamins, in *Water-Soluble Vitamin Assays in Food Analysis,* Elsevier, New York, 1988, chap. 2.

2. Budavari, S., *The Merck Index,* 12th ed., Merck and Company, Whitehouse Station, N.J., 1996.

3. Mino, M., Nakamura, H., Diplock, A. T., and Kayden, H. J., *Vitamin E,* Japan Scientific Societies Press, Tokyo, 1993.

4. Machlin, L. J., Vitamin E, in *Handbook of Vitamins,* 2nd Ed., Marcel Dekker, New York 1991, chap. 3.

Table 3.4 Compendium, Handbook, and Regulatory Methods for Vitamin E Analysis

1. United States Pharmacopeial Convention, *U.S. Pharmacopeia National Formulary,* USP 23/NF 18, Nutritional Supplements, Official Monographs, United States Pharmacopeial Convention, Rockville, MD, 1995.

2. Scottish Home and Health Department, *British Pharmacopoeia,* 15th ed., British Pharmacopoeic Commission, United Kingdom, 1993.

3. AOAC International, *Official Methods of Anaysis,* 16th ed., AOAC International, Arlington, VA, 1995.

4. Ames, S. T., Determination of vitamin E in foods and feeds—a collaborative study, *J. Assoc. Off. Anal. Chem.,* 54, 1, 1971.

5. Ames, S. R. and Drury, E. E., Identification of δ- or α-tocopherol in pharmaceuticals, food supplements, or feed supplements: a collaborative study, *J. Assoc. Off. Anal. Chem.,* 58, 585, 1975.

6. Labadie, M. P. and Boufford, C. G., Gas chromatographic assay of supplemental vitamin E acetate concentrates: collaborative study, *J. Assoc. Off. Anal. Chem.,* 71, 1168, 1988.

7. Association of Official Analytical Chemists, Changes in methods: vitamins and other nutrients, *J. Assoc. Off. Anal. Chem.,* 61, 475, 1978.

8. Tanner, J. T., Barnett, S. A., and Mountford, M. K., Analysis of milk-based infant formula. Phase V. Vitamins A and E, folic acid, and pantothenic acid: Food and Drug Administration - Infant Formula Council: collaborative study, *J. AOAC Int.,* 76, 399, 1993.

9. American Feed Ingredients Association, *Laboratory Methods Compendium,* Vol. I: *Vitamins and Minerals,* American Feed Ingredients Association, West Des Moines, IA, 197, 1991.

10. Cort, W. M., Vincente, T. S., Waysek, E. H., and Williams, B. D., Vitamin E content of feedstuffs determined by high-performance liquid chromatographic fluorescence, *J. Agric. Food Chem.,* 31, 1330, 1983.

11. Keller, H. E., *Analytical Methods for Vitamins and Carotenoids,* Hoffmann-LaRoche, Basel, 12, 1988.

12. Manz, U. and Philippi, K., A method for the routine determination of tocopherols in animal feed and human foodstuffs with the aid of high performance liquid chromatography, *Int. J. Vit. Nutr. Res.,* 51, 342, 1981.

13. Committee on Food Chemicals Codex, *Food Chemicals Codex,* 4th ed., National Academy Press, Washington, D.C., 417, 1996.

14. Brubacher, G., Müller-Mulot, W., and Southgate, D.A.T., *Methods for the Determination of Vitamins in Food,* Elsevier, New York, chaps. 8, 9, 1985.

Table 3.5   HPLC Methods for the Analysis of Vitamin E in Foods, Feeds, Pharmaceuticals, and Biologicals

Food

1. Speek, A. J., Schrijver, J., and Schreurs, W.H.P., Vitamin E composition of some seed oils as determined by high-performance liquid chromatography with fluorometric detection, *J. Food Sci.,* 50, 121, 1985.

2. Syväoja, E. L., Piironen, V., Vara, P., Koivistoinen, P., and Salminen, K., Tocopherols and tocotrienols in Finnish foods: oils and fats, *JAOCS,* 63, 328, 1986.

3. Desai, I. D., Bhagavan, H., Salkeld, R., and Dutra De Oliveira, J. E., Vitamin E content of crude and refined vegetable oils in southern Brazil, *J. Food Comp. Anal.,* 1, 231, 1988.

4. Rogers, E., Rice, S. M., Nicolosi, R. J., Carpenter, D. R., McClelland, C. A., and Romanczyk, L. J., Identification and quantitation of γ-oryzanol components and simultaneous assessment of tocols in rice bran oil, *JAOCS,*. 70, 301, 1993.

5. Chase, G. W., Jr., Akoh, C. C., and Eitenmiller, R. R., Analysis of tocopherols in vegetable oils by high-performance liquid chromatography: comparison of fluorescence and evaporative light-scattering detection, *JAOCS,* 71, 877, 1994.

6. Dionisi, F., Prodolliet, J., and Tagliaferri, E., Assessment of olive oil adulteration by reversed-phase high performance liquid chromatography/amperometric detection of tocopherols and tocotrienols, *JAOCS,* 72, 1505, 1995.

7. Gorden, M. H. and Kourjmska, L., Effect of antioxidants on losses of tocopherols during deep-fat frying, *Food Chem.,* 52, 175, 1995.

8. Woollard, D. C. and Blott, A. D., The routine determination of vitamin E acetate in milk powder formulations using high-performance liquid chromatography, *J. Micronutr. Anal.,* 2, 97, 1986.

9. Tuan, S., Lee, T. F., Chou, C. C., and Wei, Q. K., Determination of vitamin E homologues in infant formulas by HPLC using fluorometric detection, *J. Micronutr. Anal.,* 6, 35, 1989.

10. Indyk, H. E., Simplified saponification procedure for the routine determination of total vitamin E in dairy products, foods, and tissues by high-performance liquid chromatography, *Analyst,* 113, 1217, 1988.

11. Tanner, J. T., Barnett, S. A., and Mountford, M. K., Analysis of milk based infant formula. Phase V. Vitamins A and E, folic acid, and pantothenic acid: Food and Dairy Administration—Infant Formula Council: collaborative study, *J. AOAC Int.,*. 76, 399, 1993.

12. Thompson, J. N. and Hatina, G., Determination of tocopherols and tocotrienols in foods and tissues by high performance liquid chromatography, *J. Liq. Chromatogr.,* 2, 327, 1979.

13. Hogarty, C. J., Ang, C., and Eitenmiller, R., Tocopherol content of selected foods by HPLC/fluorescence quantitation, *J. Food Comp. Anal.,* 2, 200, 1989.

14. Piironen, V., Varo, P., Syväoja, E. L., Salminen, K., and Koivistoinen, P., High performance liquid chromatographic determination of tocopherols and tocotrienols and its application to diets and plasma of Finnish men, I. Analytical method, *Int. J. Vit. Nutr. Res.,* 53, 35, 1984.

15. Piironen, V., Varo, P., Syväoja, E. L., Salminen, K., Koivistoinen, P., and Arvilommi, H., High-performance liquid chromatographic determination of tocopherols and tocotrienols and its application to diets and plasma of Finnish men, II. Applications, *Int. J. Vit. Nutr. Res.,* 53, 41, 1984.

16. Piironen, V., Syväoja, E. L., Varo, P., Salminen, K., and Koivistoinen, P., Tocopherols and tocotrienols in Finnish foods: meat and meat products, *J. Agric. Food Chem.*, 33, 1215, 1985.

17. Syväoja, E. L., Salminen, K., Piironen, V., Varo, P., Kerojoki, D., and Koivistoinen, P., Tocopherols and tocotrienols in Finnish foods: fish and fish products, *JAOCS*, 62, 1245, 1985.

18. Syväoja, E. L., Piironen, V., Varo, P., Koivistoinen, P., and Salminen, K., Tocopherols and tocotrienols in Finnish foods: human milk and infant formulas, *Int. J. Vit. Nutr. Res.*, 55, 159, 1985.

19. Piironen, V., Syväoja, E. L., Varo, P., Salminen, K., and Koivistoinen, P., Tocopherols and tocotrienols in Finnish foods: vegetables, fruits and berries, *J. Agric. Food Chem.*, 34, 742, 1986.

20. Piironen, V., Syväoja, E. L., Varo, P., Salminen, K., and Koivistoinen, P., Tocopherols and tocotrienols in cereal products from Finland, *Cereal Chem.*, 63, 78, 1986.

21. Piironen, V., Varo, P., and Koivistoinen, P., Stability of tocopherols and tocotrienols in food preparation procedures, *J. Food Comp. Anal.*, 1, 53, 1987.

22. Piironen, V., Varo, P., and Koivistoinen, P., Stability of tocopherols and tocotrienols during storage of foods, *J. Food Comp. Anal.*, 1, 124, 1988.

23. Ang, C. Y. W., Searcy, G. K., and Eitenmiller, R. R., Tocopherols in chicken breast and leg muscles determined by reverse phase liquid chromatography, *J. Food Sci.*, 55, 1536, 1990

24. Yao, F., Dull, G., and Eitenmiller, R. R., Tocopherol quantification by HPLC in pecans and relationship to kernel quality during storage, *J. Food Sci.*, 57, 1194, 1992.

25. Hashim, I. B., Koehler, P. E., Eitenmiller, R. R., and Kvien, C. K., Fatty acid composition and tocopherol content of drought stressed Florunner peanuts, *Peanut Sci.*, 20, 21, 1993.

26. Hashim, I. B., Koehler, P. E., and Eitenmiller, R. R., Tocopherols in Runner and va peanut cultivars at various maturity stages, *JAOCS*, 70, 633, 1993.

27. Lehmann, J . W., Putnam, D. H., and Qureshi, A.A., Vitamin E isomers in grain Amaranths (*Amaranthus spp.*), *Lipids*, 29, 177, 1994.

28. Balz, M. K., Schulte, E., and Thier, H. P., Simultaneous determination of α-tocopheryl acetate, tocopherols and tocotrienols by HPLC with fluorescence detection in foods, *Fat Sci. Technol.*, 95, 215, 1993.

29. Ueda, T. and Igarashi, O., Evaluation of the electrochemical detector for the determination of tocopherols in feeds by high performance liquid chromatography,. *J. Micronutr. Anal.*, 1, 31, 1985.

30. Blott, A. D. and Woollard, D. C., Rapid determination of α-tocopheryl acetate in animal feeds by high performance liquid chromatography, *J. Micronutr. Anal.*, 2, 259, 1986.

31. Analytical Methods Committee, Royal Society of Chemistry, Determination of vitamin E in animal feedstuffs by high performance liquid chromatography, *Analyst*, 116, 421, 1991.

Biologicals

1. Sarzanini, C., Mentasti, E., Vincenti, M., Nerva, M., and Gaido, F., Determination of plasma tocopherols by high-performance liquid chromatography with coulometric detection, *J. Chromatogr.*, 620, 268, 1993.

2. Ueda, T., Ichikawa, H., and Igarashi, O., Determination of α-tocopherol stereoisomers in biological specimens using chiral phase high performance liquid chromatography, *J. Nutr. Sci. Vitaminol.*, 39, 207, 1993.

3. Gonzalez-Corbella, M. J., Lloberas-Blanch, N., Castellote-Bargallo, A. I., Lopez-Sabater, M. C., and Rivero-Urgell, M., Determination of α-tocopherol in plasma and erythrocytes by high performance liquid chromatography, *J. Chromatogr. B*, 660, 395, 1994.

4. Wakabayashi, H., Yamato, S., Nakajima, M., and Shimada, K., Simultaneous determination of oxidized and reduced coenzyme Q and α-tocopherol in biological samples by high performance liquid chromatography with platinum catalyst reduction and electrochemical detection, *Biol. Pharm. Bull.*, 17, 997, 1994.

5. Torrado, S., Caballero, E. R., Cardonniga, R., and Torrado, J., A selective liquid chromatography assay for the determination of dl-α-tocopherol acetate in plasma samples, *.J. Liq. Chromatogr.*, 18, 1251, 1995.

6. Koprivnjak, J. F., Lum, K. R., Sisak, M. M., and Saborowski, R., Determination of α-, γ (+ β)-, and δ-tocopherols in a variety of liver tissues by reverse-phase high pressure liquid chromatography, *Comp. Biochem. Physiol.,* 113B, 143, 1996.

7. Cooper, J., Thadwal, R., and Cooper, M., Determination of vitamin E in human plasma by high-performance liquid chromatography, *J. Chromatogr. B,.* 690, 355, 1997.

8. Kramer, J. K. G., Blais, L., Fouchard, R. C., Melnyk, R. A., and Kallury,K. M. R., A rapid method for the determination of vitamin E forms in tissues and diets by high-performance liquid chromatography using a normal-phase diol column, *Lipids,* 32, 323, 1997.

4 Vitamin K

4.1 REVIEW

The existence and basic function of vitamin K was determined in the 1930s through the efforts of several research groups. Original observations by Dam in Denmark showed that chicks developed blood with poor clotting properties along with hemorrhages when fed diets extracted with ether. Addition of the ether extract back into the diet improved the condition of the chicks. Dam named the fat-soluble, antihemorrhagic factor vitamin K from the word "koagulation." Vitamin K was isolated by Dam from alfalfa and identified as 2-methyl-3-phytyl-1,4-naphthoquinone. The designation K_1 was given along with the generic name "phylloquinone." Vitamin K_2, the menaquinone-n (Mk-n) form, was crystallized from bacterial fermented fishmeal by Doisy. The menaquinones are 2-methyl-1,4-naphthoquinones substituted at position -3 with an unsaturated isoprenyl sidechain of varying numbers of isoprenoid units. Doisy synthesized vitamin K_1 in 1939. In 1943, Dam and Doisy received Nobel Prizes for their work on the discovery of vitamin K (Dam) and its synthesis (Doisy).[1]

In the human, vitamin K deficiency commonly occurs in the newborn and is named hemorrhagic disease. The deficiency is not due to poor nutriture of the mother, but to poor placental transfer and absence of bacterial synthesis in the newborn's gut.[2] The deficiency is characterized by low plasma prothrombin concentrations resulting from the lack of biosynthesis of prothrombin by the immature liver and the lack of vitamin K. Hemorrhagic disease produces bleeding in the skin, subcutaneous tissue, GI tract, umbilical cord, and intracranium. Central nervous system damage occurs and the deficiency is often fatal.[3] Hemorrhagic disease is prevented by intramuscular injection of vitamin K_1 at birth. Breast fed infants are more likely to develop hemorrhagic disease than formula fed infants because human milk is low in vitamin K content. Infant formula is fortified at a minimum level of 4 μg per serving specified by the Infant Formula Act of 1980.[4]

Deficiency of vitamin K in the adult is rare. When it does occur, the deficiency results from fat malabsorption syndromes, liver disease, and antibiotic therapy that inhibits microbial vitamin K_2 synthesis in the gut. Anticoagulant treatment with coumarin and related compounds produces a functional or secondary vitamin K deficiency through disruption of the vitamin K cycle and inhibition of the synthesis of vitamin K dependent blood clotting proteins in the liver. Defective coagulation of the blood measured by a one-stage prothrombin time (PT) is still used to assess vitamin K status. Other biochemical markers, including quantitation of proteins induced by vitamin K deficiency (PIVKA-II), provide sensitivity to determine infants at risk for hemorrhagic disease.[5]

Information on the vitamin K content of the food supply has been greatly improved through research conducted by Sadowski and colleagues during the 1990s.[6–16] This work not only provided methodology necessary to accurately measure vitamin K_1 in foods, but presents usable food composition tables[9] and information on vitamin K_1 intake.[15] Table 4.1 summarizes vitamin K_1 intake in women's diets collected from the 1990 Food and Drug Administration Total Diet Study.[15] Major top five contributors of vitamin K were spinach, collards, broccoli, iceberg lettuce, and coleslaw with dressing. Addition of fats and oils to mixed dishes and desserts was considered an important source of vitamin K_1 in the American diet.

Leafy, green vegetables, certain legumes, and vegetable oils are considered good sources of vitamin K_1[17] Milk and dairy products, meats, eggs, cereals, fruits, and vegetables are considered low but consistent, and significant sources of vitamin K to the American diet.[18] The Recommended Dietary Allowances (RDAs) range from 5 μg/day for the infant up to 6-months of age to 80 μg/day for the adult male. The RDA for pregnant and lactating females is 65 μg/day.[18] Booth et al.[15] recently estimated that 25 to 30 year-old men and women consumed 66 μg and 59 μg per day of

TABLE 4.1

Major Contributors of Vitamin K$_1$ in Women's Diets: Data from the 1990 Total Diet Study[a]

Rank/Food Description	Vitamin K$_1$	
	% of Total	% Cumulative
1. Spinach, fresh/frozen, boiled	13.1	13.1
2. Collards, fresh/frozen, boiled	11.9	25.0
3. Broccoli, fresh/frozen, boiled	9.8	34.8
4. Iceberg lettuce, raw	6.9	41.7
5. Coleslaw with dressing, homemade	5.6	47.3
6. French salad dressing, regular	3.2	50.5
7. Cabbage, fresh, boiled	3.0	53.5
8. Green beans, fresh/frozen, boiled	2.3	55.8
9. Brussels sprouts, fresh/frozen, boiled	2.3	58.1
10. Green peas, fresh/frozen, boiled	2.1	60.2
11. Margarine, stick, regular	1.9	62.1
12. Tuna, canned in oil, drained	1.6	63.7
13. Beef chow mein, carryout	1.5	65.2
14. Asparagus, fresh/frozen, boiled	1.5	66.7
15. Mayonnaise, regular, bottled	1.4	68.1
16. Carrots, fresh, boiled	1.2	69.3
17. Eggs, scrambled	1.1	70.4
18. Apple pie, fresh/frozen, commercial	1.1	71.5
19. Taco/tostada, carryout	1.1	72.6
20. Mashed potatoes from flakes	1.0	73.6

[a]Reproduced with permission from Reference 15.

vitamin K$_1$. These levels are below recommended levels.[15] Six-month old infants had a daily intake of 77 μg/day, of which fortified infant formulas contributed 87% of the vitamin K$_1$. Throughout adulthood, vitamin K intake was above the RDA, except for the 25 to 30 year-old segment. All intakes were below 90 μg/day.[15] A Reference Daily Intake (RDI) has not been established by the Food and Drug Administration for use on nutritional labels.[19]

Metabolically, vitamin K participates in the carboxylation of glutamate to d-carboxyglutamic acid (Gla). At this time, six vitamin K-dependent proteins including prothrombin (factor II), factors VII, IX, X, protein C, and protein S have been identified as factors required for blood coagulation. Other vitamin K-dependent proteins have been identified in skeletal tissue, including osteocalcin, which most likely participates in bone mineralization. Gla is present in various other tissues; however, roles for such vitamin K-dependent proteins are not clearly understood.[2]

4.2 PROPERTIES

4.2.1 CHEMISTRY

4.2.1.1 General Properties

Chemically, vitamin K$_1$ refers to 2-methyl-1,4-naphthoquinone and all derivatives providing the antihemorrhagic activity of vitamin K$_1$, phylloquinone.[20] Figure 4.1 shows the structure of 2-methyl-1,4-naphthoquinone which is the synthetic and simplest form of vitamin K, known as menadione, or vitamin K$_3$ (Mk-o). Menadione (Figure 4.1) is the correct name for the compound which was formerly called "menaquinone." This synthetic form of vitamin K is still designated vitamin K$_3$.

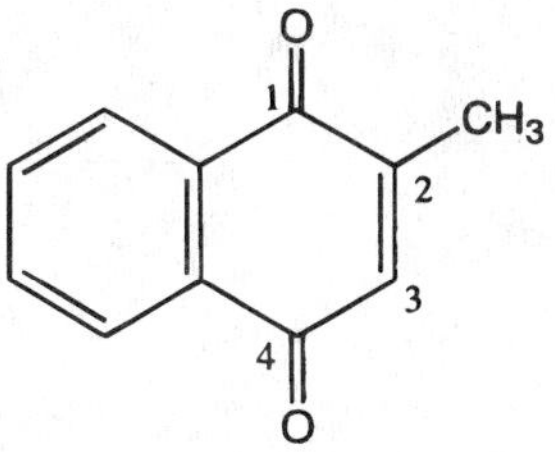

Menadione

2-methyl-1,4 naphthoquinone

MK-O, Vitamin K_3

FIGURE 4.1   Structure of menadione.

Phyloquinones or vitamin K_1 compounds (Figure 4.2) are produced by plants. Alkylation at position -3 of the 2-methyl-1,4-naphthoquinone ring with five-carbon isoprenoid units produces the vitamin K series found in nature. $K_{1(20)}$, the most common phylloquinone, contains four isoprenoid units—three of which are reduced. The reduced sidechain or "phytyl" sidechain with one double bond characterizes the phylloquinones. Phylloquinones are, therefore, classified chemically as 2-methyl-3-phytyl-1,4-naphthoquinones. USP designates vitamin K_1 as phytonadione. USP phytonadione is a mixture of E and Z isomers containing not more than 21% Z isomers. Natural phylloquinone is 2'-E,7'R and 11'R.[1]

Vitamin K compounds of the menaquinone-n series (MK-n) (Figure 4.2) have polyisoprenyl side chains at position -3. Such compounds are synthesized by bacteria and not by plants. Side chains are unsaturated and usually contain from 4 to 13 prenyl groups. The MK-n designation indicates the number of prenyl groups in the side chain. One or more of the isoprene units might be hydrogenated,[1] usually at the second isoprenoid unit from the naphthoquinone nucleus.

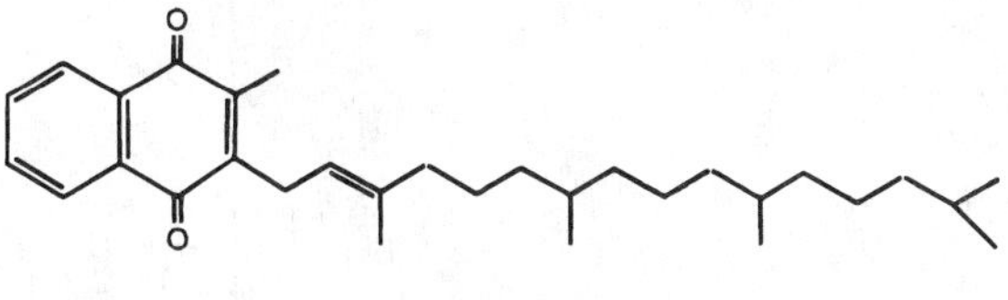

Phylloquinone

2-methyl-3-phytyl-1,4-naphthoquinone

Vitamin K_1

$K_{1\ (20)}$

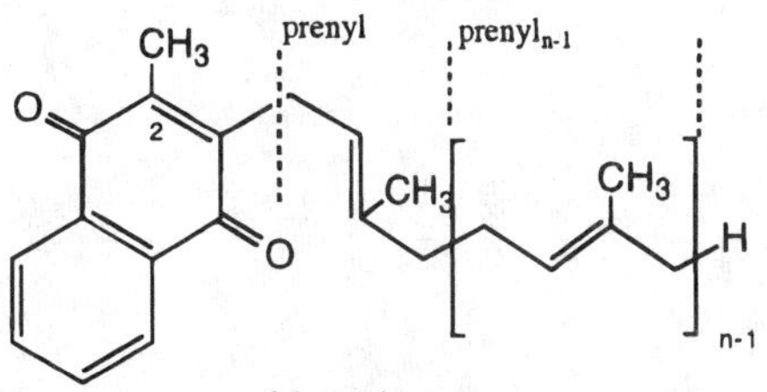

Menaquinone-n

2-methyl-3-multiprenyl-1,4-naphthoquinone (Class)

Vitamin K_2

MK-n

n=10; $K_{2(50)}$

n= 6; $K_{2(30)}$

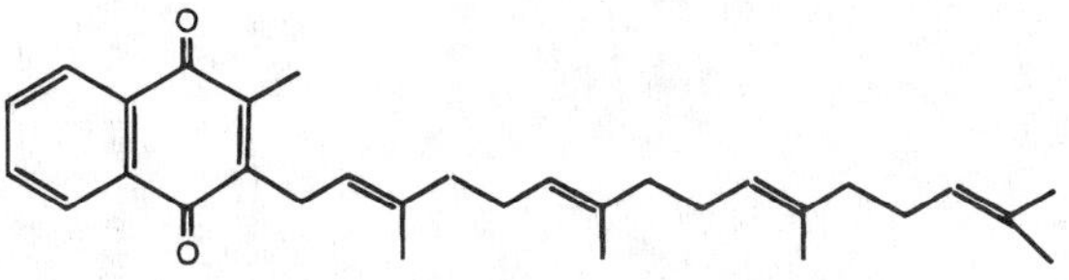

Menaquinone-4

Vitamin K_2

MK-n

2-methyl-3-tetraprenyl-1,4-naphthoquinone

FIGURE 4.2   Structures of phylloquinone (vitamin $K_{1(20)}$) and menaquinones (vitamin K_2 or Mk-4).

TABLE 4.2
Physical Properties of Vitamin K

Substance[a]	Molar Mass	Formula	Solubility	Melting Point °C	Crystal Form	Spectral Properties[b] λ max nm	Spectral Properties[b] $E^{1\%}_{1\,cm}$	Spectral Properties[b] $\varepsilon \times 10^{-3}$
Phylloquinone (Vitamin K$_1$) CAS No. 84-80-0 7536	450.71	$C_{31}H_{46}O_2$	Sparingly soluble in methanol. Soluble in ethanol, acetone, benzene, petroleum ether, hexane, CHCl$_3$, ether	—	none / yellow oil	242 248 260 269 325	396 419 383 387 68	[17.9] [18.9] [17.3] [17.4] [3.1]
Menaquinone-4 5876 Vitamin K$_1$ Mk-4	444.70	$C_{31}H_{40}O_2$		35	yellow crystals	248	439	[19.5]
Menaquinone-6 5876 Vitamin K$_2$ Mk-6	580.0	$C_{41}H_{56}O_2$		50	yellow crystals	243 248 261 270 325–328	304 320 290 292 53	[17.6] [18.6] [16.8] [16.9] [3.1]
Menaquinone-7 5876 Vitamin K$_2$ Mk-7	649.0	$C_{46}H_{64}O_2$		54	micro-yellow crystalline plates	243 248 261 270 325–328	278 195 266 467 53	[18.0] [19.1] [17.3] [30.3] [3.1]
Menadione (Vitamin K$_3$) CAS No. 58-27-5 5874	172.18	$C_{11}H_8O_2$	Insoluble in water Moderately soluble in CHCl$_3$	105–107	bright yellow crystals	325–328	48	[3.1]

[a] Common or generic name; CAS No.—Chemical Abstract Service number; bold print designates the Merck Index monograph number.

[b] In petroleum ether; values in brackets are calculated from corresponding $E^{1\%}_{1\,cm}$ values.

Budavari, S., *The Merck Index*, 12th ed., 1996.

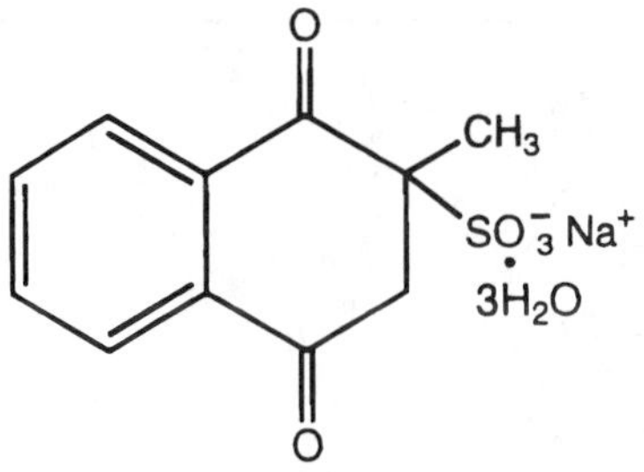

Menadione Sodium Bisulfite
MSB

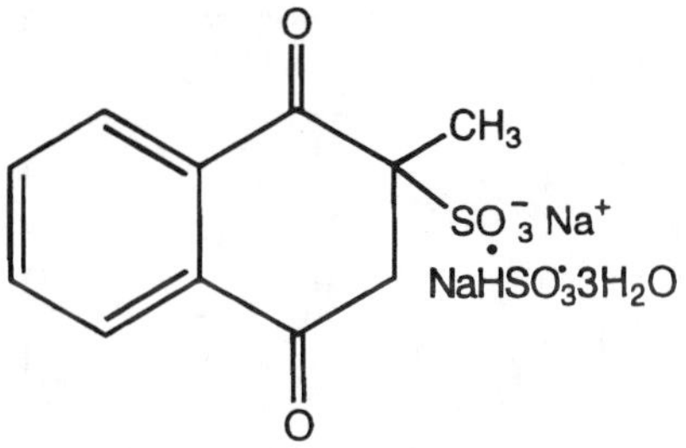

Menadione Sodium Bisulfite Complex
MSBC

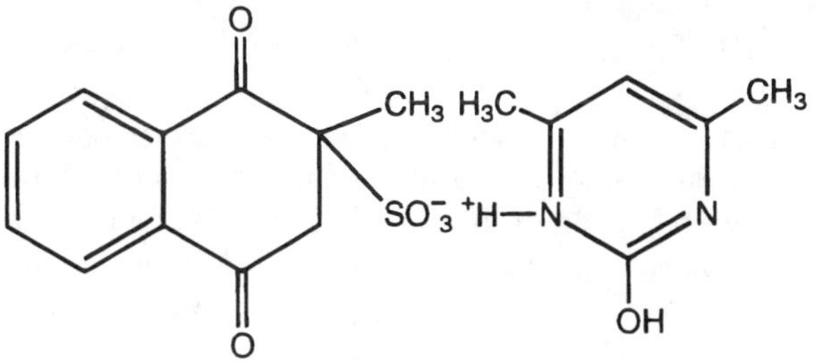

Menadione Dimethylpyrimidinol Bisulfite
MPB

Figure 4.3 Water-soluble menadione forms.

Physical properties of phylloquinone, Mk-4, Mk-6, Mk-7, and menadione are given in Table 4.2. Vitamin K compounds other than modified menadiones are soluble in lipids, ether, and other non-polar organic solvents. They are sparingly soluble in polar organic solvents. Vitamin $K_{1(20)}$ is synthesized commercially for use in infant formula, medical foods, and pharmaceuticals. Vitamin $K_{1(20)}$ is used in olestra containing products according to 21CFR171.867.[21] Menadione and its derivatives are important additives in the feed industry. Menadione is not used for human supplements owing to toxicity. Vitamin K_1 is not used in animal feed due to its cost, and menadione provides an inexpensive alternative.[22] Menadione addition to feeds is particularly important to poultry rations since chemotherapeutic agents against coccidiosis and parasitic diseases inhibit intestinal synthesis and increase the dietary requirements of the chicken.[22] Various stabilized forms of menadione that are water-soluble are available to the industry. These include menadione sodium bisulfate (MSB), menadione sodium bisulfite complex (MSBC), and menadione dimethyl-pyrimidinol bisulfite (MPB). Structures are given in Figure 4.3. MSB is the addition product formed between menadione and sodium bisulfite. The product is soluble in water and insoluble in most organic solvents. MSBC is the crystallization product of MSB as a complex in excess sodium bisulfite. MPB is the salt of MSB and dimethylpyrimindinol. The menadione salts are absorbed more efficiently than menadione because of their greater water solubility.[23] The water-soluble menadione forms show better stability to environmental and feed processing conditions compared to free menadione.[23]

4.2.1.2 Spectral Properties

Phylloquinones and menaquinone-n forms show UV spectra characteristic of the naphthoquinone ring. The UV spectrum of phylloquinone (Figure 4.4-I) shows absorption maxima at 242 nm,

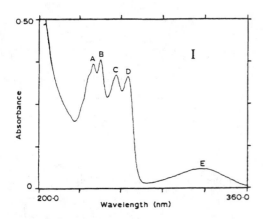

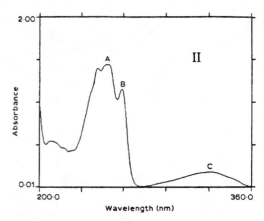

FIGURE 4.4-I   UV absorption spectrum of phylloquinone in hexane (λ max of Peak B is 248 nm).
Reproduced with permission from Reference 22.

FIGURE 4.4-II   UV absorption spectrum of
menadione in hexane (λ max of Peak A is 252 nm).
Reproduced with permission from Reference 22.

248 nm, 260 nm, 269 nm, and 325 nm. Figure 4.4-II gives the absorption spectrum of menadione. $E_{1\,cm}^{1\%}$ values are provided in Table 4.2. Vitamin K compounds do not fluoresce; however, fluorescence can be induced through reduction of the quinone to hydroquinone. This property has been incorporated into LC methodology to provide a highly specific detection system (Section 4.3.2.2.2). The hydroquinone shows maximal fluorescence at Ex λ = 244, Em λ = 418.

4.2.2   STABILITY

Vitamin K_1 is quite stable to oxidation and most food processing and food preparation procedures.[17] It is unstable to light and alkaline conditions. Instability to alkalinity prohibits the use of saponification for sample extraction and led to extensive research to develop sample clean-up procedures to overcome insufficiencies of UV detection for LC methodology (Section 4.3). Reducing agents also destroy the biological activity of vitamin K_1. Isomerization of the *trans* bond in the 2′-E, 7′R, and 11′R system to 2′-Z, 7′R, and 11′R isomer is problematic because the *cis*-isomer possesses no biological activity.[1] Presence of variable quantities of the *cis*-isomer in commercial vitamin K_1 preparations used for food fortification requires that methodology must accurately assess amounts of *cis*- and *trans*-isomers to estimate biological activity. As discussed in Section 4.3, current AOAC International methods do not meet this requirement.

Few definitive studies exist on vitamin K_1 stability owing to our past inability to accurately quantitate the vitamin. Development of excellent LC procedures has changed this situation. Methods developed in the 1980s and early 1990s have dramatically improved available vitamin K_1 assay methods. In 1992, Ferland and Sadowski[6] reported the effects of heat and light exposure on the stability of vitamin K_1 in vegetable oils. The vitamin was stable during processing and slightly unstable during heating at frying temperatures of 185°C to 190°C for 40 minutes. The significant findings of the study related to the degree of instability noted on exposure to daylight and fluorescent light. Various conditions were studied and the reader is urged to refer to the complete reference for a complete discussion of the results. However, extensive vitamin K_1 losses approaching 100% were noted in some plant oil after only two days exposure to fluorescent light. The authors stressed that from an analytical standpoint, it is necessary to work in subdued light when foods are being analyzed. For the consumer, vitamin K_1 content of oils can vary depending upon time and conditions of the marketing channel.

Recently, the Sadowski research group reported on the presence of endogenous 2′,3′,-dihydro-vitamin K_1 in hydrogenated vegetable oils.[12,13,14] The physiological importance of the conversion of vitamin K_1 to dihydro-vitamin K_1 is not known, because its biological activity is unknown.[12,13]

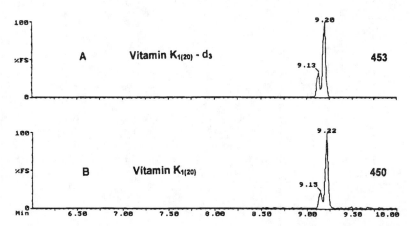

FIGURE 4.5 Single-ion recording (SIR) mass chromatograms of (B) unlabeled and (A) deuterium-labeled Vitamin $K_{1(20)}$ without derivatization. Double peaks correspond to 2'-Z (*cis-*) and 2'-E (*trans-*) isomers of vitamin K_1. The *cis*-isomers elute prior to *trans*-isomer at 9.13 and 9.15 min. Reproduced with permission from Reference 26.

Owing to the intake of hydrogenated oils, dihydro-vitamin K_1 in the U.S. diet is quite high. Booth et al.[13] reported that intake of dihydro-vitamin K_1 ranged from 12 to 24 mg per day for all age groups except infants. Vitamin K_1 intake ranges from 24 to 86 mg per day. These authors concluded that if 2',3'-dihydro-vitamin K_1 does not contribute to vitamin K_1 nutritional needs, hydrogenation of plant oils may be reducing the already low vitamin K_1 intakes.[12,15]

4.3 METHODS

Reviews on vitamin K analysis include Eitenmiller and Landen,[17] Ball,[22] Berruti,[23] and Lambert and De Leenheer.[24] Berruti's review published in 1985 is informative on older methods for menadione analysis including the titrimetric method with ceric sulfate and colorimetric assays with ethyl-cyanoacetate and 2,4-dinitro-phenylhydrazine.

Methods based on gas liquid chromatography (GC) are available for phylloquinone, menaquinone-n, and menadione analysis. Most GC procedures use adaptations of original work by Bechtold and Jahnchen[25] for the separation of vitamin $K_{1(20)}$ and Mk-4 on 3% OV-17 with electron capture detection. The low volatility of vitamin K compounds requires high column temperatures. Bechtold and Jahnchen[25] used 302°C. Recently published methods used temperature gradients up to 310°C.[26,27] GC allows direct coupling to a mass spectrometer for exact identification and sensitive quantitation. Fauler et al.[26] recently published a GC/MS method for plasma analysis that combined mass-selective detection with isotope dilution for internal standardization. The detection limit was 1.0 pg and the quantitation limit was 2.0 pg/mL. Chromatograms and mass spectra from the Fauler et al.[26] study are given in Figure 4.5 and Figure 4.6. Deuterium-labeled vitamin K_1 was synthesized for the study. The procedure quantitated both the 2'-Z and natural 2'-E isomers in standards at a ratio of 20 : 80. The 2'-Z isomer was not detected in plasma samples.

AOAC International provides a GC method for the assay of menadione sodium bisulfite in feed premixes. The method "Menadione Sodium Bisulfite (Water-Soluble Vitamin K_3) in Feed Premixes—Method 974.30" uses 2% OV-17 on Chromosorb W with FID. However, the procedure is applicable only to high concentration samples. Reviews by Ball[22] and Lambert and De Leenheer[24] give detailed information on GC methods for vitamin K analysis. Disadvantages of long retention time, high column temperatures, and the potential for on-column degradation have hindered the routine application of GC to vitamin K assay.

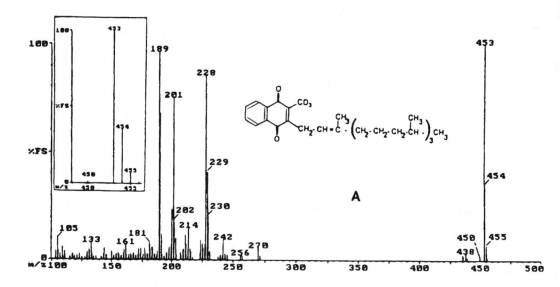

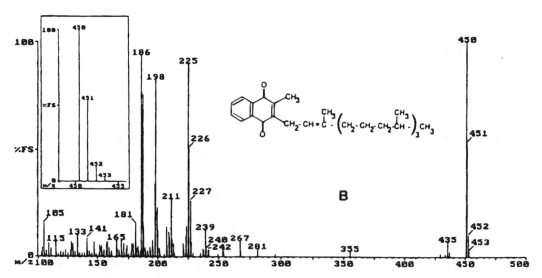

FIGURE 4.6   Electron impact (EI) mass spectra of (B) unlabeled and (A) deuterium-labeled vitamin $K_{1(20)}$. Reproduced with permission from Reference 26.

Dramatic improvements have developed for the LC determination of vitamin K in biologicals. In Ball's review (1988),[22] LC methods were presented that were primarily based upon UV detection. Lack of specificity led to poor chromatograms and, hence, to complicated and somewhat unwieldy clean-up procedures. Over the last decade, excellent methods were published incorporating reductive conversion of the quinones to highly fluorescent hydroquinones. This development (Section 4.3.1) provided a significant advance for use of the resolution power of LC for vitamin K analysis. Now, vitamin K can be accurately quantitated in most biologicals with a great deal of confidence. Table 4.3 summarizes compendium and handbook methods; however, most of these procedures have not kept abreast of more recently published procedures (Table 4.4) and should be used cautiously.

TABLE 4.3
Compendium, Regulatory, and Handbook Methods for the Analysis of Vitamin K and Related Compounds

Source	Form	Methods and Application	Approach	Most Current Cross-Reference
U.S. Pharmacopeia National Formulary, 1995, USP 23/ NF 18 Nutritional Supplements Official Monograph[1]				
1. pages 2139, 2141	Phylloquinone (K_1)	Phytonadione in oil-soluble vitamin capsules/tablets	HPLC 254 nm	None
2. pages 2142, 2145, 2147, 2151	Phylloquinone (K_1)	Phytonadione in oil- and water-soluble vitamin capsules/tablets with or without minerals	HPLC 254 nm	None
3. pages 1224–1225	Phylloquinone (K_1)	Phytonadione (NLT 97.0%, NMT 103.0%)	HPLC 254 nm	None
4. pages 1225–1226	Phylloquinone (K_1)	Phytonadione injection, tablets	HPLC 254 nm	None
5. page 948	Menadione (K_3)	Menadione injection (NLT 98.5%, NMT 101.0%)	Colorimetric 635 nm	None
British Pharmacopoeia, 15th ed., 1993[2]				
1. Vol. 1, pages 516–517	Phylloquinone (K_1)	Phytomenadione	Spectrophotometric 249 nm	None
2. Vol. II, pages 1059–1060	Phylloquinone (K_1)	Phytomenadione injection	HPLC 254 nm	None
3. Vol. II, page 1060	Phylloquinone (K_1)	Phytomenadione tablets	HPLC 254 nm	None
AOAC Official Methods of Analysis, 16th ed., 1995[3]				
1. 50.1.06	Phylloquinone (K_1)	AOAC Official Method 992.27 *Trans*-Vitamin K_1 (Phylloquinone) in Ready-To-Feed Milk-Based Infant Formula	HPLC 254 nm	*J. Assoc. Off. Anal. Chem.*, 68, 684, 1985[4] *J. AOAC Int.*, 76, 1042, 1993[5]
2. 41.1.31	Menadione (K_3)	AOAC Official Method 974.30 Menadione Sodium Bisulfate (Water-Soluble Vitamin K_3) in Feed Premixes	GC flame ionization	*J. Assoc. Off. Anal. Chem.*, 56, 1277, 1973[6]

TABLE 4.3. Continued

Source	Form	Methods and Application	Approach	Most Current Cross-Reference
American Feed Ingredients Association, *Laboratory Methods Compendium*, vol. 1, 1991[7]				
1. pages 87–89	Menadione (K₃)	Modified 2,4-dinitrophenylhydrazine Method for combined forms of Menadione (feedstuffs, concentrates, premixes) (>1 ppm)	Colorimetric 635 nm	
2. pages 91–92	Menadione (K₃)	Ethylcyanoacetate method for Water-Soluble menadione derivatives (vitamin Premixes containing water-soluble derivatives of menadione)	Colorimetric 575 nm	
3. pages 93–94	Menadione (K₃)	Reduction-oxidation method for Menadione assay (pure menadione or Derivatives-tablets, capsules, Injectibles)	Titration	USP 23/NF 18 Official Monographs, 948[1]
4. pages 215–217	Menadione (K₃)	Determination of vitamin K₃ in Complete feeds, premixes, and vitamin concentrates with the aid of HPLC (2–20 mg/kg)	HPLC 254 nm	Hoffmann-LaRoche, *Analytical Methods for Vitamins and Carotenoids in Feed*, 17[8] *Int. J. Vit. Nutr. Res.*, 52, 248, 1982[9]
5. pages 219–229	Menadione (K₃)	Determination of vitamin K₃ in Feedstuffs and premixes using HPLC (>1 mg/kg)	HPLC 251 nm	None
6. pages 221–222	Menadione (K₃)	Menadione sodium bisulfate (vitamin K) premixes (>1000 mg/kg)	GC flame ionization	AOAC Official Methods, 16th ed., 45.1.31[3]
Hoffmann-LaRoche, *Analytical Methods for Vitamins and Carotenoids in Feed*, 1988[8]				
pages 17–19	Vitamin K₃	Determination of vitamin K₃ in Complete feeds, premixes and vitamin Concentrates with the aid of HPLC (>0.5 mg/kg)	HPLC 251 nm	*Int. J. Vit. Nutr. Res.*, 52, 248, 1982[9]

TABLE 4.4
HPLC Methods for the Analysis of Vitamin K in Foods, Feed, Pharmaceuticals and Biologicals

		Sample Preparation		HPLC Parameters				
Sample Matrix	Analyte	Sample Extraction	Clean Up	Column	Mobile Phase	Detection	Quality Assurance Parameters	References

Foods
Infant Formula and Milk

Sample Matrix	Analyte	Sample Extraction	Clean Up	Column	Mobile Phase	Detection	Quality Assurance Parameters	References
1. Infant formula	K_1, other fat-soluble vitamins	Add cholesterol phenyl acetate (IS) Lipase hydrolysis Add NH_4OH, EtOH Extract with pentane		Two Zorbax-ODS in series 25 cm × 4.6 mm	Gradient MeOH : EtOAC (86 : 4) against 100% MeCN Variable flow rate	256 nm	—	*Anal. Chem.*, 52, 610, 1980[1]
2. Infant formula, milk, bovine, human	K_1	Extract with $CHCl_3$: MeOH (2 : 1)	Kieselgel 60 Semi-prep LC on silica or amino-cyano-bonded phase	a. Zorbax-ODS 25 cm × 4.6 nm b. Hypersil-ODS 25 cm × 5.0 mm	Isocratic a. MeOH : CH_2Cl_2 (8 : 2) or MeCN : CH_2Cl_2 (7 : 3) for Zorbax ODS b. MeOH : CH_2Cl_2 (9 : 1) or MeCN : CH_2Cl_2 (17 : 3) for Hypersil-ODS Flow rates not specified	250 nm or 270 nm	—	*J. Nutr.*, 112, 1105, 1982[2]
3. Infant formula	K_1	Lipase hydrolysis Add NH_4OH, EtOH Extract with pentane		μBondapak C_{18} 25 cm × 4.6 mm	Isocratic MeOH : MeCN : THF : water (39 : 39 : 16 : 6) 1.5 mL/min	254 nm	% Recovery 84–103	*J. Assoc. Off. Anal. Chem.*, 66, 1063, 1983[3]

TABLE 4.4 Continued

Sample Matrix	Analyte	Sample Preparation			HPLC Parameters			Quality Assurance Parameters	References
		Sample Extraction	Clean Up	Column	Mobile Phase	Detection			
4. Infant formula	K_1, other fat-soluble vitamins	NH_4OH, methanol Extract with CH_2Cl_2 : iOct (2 : 1) Evaporate Redissolve in iOct with 0.01% IP	Silica open-column	Apex Silica on Spherisorb ODS, 5 μm 25 cm × 4.6 mm	Isocratic a. Normal-phase iOct : CH_2Cl_2 : IP (70 : 30 : 0.02) 1 mL/min b. Reversed-phase THF : MeOH : water (27 : 67 : 6) 1 mL/min	254 nm		QL 2 μg/L as fed RSD = 4.1% % Recovery 95 ± 9	J. Assoc. Off. Anal. Chem., 68, 684, 1985[4]
5. Milk, bovine, human	K_1, K_2	Lipase hydrolysis Add NH_4OH, EtOH Extract with pentane Evaporate Redissolve in IP	Nucleosil C_{18}	a. K_1, MK-4 Partisil ODS-2, 5 μm 25 cm × 4.6 mm b. MK-6, MK-7, MK-8, MK-9, Partisil ODS-3, 5 μm 25 cm × 4.6 mm	Isocratic MeOH : EtOH : 60% perchloric acid (600 : 400 : 1.2) 0.05 M $NaClO_4$ 1 mL/min	EC— 0.45 V/ +0.35V		K_1 in cow's milk RSD = 8.3% K_1 in human milk RSD = 13%	J. Dairy Sci., 71, 627, 1988[5]
6. Infant formula	K_1, D_3	Extract lipids with CH_2Cl_2 and IP Dry with $MgSO_4$	a. GPC Four μStryagel 100Å in series b. μBondapak/NH_2 25 cm × 4.6 mm Collect K_1 fraction	Zorbax-ODS, 6 μm 25 cm × 4.6 mm	Isocratic CH_2Cl_2 : MeCN : MeOH (300 : 700 : 2) 1 mL/min	254 nm		% CV = 2.8	J .Food Comp. Anal., 2, 140, 1989[6]

No. / Sample	Vitamer	Sample preparation	Cleanup column	Analytical column	Mobile phase	Detection	Results	Reference
7. Milk, human	K_1, K_2	Add MK-7 (IS) Extract with IP : Hex (2 : 1) Centrifuge Evaporate Hex layer from 10 vol of chloroform : methanol (2 : 1) Redissolve residue in Hex Dry and redissolve in iOct	a. Silica CC-4 open-column b. Bio-Sil open-column	a. C_{18} Radial Pak, 5μm b. C_{18} Radial Pak, 10μm Collect K_1 fraction from (a) Concentrate inject on (b)	a. Convex gradient EtOH : water (90 : 10) to EtOH : Hex (90 : 10) b. Isocratic EtOH : Hex : water (90 : 6.5 : 3.5) Flow rate not specified	a. 254 nm b. EC dual glassy carbon −0.6 V reductive +0.2 V oxidative Ag/AgCl reference	% Recovery 65.2 RSD = 32.3	*Lipids,* 25, 406, 1990[7]
8. Milk, human	K_1	Add MK-5 (IS) in EtOH, albumin, sodium taurcholate, $CaCl_2$, NaCl Sonicate Lipase hydrolysis Add NH_4OH, EtOH Extract with Hex	R Sil adsorption column	RoSil, C_{18}, HL, 5 μm 15 cm × 3.2 mm	Isocratic MeOH : EtOAC (96 : 4) Containing tetramethyl ammonium octahydridotriborate as the reducing agent 0.7 mL/min	$K_{1(20)}$ and $K_{1(25)}$ reduced post-column Fluorescence Ex λ = 325 Em λ = 430	QL 35 ng/L % CV = 5.2 (within day) % CV = 5.8 (day-to-day) % Recovery = 62.5	*Clin. Chem.* 38, 1743, 1992[8]
9. Infant formula	K_1	Add NH_4OH, MeOH, CH_2Cl_2 : iOct mixture (2 : 1). Collect organic layer Evaporate	Silica over-layered with sodium sulfate	Apex I, silica, 5 μm	CH_2Cl_2 : iOct (30 : 70) containing 0.02% IP 1 mL/min	254 nm	RSD_r = 3.2% RSD_R = 16.0%	*J. AOAC Int.,* 76, 1042, 1993[9]
10–11. Infant formula, milk, bovine	K_1	Lipase hydrolysis Add EtOH : MeOH (95 : 5), potassium carbonate and cholesteryl phenylacetate (IS) Extract with Hex	Semi-prep LC Resolve Silica (8 × 10) radial compression	Resolve C_{18}, 5 μm 8 × 10 RCM	Isocratic MeOH : IP : ETOAC : Water (450 : 350 : 145 : 135) 2 mL/min	dual wavelength 269 nm 277 nm	DL (ng) on-column 1 QL 0.5 μg /100 g powder 0.1 μg /100 g fluid % Recovery 88.9 RSD_r = 1.5% RSD_R = 2.8%	*J. AOAC Int.,* 78, 719, 1995[10] *Food Chem.* 54, 403, 1995[11]

TABLE 4.4 Continued

Sample Matrix	Analyte	Sample Preparation — Sample Extraction	Clean Up	HPLC Parameters — Column	Mobile Phase	Detection	Quality Assurance Parameters	References
12. Infant formula, milk, bovine	K_1, K_2 Dihydro-K_1	Weigh 1 g powder or 10 g fluid milk Add 15 mL water (<40°C) to powder Dilute fluid to 15 mL with water (<40°C) Add 5mL phosphate buffer, 54 g KH_2PO_4 in 500 mL water, pH 7.9–8.0 Add lipase Vortex, 7 min Incubate 37°C, 2 h Add 10 mL alcohol (EtOH : MeOH) (95 : 5) Add 1 g potassium carbonate Add 30 mL Hex Shake, 7 min Centrifuge Transfer Hex layer to amber vial Evaporate under nitrogen Dissolve residue in MeOH	—	See Reference 10.	See Reference 10.	See Reference 10.	DL (pg) on-column 30 pg % Recovery > 98 RSD_R K_1 = 2.35% MK-4 = 2.32%	*Analyst,* 122, 465, 1997[12]
13. Vegetables	K_1	Add MK-6 (IS) Homogenize Extract with Hex Add water Centrifuge Evaporate Hex Redissolve in MeOH	—	Hypersil ODS, 5 μm 10 cm × 3.0 mm	Isocratic MeOH : water (92.5 : 7.5) containing 0.03 M sodium perchlorate/100 mL 0.8 mL/min	Post-column EC reduction of K_1 to K_1 hydroquinone Fluorescence Ex λ = 320 Em λ = 430	DL (pg) On-column 50 % Recovery 92.5	*Acta Aliment.,* 15, 187, 1986[13]

	Analyte	Sample preparation	Cleanup	Column	Mobile phase	Detection	Notes	Reference
14–16. a. Vegetable juice, milk	K$_1$	Add dihydrophyllo-quinone (IS), IP : Hex (3 : 2), water Sonicate, vortex, centrifuge Evaporate Hex layer Redissolve in Hex *Whole milk requires additional Hex partitioning step.	SPE Silica gel J. T. Baker, 3 ml *Whole milk residue requires additional liquid phase reductive extraction that reduces K$_1$ and IS to acetonitrile soluble hydroquinones. After extraction, hydroquinones are oxidized to Hex soluble quinones.	Hypersil ODS, 3 µm 15 cm × 4.6 mm	Isocratic MeOH : CH$_2$Cl$_2$ (90 : 10) Add 5 mL of a solution of 2 M ZnCl, 1 M HAC, and 1 M NaOAC per 100 mL 1 mL/min	Fluorescent derivatives of quinones were produced in a post-column reactor packed with Zn metal. Fluorescence Ex λ = 244 Em λ = 418	Vegetable juice % CV = 12.7 Milk % CV = 13.8	*J. Agric. Food Chem.,* 40, 1874, 1992[14], 42, 295, 1994[15] *Meth. Enzymol.,* 282, 446, 1997[16]
b. Spinach	K$_1$	Grind with sodium sulfate Add dihydrophyllo-quinone (IS) Follow (a)	SPE Silica gel J. T. Baker, 3 mL	Hypersil ODS, 3 µm 15 cm × 4.6 mm	Isocratic MeOH : CH$_2$Cl$_2$ (90 : 10) Add 5 mL of a solution of 2 M ZnCl, 1 M HAC and 1 M NaOAC per 100 mL 1 mL/min	Fluorescent derivatives of quinones were produced in a post-column reactor packed with Zn metal. Fluorescence Ex λ = 244 Em λ = 418	% CV = 7.4	*J. Agric. Food Chem.,* 42, 295, 1994[15]
c. Bread	K$_1$	Add K$_{1(25)}$ (IS) Follow (a)	SPE Silica gel J. T. Baker, 3 mL	Hypersil ODS, 3 µm 15 cm × 4.6 mm	Isocratic MeOH : CH$_2$Cl$_2$ (90 : 10) Add 5 mL of a solution of 2 M ZnCl, 1 M HAC and 1 M sodium acetate per 100 mL 1 mL/min	Fluorescent derivatives of quinones were produced in a post-column reactor packed with Zn metal. Fluorescence Ex λ = 244 Em λ = 418	% CV = 10.8	*J. Agric. Food Chem.,* 42, 295, 1994[15]

TABLE 4.4 Continued

Sample Matrix	Analyte	Sample Preparation		HPLC Parameters				
		Sample Extraction	Clean Up	Column	Mobile Phase	Detection	Quality Assurance Parameters	References
d. Ground beef	K_1	Grind with sodium sulfate. Add $K_{1(25)}$ IS Follow (a) with increased volume of water	a. SPE silica gel b. SPE C_{18}	Hypersil ODS, 3 μm 15 cm × 4.6 mm	Isocratic MeOH : CH_2Cl_2 (90 :10) Add 5 mL of a solution of 2 M $ZnCl$, 1 M HAC and 1 M NaOAC per 100 mL 1 mL/min	Fluorescent derivatives of quinones were produced in a post-column reactor packed with Zn metal. Fluorescence Ex λ = 244 Em λ = 418	% CV = 12.6	J. Agric. Food Chem., 42, 295, 1994[15]
17. Edible oils	K_1	Add dihydro-vitamin $K_{1(25)}$ IS Dissolve in Hex	SPE Silica J. T. Baker	Hypersil ODS, 3 μm 15 cm × 4.6 mm	Isocratic MeOH : CH_2Cl_2 (90 : 10) Add 5 mL of a solution of 2 M $ZnCl$, 1 M HAC and 1 M NaOAC per 100 mL 1 mL/min	Fluorescent derivatives of quinones were produced in a post-column reactor packed with Zn metal. Fluorescence Ex λ = 244 Em λ = 418		J. Agric. Food Chem., 40, 1869, 1992[17]

		Sample preparation	SPE	Column	HPLC conditions	Detection	Precision/Recovery	Reference
18. Canola oil	K_1	Add MK-4 (IS) to 2 g oil Add 1 g lipase (Sigma Type VII) Add 100 mL 0.2 M phosphate buffer, pH 7.7 Incubate with stirring, 37°C, 1.5 h Transfer hydrolysate to separatory funnel containing 5 mL 10 M NaOH and 100 mL 95% EtOH Extract with Hex Wash Hex with buffer, then water Dry over Na_2SO_4 Evaporate to dryness	Silica SPE	PartiSphere C_{18} 5 μm 15 cm × 3.9 mm	Isocratic MeCN : MeOH (150 : 850) plus 5 mL MeCN : MeOH (85 : 15) containing 2 M $ZnCl_2$, 1 M NaOAC, and 1 M HAC 1 mL/min	See Reference 15.	% CV = 2.2 % Recovery 81–95	Food Res. Int., 28, 61, 1995[18]
19. Various foods	K_1	Add dihydro-K_1 (IS) Homogenize Extract with Hex Evaporate Redissolve in Hex Add equal volume of MeOH : water (9 : 1) to Hex extract Mix, centrifuge Remove upper Hex layer Evaporate to dryness Dissolve residue in mobile phase	—	Hypersil ODS, 5 μm 25 cm × 4.6 mm	Isocratic CH_2Cl_2 : MeOH (100 : 900) containing 5 mL methanolic solution containing 1.37 g $ZnCl_2$, 0.41 g NaOAC, and 0.3 g HAC 1 mL/min 40°C	Post-column reduction Fluorescence Ex λ = 243 Em λ = 430	% CV within-run 3–98 % Recovery 95–101	Food Chem., 56, 87, 1996[19]

TABLE 4.4 Continued

Sample Matrix	Analyte	Sample Preparation		HPLC Parameters				References
		Sample Extraction	Clean Up	Column	Mobile Phase	Detection	Quality Assurance Parameters	
20. Vegetables	K_1	To 1–5 g sample, sonicate with 10 mL MeOH, 15 min / Centrifuge / Mix 2 mL extract with 4 mL sodium carbonate / Heat at 80°C, 1 h / Partition with 4 mL Hex, 3× / Evaporate Hex layer / Redissolve in MeOH	—	LiChrosorb RP-8, 10 μm 25 cm × 4.6 mm	Isocratic 100% MeOH 0.6 mL/min	247 nm and particle beam mass spectrometry	DL (ng) on-column UV—0.1 MS EI—1 PICI-5 NICI—0.1 % Recovery 82–90	Fres. J. Anal. Chem., 355, 48, 1996[20]
21. Oil, margarine, butter	K_1	Oil Add MK-4 (IS) to 0.5–1 g sample Dilute to 10 mL with Hex Butter and Margarine Extract with 1. Hex 2. IPA : Hex (1 : 1) 3. Add 2 mL water and 2 mL 25% ammonia. Shake, add 5 mL EtOH Extract with E_2O and PE Wash with water Evaporate Dissolve in Hex	Semi-Prep LC μPorasil 30 cm × 3.9 mm 5 μm	Vydac 205TP54 25 cm × 4.6 m 5 μm	Isocratic 95% MeOH : 0.05 M NaOAC, pH 3.0 1 mL/min	EC Redox Mode upstream— 1.1 V downstream— 0 V	DL (pg) K_1 = 50 MK-4 = 20 % CV 0.1–14.3 % Recovery 78–98	Food Chem., 59, 473, 1997[21]

Sample	Analyte	Extraction	Sample preparation	Column	Mobile phase	Detection	DL (ng)	Reference
22. Vitamin premix	K_1	—	Add DMSO, Heat at 65°C in ultrasonic bath, 30 min, Extract with Hex, Evaporate, Redissolve in IP for reverse-phase HPLC, Inject Hex directly for normal-phase chromatography	a. Reverse phase Rad-Pak C_{18}, 5 µm b. Normal-phase Silica Rad-Pak, 5 µm, 10 cm × 0.8 mm	Isocratic a. Reverse-phase MeOH : Water (96 : 4) b. Normal-phase Hex : IP (99.1 : 0.1) 1.0–2.5 mL/min	254 nm and Fluorescence Ex λ = 325 Em λ = 420 High intensity 150 W Xe lamp	DL (ng) On-column 10 by fluorescence	*J. Micronutr. Anal.,* 4, 61, 1988[22]

Pharmaceuticals

Sample	Analyte	Extraction	Sample preparation	Column	Mobile phase	Detection	DL (ng)	Reference
1. Intravenous lipid emulsion	K1	a. SPE Silica gel b. Liquid-phase reductive extraction	Add dihydrophyllo-quinone (IS), Extract with IP : Hex (3 : 2), Centrifuge, Evaporate Hex	Hypersil ODS	Isocratic MeOH : CH_2Cl_2 (85 : 15) containing: 10 mmol/L $ZnCl_2$, 5 mmol/L HAC, 5 mmol/L NaOAC, Flow rate not specified	Post column reduction to fluorescent hydroquinone Fluorescence Ex λ = 244 Em λ = 418	—	*JPEN,* 17, 142, 1993[1]
2. Intravenous fat emulsion, soybean oil	K_1	Sep-Pak silica	Add $K_{1(25)}$ IS, 0.9% NaCl, EtOH, Extract with Hex	XL 3 µm Octyl cartridge 7 cm × 4.7 mm	Isocratic MeCN : EtOH (95 : 5) containing 0.005 sodium perchlorate 0.8 mL/min	EC reduction followed by fluorescence detection	QL 2 ng K_1/g RSD = 4–7.1%	*J. Chromatog. A.,* 664, 189, 1994[2]

Biologicals

Sample	Analyte	Extraction	Sample preparation	Column	Mobile phase	Detection	DL (ng)	Reference
1. Rat liver	K_1	Sep-Pak silica	Add vitamin K_1 epoxide (IS), Extract with Hex, Dry with sodium sulfate, Evaporate	Hypersil-ODS, 25 cm × 5.0 mm	Isocratic MeCN : CH_2Cl_2 (17:3) 1 mL/min	254 nm	% CV = 11.1	*J. Lipid Res.,* 24, 481, 1983[1]

TABLE 4.4 Continued

| Sample Matrix | Analyte | Sample Preparation | | HPLC Parameters | | | | References |
		Sample Extraction	Clean Up	Column	Mobile Phase	Detection	Quality Assurance Parameters	
2. Plasma	K_1	Add MK-6 (IS) NaCl solution (1%), IP Extract with Hex Evaporate Redissolve in MeOH		Hypersil-MOS, 5 μm 10 cm × 3.0 mm	Isocratic MeOH : Water (92.5 : 7.5) containing 0.03 M NaClO$_4$ 1 mL/min	Post-column EC reduction of K_1 to K_1 hydroquinone Fluorescence Ex λ = 320 Em λ = 420 or amperometric or coulometric reoxidation	QL 2.3 ng/mL without clean-up by fluorescence DL (pg) On-column Fluorescence—25 Amperometric—280 Coulometric—150	J. Chromatogr., 305, 61, 1984[2]
3. Plasma	K_1, K_2, MK-4, MK-6, MK-7, MK-9, MK-10	Add water and EtOH Extract with Hex Centrifuge Evaporate Redissolve in Hex	Sep-Pak silica	Nucleosil C_{18}, 5 μm 15 cm × 4.6 mm	Isocratic EtOH : Water (92.5 : 7.5) containing 0.25% NaClO$_4$ 1 mL/min	Post-column EC reduction of K_1 and K_2 to hydroquinone derivatives Fluorescence parameters not specified	DL (pg) On-column 5 or 50 pg/mL	Chem. Pharm. Bull., 34, 845, 1986[3]
4. Plasma	K_1	Add $K_{1(25)}$ IS, EtOH Extract with Hex Evaporate Redissolve Hex : DIPE (98.5 : 1.5)	Semi-prep silica column, RoSIL 5 μm Collect K fraction Concentrate	RSIL C_{18} HL, 5 μm 15 cm × 3.2 mm	Isocratic MeOH : EtOAC(96 : 4) 0.7 mL/min	Post-column reduction by tetramethyl-ammonium octahydro-triborate Fluorescence Ex λ = 325 Em λ = 430	QL 50 pg/mL DL on-column	Anal. Biochem., 158, 257, 1986[4]

Sample	Analyte	Extraction	Cleanup	Column	Mobile phase	Detection	Performance	Reference
5. Plasma	K_1	Add dehydro-K_1 (IS), EtOH; Extract with Hex; Evaporate	a. Sep-Pak silica b. Reductive extraction c. Reconversion of K_1-hydroquinone to K_1	Hypersil-ODS, 5 μm, 25 cm × 4.6 mm	Isocratic CH$_2$Cl$_2$:MeOH (8:2) containing ZnCl$_2$, sodium acetate and HAC 1 mL/min	Post-column reduction of K_1 to K_1-hydroquinone Fluorescence Ex λ = 325 Em λ = 430	QL 0.05 μg/L % CV < 10	Clin. Chem., 32, 1925, 1986[5]
6. Plasma	K_1, K_2 MK-4 K_1 epoxide	Add water, EtOH; Extract with Hex; Evaporate; Redissolve in Hex	Sep-Pak silica	Column switching a. Precolumn TSK gel ODS-120T—5 μm 5 cm × 4.6 mm b. Analytical TSK gel ODS-120 T-5 μm 20 cm × 4.6 mm	Isocratic MeOH:MeCN (6:4) containing 0.25% NaClO$_4$ 1 mL/min	Post-column EC reduction to hydroquinones Fluorescence Ex λ = 320 Em λ = 430	DL (pg) On-column K_1 = 5 MK-4 = 5 K1 epoxide = 8 per mL plasma K_1 = 30 MK-4 = 3 K1 epoxide = 50	J. Chromatogr., 430, 21, 1988[6]
7. Umbilical cord plasma	K_1, MK-4, MK-6, MK-7	Add water, EtOH; Extract with Hex; Evaporate; Redissolve in Hex	Sep-Pak silica	Nucleosil 5 C$_{18}$, 15 cm × 4.6 mm	Isocratic MeOH:EtOH (4:1) containing 0.25% NaClO$_4$ 1 mL/min	Post-column reduction with Pt column Fluorescence Ex λ = 320 Em λ = 430	QL > 10 pg/mL DL (pg) On-column K_1 = 5 MK-4 = 5 MK-6 = 10	J. Chromatogr., 430, 143, 1988[7]
8–9. Human intestinal contents	K_1, MK-4 to MK-10	Add water: CHCl$_3$:MeOH (10:12.5:25) Centrifuge Add CHCl$_3$ and water to supernatant Evaporate lower, organic layer Redissolve in Hex	Sep-Pak silica	Novapak C$_{18}$ 15 cm × 3.9 mm	Isocratic EtOH:Water (95:5) 0.7 mL/min	Post-column reduction with 0.1% NaBH$_4$ in ethanol Fluorescence Ex λ = 320 Em λ = 430	QL 0.02 μg to 0.05 μg/g	Am. J. Gastroenterol., 87, 311, 1992[8]; Meth. Enzymol., 282, 457, 1997[9]
10. Human liver	K_1, K_1-epoxide	Add water, EtOH dihydrovitamin K_1 (IS) Extract with Hex Evaporate Redissolve in Hex	a. Sep-Pak silica b. HPTLC Silica gel-60	Chromospher C$_{18}$ 10 cm × 3 mm	Isocratic MeOH:IP:Water (450:50:7) containing tetramethyl ammonium octahydrotriborate 0.7 mL/min	Post-column EC reduction Fluorescence Ex λ = 244 Em λ = 430	Recovery = 86 ± 10% % CV = 9–16	Br. J. Haematol., 84, 681, 1993[10]

TABLE 4.4 Continued

Sample Matrix	Analyte	Sample Preparation		HPLC Parameters				References
		Sample Extraction	Clean Up	Column	Mobile Phase	Detection	Quality Assurance Parameters	
11. Bone	K_1, MK-6 MK-7 MK-8	Extract washed and dried bone powder with $CHCl_3$: MeOH (3 : 1) Evaporate Add EDTA to demineralize Reextract with $CHCl_3$: MeOH Reduce volume Extract with Hex Evaporate Hydrolyze residue with lipase Add EtOH Extract with Hex	a. Sep-Pak silica b. Spherisorb CN	Hypersil C_{18}, 5 μm 25 cm × 4.6 mm	Isocratic MeOH : NaOAC (97 : 3), containing pH 3.0, containing 0.1 mM EDTA Flow rate not specified	Dual electrode EC in redox mode upstream— 13 V downstream : 0.05 V	—	J. Bone Mineral Res., 8, 1005, 1993[11]
12–13. Rat tissue	K_1, MK-4, MK-6, MK-7, MK-8, MK-9	Add water, EtOH dihydrovitamin K_1 (IS) Extract with Hex Evaporate Redissolve in Hex	Silica 60	Chromospher C_{18}, 10 cm × 3 mm	Isocratic MeOH : IP : Water (450 : 50 : 7) containing tetramethyl ammonium octahydrotriborate Flow rate not specified	Post-column EC reduction Fluorescence Ex λ = 244 Em λ = 430	See Reference 9.	Br. J. Nutr., 72, 415, 1994[12] 75, 121, 1996[13]

	Analyte	Extraction	Partition/SPE	Column	Conditions	Detection	DL/QL	Reference
14. Rat liver	K_1, K_1-epoxide, MK-9, MK-9 epoxide	Add trans-^{3}H-phylloquinone and 6-methyl-menaquinone-9 (IS) EtOH, Et$_2$O, Extract with Hex Evaporate	a. Sep-Pak silica b. μ Porasil	Zorbax ODS, C$_{18}$ 5 μm 25 cm × 4.6 mm	Isocratic a. K1, K1 epoxide MeOH : CH$_2$Cl$_2$ (85 : 15) containing ZnCl$_2$, NaOAC, HAC 1 mL/min b. MK-9 MK-9 epoxide and 6-methyl-MK-9 (IS) increase CH$_2$Cl$_2$ to 30% in MeOH 1 mL/min	Post-column metallic Zn reduction of the vitamin K quinones and epoxides to hydroquinones Fluorescence Ex λ = 330 Em λ = 430	DL (pg) On-column K$_1$–25 K$_1$ epoxide—40 MK-9—150 MK-9 epoxide—250	PSEBM, 209, 403, 1995[14]
15. Plasma	K_1, retinol, α-T, γ-T β-carotene	Add dihydrovitamin K$_1$, EtOH Extract with Hex Centrifuge Remove Hex layer	Partition Hex with MeOH : water (9 : 1)	Hypersil ODS, 5 μm 25 cm × 4.6 mm	Isocratic MeOH : CH$_2$Cl$_2$ (9 : 1) containing ZnCl$_2$, NaOAC and HAC 0.8 mL/min	Post-column metallic Zn reduction Fluorescence Ex λ = 243 Em λ = 430	QL 0.04 μg/ml within run % CV = 5.6	Int. J. Vit. Nutr. Res., 65, 31, 1995[15]
16. Plasma	K_3	Use silicon gel glassware Add carbazole (IS) Extract with Hex Centrifuge Freeze at −76°C Pour Hex into tube containing 70% MeOH Evaporate	—	Ultrasphere ODS, 5 μm 25 cm × 4.6 mm	Isocratic MeOH : Water (70 : 30) 0.8 mL/min	265 nm	QL 10 ng/ml % Recovery 82	J. Chromatogr. B., 666, 299, 1995[16]
17. Serum	K_1	To 500 mL serum, add 1 mL of 1 ng/mL K$_2$ (IS) in IPA Vortex Extract 3 × with 2 mL Hex Centrifuge Dry under nitrogen Dissolve residue in Hex	SPE silica	Vydac 201TP54, 5 μm 25 cm × 4.6 mm	Isocratic EtOH : MeOH (40 : 60) 1 mL/min	Post-column reduction of vitamin K to hydroquinones with platinum-on-alumina catalyst/ alcohol Fluorescence Ex λ = 242 Em λ = 430	DL (pg) On-column 20 % Recovery 70 ± 34 n = 20	J. Chromatogr. B., 670, 209, 1995[17]

TABLE 4.4 Continued

| Sample Matrix | Analyte | Sample Preparation | | HPLC Parameters | | | | |
		Sample Extraction	Clean Up	Column	Mobile Phase	Detection	Quality Assurance Parameters	References
18. Human osteoblasts	MK-4 MK-4 epoxide	Extract cells with MeOH Add deuterated MK-4 (IS)	—	L-column ODS, 15 cm × 1.5 mm	Isocratic EtOH : MeOH (80 : 20) positive ion 0.15 mL/min	Mass spectrometric MK-4 = 20 pg atmospheric pressure chemical ionization (APCI) as an LC/MS interface	RSD < 10% DL On-column MK-4 epoxide = 50 pg	Anal. Sci., 13, 67, 1997[18]
19a. Plasma	K_1	To 0.5 mL plasma Add $K_{1\,(25)}$ (IS) EtOH Vortex Add water, Hex Plasma : EtOH : Hex (1 : 2 : 6)—optimal Mix, centrifuge Transfer Hex layer Evaporate Dissolve in IPA, 50°C	SPE C_{18}	BDS-Hypersil, 3 μm 15 cm × 3.0 mm Platinum-on-alumina oxygen scrubber in-line between pump and injector	Isocratic CH_2Cl_2 : MeOH (10 : 90) Add 5 mL of a solution of 2 M $ZNCl_2$, 1 M HAC, and 1 M NaOAC to each liter 0.6 mL/min	Post-column zinc reduction Fluorescence Ex λ = 244 Em λ = 418	% CV within run 5.6 % Recovery (IS) 75 QL 15 pg/mL	Meth. Enzymol., 282, 408, 1997[19]
19b. Plasma	K_1 K_1, 2, 3 epoxide	To 2.0 mL plasma Add 50 mL $K_{1\,(25)}$ (IS) 4.0 mL EtOH Vortex Add 2.0 mL water, 12 mL Hex Mix, centrifuge Transfer Hex layer Evaporate	SPE on silica followed by SPE on C_{18}	BDS-Hypersil, 5 mm 25 cm × 2.1 mm Platinum-on-alumina oxygen scrubber in-line between pump and injector	Isocratic CH_2Cl_2 : MeOH (10 : 90) Add 5 mL of a solution of 2 M $ZNCl_2$, 2 M HAC, and 1 M NaOAC Initial flow 0.25 mL/min Increase to 0.5 mL/min at 16 min Return to 0.25 mL/min at 29 min	See (a).	DL (pg) On-column K_{1-4} K_1epoxide—5	Meth. Enzymol., 282, 421, 1997[20]

		Sample prep	Semi-prep	Column	Mobile phase	Detection	DL/QL	Reference
20. Plasma	K_1	Add MK-6 (IS), Precipitate proteins with EtOH, Extract in Hex	Semi-prep LC Spherisorb CN Nitrile, 5 μm, Collect K_1 fraction, Evaporate, Dissolve in EtOH on mobile phase	Exsil C_{18} 5 μm 25 cm × 5 mm	Isocratic 0.05 M NaOAC, pH 3.0, in MeOH 1.0 mL/min	Dual-electrode cuolometric— 1.2 to 1.6 V Amperometric electrode at +0.15 to +0.20 V	DL 2 to 5 mg/L RSD% 1.6–4.1 Intrassay Precision 9.8–11.3%	Meth. Enzymol., 282, 421, 1997[20]

Vitamin K_3 in Feed

		Sample prep	Semi-prep	Column	Mobile phase	Detection	DL/QL	Reference
1. Premixes, animal feed	K_3	Add carbozol (IS), $CHCl_3$, NH_4OH : celite-sodium sulfate, Mix 30 min, Centrifuge, Dilute or concentrate $CHCl_3$ extract	—	LiChrosorb Si 60, 5 μm 25 cm × 3.2 mm	Isocratic THF : Hex (5 : 95) or $CHCl_3$: Hex (4 : 96) 1 mL/min	251 nm	DL (ng) On-column 1	Int. J. Vit. Nutr. Res., 52, 248, 1982[1]
2. Premixes, animal feed	K_3 (MSB)	Add water : EtOH (6 : 4), Mix 10 min, Add 10% tannin solution, Mix 1 min, Centrifuge supernatant, Add Hex and 10% sodium carbonate, Collect Hex layer, Evaporate	—	ODS—Hypersil 5 μm 25 cm × 4.6 mm	Isocratic EtOH : Water (6 : 4) 0.6 mL/min	Post-column reduction to 2-methyl-1,4-dihydroxy-napthalene by sodium borohydride Fluorescence Ex λ = 325 Em λ = 425	QL 0.02 μg/g	J. Chromatogr., 301, 441, 1984[2]
3. Rat chow	K_3	SFE CO_2, 8000 psi, 60°C 20 min	—	μBondapak C_{18}, 10 μm 15 cm × 3.9 mm	MeCN : 0.025 m $NaClO_4$ (90 : 10) 2 mL/min	EC reductive mode Ag electrode at −0.75 V vs calomel electrode	DL 125 pg at detector % Recovery 90.5 QL 20 μg/g product	J. Chromatogr. Sci., 26, 458, 1988[3]

TABLE 4.4 Continued

		Sample Preparation		HPLC Parameters				
Sample Matrix	Analyte	Sample Extraction	Clean Up	Column	Mobile Phase	Detection	Quality Assurance Parameters	References
4. Animal feeds	K_3	Add $CHCl_3$, NH_4OH, Celite-sodium sulfate (3 : 10) Shake 20 min Neutralize with HAC Centrifuge Dilute or concentrate $CHCl_3$ extract Extraction based on reference	—	LiChrosorb Si 60, 5 μm 25 cm × 4 mm	Isocratic CH_2Cl_2 (100%) 1.8 mL/min	251 nm	DL (ng) On-column 2.5 ng % Recovery 93–97	J. Assoc. Off. Anal. Chem., 71, 826, 1988[4]
5. Animal feed	K_3 (MSB)	Extract with water : MeOH (60 : 40) Shake 30 min Centrifuge Add 5% sodium carbonate Extract with n-pentane Evaporate Redissolve in MeOH	—	Supelcosil LC-18, 5 μm 25 cm × 4 mm	Isocratic MeOH : Water (75 : 25) 0.9 mL/min	Post-column reduction to 2-methyl-1,4-dihydroxy napthalene Fluorescence Ex λ = 325 Em λ = 425	QL 20 μg/kg % Recovery >90	J. Chromatogr., 472, 371, 1989[5]
6. Animal feed	K_1, K_2, (MK-4) K_3	Add $CHCl_3$ Shake 3 min Add 25% ammonia Shake 3 min Add celite : sodium sulfate (3 : 10) Shake 20 min Neutralize with HAC Centrifuge Filter $CHCl_3$ layer	—	LiChrosorb Si 60, 5 μm 25 cm × 4 mm	Isocratic Hex : CH_2Cl_2 30°C 1 mL/min	264 nm	QL 100 ng/g	Anal. Proc., 30, 266, 1993[6]

4.3.1 HIGH PERFORMANCE LIQUID CHROMATOGRAPHY

4.3.1.1 Extraction Procedures for Vitamin K Analysis by HPLC

The instability of vitamin K under alkaline conditions precludes the use of saponification for sample extraction. The necessity to remove other lipid components from vitamin K extracts prior to LC quantitation was a hindrance to early attempts to assay the vitamin from complex, fat-containing matrices. Extraction with water-soluble organic solvents such as ethanol, isopropanol, and acetonitrile to denature proteins followed by partitioning with non-polar solvents efficiently can be used to extract vitamin K from serum. However, when used with more complex matrices, a total fat extract is obtained that must be extensively fractionated to eliminate the fat prior to determinative chromatography. Chromatograms obtained by LC and UV detection are often complex with poor resolution of vitamin K compounds from chromatographic interferences.

Development of extraction procedures that efficiently removed fat from the initial homogenate or extract were necessary to further the application of LC to complex matrices. In 1980, Barnett et al.[28] introduced the use of lipase hydrolysis as a primary extraction step. These investigators used the non-specific lipase from the yeast *Candida cyclindraccae* to hydrolyze lipids in infant formula and dairy products as the initial step in the extraction of fat-soluble vitamins. Fatty acid hydrolyzates were then partitioned with pentane to yield an extract suitable for reversed-phase chromatography with detection at 265 nm. The Barnett et al.[28] lipase hydrolysis procedure has been incorporated into many published procedures for vitamin K analysis (Table 4.4).

Solid-phase extraction is an integral part of most current assay methods for vitamin K. As shown in Table 4.4, methods for clinical samples almost universally rely upon Sep-Pak silica for clean-up of initial solvent extracts prior to LC resolution. Of significance to AOAC International methodology, Hwang[29] applied an open-column chromatographic clean up step on silica to infant formula extracts to allow resolution of trans- and cis-isomers of vitamin K_1 by normal-phase chromatography. This work provides the basis of AOAC International Method 992.27 "*Trans*-vitamin K_1 (Phylloquinone) in Ready-To-Feed Milk-Based Infant Formula," *AOAC Official Methods of Analysis,* chap. 50.1.06. Currently, Method 992.27 is the only collaborated method offered by AOAC International for analysis of vitamin K_1 in infant formula. It is not without problems. An unacceptable deficiency is the method's inability to measure the *cis*-isomer in products formulated with corn oil owing to UV absorbing interferences masking the *cis*-isomer peak. Additionally, chromatograms of most samples tend to be complex because of lipid interferences. Overall, RSD_r values are unacceptably high at 20.9%.

The Task Force on Methods for Nutrition Analysis[30] realized the deficiencies of Method 992.27 and recommended two procedures for collaborative study to improve regulatory methods for analysis of vitamin K_1 in infant formula. A method developed by Bueno and Villalobos[31] modified the lipase hydrolysis procedure of Barnett et al.[28] in an attempt to improve chromatography. Chromatograms were still subject to UV absorbing interferences. A second method recommended by the Task Force was part of a series of papers published by Landen and colleagues that showed the power of gel permeation chromatography to fractionate fat-soluble vitamins from triacylglycerols and other lipids; thus, providing an efficient clean-up of extracts prior to determinative chromatography.[32] The procedures are discussed in detail in Chapter 5. Neither method was collaborated.

In addition to lipase hydrolysis, SPE clean up, and gel permeation chromatography, semi-preparative LC can be effectively used in vitamin K methodology. Methods by Haroon et al.[33] and Indyk et al.[34] for analysis of bovine milk and infant formula and Lambert et al.[35] for analysis of serum applied semi-preparative LC procedures for clean up of initial extracts.

4.3.1.2 Chromatography Parameters

4.3.1.2.1 Supports and Mobile Phases

Methods for vitamin K analysis were developed through the combination of adsorption chromatography for extract clean up and reversed-phase chromatography on C_{18} supports as the determinative step. Methods presented in Table 4.4 that were published since 1990 incorporate this proven approach. Mobile phases are usually isocratic based upon methanol modified with dichloromethane; however, a wide selection of mobile-phase compositions have been effective.

Mobile-phase composition is dependent upon the detection mode. Electrochemical detection requires addition of an electrolyte such as sodium acetate or perchlorate in the mobile phase to support the conductivity. Post-column reduction of the quinones to the fluorescent hydroquinones requires the addition of zinc chloride when a post-column zinc metal reduction column is used.

4.3.1.2.2 Detection

UV detection near absorption maxima can be used for high potency samples including premixes, supplements, and vitamin pills. Use of UV filters as the complexity of the sample matrix increases and concentrations of vitamin K compounds decreases to clinical levels. Problems associated with UV interfering compounds present in lipid containing extracts makes UV detection unworkable for many matrices. Detection methods based on electrochemistry or reductive formation of fluorescent hydroquinones from the quinones were largely necessitated because of the lack of sensitivity and selectivity of UV detection.

Lambert and De Leenheer[24] provide an in-depth review of electrochemical detection and reductive inducement of fluorescence by electrochemical, photodegradative, or chemical reaction for the subsequent fluorescence detection of the reduced, highly fluorescent hydroquinone forms of vitamin K. Current methods utilize techniques originally developed by Haroon et al.[36] for plasma and other biological samples. The method was based on post-column reduction of vitamin K (quinone) into fluorescent hydroquinones by use of a solid-phase reductive column packed with metallic zinc particles. The work followed studies by Langenberg and Tjaden[37] on application of an electrochemical detector for the reductive process followed by fluorescence detection for quantitation. Haroon's research showed that the solid-phase reactor offered many advantages over electrochemical reduction. Of significance, the zinc column increased reduction efficiency and simplified the instrumental set-up compared to electrochemical reduction. The zinc, post-column reduction inducement of fluorescence in vitamin K extracts forms the basis of newer, highly specific assay methods for vitamin K. Methods adapted by Sadowski's research group for vitamin K_1 and dihydro-vitamin K_1 in foods[6–16] and recently by Indyk and Woollard[38] for analysis of milk and infant formula use the solid-phase zinc reduction column methodology put forth by Haroon et al.[36] These methods are detailed in Section 4.4. The sensitivity and specificity afforded by reductive formation of the fluorescent quinones makes this methodology preferential to other analytical approaches for vitamin K. Discussions by Davidson and Sadowski[39] and Booth and Sadowski[40] further detail chromatography systems using zinc reduction column methodology. Modification of the chromatography system permits simultaneous assay of the phylloquinone and phylloquinone 2,3-epoxide in plasma.[39] These modifications are provided in Table 4.4 (Table 4.4, Biologicals, Reference 19).

Zinc reduction was adapted to a flow injection fluorometric assay of menadione sodium bisulfate (MSB).[41] The fluorescent hydroquinone derivative was formed by two coupled steps in the flow injection system. The sodium sulfite form of the menadione (K_3) was hydrolyzed by merging MSB in acetonitrile : water (9 : 1) with 0.035 M sodium hydroxide. The hydroquinone was then produced in a zinc reactor in an acidic medium formed by merging 0.08 M hydrochloric acid in acetonitrile : water (4 : 6) with the sodium hydroxide stream. The assay was applied to various pharmaceutical products. The limit of detection was 0.005 μg/mL with reproducibility of 1.6%. Seventy samples could be assayed per hour.

4.3.1.2.3 Internal Standards

The use of internal standards in the LC quantitation of vitamin K is encouraged because of the extensive clean up of extracts that is required and, in the case of reductive formation of hydroquinones for fluorescence detection, the chance for incomplete conversion of the quinone to the fluorescent form.

Internal standards that are effective include vitamin $K_{1(25)}$, Mk-5, Mk-6, Mk-7, 6-methyl-men-quinone (Mk-9) (Table 4.4). Dihydro-vitamin K_1 and vitamin K_1 epoxide quite frequently have been used as internal standards. Their use should be considered only after complete absence in the biological matrix is assured. Dihydro-vitamin K_1 has been documented to be a product of the hydrogenation of edible oils.[12,13,14] Therefore, use of dihydro-vitamin K_1 as an internal standard should be limited to biologicals and foods where its absence is documented.

4.4   METHOD PROTOCOLS
Evaluation of an HPLC Method for the Determination of Phylloquinone (Vitamin K₁) in Various Food Matrices

Principle
- After initial extraction in isopropanol and hexane, the food extracts were purified by solid-phase extraction on silica gel. The amount of K_1 was determined by LC by applying a post column chemical reduction followed by fluorescence detection of the hydroquinone.

Chemicals
- Vitamin K_1 standard
- 2,3 dihydrophylloquinone—internal standard for vegetables, milk
- 2-methyl-3-(3,7,11,15,19-pentamethyl-2-eicosenyl)-1,4-naphthalenedione ($K_{1(25)}$)—internal standard for bread, beef
- Isopropanol
- Hexane
- Dichloromethane
- Methanol
- $ZnCl_2$
- Acetic acid
- Sodium acetate

Apparatus
- Liquid chromatograph
- Fluorescence detector
- Silica gel columns (3 mL) for solid-phase extraction
- Sonicator—Soniter-cell disrupter with $\frac{1}{8}$ in. tapered microtip
- Centrifugal evaporator

Procedure

For Vegetable Juice
- Weigh prepared sample in 50 mL centrifuge tubes
- Add internal standard
- Add 15 mL isopropanol : hexane (3 : 2, V/V) followed by 4 mL H_2O
- Sonicate at 40% duty cycle for 30 s
- Aspirate hexane layer into culture tube
- Evaporate to dryness in a centrifugal evaporator
- Dissolve residue in 2 mL hexane

Solid-Phase Extraction on Silica Gel
- Precondition column by washing with 8 mL hexane/diethyl ether (93 : 3, V/V) and 8 mL hexane

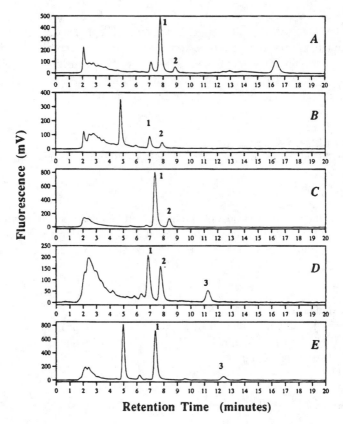

Figure 4.7   Chromatograms of extracts of vegetable juice (A), milk (B), spinach (C), bread (D), and beef (E). Peak 1—phylloquinone, Peak 2—dihydro-vitamin K_1, and Peak 3—vitamin $K_{1(25)}$. Reproduced with permission from Reference 10.

- Apply 2 mL hexane extract
- Wash with 8 mL hexane
- Elute vitamin K_1 with 8 mL hexane : diethyl ether (93 : 3, V/V)
- Collect vitamin fraction in 16 × 100 mm screw-cap culture tube
- Evaporate to dryness
- Reconstitute with 20 µL methylene chloride
- Add 180 µL methanol containing 10 mM $ZnCl_2$, 5 mM acetic acid, and 5 mM sodium acetate
- Inject 100 µL onto HPLC column

Chromatography (Figure 4.7)

Column	15.0 cm × 4.6 mm
Stationary phase	Hypersil ODS, 3 µm
Mobile phase	Methanol : methylene chloride (90 : 10, V/V). To each item add 5 mL solution containing 2 M zinc chloride, 1 M acetic acid and 1 M sodium acetate.
Column temperature	Ambient
LC post column reactor	2.0 × 50 mm packed with zinc metal
Flow	1 mL/min
Detection	Fluorescence Ex λ = 244 nm, Em λ = 418 nm

| Calculation | Internal standard, peak areas |
| Retention time | 7.5 min |

J. Agric. Food Chem., 42, 295, 1994; *J. Agric. Food Chem.,* 40, 1874, 1992; *J. Agric. Food Chem.,* 40, 1878, 1992; *Clin. Chem.,* 32, 1925, 1986

Vitamin K in Milk and Infant Formulas: Determination and Distribution of Phylloquinone and Menaquinone-4.

Principle
- Phylloquinone and menaquionone-4 are extracted by lipase digestion, protein denaturation with potassium carbonate, pH adjustment and alcohol, and hexane partitioning. Analytes are resolved by reversed-phase LC with fluorescence detection after zinc post-column reduction.

Chemicals
- Vitamin K_1 standard (USP)
- Mk-4 standard
- Ethanol
- Methanol
- Sodium hydroxide
- Potassium carbonate
- Potassium phosphate
- Zinc chloride
- Sodium acetate
- Acetic acid
- Hexane
- Dichloromethane
- Lipase, Type VII (Sigma)
- Zinc powder

Apparatus
- Liquid chromatograph
- Fluorescence detector
- Stainless-steel reductive column (20 × 4 mm)

Procedure

Extraction
- Weigh 1.0 g powdered milk or infant formula or 10 g fluid milk
- Add 15 mL warm H_2O (< 40°C)
- Add 5.0 mL phosphate buffer
- Add 1.0 g lipase
- Vortex and shake for 7 min
- Incubate at 37°C for 120 min (shaking each 20 min)
- Cool to ambient
- Add 10 mL reagent alcohol (EtOH + CH_3OH (95 + 5)
- Add 1.0 g K_2CO_3
- Mix
- Add 30.0 mL hexane
- Shake for 7 min
- Centrifuge at 1000 rpm/min for 10 min
- Transfer 0.5 mL hexane layer (supplemental formula) to glass vial

- Evaporate hexane
- Dissolve residue in 1.0 mL CH_3OH
- Filter (0.45 μm)

Chromatography

Column	Radial compression module, 10 cm × 8 mm
Stationary phase	C_{18} resolve cartridge
Mobile phase	Dichloromethane + methanol (900 + 100) + 5 mL methanolic solution of $ZnCl_2$ (1.37 g) + sodium acetate (0.41 g) + glacial acetic acid (0.3 g)

Flow	1.5 mL/min
LC post column reactor	20 × 4 mm stainless-steel column packed with Zn powder
Detection	Fluorescence, Ex λ = 243, Em λ = 430
Calculation	External standard, peak area

Analyst, 122, 465, 1997

4.5   REFERENCES

Text

1. Friedrich, W., in *Vitamins*, Walter de Gruyter, Berlin, 1988, chap. 5.
2. Suttie, J. E., Vitamin K, in *Present Knowledge in Nutrition*, 7th ed., Ziegler, E. E. and Filer, C. J., Jr., Eds., ILSI Press, Washington, DC, 1996, chap. 14.
3. Olson, R. E. and Munson, P. L., Fat-soluble vitamins, in *Principles of Pharmacology*, Munson, P. L., Mueller, R. A., and Breese, G. R., Eds., Chapman and Hall, New York, 1994, chap. 58.
4. *The Infant Formula Act of 1980* (Public Law 96-359, 94 Stat. 1190-1195), Section 412, 21 United States Code 350a, 21 CFR107.100.
5. Cornelissen, E., Kollee, L., DeAbreu, R., van Baal, J., Motohara, K., Verbruggen, B., and Monnens, L., Effects of oral and intramusclar vitamin K prophylaxis on vitamin K_1 PIVKA-II, and clotting factors in breast fed infants, *Arch. Dis. Child.*, 67, 1250, 1992.
6. Ferland, G. and Sadowski, J. A., Vitamin K_1 (phylloquinone) content of edible oils: effects of heating and light exposure, *J. Agric. Food Chem.*, 40, 1869, 1992.
7. Ferland, G. and Sadowski, J. A., Vitamin K_1 (phylloquinone) content of green vegetables: effects of plant maturation and geographical growth location, *J. Agric. Food Chem.*, 40, 1874, 1992.
8. Ferland, G., MacDonald, D. L., and Sadowski, J. A., Development of a diet low in vitamin K_1 (phylloquinone), *J. Am. Diet. Assoc.*, 92, 593, 1992.
9. Booth, S. L., Sadowski, J. A., Weihrauch, J. L., and Ferland, G., Vitamin K_1 (phylloquinone) content of foods: a provisional table, *J. Food Comp. Anal.*, 6, 109, 1993.
10. Booth, S. L., Davidson, K. W., and Sadowski, J. A., Evaluation of an HPLC method for the determination of phylloquinone (vitamin K_1) in various food matrices, *J. Agric. Food Chem.*, 42, 295, 1994.
11. Booth, S. L., Madabushi, H. T., Davidson, K. W., and Sadowski, J. A., Tea and coffee brews are not dietary sources of vitamin K_1 (phylloquinone), *J. Am. Diet. Assoc.*, 95, 82, 1995.
12. Booth, S. L., Davidson, K. W., Lichtenstein, A. H., and Sadowski, J. A., Plasma concentrations of dihydro-vitamin K_1 following dietary intake of a hydrogenated vitamin K_1-rich vegetable oil, *Lipids*, 31, 709, 1996.
13. Booth, S. L., Pennington, J. A. T., and Sadowski, J. A., Dihydro-vitamin K_1: primary food sources and estimated dietary intakes in the American diet, *Lipids*, 31, 715, 1996.
14. Davidson, K. W., Booth, S. L., Dolnikowski, G. G., and Sadowski, J. A., Conversion of vitamin K_1 to 2′,3′-dihydrovitamin K_1 during the hydrogenation of vegetable oils, *J. Agric. Food Chem.*, 44, 980, 1996.
15. Booth, S. L., Pennington, J. A. T., and Sadowski, J. A., Food sources and dietary intakes of vitamin K_1 (phylloquinone) in the American diet: data from the FDA Total Diet Study, *J. Am. Diet. Assoc.*, 96, 149, 1996.

16. Booth, S. L., Charnley, J. M., Sadowski, J. A., Saltzman, E., Bovill, E. G., and Cushman, M., Dietary vitamin K_1 and stability of oral anticoagulation: proposal of a diet with constant vitamin K_1 content, *Thromb. Haemo.*, 77, 504, 1997.

17. Eitenmiller, R. R. and Landen, W. O., Jr., Vitamins, in *Analyzing Food for Nutrition Labeling and Hazardous Contaminants*, Jeon, I. J. and Ikins, W. G., Eds., Marcel Dekker, New York, 1995, chap. 9.

18. National Research Council, *Recommended Dietary Allowances*, 10th ed., National Academy of Sciences, Washington, D.C., 1989, chap. 8.

19. Nutritional Labeling and Education Act of 1990, *Fed. Reg.*, 58, 2070, 1993.

20. **Anon.**, Nomenclature policy: generic descriptions and trivial names for vitamins and related compounds, *J. Nutr.*, 120, 12, 1990.

21. *21 CFR 172.867*, Olestra.

22. Ball, G. F. M., Chemical and biological nature of fat-soluble vitamins, in *Fat-Soluble Vitamin Assays in Food Analysis*, Elsevier, New York, 1988, chap. 2.

23. Berruti, R., Vitamin K, in *Methods of Vitamin Assay*, 4th ed., Augustin, J., Klein, B. P., Becker, D. A., and Venugopal, P. B., Eds., John Wiley and Sons, New York, 1985, chap. 11.

24. Lambert, W. E. and De Leenheer, A. P., Vitamin K, in *Modern Chromatographic Analysis of Vitamins*, 2nd ed., De Leenheer, A. P., Lambert, W. E., and Nelis, H. J., Eds., Marcel Dekker, New York, 1992, chap. 4.

25. Bechtold, H. and Jahnchen, E., Quantitative analysis of vitamin K_1 and vitamin K_1 2,3-epoxide in plasma by electron-capture gas-liquid chromatography, *J. Chromatogr.*, 164, 85, 1979.

26. Fauler, G., Leis, H., Schalamon, J., Muntean, W., and Gleispach, H., Method for the determination of vitamin $K_{1(20)}$ in human plasma by stable isotope dilution/gas chromatography/mass spectrometry, *J. Mass Spectr.*, 31, 655, 1996.

27. Imanaka, M., Kadota, M., Kumashiro, K., and Mori, T., Identification of phylloquinone (vitamin K_1) as an unknown peak in electron capture detection gas chromatograms of pyrethroid insecticide residues, *J. AOAC Int.*, 79, 538, 1996.

28. Barnett, S. A., Frick, L. W., and Baine, H. M., Simultaneous determination of vitamins A, D_2 or D_3, E, and K_1 in infant formulas and dairy products by reversed-phase liquid chromatography, *Anal. Chem.*, 52, 610, 1980.

29. Hwang, S. M., Liquid chromatographic determination of vitamin K_1 *trans-* and *cis-*isomers in infant formula, *J. Assoc. Off. Anal. Chem.*, 68, 684, 1985.

30. AOAC International, Report of the AOAC International Task Force on Methods for Nutrient Labeling Analyses, *J. AOAC Int.*, 76, 180A, 1993.

31. Bueno, M. P. and Villalobos, M. C., Reverse phase high pressure liquid chromatographic determination of vitamin K_1 in infant formula, *J. Assoc. Off. Anal. Chem.*, 66, 1063, 1983.

32. Landen, W. O., Jr., Eitenmiller, R. R., and Soliman, A. M., Vitamin D_3 and vitamin K_1 levels in infant formula produced in the United States, *J. Food Comp. Anal.*, 2, 140, 1989.

33. Haroon, Y., Shearer, M. J., Rahim, S., Gunn, W. G., McEnery, G., and Barkhan, P., The content of phylloquinone (vitamin K_1) in human milk, cow's milk and infant formula foods determined by high-performance liquid chromatography, *J. Nutr.*, 112, 1105, 1982.

34. Indyk, H. E., Littlejohn, V. C., Lawrence, R. J., and Woollard, D. C., Liquid chromatographic determination of vitamin K_1 in infant formulas and milk, *J. AOAC Int.*, 78, 719, 1995.

35. Lambert, W. E., De Leenheer, A. P., and Baert, E. J., Wet-chemical post-column reaction and fluorescence detection analysis of the reference interval of endogenous serum vitamin $K_{1(20)}$, *Anal. Biochem.*, 158, 257, 1986.

36. Haroon, Y., Bacon, D. S., and Sadowski, J. A., Liquid-chromatographic determination of vitamin K_1 in plasma, with fluorometric detection, *Clin. Chem.*, 32, 1925, 1986.

37. Langenberg, J. P. and Tjaden, U. R., Determination of (endogenous) vitamin K_1 in human plasma by reversed-phase high performance liquid chromatography using fluorometric detection after post column electrochemical reduction. Comparison with ultraviolet, single, dual electrochemical detection, *J. Chromatogr.*, 305, 61, 1984.

38. Indyk, H. E. and Woollard, D. C., Vitamin K_1 in milk and infant formulas: determination and distribution of phylloquinone and menaquinone-4, *Analyst*, 122, 465, 1997.

39. Davidson, K. W. and Sadowski, J. A., Determination of vitamin K compounds in plasma or serum by high-performance liquid chromatography using post column chemical reduction and fluorometric detection, *Meth. Enzymol.,* 282, 408, 1997.

40. Booth, S. L. and Sadowski, J. A., Determination of phylloquinone in foods by high-performance liquid chromatography, *Meth. Enzymol.,* 282, 446, 1997.

41. Torro, I. G., Garcia Mateo, J. V., and Martinez Calatayud, J., Spectrofluorometric determination of vitamin K₃ by a solid-phase zinc reactor immobilized in a flow injection assembly, *Analyst,* 122, 139, 1997.

Table 4.3 Compendium, Regulatory and Handbook Methods for the Analysis of Vitamin K and Related Compounds

1. The United States Pharmacopeial Convention, Inc., *U.S. Pharmacopeia National Formulary,* USP/NF18, Nutritional Supplements, Official Monographs, United States Pharmacopeial Convention, Rockville, MD, 1995.
2. Scottish Home and Health Department, British Pharmacopoeia, 15th ed., British Pharmacopoeia Commission, United Kingdom, 1993.
3. AOAC International, *Official Methods of Analysis,* 16th ed., AOAC International, Arlington, VA, 1995.
4. Hwang, J. S. M., Liquid chromatographic determination of vitamin K, *trans-* and *cis-*isomers in infant formula, *Assoc. Off. Anal. Chem.,* 68, 684, 1985.
5. Tanner, J. T., Barnett, S. A., and Mountford, M. K., Analysis of milk-based infant formula. Phase IV. Iodine, linoleic acid, and vitamins D and K, U.S. Food and Drug Administration—Infant Formula Council: collaborative study, *J. AOAC Int.,* 76, 1042, 1993.
6. Winkler, V. W., Collaborative study of a gas-liquid chromatographic method for the determination of water soluble menadione (vitamin K₃) in feed premixes, *J. Assoc. Off. Anal. Chem.,* 56, 1277, 1973.
7. American Feed Ingredients Association, *Laboratory Methods Compendium,* vol. 1: *Vitamins and Minerals,* American Feed Ingredients Association, West Des Moines, IA, 1991, 153.
8. Keller, H. E., *Analytical Methods for Vitamins and Carotenoids,* Hoffmann-LaRoche, Basel, 1988, 17.
9. Manz, U. and Maurer, R., A method for the determination of vitamin K₃ in premixes and animal feedstuffs with the aid of high performance liquid chromatography, *Int. J. Vit. Nutr. Res.,* 52, 248, 1982.

Table 4.4 HPLC Methods for the Analysis of Vitamin K in Foods, Feed, Pharmaceuticals and Biologicals

Foods

1. Barnett, S. A., Frick, L. W., and Baine, H. M., Simultaneous determination of vitamin A, D₂ or D₃, E and K₁ in infant formula and dairy products by reversed phase liquid chromatography, *Anal. Chem.,* 52, 610, 1980.
2. Haroon, Y., Shearer, M., Rahim, S., Gunn, W., McEnery, G., and Barkhan, P., The content of phylloquinone (vitamin K₁) in human milk, cow's milk, and infant formula foods determined by high-performance liquid chromatography, *J. Nutr.,* 112, 1105, 1982.
3. Bueno, M. P. and Villalobos, M. C., Reverse phase high pressure liquid chromatographic determination of vitamin K₁ in infant formula, *J. Assoc. Off. Anal. Chem.,* 66, 1063, 1983.
4. Hwang, S. M., Liquid chromatographic determination of vitamin K₁ *trans-* and *cis-*isomers in infant formula, *J. Assoc. Off. Anal. Chem.,* 68, 684, 1985.
5. Isshiki, H., Suzuki, Y., Yonekubo, A., Hasegawa, H., and Yamamoto, Y., Determination of phylloquinone and menaquinone in human milk using high performance liquid chromatography, *J. Dairy Sci.,* 71, 627, 1988.
6. Landen, W. O., Jr., Eitenmiller, R. R., and Soliman, A. M., Vitamin D₃ and vitamin K₁ levels in infant formula produced in the United States, *J. Food Comp. Anal.,* 2, 140, 1989.
7. Canfield, L. M., Hopkinson, J. M., Lima, A. F., Martin, G. S., Sugimoto, K., Burr, J., Clark, L., and McGee, D. L., Quantitation of vitamin K in human milk, *Lipids,* 25, 406, 1990.

8. Lambert, W. E., Vanneste, L., and De Leenheer, A. P., Enzymatic sample hydrolysis and HPLC in a study of phylloquinone concentration in human milk, *Clin. Chem.,* 38, 1743, 1992.
9. Tanner, J. T., Barnett, S.A., and Mountford, M. K., Analyses of milk-based infant formula. Phase IV. Iodide, linoleic acid, and vitamin D and K; U.S. Food and Drug Administration—Infant Formula Council: collaborative study, *J. AOAC Int.,* 76, 1042, 1993.
10. Indyk, H. E., Littlejohn, V. C., Lawrence, R. J., and Woollard, D. C., Liquid chromatographic determination of vitamin K_1 in infant formulas and milk, *J. AOAC Int.,* 78, 719, 1995.
11. Indyk, H. E. and Woollard, D. C., The endogenous vitamin K_1 content of bovine milk: temporal influence of season and lactation, *Food Chem.,* 54, 403, 1995.
12. Indyk, H. E. and Woollard, D. C., Vitamin K_1 in milk and infant formula: determination and distribution of phylloquinone and menaquinone-4, *Analyst,* 122, 465, 1997.
13. Langenberg, J. P., Tjaden, U. R., DeVogel, E. M., and Langerak, D. I., Determination of phylloquinone (vitamin K_1) in raw and processed vegetables using reversed phase HPLC with electrofluorometric detection, *Acta Aliment.,* 15, 187, 1986.
14. Ferland, G. and Sadowski, J. A., Vitamin K_1 (phylloquinone) content of green vegetables: effects of plant maturation and geographical growth location, *J. Agric. Food Chem.,* 40, 1874, 1992.
15. Booth, S. L., Davidson, K. W., and Sadowski, J. A., Evaluation of an HPLC method for determination of phylloquinone (vitamin K_1) in various food matrices, *J. Agric. Food Chem.,* 42, 295, 1994.
16. Booth, S. L. and Sadowski, J. A., Determination of phylloquinone in foods by high-performance liquid chromatography, *Meth. Enzymol.,* 282, 446, 1997.
17. Ferland, G. and Sadowski, J. A., Vitamin K_1 (phylloquinone) content of edible oils: effects of heating and light exposure, *J. Agric. Food Chem.,* 40, 1869, 1992.
18. Gao, Z. H. and Ackman, R. G., Determination of vitamin K_1 in canola oils by high performance liquid chromatography with menaquinone-4 as an internal standard, *Food Res. Int.,* 28, 61, 1995.
19. Jakob, E. and Elmadfa, I., Application of a simplified HPLC assay for the determination of phylloquinone (vitamin K_1) in animal and plant food items, *Food Chem.,* 56, 87, 1996.
20. Careri, M., Mangia, A., Manini, P., and Taboni, N., Determination of phylloquinone (vitamin K_1) by high performance liquid chromatography with UV detection and with particle beam-mass spectrometry, *Fres. J. Anal. Chem.,* 355, 48, 1996.
21. Piironen, V., Koivu, T., Tammisalo, O., and Mattila, P., Determination of phylloquinone in oils, margarines and butter by high performance liquid chromatography with electrochemical detection, *Food Chem.,* 59, 473, 1997.
22. Indyk, H., The photoinduced reduction and simultaneous fluorescence detection of vitamin K_1 with HPLC, *J. Micronutr. Anal.,* 4, 61, 1988.

Pharmaceuticals

1. Lennon, C., Davidson, K. W., Sadowski, J. A., and Mason, J. B., The vitamin K content of intravenous lipid emulsions, *JPEN,* 17, 142, 1993.
2. Moussa, F., Depasse, F., Lompret, V., Hautem, J. Y., Girardet, J., Fontaine, J., and Aymard, P., Determination of phylloquinone in intravenous fat emulsions and soybean oil by high performance liquid chromatography, *J.Chromatogr. A,* 664, 189, 1994.

Biologicals

1. Haroon, Y. and Hauschka, P. V., Application of high-performance liquid chromatography to assay phylloquinone (vitamin K_1) in rat liver, *J. Lipid Res.,* 24, 481, 1983.
2. Langenberg, J. P. and Tjaden, U. R., Determination of (endogenous) vitamin K_1 in human plasma by reversed-phase high performance liquid chromatography using fluorometric detection after post column electrochemical reduction. Comparison with ultraviolet, single, and dual electrochemical detection, *J. Chromatogr.,* 305, 61, 1984.
3. Hirauchi, K., Sakano, T., and Morimoto, A., Measurement of K vitamins in human and animal plasma by high-performance liquid chromatography with fluorometric detection, *Chem. Pharm. Bull.,* 34, 845, 1986.
4. Lambert, W. E., De Leenheer, A. P., and Baert, E. J., Wet-chemical post column reaction and fluorescence detection analysis of the reference interval of endogenous serum vitamin $K_{1(20)}$, *Anal. Biochem.,* 158, 257, 1986.

5. Haroon, Y., Bacon, D. S., and Sadowski, J. A., Liquid-chromatographic determination of vitamin K_1 in plasma, with fluorometric detection, *Clin. Chem.,* 32, 1925, 1986.

6. Hirauchi, K., Sakano, T., Nagaoka, T., and Morimoto, A., Simultaneous determination of vitamin K_1, vitamin K_1 2,3-epoxide and menaquinone-4 in human plasma by high performance liquid chromatography with fluorometric detection, *J. Chromatogr.,* 430, 21, 1988.

7. Hiraike, H., Kimura, M., and Itokawa, Y., Determination of K vitamins (phylloquinone and menaquinones) in umbilical cord plasma by a platinum-reduction column, *J. Chromatogr.,* 430, 143, 1988.

8. Conly, J. M. and Stein, K., Quantitative and qualitative measurements of K vitamins in human intestinal contents, *Am. J. Gastroenterol.,* 87, 311, 1992.

9. Conly, J. M., Assay of menaquinones in bacterial cultures, stool samples, and intestinal contents, *Meth. Enzymol.,* 282, 457, 1997.

10. Thijssen, H. H. W. and Drittij-Reijnders, M. J., Vitamin K metabolism and vitamin K_1 status in human liver samples: a search for inter-individual differences in warfarin sensitivity, *Brit. J. Haematol.,* 84, 681, 1993.

11. Hodges, S. J., Bejui, J., Leclercq, M., and Delmas, P. D., Detection of vitamins K_1 and K_2 in human cortical and trabecular bone, *J. Bone Miner. Res.,* 8, 1005, 1993.

12. Thijssen, H. H. W. and Drittij-Reijnders, M. J., Vitamin K distribution in rat tissues: dietary phylloquinone is a source of tissue menaquinone, *Br. J. Nutr.,* 72, 415, 1994.

13. Thijssen, H. H. W. and Drittij-Reijnders, M. J., Vitamin K status in human tissues: tissue-specific accumulation of phylloquinone and menaquinone-4, *Br. J. Nutr.,* 75, 121, 1996.

14. Reedstrom, C. K. and Suttie, J. W., Comparative distribution, metabolism, and utilization of phylloquinone and menaquinone-9 in rat liver, *PSEBM,* 209, 403, 1995.

15. Jacob, E. and Elmadfa, I., Rapid HPLC assay for the assessment of vitamin K, A, E, and β-carotene status in children (7–19 years), *Int. J. Vit. Nutr. Res.,* 65, 31, 1995.

16. Hu, O. Y. P., Wu, C. Y., Chan, W. K., and Wu, F. Y. H., Determination of anticancer drug vitamin K_3 in plasma by high performance liquid chromatography, *J. Chromatogr. B,* 666, 299, 1995.

17. MacCrehan, W. A. and Schönberger, E., Determination of vitamin K_1 in serum using catalytic-reduction liquid chromatography with fluorescence detection, *J. Chromatogr. B,* 670, 209, 1995.

18. Sano, Y., Kikuchi, K., Tadano, K., Hoshi, K., and Koshihara, Y., Simultaneous determination of menaquinone-4 and its metabolite in human osteoblasts by high-performance liquid chromatography/atmospheric pressure chemical ionization tandem mass spectrometry, *Anal. Sci.,* 13, 67, 1997.

19. Davidson, K. W. and Sadowski, J. A., Determination of vitamin K compounds in plasma or serum by high-performance liquid chromatography using post chemical reduction and fluorimetric detection, *Meth. Enzymol.,* 282, 408, 1997.

20. McCarthy, P. T., Harrington, D. J., and Shearer, M. J., Assay of phylloquinone in plasma by high performance liquid chromatography with electrochemical detection, *Meth. Enzymol.,* 282, 421, 1997.

Feed

1. Manz, U., and Maurer, R., A method for the determination of vitamin K_3 in premixes and animal feedstuffs with the aid of high performance liquid chromatography, *Int. J. Vit. Nutr. Res.,* 52, 248, 1982.

2. Speek, A. J., Schrijver, J., and Schreurs, W. H. P., Fluorometric determination of menadione sodium bisulphite (vitamin K_3) in animal feed and premixes by high-performance liquid chromatography with post-column derivatization, *J. Chromatogr.,* 301, 441, 1984.

3. Schneiderman, M. A., Sharma, A. K., and Locke, D. C., Determination of menadione in an animal feed using supercritical fluid extraction and HPLC with electrochemical detector, *J. Chromatogr. Sci.,* 26, 458, 1988.

4. Laffi, R., Marchetti, S., and Marchetti, M., Normal-phase liquid chromatographic determination of menadione in animal feeds, *J. Assoc. Off. Anal. Chem.,* 71, 826, 1988.

5. Billedeau, S. M., Fluorometric determination of vitamin K_3 (menadione sodium bisulfite) in synthetic animal feed by high performance liquid chromatography using a post-column zinc reducer, *J. Chromatogr.,* 472, 371, 1989.

6. White, S., Determination of vitamin K_1, K_2, (Mk-4) and K_3 in animal feeds by high-performance liquid chromatography, *Anal. Proc.,* 30, 266, 1993.

5 MULTI-ANALYTE METHODS FOR ANALYSIS OF FAT-SOLUBLE VITAMINS

5.1 REVIEW

With the development of HPLC into the primary technique for fat-soluble vitamin analysis, efforts increased to develop methods to simultaneously assay two or more vitamins. Implementation of multi-analyte procedures can result in assay efficiency with savings in time and materials. To be useful, a simultaneous assay must not lead to loss of assay sensitivity, accuracy, and precision when compared to methods that accurately quantify single vitamins.

Difficulty exists for assay of fat-soluble vitamins simultaneously because of the complexity of the analytes. Specific problems include:

1. The vitamins are present in nature as structurally-related vitamers.
   A. Carotenoids represent a truly challenging analytical area due to the numbers and diversity present in fruits and vegetables. Often, *cis*-isomers must be resolved from the natural *trans*-isomers.
   B. Vitamin E includes eight homologs that vary in biological activity (α-, β-, γ-, and δ-tocopherol and the corresponding tocotrienols).
   C. Vitamin D analysis is complicated due to the potential presence of pre-D forms and structurally related sterols.
2. The presence of synthetic forms or metabolites can complicate quantitation.
   A. Milk is fortified with retinyl palmitate and total vitamin A activity includes natural retinol and provitamin A carotenoids. *Cis*-isomers vary in biological activity from the *trans*-isomers.
   B. All-rac-α-tocopheryl acetate is the primary fortification form of vitamin E. After saponification, all-rac-α-tocopherol cannot be resolved from RRR-α-tocopherol. The biological activity of all-rac-α-tocopherol is only 74% that of the natural vitamin. Therefore, accurate methods must quantitate the synthetic form in addition to the natural forms of vitamin E.
   C. Fortified foods can contain both vitamin D_2 and vitamin D_3.
3. Concentrations of the various vitamins differ considerably in biologicals, pharmaceuticals, foods, feeds, and fortified products. Even in fortified foods, vitamin D is present at such low concentrations that extensive clean-up and/or concentration is often necessary before determinative assay.
4. Each fat-soluble vitamin requires specific detection parameters. No one detection mode is ideal for all of the vitamins. Simultaneous detection requires multiple detectors in series, programmable detectors, sensitive photodiode array detectors (PDA), or combinations of such detectors.
5. Stability differences among fat-soluble vitamins often complicate extractions. Vitamin K cannot withstand saponification.

6. Co-eluting interferences often lead to the need for specialized sample clean-up approaches.
7. Initial set-up costs can be expensive.

A single method that is universally applicable to the analyses of vitamins A, D, E and K, their synthetic forms, and metabolites is not available. Increased capability of UV/visible, fluorescence, and PDA detectors have greatly influenced this area over the past decade, and useful methods are available to complete simultaneous assays of multiple analytes. This chapter provides information on applications of multi-analyte fat-soluble assay methods for several matrices of interest to the vitamin chemist.

5.2   FOOD, FEED, AND PHARMACEUTICALS

Ball[1,2] reviewed the literature on fat-soluble vitamin analysis of food and feed through 1987. Only two procedures were categorized as concurrent assays for vitamin A and vitamin D (assays using the same extract but separate LC injections). Six simultaneous assays (assays using the same extract and a single LC injection) were identified for various fat-soluble vitamins from a variety of matrices. Multi-analyte procedures were largely limited at this point in time owing to limitations posed by the difficulties presented in Section 5.1. Also, programmable UV/visible and fluorescence detectors were not in common use and PDA detectors, while commonly available, lacked the sensitivity present in the current generation of PDA detectors. During the 1990s, significant improvements on all types of detectors have made simultaneous assays somewhat easier to develop and incorporate into routine analysis programs. Multi-analyte assays developed in the present decade together with some histori-cally significant methods for food, feed, and pharmaceutical analysis are provided in Table 5.1.

5.2.1   BUTTER, MARGARINE, AND OILS

Margarine is a primary vehicle for the delivery of vitamin A activity and provides a significant source of vitamin E in diets where it is commonly used. It is fortified with retinyl palmitate, or in some cases, with retinyl acetate, and colored with β-carotene, which provides additional vitamin A activ-ity. Because of the significance of the product, it was one of the earliest foods for which multi-ana-lyte methods were developed. Thompson and Maxwell[3] provided a method to assay retinol and β-carotene in margarine following saponification and hexane extraction. This procedure used dif-ferent LC systems and separate injections, representing a concurrent assay. The first simultaneous method to assay total vitamin A in margarine was provided by Landen and Eitenmiller[4] in 1979. The method also introduced the use of high performance gel permeation chromatography (HP-GPC) to isolate the fat-soluble vitamins from the lipid fraction prior to determinative chromatography. This approach allowed simultaneous chromatography of β-carotene and quantitated the specific vitamin A forms in the food. Chromatography is shown in Figures 5.1-I and 5.1-II.

Thompson et al.[5] also presented a simultaneous analysis of retinyl palmitate and β-carotene in margarine that avoided saponification. The method was based on direct extraction of the analytes with hexane. Five grams of sample were dissolved in hexane, insoluble material was allowed to set-tle, and 5 mL of the clear solution was shaken with 5 mL of 60% ethanol. After centrifugation, retinyl palmitate and β-carotene were quantified by direct injection of the extract onto a Si60 column using ethyl ether : hexane (2 : 98) for elution. Retinyl palmitate and β-carotene were detected at 325 nm and 453 nm, respectively. This method has been used very successfully by the authors. It is highly reliable for routine vitamin A analysis of margarine and fluid milks. A study by Zonta et al.[6] pub-lished in 1982 was one of the first simultaneous analysis procedures to utilize a programmable UV/visible detector. The method quantitated vitamins D_2 and D_3 and the previtamin D forms, β-carotene, all-*trans*-retinol, and all-rac-α-tocopherol. Detection wavelengths were 265 nm for vitamin D_2 and D_3, 295 nm for the previtamin D forms, 450 nm for β-carotene, 325 nm for retinol and 295 nm for α-tocopherol. Vitamin K_1 was extracted after lipase hydrolysis and quantitated at 270 nm.

TABLE 5.1
Multi-Analyte Assays for Fat-Soluble Vitamins in Foods, Feed, and Pharmaceuticals

Sample Matrix	Analyte	Sample Preparation — Sample Extraction	Clean Up	HPLC Parameters — Column	Mobile Phase	Detection	Quality Assurance Parameters	References
Margarine, milk	Retinyl palmitate, β-carotene	Dissolve in Hex Shake with 60% EtOH Centrifuge Inject directly	—	LiChrosorb Si60 5 μm, 25 cm × 3.2 mm 2 mL/min	Isocratic Wet Hex : Dry Hex : EtO_2 (49 : 49 : 2)	Retinyl palmitate 325 nm β-carotene 453 nm 436 nm	—	J. Assoc. Off. Anal. Chem., 63, 894, 1980 (5)[a]
Infant formula	K_1, other fat-soluble vitamins	Add cholesterol phenyl acetate (IS) Lipase hydrolysis Add NH_4OH, EtOH Extract with pentane	—	Two Zorbax-ODS in series, 25 cm × 4.6 mm	Gradient MeOH : EtOAC (86 : 14) Against 100% MeCN Variable flow rate	265 nm	—	Anal. Chem., 52, 610, 1980 (13)
Margarine, oils, infant formula, milk, cereals	all-rac-α-tocopheryl acetate, retinyl palmitate, β-carotene, vitamin D_2 or D_3, vitamin K_1	Homogenization in mixture of IPA and CH_2Cl_2 with $MgSO_4$ added to remove water	Fractionate vitamins from lipids by HP-GPC Four μStyragel columns in series, 100Å	Zorbax ODS, 6 μm 25 cm × 4.6 mm	Isocratic CH_2Cl_2 : MeCN : MeOH (300 : 700 : 2) 1 mL/min	Retinyl palmitate 325 nm β-Carotene 436 nm D_2 or D_3 280 nm Vitamin E 280 nm Vitamin K_1 280 nm	—	J. Assoc. Off. Anal.Chem., 62, 283, 1979 (4), 63, 131, 1980 (29), 65, 810, 1982 (9), 68, 509, 1985 (28) J. Food Comp. Anal., 2, 140, 1989 (30)

TABLE 5.1 Continued

| Sample Matrix | Analyte | Sample Preparation | | HPLC Parameters | | | | |
		Sample Extraction	Clean Up	Column	Mobile Phase	Detection	Quality Assurance Parameters	References
Milk, human	α-T, γ-T, retinyl esters	Add α-tocopheryl acetate (IS) Dilute with EtOH Extract with Hex Evaporate Dissolve in Hex containing 0.1% BHT	—	Rad-Pak silica cartridge, 10 μm 5 mm, id	Isocratic Hex : DIPE (95 : 15) 2 mL/min	280 nm	—	*Nutr. Res.*, 6, 849, 1986 (11)
Rodent feed	α-T, all-*trans*-retinol, all-*trans*-retinyl acetate	Saponification, overnight, ambient Extract with Hex Centrifuge	—	Supelco LC-CN, 5 μm 25 cm × 4.6 mm	Isocratic Hex : IPA : HAC (990 : 10 : 0.2) 2 mL/min	265 nm	—	*J. Agric. Food Chem.*, 39, 296, 1991 (24)
Forty foods of animal origin	all-*trans*-retinol, α-carotene, β-carotene, lycopene	Saponification, heating mantle, 30 min Extract with Hex (4×) Dry, Na$_2$SO$_4$ Evaporate Dilute with Hex	—	μBondapack C$_{18}$ 10 μm 30 cm × 3.9 mm	MeCN : MeOH : EtOAC (88 : 10 : 2) 2 mL/min	Carotenoids 436 nm Retinol 313 nm	—	*Food Chem.*, 45, 289, 1992 (27)
Eggs, feeds, tissues	all-*trans*-retinol, β-carotene, α-T	Extract with Hex : A : T : EtOH (10 : 7 : 7 : 6) Saponify extract, ambient, overnight Extract with Hex Evaporate Dissolve in Hex : EtOAC (85 : 15)	—	Nova-Pak silica, 4 μm 15 cm × 3.9 mm	Gradient 0–10 min Hex : EtOAC (85 : 15) + (70 : 30) 1–2 mL/min 11–15 min Hex : EtOAC (70 : 30) 2 mL/min	Retinol— 325 nm β-carotene, 445 nm α-T, 294 nm	QL (μg/L) retinol—9.4 β-carotene—0.1 α-T—117	*Poultry Sci.*, 73, 1137, 1994 (23) 74, 407, 1995 (25)

Matrix	Analytes	Sample preparation	Cleanup	Column	Mobile phase	Detection	DL (ng)	Reference
Pediatric parenterals	K_1, all-*trans*-retinol, all-rac-α-tocopheryl acetate, D_2	Extract with HEX, Evaporate, Dissolve in EtOH	—	Spherisorb ODS-2, 3 µm	Isocratic 100% MeOH 0.2 mL/min	Multi-wavelength retinol 325 nm, D_2—265 nm, E—284 nm, K_1—250 nm	On-column retinol—0.75, D_2—0.95, E—4.86, K_1—0-.95	*J. Liquid Chromatogr.,* 17, 4513, 1994 (20)
Italian cheese	α-, β-, γ-, δ-T, β-carotene all-*trans*-retinol	Saponification, 70°C, 30 min, Extract with Hex : EtOAC (90 : 10), Evaporate, Dissolve in mobile phase	—	Ultrasphere Si, 5 µm, 25 cm × 4.6 mm	a. Isocratic Hex : IPA (99 : 1) 1.5 mL/min b. Gradient Multi-linear Pump A Hex : IPA (99 : 1) Pump B Hex, 100%, 1.5 mL/min	a. Tocopherols Fluorescence Ex λ = 290 nm Em λ = 330 nm b. Retinol Fluorescence Ex λ = 290 nm Em λ = 330 nm c. β-carotene 450 nm	On-column α-T—0.9, β-T—0.73, γ-T—0.55, δ-T—0.56, 13-*cis*-retinol —0.09, all-*trans*-retinol—0.32, β—0.16	*Analyst,* 119, 1161, 1994 (17)
Milk, milk powder	D_3, all-*trans*-retinol, α-T	Saponification (on-line), Neutralization (on-line), Sep-Pak Plus C_{18} cartridge (on-line concentration)	Washing of C_{18} cartridge with water : MeOH (60 : 40)	Brownlee OD-224 RP 18, 5 µm, 22 cm × 4.6 mm	HAC : NaOAC (2.5 mM) in MeOH : water (99 : 1) 1 mL/min	a. 280 nm b. EC + 1300 mV	On-column retinol—0.10, D_3—6.8, E—1.34	*J. Chromatogr. A.,* 694, 399, 1995 (16)
Milk, milk powder	α-T, all-*trans*-retinol, K_1	a. α-T, retinol Saponification, overnight, ambient Extract with Hex Evaporate Dissolve in MeOH b. K_1	a. — b. Sep-Pak silica	a. OD-224 RP 18, 5 µm, 22 cm × 4.6 mm b. Brownlee OD-224 RP 18	a. Isocratic MeOH : Water (99 : 1) containing 2.5 mmol/L HAC 1.25 mL/min b. Isocratic	a. EC Dual-amperometric Glassy carbon −1100 mV + 700 mV Vs Ag/AgCl	On-column α-T—0.19, retinol—0.06, K_1—3.1	*J. Chromatogr.,* 623, 69, 1992 (14) *Analyst,* 120, 2489, 1995 (15)

TABLE 5.1 Continued

Sample Matrix	Analyte	Sample Preparation		HPLC Parameters				References
		Sample Extraction	Clean Up	Column	Mobile Phase	Detection	Quality Assurance Parameters	
		Lipase hydrolysis Add alcoholic sodium hydroxide and immediately extract with Hex			MeOH : Water (99 : 1) containing 2.5 mm HAC-NaOAC 1.25 mL/min	b. EC Dual amperometric glassy carbon— −1100 mV reductive + 700 mV oxidative Ag/AgCl reference		
Cosmetic creams	all-rac-α-tocopheryl acetate, retinyl palmitate	Supercritical fluid extraction CO$_2$ a. Dynamic, 250 atm, 40°C, 30 min b. Restrictor 100°C Flow rate 190–200 mL/min Collect into THF : methanol (4 : 1)	—	μBondapak C$_{18}$, 10 μm 30 cm × 3.9 mm 1.5 mL/min	Isocratic MeOH : MeCN (75 : 25) retinyl palmitate 325 nm	α-tocopheryl acetate 280 nm	—	J. Pharm. Biomed. Anal., 13, 273, 1995 (19)

[a] Number in ( ) is reference citation number.

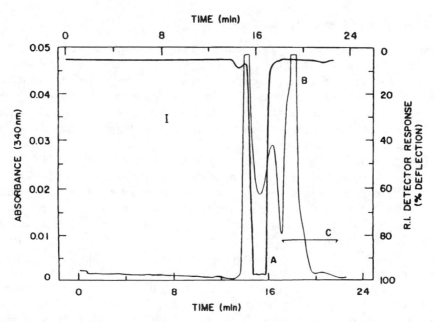

Figure 5.1.I Typical chromatogram of margarine (25 mg injected, 10% in methylene chloride containing 0.01% BHA and 0.001% triethylamine) on μStryagel, using methylene chloride containing 0.001% triethylamine at a flow rate of 0.7 mL/min. Vitamin fraction was monitored at 340 nm and oil fraction was monitored by refractive index (RI). Peak A, oil; Peak B, vitamin fraction; Peak C, collected region. Reproduced with permission from Reference 4.

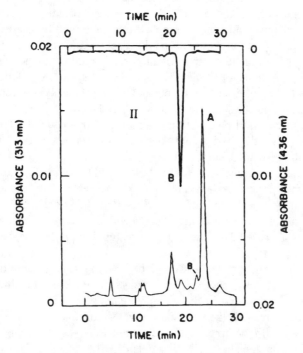

Figure 5.1.II Chromatogram of vitamin fraction from margarine after 2 passes through μStyragel on a C_{18} reverse-phase column. Mobile phase was methylene chloride-acetonitrile (30 + 70) at flow rate of 1.0 mL/min. Retinyl palmitate was monitored at 313 nm and β-carotene was monitored at 436 nm. Peak A, retinyl palmitate (150 ng); Peak B, β-carotene (60 ng). Reproduced with permission from Reference 4.

5.2.2 MILK, INFANT FORMULA, AND CHEESE

Fluid milk is fortified with vitamin A and vitamin D. Long-standing recognition of analytical problems associated with the analysis of these vitamins, particularly vitamin D, and the need for rapid, precise methods led to much method development research for their analysis from milk and infant formula. The low concentration of vitamin D, even in fortified products, continues to pose analytical problems. The low concentration and poor detection properties of the vitamin usually require analyte concentration or extensive clean-up procedures that limit application of procedures developed or applicable to other fat-soluble vitamins.

The first simultaneous assay for vitamin A and vitamin D was reported in 1979.[7] The procedure combined aspects of methods developed by Thompson and Maxwell[3] and Henderson and Wickroski.[8] One milliliter of milk was saponified, and the vitamins were extracted with hexane. After evaporation to dryness, the residue was dissolved in methanol and injected onto a Vydac C_{18} column and eluted with a mobile phase of acetonitrile : methanol (90 : 10). Retinol and vitamin D were assayed at 325 nm and 265 nm, respectively, by detectors in series. The AOAC International does not provide an official method for the simultaneous analysis of vitamin A and vitamin D in milk or infant formula. Few other methods have been published that deal with the specific analysis of vitamin A and vitamin D from milk or infant formula. Methods that assay additional vitamins with vitamin A and vitamin D are discussed later in the chapter.

Analysis of vitamin A activity together with vitamin E activity in milk and infant formula poses fewer problems compared to inclusion of vitamin D in the analysis. Landen[9] adapted the nondestructive fat-soluble vitamin isolation technique by gel permeation chromatography[4] to the simultaneous analysis of retinyl palmitate and all-rac-α-tocopheryl acetate in infant formula. Application of the technique originally developed for margarine analysis resulted in the development of a lipid extraction procedure utilizing a mixture of isopropanol and methylene chloride. After initial extraction steps, $MgSO_4$ was added to remove water. This extraction procedure is applicable to other matrices in addition to fluid milk and infant formulas. Landen's modified procedure[9] added a third μStyragel to the HP-GPC clean-up system. The third gel permeation column provided essentially complete lipid removal from the fat-soluble vitamin fraction, eliminating rechromatography of the isolated vitamin fraction. Methanol (2 mL) was added per liter to the mobile phase of methylene chloride : acetonitrile (30 : 70). Addition of methanol to the solvent system for C_{18} chromatography improves peak resolution and eliminates peak tailing caused by exposed SiOH groups on the bonded stationary phase.[10] After reversed-phase chromatography, retinyl palmitate and all-rac-α-tocopheryl acetate were simultaneously detected using two detectors in series set at 313 nm for retinyl palmitate and 280 nm for all-rac-α-tocopheryl acetate.

A method for simultaneous analysis of retinyl esters and tocopherols in human milk used direct hexane extraction of the vitamins from the milk matrix.[11] The extract was evaporated to dryness, and the residue dissolved in hexane was injected on a silica Radial-Pak® cartridge without further clean-up. Elution was with hexane : isopropylether (95 : 5) with detection at 280 nm. Natural ester forms of vitamin A eluted as a single peak. The method was rapid, reproducible, and applicable to other biological samples.

Normal-phase chromatography on LiChrosorb Si60 was used to simultaneously assay total carotene and retinol isomers from cheese.[12] Overnight saponification at ambient temperatures with hexane extraction was used to extract the vitamins. Chromatography with methyl ethyl ketone : hexane (10 : 90) did not resolve the individual carotenoids but all-*trans*-retinol, 13-*cis*-retinol, 11,13-di-*cis*-retinol, 9,13-di-*cis*-retinol and 9-*cis*-retinol were resolved. The method incorporated azobenzene and 2-nitrofluorene as internal standards. The saponification procedure from this method has been used by many investigators for extraction of retinol and carotenoids from many matrices.

Several useful simultaneous methods have been developed for milk and infant formula assay that have the capability to assay more than two fat-soluble vitamins. A non-aqueous reversed-phase chromatography system with two Zorbax ODS columns in series was utilized by Barnett et al.[13] to resolve all-*trans*-retinol, retinyl palmitate, vitamin D_2 or vitamin D_3, RRR-α-tocopherol, all-rac-α-tocopheryl acetate, vitamin K_1, and cholesterol phenyl acetate (IS). Gradient elution with methanol : ethyl acetate (86 : 14) against acetonitrile achieved baseline resolution of the analytes (Figure 5.2). A microprocessor controlled variable wavelength UV detector monitored the elution. Retinol was monitored at 325 nm and the other analytes were monitored at 365 nm. The extraction procedure was based upon lipid removal by hydrolysis with lipase from *Candida cyclindraccae*. Free fatty acids were removed from the hydrolysis mixture by alkali precipitation. Vitamins were extracted with *n*-pentane following fatty acid removal. The elimination of saponification avoids isomerization of vitamins D_2 and D_3 and destruction of vitamin K_1. Although the chromatography run time was in excess of 50 min, the RSD's for all analytes were less than 5%. The Barnett et al.[13] method provided another approach to non-destructive extraction which allows the analysis of vitamin K_1 together with other fat-soluble vitamins. Previous methods[4,5] and the lipase hydrolysis technique are not only useful for inclusion of vitamin K_1 and D_2 and D_3 in multi-analyte methodology but provide for assay of specific esters of retinol and α-tocopherol from fortified foods.

Zamarreño et al.[14,15] used electrochemical detection for the simultaneous analysis of fat-soluble vitamins, milk, and milk powder. Amperometric detection with a glassy carbon electrode at +1050 mV gave low ng detection limits. The earlier method[14] assayed vitamin D_3 in unenriched milk without preconcentration. The 1995 method[15] assayed vitamin K_1, all-*trans*-retinol, and RRR-α-tocopherol in milk after extraction by lipase hydrolysis. Hexane extraction after saponification was used in the procedure published in 1992[14] which destroyed vitamin K_1. The overall method was adapted

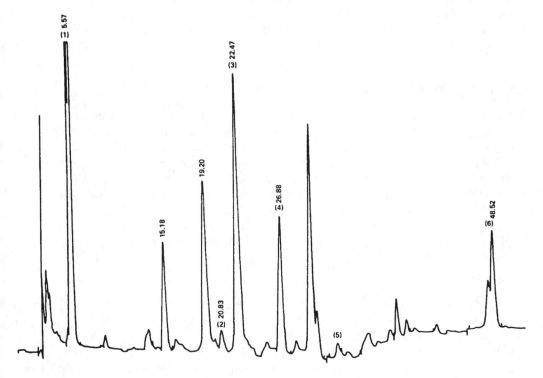

Figure 5.2   Chromatogram of a soy-base infant formula product after alkaline hydrolysis. Two Zorbax ODS 25 cm columns were used in series. Gradient elution was with methanol : ethyl acetate (86 : 14) against acetonitrile. Peak 1, vitamin A alcohol; Peak 2, vitamin D_2; Peak 3, vitamin E alcohol; Peak 4, all-rac-α-tocopheryl acetate; peak 5, vitamin K_1 (degraded); Peak 6, vitamin A palmitate. Reproduced with permission from Reference 13.

to an on-line system for the simultaneous analysis of all-*trans*-retinol, α-tocopherol, and vitamin D_3 from milk and powdered milk.[16] The on-line system linked saponification, preconcentration, and clean up on C_{18} Sep Pak and injection onto a Brownlee OD-224 RP18 column.

Panfili et al.[17] saponified cheese and extracted the digest with hexane : ethyl acetate (9 : 1) using a procedure modified from work by Ueda and Igarashi[18] for the analysis of the tocopherols, β-carotene, and *cis*- and *trans*-isomers of retinol. The extract was directly injected onto an Ultrasphere Si column. Gradient elution with hexane : isopropanol (99 : 1) and hexane provided excellent resolution of the analytes. The detection system included programmable UV/visible and fluorescence detectors in series. Visible detection at 450 nm was used for the carotenoids and fluorescence for tocopherols (Ex λ = 280, Em λ = 325) and retinols (Ex λ = 325, Em λ = 475). The procedural details for the method are given in Section 5.4.

5.2.3　PHARMACEUTICALS

5.2.3.1　Cosmetic Creams

Scalia et al.[19] successfully used supercritical fluid extraction (SFE) to isolate retinyl palmitate and all-rac-α-tocopheryl acetate from cream and lotions. SFE conditions were 30 min with supercritical carbon dioxide at 40°C and 250 atmospheres. Recoveries greater than 91.6% were achieved. The SFE minimized sample handling and the use of harmful solvents. The extracted vitamins were collected at the restrictor into 4 mL of THF : methanol (4 : 1) in a glass vial held at 0°C. The contents of the vial were diluted to 5 mL and directly injected into the LC. Chromatography was completed on a μBondapak C_{18} column and eluted with methanol : acetonitrile (75 : 25). A programmable UV/visible detector monitored retinyl palmitate at 325 nm and all-rac-α-tocopheryl acetate at 280 nm.

5.2.3.2　Parenteral Solutions

Blanco et al.[20] applied narrow-bore (2.1 mm i.d.), small particle (3μm) C_{18} columns to the simultaneous analysis of all-*trans*-retinol, vitamin D_2, all-rac-α-tocopheryl acetate, and vitamin K_1 in pediatric parenteral solutions. The narrow-bore columns gave detection limits of less than 1 ng on-column for retinol, vitamin D_2, and vitamin K_1, which are lower than most obtained with conventional columns. For all-rac-α-tocopheryl acetate, the detection limit was 4.85 ng which is excellent for UV detection. A multi-channel UV/visible detector was used with wavelengths set at 325 nm (retinol), 265 nm (vitamin D_2), 284 nm (α-tocopheryl acetate), and 250 nm (vitamin K_1). Mobile phase was 100% methanol pumped at 0.2 mL/min. Resolution was obtained within 13 min. The narrow-bore columns resulted in significant savings in mobile phase and, thus, cost savings.

5.2.4　MISCELLANEOUS PRODUCTS

Multi-analyte methods for specific food matrices have been developed since the late 1970s. Widicus and Kirk[21] assayed retinyl palmitate and all-rac-α-tocopheryl acetate in fortified cereal products. Lipids were extracted with methylene chloride and 95% ethanol. The extract was filtered through sodium sulfate to remove water and evaporated. The residue was redissolved in the mobile phase of hexane : chloroform (85 : 15) and directly injected onto μPorasil. The method is rapid and gave recoveries in excess of 95% for both analytes. Other simultaneous methods for foods include retinol, vitamin D_3, and α-tocopherol in albacore[22]; α-tocopherol, β-carotene, and retinol in eggs[23]; retinol and α-tocopherol in feed[24,25]; and synthetic and natural fat-soluble vitamins from paprika,[26] and retinol, α- and β-carotene, and lycopene in Malaysian foods.[27]

The analyst's ability to integrate various chromatography modes (normal, reversed-phase, gel permeation), various supports and mobile phases, and detection techniques together with increasingly sophisticated software packages for computer controlled instrument operations and data management can lead to integrated systems for vitamin assay from varied matrices. An integrated system that developed from several years of methodology research at the Atlanta Center for Nutrient Analysis (ACNA), Southeast Regional Laboratory, Food and Drug Administration, is shown in Figure 5.3. The system was developed for fat-soluble vitamin analysis of foods fortified with all-*trans*-retinol esters, vitamins D_2 and D_3, all-rac-α-tocopheryl acetate, β-carotene, and vitamin K_1. Additionally, natural tocopherols, α-carotene, and β-apo-8′-carotenal can be assayed. Primary applications included analysis of retinyl palmitate and β-carotene in margarine,[4] retinyl palmitate and all-rac-α-tocopheryl acetate in infant formula[9,28] and breakfast cereals,[29] and vitamin D and vitamin K_1 in infant formula and fortified milk.[30] The analysis system is useful for most fortified foods, medical foods, and pharmaceuticals.

The approach is centered on gel permeation chromatography (HP-GPC) for lipid removal and isolation of the fat-soluble vitamin fraction. The combination of HP-GPC and non-aqueous reversed-phase (NARP) chromatography has the following advantages:

1. The nondestructive extraction uses small volumes of solvent and requires no heat or saponification. Potential for vitamin degradation is decreased and production of previtamin D forms is minimized.
2. The fat-soluble vitamins can be completely resolved from the lipid fraction by HP-GPC.

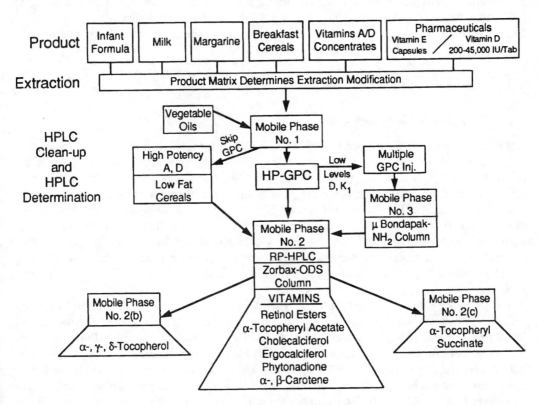

Figure 5.3 Integrated system for quantification of fat-soluble vitamins. Mobile phase compositions: No. 1—methylene chloride, No. 2(a)—acetylnitrile : methylene chloride : methanol (700 : 300 : 2), No. 2(b)—acetylnitrile : methylene chloride : methanol (700 : 300 : 50), No. 2(c)—acetylnitrile : methylene chloride (700 : 300) containing 2% v/v acetic acid, No. 3—methylene chloride : isooctane : isopropanol (600 : 400 : 1). (Unpublished).

3. Vitamin A levels in the sample can be estimated prior to the quantitative step by monitoring absorbance of HP-GPC eluates at 313 to 325 nm.
4. β-carotene, vitamin A esters, and vitamin E esters can be assayed simultaneously following HP-GPC clean up with NARP chromatography.
5. Modification of the NARP mobile phase allows resolution of α-, γ- and δ- tocopherols.

Quantitation of vitamin D and vitamin K requires an additional clean-up step on μBondapak-NH$_2$ to remove UV absorbing interferences and plant sterols in infant formula and cholesterol in milk from the fat-soluble vitamin fraction isolated by HP-GPC. The integrated system shown in Figure 5.3 is an efficient analytical approach to the analysis of products fortified at varying levels. Most advantageous to regulatory analysis, the non-destructive extraction quantitates the specific forms of the vitamins added in the formulations. Problematic to regulatory activities, the procedure was not collaborated through AOAC International.

5.3   SERUM AND PLASMA

Methodology for simultaneous analysis of fat-soluble vitamins in clinical samples continues to advance with improvements in detector sensitivity, availability of narrow-bore columns, small particle supports, and better computerization with versatile data management systems. In the 1980s, availability of electrochemical detectors provided increased sensitivity to methods previously based on UV/visible detection.[31] More recently, clinical chemists have efficiently used multi-channel UV/visible detectors and newer, highly sensitive PDA detectors to further advance simultaneous assay of multiple analytes in serum and plasma. Methodology for simultaneous assay of fat-soluble vitamins in serum or plasma is summarized in Table 5.2.

5.3.1   METHODS FOR TWO ANALYTES

5.3.1.1   Retinol and α-tocopherol

Simultaneous methods for all-*trans*-α-retinol and RRR-α-tocopherol in plasma and serum were developed in 1979 by Bieri et al.[32] and De Leenheer et al.[33] Both procedures used C$_{18}$ reversed-phase chromatography with methanol or methanol : water (95 : 5) mobile phases with UV detection. Internal standards were retinyl acetate,[32] all-rac-α-tocopheryl acetate[32] and tocol.[33] The Bieri et al.[32] method quantitated RRR-α-tocopherol, α-tocopheryl quinone and β-+γ-tocopherol. Ethanol was used to denature blood proteins and the vitamins were extracted with hexane. The detection limits were <100 μg/L for retinol and <0.8mg/L for RRR-α-tocopherol. Various studies have modified the original procedures since their introduction, but improvements have been inconsequential to their overall usefulness. Details of the Bieri et al.[32] and De Leenheer et al.[33] procedures are provided in Table 5.2.

Fluorescence detection provides increased sensitivity for quantitation of retinol and vitamin E homologs. Rhys Williams[34] incorporated a programmable fluorescence detector to serum analysis for all-*trans*-retinol and RRR-α-tocopherol. The sensitivity was such that 25 to 50 μL of serum could be assayed, compared with 200 μL samples normally used for procedures based upon UV detection. With the programmable detector, the α-tocopherol which eluted at 2.0 min from the normal-phase silica column was monitored at Ex λ = 295, Em λ = 390. After 2.5 min, the wavelengths were changed to Ex λ = 325, Em λ = 480 to monitor retinol.

Vandewoude et al.[35] and Chou et al.[36] first applied electrochemical detection to α-tocopherol analysis of plasma. Huang et al.[37] simultaneously assayed α-tocopherol and retinol in serum. The method used electrochemical detection for α-tocopherol and UV detection for retinol. On-column detection limits were 1.0 ng for both analytes. β-, γ-, and δ-tocopherols were also detectable with

TABLE 5.2
Multi-Analyte Assays for Fat-Soluble Vitamin Assays in Serum and Plasma

Sample Matrix	Analyte	Sample Preparation		HPLC Parameters			Quality Assurance Parameters	References
		Sample Extraction	Clean Up	Column	Mobile Phase	Detection		
Retinol and α-tocopherol								
Plasma	all-*trans*-retinol, α-T, β- + γ-	Add retinyl acetate (IS) and all-rac-α-tocopherol acetate (IS) Deproteinize with EtOH Extract with Hex or Hep Evaporate Dissolve Residue in EtO2 : MeOH (1 : 3)	—	μBondpak C_{18}, 30 cm × 3.9 mm	Isocratic MeOH : water (95 : 5) 2.5 mL/min	280 nm	CV% Retinol — 4.4 α-T — 2.0 % Recovery Retinol — 103.4 α-T — 100.7	*Am. J. Clin. Nutr.*, 32, 2143, 1979 (32)[a]
Plasma, serum	all-*trans*-retinol, α-T	Add tocol (IS) Deproteinize with EtOH Extract with Hex Evaporate Dissolve residue in MeOH	—	RSIL C_{18}, 10 mm 25 cm × 4.6 mm	Isocratic MeOH 2 mL/min	292 nm	QL Retinol—60 μg/L α-T—0.6 mg/L CV % Retinol—2.47 α-T—1.62 % Recovery Retinol—96.8 α-T—95.5	*J. Chromatogr.*, 162, 408, 1979 (33)
Serum	all-*trans*-retinol, α-T	Deproteinize with EtOH Extract with mobile phase Centrifuge Inject clear, top organic phase	—	HS-3 3 μm silica 100 cm × 4.6 mm	Isocratic Hex : EtOH (99 : 1) 2 mL/min	Fluorescence Retinol Ex λ = 325 Em λ = 480 α-T Ex λ = 295 Em λ = 390	QL (μmol/L) Retinol — 0.02 α-T — 0.37 CV% Retinol — 2.0 α-T — 4.9 % Recovery Retinol — 96.9 α-T — 98.5	*J. Chromatogr.*, 341, 198, 1985 (34)

TABLE 5.2 Continued

Sample Matrix	Analyte	Sample Preparation			HPLC Parameters			References
		Sample Extraction	Clean Up	Column	Mobile Phase	Detection	Quality Assurance Parameters	
Vitamin K_1 and α-Tocopherol								
Serum	α-T, K_1	Add all-rac-α-tocopheryl acetate (IS) and cetyl napthoate (IS) Deproteinize with EtOH Extract with Hex Wash Evaporate Dissolve residue in IPA	Wash Hex layer with MeOH : water (9 : 1)	Resolve C_{18}, 5 μm 15 cm × 3.9 mm	Isocratic EtOH : water (92 : 8)	α-T—292 nm K_1 Fluorescence After reduction Ex λ = 320 nm Em λ = 430 nm	DL (ng) On-column α-T—5 K_1—0.03 CV% α-T—3.5-6 K_1—8.1-12.9 % Recovery α-T—93 K_1—80	Clin. Chem., 35, 2285, 1989 (38)
Multi-Analytes								
Serum	all-trans-retinol, retinol palmitate, all-trans-β-carotene, lutein, zeaxanthin, cryptoxanthin, α-T, γ-T	Add tocol (IS) EtOH (BHT, 15 mg/L) Vortex Extract with Hex Centrifuge Reextract Evaporate Dissolve in EtOH containing BHT	—	Vydac 201TP C_{18} 5 μm 25 cm × 4.6 mm	Gradient 0–3 min water : MeOH : B (15 : 75 : 10) to 2 : 88 : 10 in 15 min Hold for 17 min 1.5 mL/min or Isocratic water : MeOH : B (2.6 : 8.74 : 10) 1.5 mL/min for 10 min then 3.0 mL/min	Multwavelength retinol — 325 nm β-carotene — 450 nm α-T — 295 nm EC Amperometric Ag/AgCl Reference +900 mV	QL-UV (μg/L) retinol—6 α-T—96 β-carotene—29 QL-EC (mg/L) retinol — 4.1 α-T — 0.65 β-carotene — 2.1	Clin. Chem., 33, 1585, 1987 (39)

Sample	Analytes	Sample preparation		Column	Mobile phase	Detection	Performance	Reference
Plasma, serum	all-*trans*-retinol, all-*trans*-β-carotene, all-*trans*-α-carotene, lycopene, β-cryptoxanthin, α-T	Add EtOH containing all-rac-α-tocopheryl acetate (IS) Extract with heptane containing BHT (0.5 g/L) Evaporate Dissolve in mobile phase	—	Spherisorb ODS-2, 3 μm 10 cm × 4.6 mm	Isocratic MeCN : MeOH : CHCl$_3$ (47 : 47 : 6) 1.5 mL/min	Multiwavelength retinol—325 nm carotenoids—450 nm α-T — 292 nm	CV% retinol—1.7 α-T—2.3 β-carotene—4.1 α-carotene— 10.4 β-cryptoxanthin—3.4	*Clin. Chem.*, 34, 377, 1988 (40)
Serum, vegetables	α-, β-, γ-, δ-T, all-rac-α-tocopheryl acetate, 10 carotenoids, 3 retinoids	a. Serum Add EtOH containing all-rac-α-tocopheryl acetate (IS) and retinyl acetate (IS) Extract with Hex (2×) Exaporate Dissolve in THF containing (BHT) b. Vegetables	—	Spheri-5-RP-18, 5μm, 22 cm × 4.6 mm	Isocratic a. MeCN : CH$_2$C$_{12}$: MeOH (70 : 20 : 10) 1.8 mL/min b. MeCN : MeOH (85 : 15) 1.8 mL/min increased to 2.5 mL/min	Multiwavelength carotenoids— 450 nm retinoids— 313 nm α-T, α-tocopheryl acetate— 280 nm	DL (ng) On-column carotenoids 0.2–0.3 retinoids 0.3–1.2 α-T, α-tocopheryl acetate—15	*J. Liq. Chromatogr.*, 13, 1455, 1990 (41) *Food Chem.*, 45, 205, 1992 (42)
Plasma	all-*trans* α-, β-carotene, *cis*-β-carotene, lutein, zeaxanthin, β-cryptoxanthin, lycopene, retinol, phytofluene, α-, γ-, δ-T	Add water, EtOH Extract with Hex Evaporate Dissolve in EtOH : dioxane (1 : 1), then add MeCN	—	Ultrasphere ODS, 5 μm 25 cm × 4.6 mm	Isocratic MeCN : THF : MeOH : 1% NH$_3$OAC (684 : 220 : 68 : 28) 1.5 mL/min	Multiwavelength α-β-carotene, β-cryptoxanthin—450 nm lycopene— 452 nm; Fluorescence α-, γ-, δ-T Ex λ = 298 Em λ = 328; Phytofluene Ex λ = 349 Em λ = 480	QL (mg/L) α-, β-carotene— 10 β-cryptoxanthin— 10 lycopene—5 retinol—20 α-, γ-T—0.05	*Int. J. Vit. Nutr. Res.*, 61, 232, 1991 (43)

TABLE 5.2 Continued

Sample Matrix	Analyte	Sample Preparation		HPLC Parameters				References
		Sample Extraction	Clean Up	Column	Mobile Phase	Detection	Quality Assurance Parameters	
Serum	all-*trans*-retinol, all-*trans*-α- and β-carotene, α-T	Add EtOH containing all-rac-α-tocopheryl acetate (IS) Extract with Hex Dissolve in mobile phase	—	Ultrasphere ODS 5 μm 15 cm × 4.6 mm	Isocratic Evaluation of 18 mobile phases Optimal MeCN : CH_2Cl_2 : MeOH (70 : 20)10 1.2 mL/min	Multiwavelength retinol— 325 nm β-carotene— 450 nm α-T, α-tocopheryl acetate— 291 nm	DL (mM) On-column retinol—0.115 β-carotene—0.29 α-T—1.55	*J. Chromatogr.*, 572, 103, 1991 (44)
Plasma, tissue	all-*trans*-retinol, α-, β-carotene, lutein, β-cryptoxanthin, lycopene, α-T	a. Plasma Add ethanol containing ascorbic acid (1 g/L) Add dl-α-tocopheryl nicotinate (IS) in MeCN Extract with Hex (3×) Evaporate 1 mL Dissolve in EtOH containing ascorbic acid Add mobile phase	—	Ultracarb ODS, 5 μm 25 cm × 4.6 mm	Isocratic MeCN : THF : MeOH : NH_4OAC (65 : 25 : 6 : 4) 1.7 mL/min	Multiwavelength retinol—325 nm carotenoids— 450 nm α-T—292 nm	QL (nmol/L) retinol—42 α-carotene—22 β-carotene—33 lutein—7 β-cryptoxanthin—14 lycopene—34 α-T—1.4 μmol/L	*Am. J. Clin. Nutr.*, 56, 417, 1992 (45)

Sample	Analytes	Procedure	Column	Mobile phase	Detection	QL	Reference
b. Tissue		Digest with lipase and collagenase; Homogenize; Add dl-α-tocopheryl nicotinate (IS) in MeCN; Extract with Hex (2×); Evaporate; Redissolve in EtOH containing ascorbic acid				—	Anal. Chem., 64, 2111, 1992 (46)
Plasma	18 carotenoids all-trans-retinol, RRR-α- and γ-tocopherol	Deproteinize with EtOH; Add ethyl β-apo-8'-carotenoate (IS) and (3R)-8'-apo-β-carotene-3,8'-diol (IS); Mix and centrifuge; Extract residue 2× with EtO₂; Wash EtO₂ extract with 5% NaCl; Dry over Na₂SO₄; Evaporate to dryness; Dissolve residue in CH₂Cl₂; Filter, evaporate; Dissolve residue in Eluent B	a. Microsorb C₁₈, 5 μm 25 cm × 4.6 μm; b. Silica-based nitrile, 5 μm 25 cm × 4.6 mm	Gradient a. MeCN : MeOH : CH₂Cl₂ : Hex (85 : 10 : 2.5 : 2.5) 0–10 min Isocratic 10–40 min (linear gradient) to MeCN : MeOH : CH₂Cl₂ : Hex (40 : 10 : 22.5 : 22.5) 0.7 mL/min b. Isocratic CH₂Cl₂ : MeOH : N, N-diisopropyl-ethylamine (74.65 : 25 : 0.25 : 0.1) 1 mL/min	PDA 470, 445, 400, 350, 290 nm	—	
Plasma	all-trans-retinol, α-, β-carotene, β-cryptoxanthin, lutein/zeaxanthin, lycopene, α-T	Add ethanol containing retinyl acetate (IS) and echinenone (IS); Extract with Hex (2×); Evaporate	Spherisorb ODS-1, 5 μm 25 cm × 4.6 mm	Gradient a. NH₄OAC (100 mmol/L) in MeOH : MeCN (80 : 20)	Multiwave-length retinol 325 nm carotenoids 450 nm	QL (μmol/L) retinol—0.35 α-, β-carotene—0.13	Clin. Chem., 39, 2229, 1993 (47)

TABLE 5.2 Continued

| | Sample Preparation | | HPLC Parameters | | | | |
Sample Matrix	Sample Extraction	Clean Up	Column	Mobile Phase	Detection	Quality Assurance Parameters	References
	Dissolve in THF Dilute with EtOH			b. NH_4OAC (100 mmol/L in water) Equilibrate with a : b mixture (90 : 10) Run 12 min linear gradient to 100% a Maintain for 10 min	α-T—292 nm	β-cryptoxanthin—0.13 lycopene—0.28 α-T—5.8	*J. Nutr. Biochem.*, 4, 58, 1993 (48)
Serum	all-*trans*-retinol, all-*trans*-α-, β-carotene, *cis*-β-carotene, lutein, β-cryptoxanthin, lycopene, canthaxanthin	Add $CHCl_3$: MeOH (2 : 1) and saline Add retinyl acetate (IS) and γ-carotene (IS) in EtOH Centrifuge Transfer $CHCl_3$ layer Reextract with Hex Combine with $CHCl_3$ extract Evaporate Dissolve in EtOH	—	Pecosphere C_{18}, 3 μm 8.3 cm $\times$ 4.6 mm	Gradient a. MeCN : THF : water (50 : 20 : 30) b. MeCN : THF : water (50 : 44 : 6) 60% a + 40% b for 1 min 9 min linear gradient to 83% b Hold 4 min 2 min linear gradient to 100% b 2 min reequilibration	Multiwave-length retinoids— 340 nm carotenoids— 450 nm	—
Serum	all-*trans*-retinol 17 carotenoids, α-, γ-T	a. Add all-*trans*-α-tocopheryl acetate (IS), canthaxanthin (IS), retinoic acid (IS), (retinyl hexanoate or β-apo-8'-carotenyl decanoate can be used as IS)	—	Resolve C_{18}, 5 μm 30 cm $\times$ 3.9 mm	Isocratic a. MeCN : CH_2Cl_2 : MeOH : 1-octanol (90 : 15 : 10 : 0.1) b. MeCN : CH_2Cl_2 : MeOH : water containing 0.1% NH_4OAC (90 : 10 : 5 : 2)	Multiwave-length and PDA retinol—325 nm retinoic acid— 350 nm phytofluene— 350 nm δ-carotene— 400 nm	*Food Chem.*, 46, 419, 1993 (49) *J. Chromatogr.*, 617, 257, 1993 (50)

Sample	Analytes	Sample preparation	Column	Mobile phase	Detection	Reference
		Add EtOH and EtOAC Centrifuge Reextract (2×) Extract pellet with Hex Add water to extract Centrifuge Remove organic layer Evaporate Dissolve in CH_2Cl_2 : CH_3OH (1 : 2) b. Add IPA and CH_2Cl_2 Add all-rac-α-tocopheryl acetate (IS), canthaxanthin (IS), retinoic acid (IS) Centrifuge Remove supernatant Dilute with IPA : CH_2Cl_2 (2 : 1)	—	c. MeCN : CH_2Cl_2 : MeOH containing 0.05% NH_4OAC	other carotenoids— 450 nm lycopene— 470 nm tocopherols— 290 nm	
Serum, foods	α-, γ-, δ-T 6 carotenoids retinal retinyl palmitate	Add tocol (IS) and trans-β-apo-10'-carotenal-oxime (IS), EtOH (BHT) Extract with Hex Evaporate Dissolve in EtOH containing BHT Sonicate Transfer to autosampler vial	Bakerbond C_{18}, 5 μm 25 cm × 4.6 mm	Gradient a. MeCN b. MeOH c. EtOH solvents contain 0.05 M NH_4OAC 1. 98% a—2% b to 75% a—18% B 7% c in 10 min 2. To 68% A—25% B, 7% c in 5 min Hold 10 min 3. Return to step 1 in 5 min Hold 10 min	1. Tocopherols Fluorescence Ex λ = 295 nm Em λ = 335 nm 2. Retinol— 325 nm 3. Carotenoids— 425 nm	J. Chromatogr., 619, 37, 1993 (51)

TABLE 5.2 Continued

	Sample Preparation			HPLC Parameters				
Sample Matrix	Analyte	Sample Extraction	Clean Up	Column	Mobile Phase	Detection	Quality Assurance Parameters	References
Plasma	25-OH-D$_2$, D$_3$ retinol, α-T	Add [^{3}H]-25-OH-D$_3$ in ethanol for recovery Add retinyl acetate (IS) and all-rac-α-tocopheryl acetate (IS) in MeOH : IPA (80 : 20) Extract with Hex Centrifuge Transfer Hex layer to autosampler vial Evaporate Dissolve in MeOH	—	SupelcoSil LC-18, 5 μm 25 cm × 4.6 mm	Solvent Switching 1. MeOH : water (85 : 15) 10 min 2.5 mL/min MeOH : Water (98 : 2) 20 min 2.5 mL/min	265 nm	QL (mmol/L) 25-OH-D$_2$—6 25-OH-D$_3$—6 retinol—0.035 α-T—1.5	J. Ped. Gastroenterol. Nutr., 18, 339, 1994 (52)
Plasma	all-*trans*-retinol, all-*trans*-α-, β-carotene, *cis*-β-carotene, lutein, lycopene, α-T	Add ethanol containing retinyl acetate (IS) Extract with Hex containing BHT (0.4 g/L) Centrifuge Evaporate Dissolve in mobile phase without aqueous solvent	—	Nucleosil 100-S C$_{18}$, 5 μm 25 cm × 4.6 mm	MeCN : THF : MeOH : 1% NH$_4$OAC (68 : 22 : 7 : 3) 1.5 mL/min	Multiwavelength retinol— 325 nm carotenoids— 450 nm lycopene— 470 nm α-T—290 nm	QL (μg/L) retinol—10 lutein—5 lycopene—10 α-carotene—20 β-carotene—20 α-T—200	J. Chromatogr., B, 654, 129, 1994 (53)

Sample	Analytes	Extraction	Cleanup	Column	Mobile phase	Detection	DL/QL	Reference
Serum	α-T, all-*trans*-retinol, 4 retinyl esters, 6 carotenoids	Add EtOH containing non-apreno-β-carotene (IS) and retinyl butyrate (IS) Extract with Hex Centrifuge Evaporate Hex Dissolve in EtOH Add MeCN	—	Ultramex ODS C$_{18}$, 5 μm 15 cm × 4.6 mm	Isocratic EtOH : MeCN (1 : 1) containing 0.1 mm DEAL/L 1 mL/min 29°C	Diode array α-T—300 nm retinol—325 nm retinyl esters—325 nm carotenoids—425 nm	DL (ng/L) On-column α-T—60 retinol—0.15 retinyl esters—0.19–0.31 β-carotene—0.2 other carotenoids—0.13–0.19	*Clin. Chem.*, 40, 411, 1994 (54)
Serum, tissues, plants	α-T, γ-T 20 carotenoids 5 retinoids	Add EtOH Extract with Hex Evaporate Dissolve in MeCl$_2$	—	Vydac 201 TP54	Isocratic MeOH : MeCN (9 : 1) 1.0 mL/min	PDA 200–800 nm	—	*J. Liq. Chromatogr.*, 18, 2813, 1995 (55)
Plasma	K$_1$, all-*trans*-retinol, α-T, γ-T, β-carotene	Add dihydrovitamin K$_1$, EtOH Extract with Hex Centrifuge Remove Hex layer	Partition Hex with MeOH : water (9 : 1)	Hypersil ODS, 5 μm 25 cm × 4.6 mm	Isocratic MeOH : CH$_2$Cl$_2$ (9 : 1) containing ZnCl$_2$, NaOAC and HAC 0.8 mL/min	Post-column metallic Zn reduction Fluorescence Ex λ = 243 Em λ = 430	QL (ng/mL) 0.04 within run CV = 5.6%	*Int. J. Vit. Nutr. Res.*, 65, 31, 1995 (56)
Plasma, neonatal	β-carotene, β-cryptoxanthin, α-T, γ-T	Add γ-tocotrienol (IS) and ethyl-β-apo-8'-carotenate (*trans*) Add BHT in EtOH Extract with Hex Evaporate Dissolve in EtOH : MeOH (1 : 1)	—	Super Pac Prep-5 C$_2$/C$_{18}$, 5 μm 25 cm × 4.0 mm	13.4 mM lithium perchlorate in MeOH : EtOH : IPA (88 : 24 : 10) 1.2 mL/min	EC coulometric conditioning cell—0.6 V followed by detection at the amperometric second electrode Electrode 1 −0.15 V Electrode 2 +0.6 V	DL (fmol) On-column 21–60	*Anal. Biochem.*, 232, 210, 1995 (57)

TABLE 5.2 Continued

| Sample Matrix | Sample Preparation | | | HPLC Parameters | | | | |
	Analyte	Sample Extraction	Clean Up	Column	Mobile Phase	Detection	Quality Assurance Parameters	References
Serum	all-*trans*-retinol, α-, β-, γ-carotene, lycopene, β-cryptoxanthin, lutein	Add water and EtOH, Extract with PE, Assay top layer directly	—	μBondapak C_{18}, 30 cm × 3.9 mm	MeCN : MeOH : EtOAC (88 : 10 : 2), 2 mL/min	retinol—325 nm, carotenoids—436 nm	—	Int. J. Food Sci. Nutr., 45, 147, 1994 (58), Food Chem., 49, 21, 1996 (59)
Plasma	all-*trans*-retinol, α-, γ-, δ-tocopherol	Add EtOH (0.625% BHT), Vortex, Add Hex (0.005% BHT), Shake, centrifuge, Evaporate aliquot, Repeat extraction 2×, Dissolve in tocol (IS) solution	—	LiChrosphere 100, 5 μm, 25 cm × 3 mm	Isocratic, MeCN : THF : MeOH : 1% NH_4OAC (684 : 220 : 68 : 28), 0.65 mL/min	retinol—325 nm, tocol—292 nm, tocopherols Fluorescence Ex λ = 298 Em λ = 330	RSD <5%, QL (mmol/L) retinol 0.192, δ-T 0.617, γ-T 0.878, α-T 2.37	J. Chromatogr. B, 668, 57, 1997 (62)

[a] Number in ( ) is reference citation number.

the amperometric detector. The method used tocol as an internal standard because low quantities of δ-tocopherol were found in normal serum. δ-tocopherol had been used in earlier studies as an internal standard to quantitate α-tocopherol by UV detection.[35,36]

5.3.1.2 Vitamin K$_1$ and α-Tocopherol

Cham et al.[38] used post-column reduction of vitamin K$_1$ with sodium borohydride to assay vitamin K$_1$ with RRR-α-tocopherol. Vitamin K$_1$ methods had previously been developed as single analyte methods (see Chapter 4). Interfering lipids in the serum were removed after hexane extraction by washing the hexane layer with methanol : water (9 : 1). This step removed sufficient lipid to allow vitamin K$_1$ analysis without further concentration or purification. HPLC was on a C$_{18}$ Resolve column with elution by ethanol : water (98 : 2). Details of the method are given in Table 5.2.

5.3.2 METHODS FOR MULTI-ANALYTES IN SERUM OR PLASMA

Numerous studies conducted in the 1980s modified methods for analysis of retinol and α-tocopherol in plasma to include β-carotene and other carotenoids. Most methods used reversed-phase chromatography on C$_{18}$ with isocratic or gradient elution. Earlier multi-fat-soluble vitamin methods including MacCrehan and Schönberger,[39] and Thurnham et al.[40] are summarized in Table 5.2. Improvements in detector sensitivity and data management systems have led to simultaneous procedures including all of the fat-soluble vitamins and many non-vitamin A active carotenoids present in serum at low, but detectable levels. Selected methods published since 1990 are summarized in Table 5.2.

Several research groups utilized programmable multi-channel UV/visible detectors to expand the number of analytes from serum that could be simultaneously assayed.[40,41,42,44,45,47,48,51,53,54] Other recent studies used UV/visible detectors in series,[58,59,62] fluorescence[56] or UV[52] only, UV and fluorescence detectors in series,[43] and electrochemical detection.[57] Representative of these methods, Sowell et al.[54] used multi-wavelength detection to assay all-trans-retinol, four retinyl esters, RRR-α- and RRR-γ-tocopherol, all-*trans*-β-carotene, 13-*cis*-β-carotene, α-carotene, lycopene, lutein, β-cryptoxanthin, and zeaxanthin in serum. The method was based upon use of non-apreno-β-carotene and retinyl butyrate as internal standards. The procedure clearly shows the power of an LC system based upon current detector capability and an advanced data handling system (Maxima Software, Waters, Inc.) to simultaneously assay several fat-soluble vitamins and related analytes. The Sowell et al.[54] procedure is outlined in Section 5.4.

A PDA detector can be aligned in series with a fluorescent detector to complete simultaneous assays using UV, visible and fluorescence properties of the analytes. Figure 5.4 shows the capability of such a set-up to efficiently quantitate tocopherols, tocotrienols, all-*trans*-retinol, retinyl palmitate, and all-*trans*-β-carotene. The sample analysis shown in Figure 5.4 is rice bran oil containing added retinol, retinyl palmitate, and β-carotene. The LC system consisted of a Waters Separation Module 2690, a Shimadzu RF-10A fluorescence detector and a Waters PDA, Model 996. Data was processed by Waters Millennium software. Chromatography parameters included a LiChrosorb Si60 column (25 cm × 4.6 mm) protected with a LiChrosorb (5 μm) guard column, a linear flow gradient from 0.9% to 1.2% isopropyl alcohol in hexane, and a flow gradient that changed from 1.2 mL to 0.9 mL over the course of the chromatographic run. Vitamin E homologs were detected fluorometrically (Ex λ = 290, Em λ = 330), retinol and retinyl palmitate at 326 nm, and β-carotene at 450 nm (unpublished).

Miller and Yang[60] used a Hewlett-Packard 1040A PDA for quantitation of all-*trans*-retinol, RRR-α-tocopherol, all-*trans*-β-carotene, α-carotene and lycopene from serum or plasma. This was one of the earliest simultaneous methods for fat-soluble vitamin analysis of serum using PDA technology. Chromatography was on C$_{18}$ Radial-Pak with gradient elution with methanol : acetonitrile : chloroform (47 : 42 : 11) preceded with 100% methanol. Another early study using PDA detection was completed by Milne and Botnen.[61]

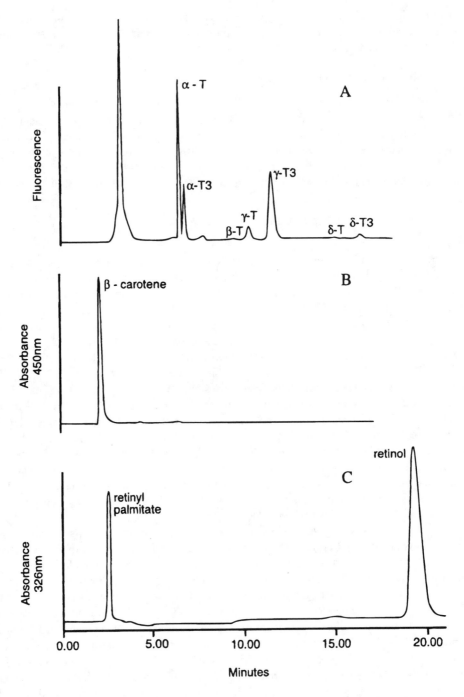

FIGURE 5.4 Chromatograms of human serum with detection at 450, 325, and 300 nm (a). Enlargement of the 450 and 325, showing the retinyl esters (b). 1. Lutein/zeaxanthin, 2. 2,2′,3′-Anhydrolutein, 3. Mixed carotenoids, 4. α-cryptoxanthin, 5. β-cryptoxanthin, 6. Lycopene, 7. α-Carotene, 8. *trans*-β-carotene, 9. 13-*cis*-β-carotene, 10. Non-apreno-β-carotene, 11. Retinol, 12. Retinyl butyrate, 13. γ-tocopherol, 14. α-tocopherol, 15. Retinyl oleate, 16. Retinyl palmitate, 17. Retinyl stearate. Reproduced with permission from Reference 54.

Khachik et al.[46] showed the versatility of PDA detection in a study of plasma carotenoids and carotenoid oxidation products. Eighteen carotenoids were resolved and identified using reversed-phase chromatography on C_{18} and chromatography on silica-based nitrile columns. Carotenoids were identified by mass spectroscopy with an LC/MS system interconnected by a particle beam interface. The study represents one of the most intense identification and quantitative studies completed on carotenoids in plasma. Additionally, the procedure quantitated retinol and α- and γ-tocopherol along with the carotenoids. Carotenoids identified in plasma by Khachik et al.[46] are given in Table 5.3.

Sensitivity of PDA detectors, once an impediment to routine applications, has been greatly increased in new models. Recent methods designed to simultaneously quantitate fat-soluble vitamins in serum and other low concentration samples rely on the capability of the PDA. Barua et al.[49,50] identified 17 carotenoids and measured all-*trans*-retinol and RRR-α- and RRR-γ-tocopherol in serum. Chromatography was on C_{18}. Resolve and quantitation of the analytes using PDA was at 290, 325, and 450 nm. Chromatographic data obtained in the study is given in Table 5.4. The procedure is summarized in Table 5.2 and more fully described in Section 5.4. In 1995, Ben-Amotz.[55] developed an LC system for the simultaneous separation and identification of 20 carotenoids, retinol, other retinoids, and α- and γ- tocopherol from serum. The method was based on chromatography on Vydac C_{18} and on-line monitoring with a PDA. The method was applied to plant and algae tissue in addition to human serum. Identified compounds in serum and their absorption maxima are given in Table 5.5.

TABLE 5.3

Carotenoids Identified in Human Serum and Their Absorption Maxima

Plasma Carotenoids[a,b]	Absorption Maxima (nm)[c]
Eluent B	
ε,ε-carotene-3,3'-dione	420, 442, 472
3'-hydroxy-ε,ε-caroten-3-one	(422–424), 442, 472
(all-E)-5,6-dihydroxy-5,6-dihydro-ψ,ψ-carotene	436, 460, 492
(5,6-dihydroxy-5,6-dihydrolycopene)	
(Z)-5,6-dihydroxy-5,6-dihydro-ψ,ψ-carotene	434, 458, 490
3-hydroxy-β,ε-carotene-3'-one	(422–424), 448, 476
(Z)-3-hydroxy-β,ε-caroten-$\overline{3}$ one	(418–420), 442, 470
(all-E,3R,3'R)-β,ε-carotene-3,3'diol	
((all-E)-lutein)	(422–424), 448, 476
(all-E,3R,3'R)-β,β-carotene-3,3'diol ((all-E)-3'-zeaxanthin)	(428), 454, 482
(all-E,3R,3'S,6'R)-β,ε-carotene-3,3'diol ((all-E)-3'-epilutein)	(422–424), 448, 476
(9Z)-lutein	334, 420, 442, 470
(9'Z)-lutein	332, (420), 444, 472
(all-E,3R)-8' apo-β-carotene-3,8'diol	
(internal std)	(408), 427, 454
(Z,3R)-8'apo-β-carotene-3,8'diol	(405), 424, 450
(13Z)-lutein + (13'Z)-lutein	334, (418), 440, 468
(9Z)-zeaxanthin	340, (424), 450, 474
(13Z)-zeaxanthin	338, (419), 446, 470
(15Z)-zeaxanthin	338, (426), 450, 478

(*continued*)

TABLE 5.3 Continued

Eluent A

(*all-E*)-3-hydroxy-2′-3′-didehydro-β,ε-carotene	(424), 446, 474
((*all-E*)-2′,3′-anhydrolutein)	
(Z)-2′,3′-anhydrolutein	332, (420), 440, 468
ethyl β-apo-8′-carotenoate (IS)	444, (468)
β,ε-caroten-3-ol (α-cryptoxanthin)	(424), 446, 476
3-hydroxy-β-carotene (β-cryptoxanthin)	(428–430), 454, 480
(*all-E*)-ψ,ψ-carotene ((*all-E*)-lycopene)	446, 472–474, 502
(Z)-ψ,ψ-carotene ((Z)-lycopene)	346, 360, 442, 468, 498
7,8-dihydro-ψ,ψ-carotene (neurosporene)	(420–422), 440, 468
β,ψ-carotene (γ-carotene)	(440), 462, 492
7,8,7′,8′-tetrahydro-ψ,ψ-carotene	
(ζ-carotene)	378, 400–402, 426
β,ε-carotene (α-carotene)	(428), 446–448, 474
(*all-E*)-β,β-carotene	(430), 454, 478
(Z)-β,β-carotene	334, (422), 446, 474
(*all-E*)- or (Z)-7,8,11,12,7′,8′-bexahydro ψ,ψ-carotene	332–334, 350, 368
((*all-E*)- or (Z)-phytofluene)	
(Z)- or (*all-E*)-phytofluene	332–334, 350, 368
7,8,11,12,7′,8′,11′,12′-octahydro-ψ,ψ-carotene (phytoene)	(276), 286, (295)

[a] (Z)-Carotenoids have been designated the same number as their *all-E*-isomers, but distinguished from their *all-E*-compounds by prime symbols.

[b] Common names for certain carotenoids are shown in parentheses.

[c] Values in parentheses represent points of inflection.

Table adapted from Reference 46.

TABLE 5.4
Chromatographic Characteristics of Retinoids, Tocopherols and Carotenoids

Compound	Chromatographic Characteristics		Limit of Detection		Reported Range for Humans	
	Capacity Factor	Relative Retention Index[a]	pmol	ng	μmol liter^{-1}	ng ml^{-1}
Retinol	0.70	1664	0.21	0.06	1.6–3.4	456–973
γ-Tocopherol	2.58	2325	3.6	1.50		
α-Tocopherol	3.02	2410	6.4	2.70	16–36	6,800–15,600
Retinyl palmitate	8.59	2966	1.8	0.50		
Lutein	0.96	1858	ND			
Zeaxanthin	1.43	2006	ND			
β-Cryptoxanthin	3.43	2468	ND			
Lycopene	3.99	2563	ND			
α-Carotene	6.61	2835	0.8	0.45		
β-Carotene	7.28	2885	0.8	0.45	0.31–1.1	151–616
Internal Standards						
Retinyl hexanoate	1.41	2030				
β-Apo-8′-carotenyl decanoate	4.88	2660	0.6	0.25		

[a] Retention relative to alkylphenone standards; acetophenone = 800.

ND = Not determined.

Table adapted from Reference 49.

TABLE 5.5

Carotenoids, Retinoids and Tocopherols Assayed by HPLC Photodiode Array in Comparison to Literature Data

Carotenoid and Origin	Retention Time (min)	Absorption Maxima (nm) Waters 3-D system	Absorption Maxima (nm) Literature
β-apo-8′-carotenal (synthetic)	9.3	269.9, *465*	*463*
canthaxanthin (synthetic)	9.1	*475.2*	474–478
all-*trans*-α-carotene (synthetic)	18.0	269.9, 331.9, 431.5, *441.2*, 467.0	422, *442*, 471
all-*trans*-α-carotene (carrots)	16.5	269.9, 436.4, 446.0, *475.2*	—
all-*trans*-β-carotene (synthetic)	18.5	275.4, 417.0, *450.8*, 475.1	429, *449*, 475
9-*cis*-β-carotene (*Dunaliella*)	20.7	268.4, 341.5, 436.4, *446.0*, 472.7	*445*
15-*cis*-β-carotene (synthetic)	21.8	336.6, *450.9*, 470.3	*448*
9,15-di-*cis*-β-carotene (synthetic)	19.7	284.2, 336.6, *446.0*, 465.2	—
all-*trans* γ-carotene (synthetic)	21.4	280.3, 441.0, *463.0*, 490.2	437, *460*, 490
all-*trans*-ζ-carotene (*Dunaliella*)	18.3	236.2, 378.0, *399.6*, 424.1	295, 377, *398*, 422
9-*cis*-ζ-carotene (*Dunaliella*)	19.5	236.1, 374.1, 395.2, 420.1	295, 374, *395*, *419*
β-cryptoxanthin (synthetic)	10.5	274.7, 426.8, 450.8, 480.1	425, *449–452*, 473–8
echinenone (synthetic)	11.6	299.4, *465.5*	457–461
lutein (alfalfa)	5.0	269.9, 331.9, *446.1*, 475.2	422, *443*, 470
lycopene (tomato)	25.3	293.7, 263.9, 446.1, *470.3*, *504.4*	444, *470*, 502
all-*trans*-phytoene (*Dunaliella*)	18.9	277.8, 286.1, 296.0	276, *286*, 297
9-*cis*-phytoene (*Dunaliella*)	18.0	277.8, 286.1, 296.0	276, *284*, 294
phytofluene, all-*trans*-and 9-*cis*- (*Dun*)	18.8, 19.2	331.4, *348.2*, 368.2	329, *346*, 365
Violaxanthin (*Dunaliella*)	4.8	267.5, 329.4, *443.6*, 471.0	414, *441*, 471
Zeaxanthin (*Dunaliella*)	5.3	276.1, 425.9, *450.3*, 477.3	341, 427, *448*, 475
Retinoids:			
Retinol (synthetic)	3.8	*327.1*	—
Retinol (serum)	3.8	*323.5*	325
9-*cis*-retinol (synthetic)	3.85	*322.3*	—
all-*trans*-retinoic acid (synthetic)	3.0	*336.6*	—
13-*cis*-retinoic acid (synthetic)	3.2	*341.4*	—
Vitamin E:			
α-tocopherol (synthetic)	6.9	291.3	292
γ-tocopherol (synthetic)	6.2	294.8	294

Table adapted from Reference 55.

5.4   METHOD PROTOCOLS
New Simplified Procedures for the Extraction and Simultaneous High-Performance Liquid Chromographic Analysis of Retinol, Tocopherols and Carotenoids in Human Serum

Principle
- Retinol, tocopherols, and carotenoids are extracted by a simplified extraction procedure and quantitated by reversed-phase chromatography on Resolve C_{18}. PDA detection was used to quantitate and confirm the identity of the analytes.

Chemicals
- Acetonitrile
- Methanol
- Dichloromethane
- Dichloroethane
- Isopropanol
- 1-Octanol
- Argon

Apparatus
- Liquid chromatograph
- PDA
- Automated injector
- Data management system

Procedure

Extraction
- Extract 20–500 μL serum with 2 × volume ethanol and 1 mL ethyl acetate
- Add all-rac-α-tocopheryl acetate (IS) and/or canthaxanthin (IS) and/or retinoic acid (IS)
- Vortex, 30 s
- Centrifuge, 30 s
- Remove supernatant, break pellet
- Re-extract 2× with ethyl acetate (0.5-1 mL)
- Re-extract with hexane (0.5-1 mL)
- Centrifuge, combine supernatants
- Add 50 μL water
- Vortex, centrifuge
- Remove organic layer, evaporate to dryness with argon stream
- Dissolve residue in 100 mL dichloromethane : methanol (1 : 2)
- Filter, inject

Chromatography

Column	39 cm × 3.9 mm
Stationary phase	Resolve C_{18}, 5 μm
Mobile phase	(A) Acetonitrile : dichloromethane : methanol : 1-octanol (90 : 15 : 10 : 0.1)
	(B) Acetonitrile : dichloromethane : methanol (85 : 10 : 5)
Column temperature	Ambient
Flow	(A) 1 mL/min
	(B) 1.5 mL/min
Detection	PDA
	Carotenoids 450 nm
	Retinoids 325 nm
	Tocopherols 290 nm
Calculation	Peak area, IS

Note: All sample extractions completed cold and under yellow light.

J. Chromatogr., 617, 257, 1993

High Performance Liquid Chromatographic Method for the Simultaneous Determination of Tocopherols, Carotenes, and Retinol and its Geometric Isomers in Cheese and Milk,

Principle
- α-, β-, γ-, and δ-tocopherol, *cis*- and *trans*-isomers of retinol and total carotenes are saponified and extracted with hexane : ethyl acetate (9 : 1). Analytes are resolved on Ultrasphere Si and detected with programmable UV/visible and fluorescence detectors in series.

Chemicals
- Potassium hydroxide (60%)
- Ethanol (95%)
- Sodium chloride
- Pyrogallol
- Isopropanol
- Hexane

Apparatus
- Liquid chromatograph
- Programmable UV/visible detector
- Programmable fluorescence detector

Procedure

Extraction
- Saponify 0.5 g cheese with 2 mL 60% KOH, 2 mL 95% ethanol, 1 mL 1% NaCl and 5 mL 6% ethanolic pyrogallol
- Flush tube with nitrogen
- Reflux at 70°C, 30 min
- Cool, icebath
- Add 15 mL 1% NaCl
- Extract 2 × with 15 mL portions of hexane : ethyl acetate (9 : 1)
- Evaporate organic layer
- Dissolve residue in 2 mL mobile phaes
- Filter, inject

Chromatography

Column	25 cm × 4.6 mm
Stationary phase	Ultrasphere Si, 5 μm
Mobile phase	(A) 1% isopropanol in hexane
	(B) Hexane
	Gradient

Time (min)	%A	%B
0	50	50
11	90	10
19	50	50

Column temperature	Ambient	
Flow	1.5 mL/min	
Detection	Carotenes	450 nm
	Tocopherols	Fluorescence Ex λ = 280, Em λ = 325
	Retinoids	Fluorescence Ex λ = 325, Em λ = 475
Calculation	Peak area, linear regression	

Note: Method does not resolve individual carotenoids. Authors state that carotenoids other than all-*trans*-β-carotene negligibly contribute to the vitamin A activity in cheese.

Analyst, 119, 1161, 1994

Retinol, α-Tocopherol, Lutein/Zeaxanthin, β-Cryptoxanthin, Lycopene, α-Carotene, *trans*-β-Carotene and Four Retinyl Esters in Serum Determined Simultaneously by Reversed-Phase HPLC with Multiwavelength Detection

Principle
- Fat-soluble vitamins and carotenoids were extracted from serum with hexane after ethanol deproteinization. Analytes are quantitated isocratically with elution from C_{18} support. Multiwavelength detection was used to monitor the analytes.

Chemicals
- Acetonitrile
- Hexane
- Ethanol (95%)
- Non-apreno-β-carotene (IS)
- Retinyl butyrate (IS)

Apparatus
- Liquid chromatograph
- Multiwavelength detector
- Autosampler
- Column heater
- Data management system

Procedure

Extraction
- Add 200 μL ethanol containing retinyl butyrate (IS) and non-apreno-β-carotene (IS)
- Vortex 10 s
- Add 1.0 mL hexane
- Vortex, 30 s
- Centrifuge, 1500 × g, 5 min
- Transfer hexane layer
- Dry under reduced pressure without heat to waxy consistency
- Add 100 μL ethanol
- Add 100 μL acetonitrile
- Vortex
- Filter (0.45 μm)

Chromatography

Column	15 cm × 4.6 mm
Stationary phase	Ultramex C_{18}, 5 μm
Mobile phase	Ethanol : acetonitrile (1 : 1) containing 0.1 mL diethylamine per L
Column temperature	29°C
Flow	0.9 mL/min
Detection	β-carotene 450 nm
	Retinoids 325 nm
	Tocopherols 300 nm
Calculation	Peak height, IS

Clin. Chem., 40, 411, 1994

Application of Gel Permeation Chromatography and Nonaqueous Reverse Phase Chromatography to High Performance Liquid Chromatographic Determination of Retinyl Palmitate and α-Tocopheryl Acetate in Infant Formulas

Principle

- The lipid-soluble components were extracted from the aqueous phase by homogenizing in isopropanol and methylene chloride with $MgSO_4$ added to remove water. Retinyl palmitate, β-carotene and α-tocopheryl acetate were fractionated from the lipid material using gel permeation chromatography (HP-GPC) with quantitation by reversed-phase LC and multiple wavelength detection (280, 313, 436 nm).

Chemicals

- Methanol
- Isopropanol
- α-tocopheryl acetate standard
- Retinyl palmitate standard
- β-carotene standard
- Compressed helium

Apparatus

- Rotary flash evaporator with −10°C cold trap
- Liquid chromatographs for GPC lipid removal and analytical chromatograph
- Closed evaporation system, Reactiware® vials, vacuum adapter and microconnectors
- 3-port switching valve for vitamin fraction collection

Procedure

Extraction

- Weigh sample in 100 mL graduated cylinder (low form)
- Add 15 mL isopropyl alcohol and 6.5 g $MgSO_4$ and 35 mL CH_2Cl_2
- Homogenize for 1 min
- Filter sample and wash solid material with two 15 mL portions CH_2Cl_2
- Transfer solid material to original cylinder and repeat homogenization with 25 mL CH_2Cl_2
- Filter and combine filtrates
- Evaporate to dryness using rotary flash evaporator
- Transfer oil residue to 5 μL volumetric flask and dilute to volume with CH_2Cl_2
- HP-GPC — Inject 250 μL and collect vitamin fraction (3.5 mL) based on UV detector response after oil elution as monitored by refractive index detector
- Evaporate to dryness and dissolve residue in reverse-phase mobile phase
- RP-LC — Inject 100 μL

Chromatography

Clean Up

Column	Three μ Styragel (100Å) 30 cm × 7.8 mm
Mobile phase	Methylene chloride containing 0.001% TEA
Column temperature	Ambient
Flow	1 mL/min
Detector	340 nm
Refractive Index Detection	Lipids

Analytical

Column	Zorbax ODS, 6 mm, 25 cm × 4.6 mm
Mobile phase	Methylene chloride + acetonitrile (300 +700) + 2 mL methanol

Column temperature	Ambient
Flow	1 mL/min
Detector	280/313/436 nm
Standard curve	3 point standard curve for each analyte
Standard concentrations	Vitamin A 0.25–1.2 µg/mL
	Vitamin E 2.5–12.5 µg/mL
	β-carotene 0.04–0.32 µg/mL
Retention times	Vitamin E 9 min
	Vitamin A 16 min
	β-carotene 18 min
Calculation	External standards, peak areas, 3 point-standard curve, linear regression

J. Assoc. Off. Anal. Chem., 65, 810, 1982

5.5 REFERENCES

1. Ball, G. F. M., Applications of HPLC to the determination of fat-soluble vitamins in foods and feeds (A Review 1977–1987), *J. Micronutr. Anal.*, 4, 255, 1988.
2. Ball, G. F. M., *Fat-Soluble Vitamin Assays in Food Analysis*, Elsevier, New York, 1988.
3. Thompson, J. N. and Maxwell, W. B., Reverse phase liquid chromatography of vitamin A in margarine, infant formula, and fortified milk, *J. Assoc. Off. Anal. Chem.*, 60, 766, 1977.
4. Landen, W. O., Jr. and Eitenmiller, R. R., Application of gel permeation chromatography and non-aqueous reverse phase chromatography to high pressure liquid chromatographic determination of retinyl palmitate and β-carotene in oil and margarine, *J. Assoc. Off. Anal. Chem.*, 62, 283, 1979.
5. Thompson, J. N., Hatina, G. and Maxwell, W. B., High performance liquid chromatographic determination of vitamin A in margarine, milk, partially skimmed milk and skimmed milk, *J. Assoc. Off. Anal. Chem.*, 63, 894, 1980.
6. Zonta, F., Stancher, B. and Bielawny, J., Separation and identification of vitamins D_2 and D_3 and their isomers in food samples in the presence of vitamin A, vitamin E and carotene, *J. Chromatogr.*, 246, 105, 1982.
7. Henderson, S. K. and McLean, L. A., Screening method for vitamins A and D in fortified skim milk, chocolate mik and vitamin D liquid concentrates, *J. Assoc. Off. Anal. Chem.*, 62, 1358, 1979.
8. Henderson, S. K. and Wickroski, A. L., Reverse phase high presure liquid chromatographic determination of vitamin D in fortified milk, *J. Assoc. Off. Anal. Chem.*, 61, 1130, 1978.
9. Landen, W. O., Application of gel permeation chromatography and nonaqueous reverse phase chromatography to high performance liquid chromatographic determination of retinyl palmitate and α-tocopheryl acetate in infant formulas, *J. Assoc. Off. Anal. Chem.*, 65, 810, 1982.
10. Landen, W. O., Jr., Resolution of fat-soluble vitamins in high-performance liquid chromatography with methanol-containing mobile phases, *J. Chromatogr.*, 211, 155, 1981.
11. Chappell, J. E., Francis, T. and Clandinin, M. T., Simultaneous high performance liquid chromatography analysis of retinol ester and tocopherol isomers in human milk, *Nutr. Res.*, 6, 849, 1986.
12. Stancher, B. and Zonta, F., High-performance liquid chromatographic determination of carotene and vitamin A and its geometric isomers in foods, *J. Chromatogr.*, 238, 217, 1982.
13. Barnett, S. A., Frick, L. W. and Baine, H. M., Simultaneous determination of vitamins A, D_2 or D_3, E and K_1 in infant formulas and dairy products by reversed-phase liquid chromatography, *Anal. Chem.*, 52, 610, 1980.
14. Zamarreño, M. M. D., Perez, A. S., Perez, M. C. G., and Mendez, J. H. High performance liquid chromatography with electrochemical detection for the simultaneous determination of vitamin A, D_3 and E in milk, *J. Chromatogr.*, 623, 69, 1992.

15. Zamarreño, M. M. D., Perez, A. S., Perez, M. C. G., Moro, M. A. F. and Mendez, J. H., Determination of vitamins A, E, and K_1 in milk by high-performance liquid chromatography with dual amperometric detection, *Analyst*, 120, 2489, 1995.

16. Zamarreño, M. M. D., Perez, A. S., Perez, M. C. G. and Mendez, J. H., Directly coupled sample treatment—high-performance liquid chromatography for on-line automatic determination of liposoluble vitamins in milk, *J. Chromatogr. A*, 694, 399, 1995.

17. Panfili, G., Manzi, P. and Pizzoferrato, C., High-performance liquid chromatographic method for the simultaneous determination of tocopherols, carotenes, and retinol and its geometric isomers in Italian cheeses, *Analyst*, 119, 1161, 1994.

18. Ueda, T. and Igarashi, O., Effect of coexisting fat on the extraction of tocopherols from tisues after saponification as a pretreatment for HPLC determination, *J. Micronutr. Anal.*, 3, 15, 1987.

19. Scalia, S., Renda, A., Ruberto, G., Bonina, F. and Menegatti, E., Assay of vitamin A palmitate and vitamin E acetate in cosmetic creams and lotions by supercritical fluid extraction and HPLC, *Pharm. Biomed. Anal.*, 13, 273, 1995.

20. Blanco, D., Pajares, M., Escotet, V. J. and Gutierrez, M. D., Determination of fat-soluble vitamins by liquid chromatography in pediatric parenteral nutritions, *J. Liq. Chromatogr.*, 17, 4513, 1994.

21. Widicus, W. A. and Kirk, J. R., High pressure liquid chromatographic determination of vitamin A and E in cereal products, *J. Assoc. Off. Anal. Chem.*, 62, 637, 1979.

22. Pozo, R. G., Saitua, E. S., Uncilla, I. and Montoya, J. A., Simultaneous determination by HPLC of fat-soluble vitamins in Albacore *(Thunnus alalunga)*, *J. Food Sci.*, 55, 77, 1990.

23. Jiang, Y. H., McGeachin, R. B. and Bailey, C. A., α-tocopherol, β-carotene, and retinol enrichment of chicken eggs, *Poultry Sci.*, 73, 1137, 1994.

24. Rushing, L. G., Cooper, W. M. and Thompson, H. C., Simultaneous analysis of vitamins A and E in rodent feed by high-pressure liquid chromatography, *J. Agric. Food Chem.*, 39, 296, 1991.

25. McGeachin, R. B. and Bailey, C. A., Determination of carotenoid pigments, retinol, and α-tocopherol in feeds, tissues, and blood serum by normal phase high performance liquid chromatography, *Poultry Sci.*, 74, 407, 1995.

26. Vinas, P., Campillo, N., Garcia, I. L. and Cordoba, M. H., Liquid chromatographic determination of fat-soluble vitamins in paprika and paprika oleoresin, *Food Chem.*, 45, 349, 1992.

27. Tee, E.-S. and Lim, C.L., Re-analysis of vitamin A values of selected Malaysian foods of animal origin by the AOAC and HPLC methods, *Food Chem.*, 45, 289, 1992.

28. Landen, W. O., Hines, D. M., Hamill, T. W., Martin, J. I., Young, E. R., Eitenmiller, R. R. and Soliman, A.-G. M., Vitamin A and vitamin E content of infant formulas produced in the United States, *J. Assoc. Off. Anal. Chem.*, 68, 509, 1985.

29. Landen, W. O., Jr., Application of gel permeation chromatography and nonaqueous reverse phase chromatography to high pressure liquid chromatographic determination of retinyl palmitate in fortified breakfast cereals, *J. Assoc. Off. Anal. Chem.*, 63, 131, 1980.

30. Landen, W. O., Jr., Eitenmiller, R. R. and Soliman, A. M., Vitamin D_3 and vitamin K_1 levels in infant formula produced in the United States, *J. Food Comp. Anal.*, 2, 140, 1989.

31. De Leenheer, A. P., Nelis, H. J., Lambert, W. E. and Bauwens, R. M., Chromatography of fat-soluble vitamins in clinical chemistry, *J. Chromatogr.*, 429, 3, 1988.

32. Bieri, J. G., Tolliver, T. J. and Catignani, G. L., Simultaneous determination of α-tocopherol and retinol in plasma or red cells by high pressure liquid chromatography, *Am. J. Clin. Nutr.*, 32, 2143, 1979.

33. De Leenheer, A. P., Veerle, O. R. C., DeBevere, M. DeRuyter, G. M. and Claeys, A. E., Simultaneous determination of retinol and α-tocopherol in human serum by high-performance liquid chromatography, *J. Chromatogr.*, 162, 408, 1979.

34. Rhys Williams, A. T., Simultaneous determination of serum vitamin A and E by liquid chromatography with fluorescence detection, *J. Chromatogr.*, 341, 198, 1985.

35. Vanderwoude, M., Claeys, M. and DeLeeuw, I., Determination of α-tocopherol in human plasma by high-performance liquid chromatography with electrochemical detection, *J. Chromatogr.*, 311, 176, 1984.

36. Chou, P. P., Jaynes, P. K. and Bailey, J. L., Determination of vitamin E in microsamples of serum by liquid chromatography with electrochemical detection, *Clin. Chem.*, 31, 880, 1985.

37. Huang, M. L., Burckart, G. J. and Venkataramanan, R., Sensitive high-performance liquid chromatographic analysis of plasma vitamin E and vitamin A using amperometric and ultraviolet detection, *J. Chromatogr.*, 380, 331, 1986.

38. Cham, B. E., Roeser, H. P. and Kamst, T. W., Simultaneous liquid chromatographic determination of vitamin K_1 and vitamin E in serum, *Clin. Chem.*, 35, 2285, 1989.

39. MacCrehan, W. A. and Schönberger, E., Determination of retinol, α-tocopherol, and β-carotene in serum by liquid chromatography with absorbance and electrochemical detection, *Clin. Chem.*, 33, 1585, 1987.

40. Thurnham, D. I., Smith, E. and Flora, P. S., Concurrent liquid chromatographic assay of retinol, α-tocopherol, β-carotene, α-carotene, lycopene, and β-cryptoxanthin in plasma, with tocopherol acetate as internal standard, *Clin. Chem.*, 34, 377, 1988.

41. Olmedilla, B., Granado, F., Rojas-Hidalgo, E. and Blanco, I., A rapid separation of ten carotenoids, three retinoids, α-tocopherol, and d-α-tocopherol acetate by high performance liquid chromatography and its application to serum and vegetable samples, *J. Liq. Chromatogr.*, 13, 1455, 1990.

42. Olmedilla, B., Granado, F., Blanco, I., and Rojas-Hidalgo, E., Determination of nine carotenoids, retinol, retinyl palmitate, and α-tocopherol in control human serum using two internal standards, *Food Chem.*, 45, 205, 1992.

43. Hess, D., Keller, H. E., Oberlin, B., Bonfanti, R. and Schüep, W., Simultaneous determination of retinol, tocopherols, carotenes and lycopene in plasma by means of high-performance liquid chromatography on reversed phase, *Int. J. Vit. Nutr. Res.*, 61, 232, 1991.

44. Arnaud, J., Fortis, I., Blachier, S., Kia, D. and Favier, A., Simultaneous determination of retinol, α-tocopherol and β-carotene in serum by isocratic high performance liquid chromatography, *J. Chromatogr.*, 572, 103, 1991.

45. Nierenberg, D. W. and Nann, S. L., A method for determining concentrations of retinol, tocopherol, and five carotenoids in human plasma and tissue samples, *Am. J. Clin. Nutr.*, 56, 417, 1992.

46. Khachik, F., Beecher, G. R. and Goli, M. B., Separation and identification of carotenoids and their oxidation products in the extracts of human plasma, *Anal. Chem.*, 64, 2111, 1992.

47. Zaman, Z., Fielden, P. and Frost, P. G., Simultaneous determination of vitamins A and E and carotenoids in plasma by reversed-phase HPLC in elderly and younger subjects, *Clin. Chem.*, 39, 2229, 1993.

48. Tang, G., Dolnikowski, G. G., Blanco, M. C., Fox, J. G. and Russell, R. M., Serum carotenoids and retinoids in ferrets fed canthaxanthin, *J. Nutr. Biochem.*, 4, 58, 1993.

49. Barua, A. B., Furr, H. C., Janick-Buckner, D. and Olson, J. A., Simultaneous analysis of individual carotenoids, retinol, retinyl esters, and tocopherols in serum by isocratic non-aqueous reversed-phase HPLC, *Food Chem.*, 46, 419, 1993.

50. Barua, A. B., Kostic, D. and Olson, J. A., New simplified procedures for the extraction and simultaneous high-performance liquid chromatographic analysis of retinol, tocopherols and carotenoids in human serum, *J. Chromatogr.*, 617, 257, 1993.

51. Epler, K. S., Ziegler, R. G. and Craft, N. E., Liquid chromatographic method for the determination of carotenoids, retinoids and tocopherols in human serum and in food, *J. Chromatogr.*, 619, 37, 1993.

52. Aksnes, L., Simultaneous determination of retinol, α-tocopherol, and 25-hydroxyvitamin D in human serum by high-performance liquid chromatography, *J. Ped. Gastroenterol. Nutr.*, 18, 339, 1994.

53. Bui, M. H., Simple determination of retinol, α-tocopherol and carotenoids (lutein, all-*trans*-lycopene, α- and β-carotenes) in human plasma by isocratic liquid chromatography, *J. Chromatogr. B*, 654, 129, 1994.

54. Sowell, A. L., Huff, D. L., Yeager, P. R., Caudill, S. P. and Gunter, E. W., Retinol, α-tocopherol, lutein/zeaxanthin, β-cryptoxanthin, lycopene, α-carotene, *trans*-β-carotene, and four retinyl esters in serum determined simultaneously by reversed-phase HPLC with multiwavelength detection, *Clin. Chem.*, 40, 411, 1994.

55. Ben-Amotz, A., Simultaneous profiling and identification of carotenoids, retinols, and tocopherols by high performance liquid chromatography equipped with three-dimensional photodiode array detection, *J. Liq. Chromatogr.*, 18, 2813, 1995.

56. Jakob, E. and Elmadfa, I., Rapid HPLC assay for the assessment of vitamin K_1, A, E, and β-carotene status in children (7–19 years), *Int. J. Vit. Nutr. Res.*, 65, 31, 1995.
57. Finckh, B., Kontush, A., Commentz, J., Hübner, C., Burdelski, M. and Kohlschütter, A., Monitoring of Ubiquinol-10, Ubiquinone-10, carotenoids, and tocopherols in neonatal plasma microsamples using high-performance liquid chromatography with coulometric electrochemical detection, *Anal. Biochem.*, 232, 210, 1995.
58. Tee, E. S., Lim, C. L. and Chong, Y. H., Carotenoid profile and retinol content in human serum—simultaneous determination by high-pressure liquid chromatography (HPLC), *Int. J. Food Sci. Nutr.*, 45, 147, 1994.
59. Tee, E. S., Lim, C. L., Chong, Y. H. and Khor, S. C., A study of the biological utilization of carotenoids of carrot and swamp cabbage in rats, *Food Chem.*, 49, 21, 1996.
60. Miller, K. W. and Yang, C. S., An isocratic high performance liquid chromatography method for the simultaneous analysis of plasma retinol, α-tocopherol and various carotenoids, *Anal. Biochem.*, 145, 21, 1985.
61. Milne, D. B. and Botnen, J., Retinol, α-tocopherol, lycopene and α- and β-carotene simultaneously determined in plasma by isocratic liquid chromatography, *Clin. Chem.*, 32, 874, 1986.
62. Göbel, Y., Schaffer, C. and Koletzko, B., Simultaneous determination of low plasma concentrations of retinol and tocopherols in preterm infants by a high-performance liquid chromatographic micromethod, *J. Chromatogr. B*, 688, 57, 1997.

Water-Soluble Vitamins

6 Ascorbic Acid

Vitamin C

6.1 REVIEW

Scurvy is the centuries old name for vitamin C deficiency. Like many other nutritional deficiencies, scurvy was recognized long before the active nutritional component was known and understood. With scurvy, associations were made with the curative and preventative effects of various foods. In 1747, James Lind, a British naval physician, documented the role of citrus fruits in curing British sailors suffering from scurvy. His work, representing the first controlled therapeutic medical trial, established citrus fruits as a curative food.[1] Essentially, no further advances were made until the disease was induced in guinea pigs in 1907. An animal assay based upon the guinea pig's response was developed in 1917 to test the antiscorbutic activity of foods. Ascorbic acid was isolated from natural sources, shown to be the antiscorbutic factor and structurally characterized by Szent-Györgyi and Haworth and King in the early 1930s. The vitamin was synthesized by Reichstein in 1933. In 1937, Szent-Györgyi and Haworth were awarded the Nobel Prize for their research on ascorbic acid.[2]

Olson[1] categorized scurvy symptoms as systemic, hemorrhagic, psychologic, secretory, neurologic, hematologic, and connective tissue related. The symptoms are more fully described in Table 6.1. Serum and leukocyte ascorbic acid concentrations are frequently used to assess human ascorbic acid status. Leukocyte concentrations are more reliable status indicators than serum, erythrocyte, or

TABLE 6.1
Signs of Ascorbic Acid Deficiency

	Symptom
Systemic	Fatigue
	Lassitude
Hemorrhagic	Petechiae
	Perifollicular hemorrhage
	Ecchymoses
	Bleeding gums
Psychologic	Depression
	Hypochondriasis
	Hysteria
Secretory	Dry Skin ⎫
	Xerophthalmia ⎬ Sjögren's Syndrome
	Xerostomia ⎭
	Follicular hyperkeratosis
Vasomotor instability	Altered neurotrophic amine metabolism
Hematologic	Impaired iron absorption
	Impaired folate metabolism
Connective tissue	Scorbutic arthritis
	Impaired wound healing

Adapted from Reference 1.

whole blood levels since short-term fluctuations in intake affect the leukocyte concentration to a lesser degree.[3] Urinary excretion decreases as intake decreases and is highly reflective of recent intake. Even with 24 h urine collections, urinary levels are not a sensitive index of status. Chemical and liquid chromatographic techniques provide highly reliable measures of ascorbic acid in clinical samples. Ascorbic acid plasma levels plateau at 1.2 to 1.5 mg/100 mL.

Ascorbic acid is present in all animals and higher plants, but only humans and a few other vertebrates have specific requirements. Other species synthesize the compound. Vegetables and fruits are the primary dietary sources for the human. Citrus and various vegetables including peppers, tomatoes, potatoes, and leafy greens are excellent sources. Dairy products, meats, and cereal grains are poor sources of vitamin C. The adult Recommended Dietary Allowance (RDA) for vitamin C is 60 mg.[4] The RDA increases to 70 mg during pregnancy and 95 mg and 90 mg, respectively, during the first and second six months of lactation. RDA's from infancy through adolescence range from 30 to 50 mg. The Reference Daily Intake (RDI) set in the Nutritional Labeling and Education Act of 1990 is 60 mg.[5]

L-ascorbic acid is the active form of vitamin C. Its stereoisomer, D-isoascorbic acid, has only minimal biological activity. Biochemical functions are largely based upon the oxidation-reduction properties of the vitamin. L-ascorbic acid is a cofactor in the procollagen proline hydroxylase reaction which converts proline in procollagen to hydroxyproline in collagen. The enzyme requires Fe^{+2}, L-ascorbic acid, oxygen, and α-ketoglutarate. α-ketoglutarate is oxidized to succinate with the release of carbon dioxide. The involvement of L-ascorbic acid in collagen synthesis is directly related to the etiology of scurvy. L-ascorbic acid functions in many hydroxylase reactions. All enzymes that require L-ascorbic acid are Fe or Cu metalloenzymes. Monoxygenases like dopamine-β-hydroxylase incorporate one oxygen atom into a product with concomitant reduction of the other oxygen atom into water. Dopamine-β-hydroxylase functions in the conversion of dopamine into norepinephrine in catecholamine synthesis. In this class of enzymes, two substrates are oxidized and the term mixed-function oxidase is applicable. L-ascorbic acid also functions with dioxygenases that require α-ketoglutarate as a cosubstrate. In these reactions, one oxygen atom is incorporated into succinate and one into the product. The procollagen proline hydroxylase conversion of proline into hydroxyproline characterizes this class of reactions. The co-enzyme roles of L-ascorbic acid were recently discussed in detail by Basu and Dickerson.[6]

Vitamin C's role as an *in vivo* antioxidant has received much attention over the past decade. In this respect, it is included in the antioxidant complex including vitamin E, β-carotene, and other non-provitamin A carotenoids such as lutein and lycopene, flavonoids, and selenium. While significant press has been given to the antioxidant components of the diet, definitive clinical results are largely lacking. Like vitamin E, L-ascorbic acid is a primary defensive nutrient through its function as a free-radical scavenger. It can react in aqueous media against *in vivo* peroxidations, including quenching of singlet oxygen species. L-ascorbic acid also functions in immune response, steroid and drug metabolism, iron bioavailability, antihistamine reactions, and possibly as an anticarcinogen.[7]

6.2 PROPERTIES

6.2.1 CHEMISTRY

6.2.1.1 General Properties

L-ascorbic acid ($C_6H_8O_6$) is the trivial name for vitamin C which is the accepted IUPAC-IUB Commission on Biochemical Nomenclature name.[8] The systematic chemical designation is 2-oxo-L-threo-hexono-1,4-lactone-2,3-enediol. The structure is given in Figure 6.1. L-ascorbic acid is the USP standard. Vitamin C refers to compounds exhibiting full or partial biological activity of

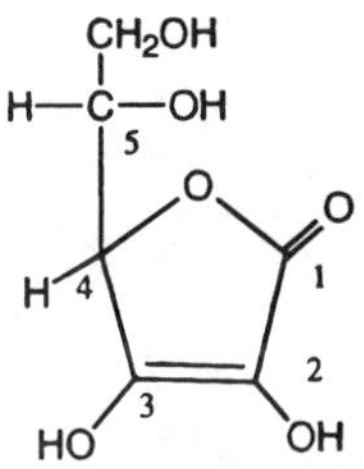

L-Ascorbic Acid
2-oxo-L-threo-hexono-1,4-lactone-2,3-enediol
Vitamin C

FIGURE 6.1 Structure of L-ascorbic acid.

L-ascorbic acid. These include esters of ascorbic acid such as ascorbyl palmitate, 100% relative activity, synthetic forms such as 6-deoxy-L-ascorbic acid with 33% relative activity and the primary oxidized form of L-ascorbic acid, dehydroascorbic acid with 80% relative activity.[7] L-ascorbic acid and dehydroascorbic acid are the primary dietary sources of vitamin C.[8] Use of ascorbyl palmitate as a component in commercial antioxidant preparations is increasing. Since animals efficiently reduce dehydroascorbic acid to L-ascorbic acid, both forms must be measured to accurately quantitate "total" vitamin C activity of food or other biological samples.[9]

L-ascorbic acid has chiral centers at carbons 4 and 5 and can exist in four stereoisomeric forms. Enantiomeric pairs are L- and D-ascorbic acid and L- and D-araboascorbic acid. L-ascorbic acid and D-araboascorbic acid (more commonly known as D-isoascorbic acid) or erythorbic acid, are epimers differing in orientation of the hydrogen and hydroxyl on carbon 5.[10] We will use the term isoascorbic acid throughout this chapter. Structures of various ascorbic acid forms are given in Figure 6.2. Isoascorbic acid is not present in foods but is synthesized commercially for its antioxidant properties. The stereoisomers have no biological activity other than a small amount from isoascorbic acid (2.5 to 5% relative to L-ascorbic acid).[8] The use of isoascorbic acid as an antioxidant in foods, usually processed meats, and its low biological activity led to the development of LC methods capable of quantitating the individual isomers. Most other assay techniques will not differentiate the epimers. Because isoascorbic acid is used in some processed foods, erroneously high vitamin C values will be found if improper methodology is used.

Physical properties of L-ascorbic acid, its salts, and ascorbyl palmitate are given in Table 6.2. L-ascorbic acid is a white to slightly yellow crystalline powder with high water solubility (30 g/100 mL) at ambient temperature. Its salts have higher water solubility. All commercial forms except fatty acid esters such as ascorbyl palmitate are insoluble in fats and oils. L-ascorbic acid is a widely-used food additive with many functional roles, many of which are based upon its oxidation-reduction properties. Its functional roles include its uses as a nutritional food additive, antioxidant, browning inhibitor, reducing agent, flavor stabilizer, modifier and enhancer, color stabilizer, dough modifier and in many other capacities. Ascorbyl palmitate was developed to provide an ascorbic acid form with greater lipid solubility for use in antioxidant preparations. Ascorbyl palmitate is highly effective synergistically with primary antioxidants including phenols and tocopherols.

6.2.1.2 Spectral Properties

Absorption properties are dependent upon the ionic species present and, therefore, dependent upon the pH of the aqueous media. Ball[10] provides an excellent review of the spectral properties of L-ascorbic acid. The spectra of L-ascorbic acid at pH 2.0 and pH 6.0 and dehydroascorbic acid at pH 3.1 are given in Figure 6.3. $E_{1\,cm}^{1\%}$ values for L-ascorbic acid are 695 at pH 2.0 and 940 at pH 6.0 (Table 6.2). Above pH 5.0, L-ascorbic acid exists predominantly as the monoanion and has maximal

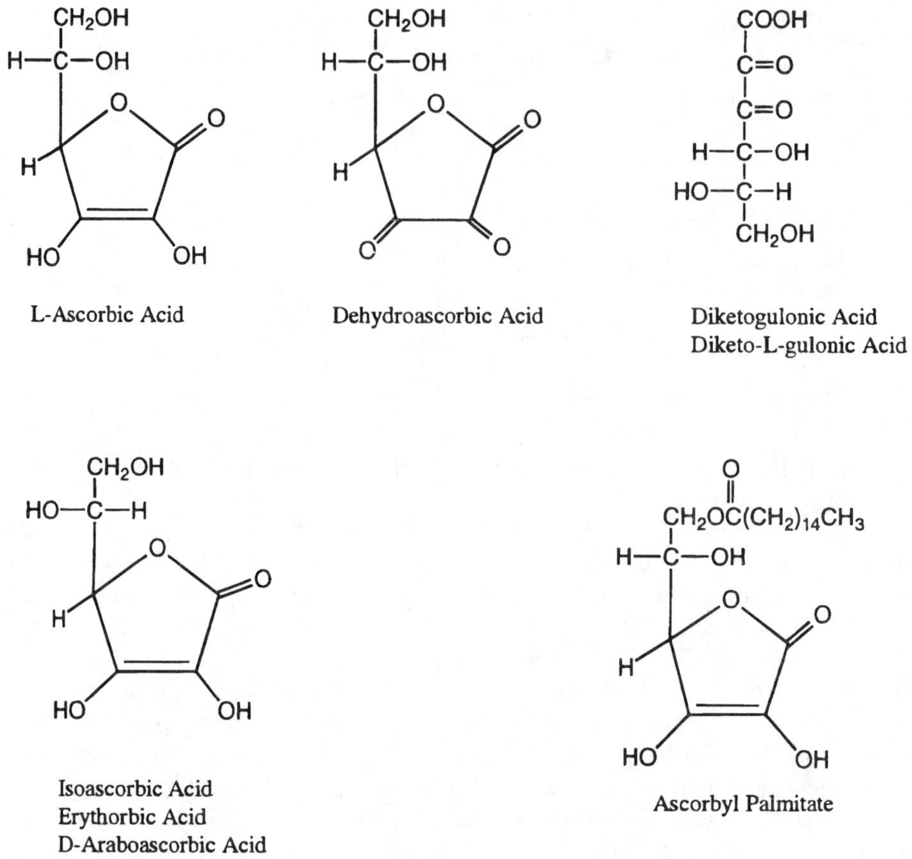

FIGURE 6.2   Structures of L-ascorbic acid and related compounds.

absorption at 265 nm. Undissociated, at more acid pH levels, maximal absorption occurs at 244 to 245 nm. Fully dissociated, above pH 12.0, maximal absorption occurs at 300 nm.

L-ascorbic acid does not fluoresce; however, derivatization with o-phenylenediamine to form a highly fluorescent product is used advantageously in chemical and LC methods discussed in Section 6.3.

6.2.2   STABILITY

Crystalline L-ascorbic acid is highly stable in the presence of oxygen when water activity remains low.[9] In solution, the strong reducing properties of the vitamin can lead to rapid and excessive oxidative changes with conversion to dehydroascorbic acid. Irreversible hydrolysis of dehydroascorbic acid produces the biologically inactive 2,3-diketo-L-gulonic acid. Reducing agents can convert the dehydro form back to L-ascorbic acid in biological systems. Enzymatic conversion of dehydroascorbate to L-ascorbic acid by glutathione dehydrogenase is an important biological defense against oxidative stress. Oxygen, temperature, light, metal catalysts, pH, and the possible presence of ascorbic acid oxidase in biological systems interact to produce a complex set of interactions influencing oxidative stability. Metal catalysts can increase degradation rates compared to uncatalyzed oxidation. Rates increase as pH increases through pK_1 (4.04).[11]

L-ascorbic acid can oxidize through one- or two-electron transfers. One-electron reductions utilize the transition through the L-ascorbic acid free radical (semi-dehydroascorbic acid or monodehydroascorbic acid). At physiological pH, a bicyclic radical is formed with the loss of a proton. The

TABLE 6.2
Physical Properties of L-Ascorbic Acid and Related Compounds

Substance[a]	Molar Mass	Formula	Solubility	Melting Point °C	Crystal Form	Absorbance[b]			Solvent
						λ max nm	$E_{1\,cm}^{1\%}$	$\epsilon \times 10^{-3}$	
Ascorbic Acid CAS No. 50-81-7 **867**	176.13	$C_6H_8O_6$	Sol in water 30 g/100 mL; Sl sol in alcohol; Insol in ether, $CHCl_3$, benzene, petroleum ether, oils and fats	190–192 (dec.)	Monoclinic platelets and needles; White or yellow	245 265	695 940	[12.2] [16.6]	Water, pH 2.0 Water, pH 6.4
Na Ascorbate CAS No. 134-03-2 **8723**	198.11	$C_6H_7O_6Na$	Sol in water 90 g/100 g	—	White to sl yellow powder	—	—	—	—
Ca Ascorbate CAS No. 5743-27-1 **1688**	390.31	$(C_6H_7O_6)_2Ca$	Sol in water 5 g/100 g; Sl sol in alcohol; Insol in ether	—	White to sl yellow crystalline powder	—	—	—	—
Ascorbyl Palmitate	414.54	$C_{22}H_{38}O_7$	Sl sol in oils; Sol in alcohol 22 g/100 mL	—	White to sl yellow powder	—	—	—	—

[a] Common or generic name; CAS No.—Chemical Abstract Service number, bold print designates the Merck Index monograph number.
[b] Values in brackets are calculated from corresponding $E_{1\,cm}^{1\%}$ values.

Budavari, S. *The Merck Index.* 1996.[1]
Friedrich, W., *Vitamins.*[2]
Food Chemicals Codex.[3]

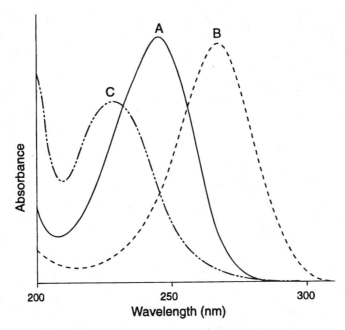

FIGURE 6.3 UV absorption spectra of L-ascorbic acid and dehydroascorbic acid. Solid line—L-ascorbic acid in 0.1 M phosphate buffer, pH 2.0; Broken line—L-ascorbic acid in 0.1 M phosphate buffer, pH 6.0; Discontinuous line—Dehydroascorbic acid, water, pH 3.1. λ max—A = 244 nm, B = 265 nm, C = 223nm. Spectra reproduced with permission from Reference 10.

anion radical is the intermediate in the reversible redox system formed by ascorbic acid and dehydroascorbic acid. Reducing agents and glutathione dehydrogenase convert dehydroascorbic acid back to ascorbic acid, completing the oxidation-reduction cycle. Classic free radical termination occurs by reduction of a free-radical with L-ascorbate. An electron is transferred to the free radical from ascorbate, producing an ascorbate radical which acts as a redox agent. The ascorbate radical interacts with itself, forming a 1 : 1 mixture of L-ascorbic acid and dehydroascorbic acid.[12]

Two-electron reductions occur when transition metals catalyze L-ascorbic acid oxidation. A ternary complex forms between the metal, L-ascorbic acid and oxygen, and two π electrons shift from L-ascorbic acid to oxygen through the transition metal.[13] The complex then dissociates with the formation of dehydroascorbic acid, hydrogen peroxide and metal ion. Unless converted back to L-ascorbic acid, dehydroascorbic acid can be quickly hydrolyzed to biologically inactive 2,3-diketo-L-gulonic acid.

In foods, pH greatly influences oxidative stability. At low pH levels, the fully protonated form is quite stable. As the pH approaches pK_1 (4.04), stability decreases. Maximal stability usually occurs between pH 4 and 6[8]; however, degradation rates are dependent on oxygen availability, the presence of antioxidants, thermal processing conditions, transition metal catalysis, oxidizing lipid effects, presence of reducing substances, the presence of ascorbic acid oxidase, and the multitude of possible interactions. Cooking losses depend upon degree of heating, leaching into the cooking medium, surface area exposed to water and oxygen, pH, presence of transition metals, and any other factors that facilitate the oxidation of L-ascorbic acid and its conversion into non-biologically active forms. L-ascorbic acid is a characteristic reductone and enters into the non-enzymatic Maillard browning reaction. Browning in a food product can significantly reduce vitamin C content.

The quite extreme lability of L-ascorbic acid at or near physiological pH is a primary consideration in all analytical procedures. Specific extraction procedures designed to stabilize the vitamin are discussed in Section 6.3.

6.3   METHODS

Vitamin C is the only water-soluble vitamin not assayed microbiologically. Rapid advances were made in vitamin C analysis after the guinea pig bioassay was developed in 1922 to measure antiscorbutic activity.[14] Methodology has advanced from the bioassay approach to titrations using redox indicators, derivatization procedures, enzymatic methods, and electrochemical procedures. Now, excellent LC procedures are commonly available and capillary electrophoretic techniques are showing excellent potential for vitamin C assay. Each of these techniques will be discussed in detail.

Recent reviews covering the many different aspects of vitamin C analysis were published by Pelletier,[15] Pachla et al.,[16] Lumley,[17] Parviainen and Nyyssönen,[18] Ball,[10] and Eitenmiller and Landen.[9] Published handbook and compendium procedures are summarized in Table 6.3. Several of these procedures are discussed in the following sections as they represent the more traditional approaches to vitamin C analysis. Pachla et al.[16] in 1985 classified vitamin C methods into spectroscopic, electrochemical, enzymatic, and chromatographic classes. With the development of capillary electrophoretic methods and their successful application to vitamin C analysis, this technique must be added to the analytical approaches available for biological sample analysis.

6.3.1   EXTRACTION PROCEDURES

Due to the labile nature of vitamin C, extraction procedures are designed to stabilize the vitamin. Cooke and Moxon[19] reviewed the literature up to 1981 and found that 20 or more extraction solutions were used by various researchers working with a large number of biological matrices. Extraction solutions should maintain an acidic environment, chelate metals, inactivate ascorbic acid oxidase, and precipitate starch and proteins. Choice of the extraction solution depends upon the sample matrix and the determinative procedure. Extractants that usually limit L-ascorbic acid destruction to less than 5% include 3 to 6% metaphosphoric acid containing acetic or sulfuric acid or 0.005 M ethylenediaminetetraacetic acid (EDTA).[19] Metaphosphoric acid, while not compatible to some HPLC procedures, has been the most commonly used extractant. Metaphosphoric acid inhibits L-ascorbic acid oxidase, inhibits metal catalysis, and precipitates proteins which aids in extract clarification.[15] Starch is problematic in that it interferes with colorimetric titrations and fluorometric assays. Addition of ethanol or acetone to the metaphosphoric extract precipitates solubilized starch.[20,21] This step is necessary for analysis of many vegetables including potatoes, legumes, and corn by spectroscopic methods. Acetone is also useful to remove metabisulfite and sulfur dioxide from dehydrated fruit products and fruit juices. These reducing agents interfere with the 2,6-dichloroindophenol titration based on reduction of the oxidized dye. EDTA is active as a chelator in vitamin C extractants. It is effective for copper chelation in metaphosphoric acid and trichloroacetic acid, but ineffective for oxalic acid chelation.

All extraction procedures should be completed rapidly in subdued light to limit light catalyzed oxidative reactions. Particle size reduction methods should avoid heat build up. Whenever possible, the sample should be overlayered with nitrogen during initial sample compositing procedures.[9] Freeze drying is not recommended for sample concentration or preservation since vitamin C stability decreases in the porous matrix.[19] When high moisture samples are blended, the stabilizing extractant should be added prior to blending.

6.3.2   SPECTROSCOPIC

6.3.2.1   Oxidation-Reduction Methods

6.3.2.1.1   2,6-Dichloroindophenol Titration

The 2,6-dichloroindophenol (DCIP) titration was introduced by Tillmans in 1930[22]. DCIP is reduced by L-ascorbic acid to a colorless solution from the deep blue color of the oxidized dye (Figure 6.4). L-ascorbic acid is oxidized to dehydroascorbic acid and excess dye remains pink in acid solution,

TABLE 6.3
Compendium, Regulatory, and Handbook Methods of Analysis for Ascorbic Acid

Source	Form	Methods and Application	Approach	Most Current Cross-Reference
U.S. Pharmacopeia, National Formulary, 1995, USP 23/NF 18 Nutritional Supplements Official Monographs[1]				
1. pages 1674, 2141, 2145, 2147, 2152	Ascorbic acid	Ascorbic acid in oil- and water-soluble vitamin capsules/tablets w/wo minerals	Titration Dichlorophenolindolphenol or automated fluorescence Ex λ = 335 Em λ = 426	None
2. pages 1674, 2159, 2162, 2169, 2171	Ascorbic acid	Ascorbic acid in water-soluble vitamin capsules/tablets w/wo minerals	Titration Dichlorophenolindolphenol or automated fluorescence Ex λ = 335 Em .λ = 426	None
3. page 130	Ascorbic acid	Ascorbic acid (NLT 99.0%, NMT 100.5%)	Titration, iodine	None
4. pages 130-131	Ascorbic acid	Ascorbic acid injection, oral solution, tablets	Titration, Dichlorophenolindolphenol	None
5. pages 245-246	Calcium ascorbate	Calcium ascorbate	Titration, iodine	None
British Pharmacopoeia, 15th ed., 1993[2]				
vol. I, pages 53–54	Ascorbic acid	Ascorbic acid	Titration	None
vol. II, page 778	Ascorbic acid	Ascorbic acid injection	Titration	None
vol. II, page 778	Ascorbic acid	Ascorbic acid tablets	Titration	None
addend., 1994, page1293	Ascorbyl palmitate	Ascorbyl palmitate	Titration	None
AOAC Official Methods of Analysis, 16th ed., 1995[3]				
1. 45.1.14	Ascorbic acid	AOAC Official Method 967.21 Vitamin C in Juices and Vitamin Preparations	Titration, dichlorophenolindolphenol	*J. Assoc. Off. Anal. Chem.*, 50, 798, 1967[4]

	Analyte	Method	Technique	Reference
2. 45.1.15	Ascorbic acid	AOAC Official Method 967.22 Vitamin C in Vitamin Preparations	Fluorescence Ex λ = 350 Em λ = 430	J. Assoc. Off. Anal. Chem., 48, 1248, 1965[5]; 50, 798, 1967[4]
3. 45.1.16	Ascorbic acid	AOAC Official Method 984.26 Vitamin C in Foods	Semiautomated Fluorescence Ex λ = 365 Em λ = 440	J. Assoc. Off. Anal. Chem., 66, 1371, 1983[6]
4. 50.1.09	Ascorbic acid	AOAC Official Method 985.33 Vitamin C in Ready-To-Feed Milk-Based Infant Formula	Titration, dichlorophenolindolphenol	J. Assoc. Off. Anal. Chem., 68, 514, 1985[7]
American Association of Cereal Chemists *Approved Methods*, vol. 2, 1996[8]				
1. AACC 86-10	Ascorbic acid	Ascorbic acid in cereal products	Spectrophotometric 500 nm	J. Biol. Chem., 160, 217, 1945[9] AOAC International, 16th ed., 1995, 45.1.14[3]
American Feed Ingredients Association, *Laboratory Methods Compendium*, vol. 1, 1991[10]				
1. pages 61–62	Ascorbic acid	Ascorbic acid in complete feeds, premixes, and vitamin concentrates (>40 mg/kg)	Titration, dichlorophenolindolphenol	Fresen. Zeits. Anal. Chem., 253, 271, 1971[11]
2. pages. 63–64	Ascorbic acid	HPLC of ascorbic acid, nicotinic acid, calcium pantothenate and panthenol in liquid and solid vitamin mixtures (>50 mg/kg)	HPLC 245 nm	None
Food Chemicals Codex, 4th ed., 1996[12]				
1. pages 33–34	Ascorbic acid	Ascorbic acid (NLT 99.0%, NMT 100.5%)	Titration, iodine	None
2. page 34	Ascorbyl palmitate	Ascorbyl palmitate (NLT 95.0%)	Titration, iodine	None
Hoffmann-LaRoche, *Analytical Methods for Vitamins and Carotenoids in Feed*, 1988[13]				
pages 20–22	Ascorbic acid	Determination of ascorbic acid in complete feeds, premixes and vitamin concentrates (>240 mg/kg)	Titration Dichlorophenolindolphenol, visual or potentiometrically	Fres. Zeits. Anal. Chem., 253, 271, 1971[11]

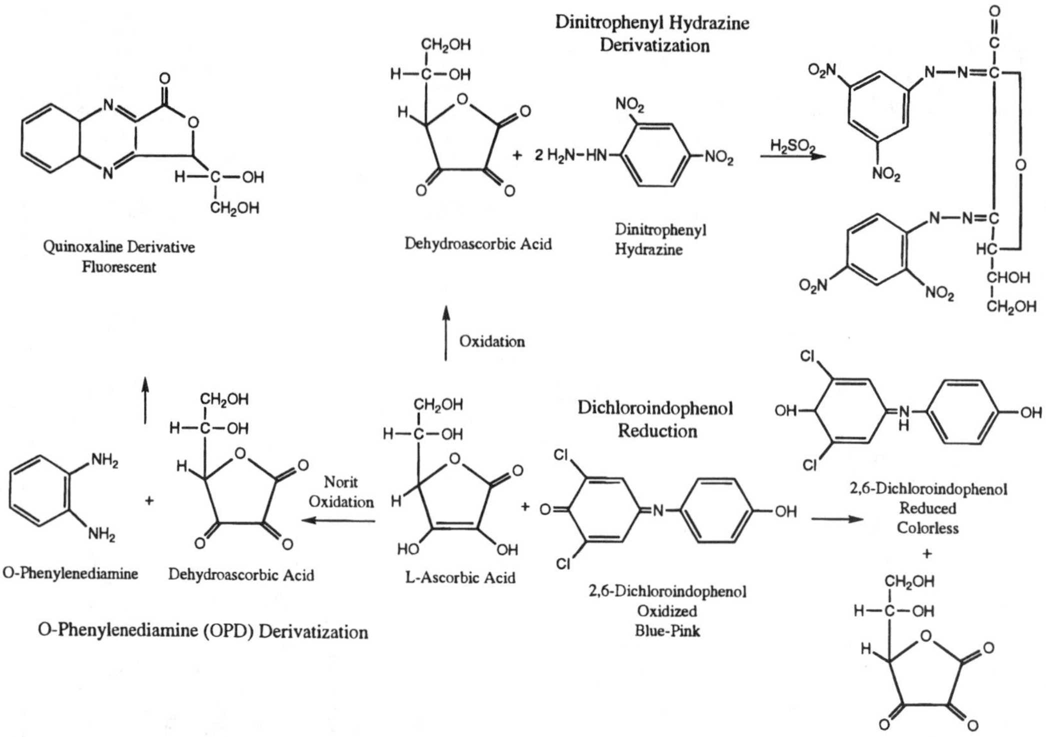

FIGURE 6.4 L-ascorbic acid reactions important to vitamin C analysis. Figure adapted with permission from Reference 9.

forming the visual endpoint of the titration. Absorbance at 518 nm can be used alternatively to visual end point determination.

Several important deficiencies exist with the method. Most importantly, the titration is limited to quantitation of L-ascorbic acid. Dehydroascorbic acid will not be measured unless it is reduced to ascorbic acid. The titration will not distinguish between L-ascorbic acid and isoascorbic acid. The method cannot be used for vitamin C analysis of processed and cured meats containing isoascorbic acid. DCIP titration can be used for fresh juices and multivitamins that do not contain excessive amounts of copper or iron.[15] For processed or cooked foods known to contain copper, iron, or tin, other methods capable of measuring dehydroascorbic acid in addition to L-ascorbic acid should be used to quantitate total vitamin C.[9] Highly colored extracts from fruit and vegetables can mask the color change at the titration's end point.

Reduction of DCIP is not limited to L-ascorbic acid and any reducing substance present in the sample can reduce the dye. Such interferences can lead to erroneously high measurements, if not recognized. Substances that can interfere include cuprous, ferrous, and stannous ions, sulfite, thiosulfate, tannins, betanin, cysteine, glutathione, and reductones generated by non-enzymatic browning. Several method modifications have been introduced to eliminate or minimize the effects of interferences on the DCIP titration.[15,16,19]

Recently, a solid-phase extraction (SPE) procedure was developed that expands the DCIP titration to highly colored multivitamins, soft drinks, and fruit and vegetables.[23] Further, the clean-up step removes copper, iron, sulfite, and other interfering reducing substances, like cysteine and glutathione. C_{18} silica impregnated with 2,2'-bipyridyl-2,9-dimethyl-1,10-phenathroline (neocuproine) and N-ethylmaleimide removes Fe (II) and Cu (I) and sulfhydryl compounds, respectively. The method provides for determination of L-ascorbic acid and dehydroascorbic acid by reducing the dehydroascorbic acid back to L-ascorbic acid with cysteine prior to the SPE step. This procedure is simple and increases the sensitivity of the DCIP procedure. Incorporation of the SPE step into existing regulatory methods could decrease problems associated with existing titration procedures.

AOAC Official Method 967.21[24], Ascorbic Acid in Vitamin Preparations and Juices, 2,6-Dichloroindophenol Titrimetric Method, AOAC Official Methods of Analysis 45.1.14— AOAC Method 967.21 was recommended for the analysis of L-ascorbic acid in beverages and juices for nutritional labeling purposes.[25] However, the method is routinely applied world-wide to other food matrices due to its simplicity. If the deficiencies of the method are recognized by the analyst, the procedure provides reliable measures for L-ascorbic acid provided that the food does not contain appreciable quantities of reducing substances and dehydroascorbic acid.[9] Application of the SPE clean up discussed previously could greatly expand the use of the DCIP titration since many laboratories still must rely on simple, non-instrumental approaches to food analysis.

The method includes the following steps:

1 Extraction—L-ascorbic acid is extracted from dry materials with metaphosphoric acid containing glacial acetic acid. The solution is stable for seven to ten days when refrigerated. The extractant is used to dilute juices or other liquid samples. For analysis of highly basic materials, the extractant is prepared by replacing water in the extractant with 0.3 N H_2SO_4. When whole food products are extracted, the food should be blended in the metaphosphoric acid extractant. Following filtration or centrifugation, the residue should be extracted at least one additional time by blending in the extractant. Proper extraction including light protection, speed, and quantitative techniques result in recoveries greater than 95% with minimal formation of dehydroascorbic acid.[9]

2 Titration—Clarified extracts are titrated with standard dye prepared by dissolving 50 mg DCIP Na salt (Eastman Kodak No. 3463) in 50 mL water containing 42 mg $NaHCO_3$, with dilution to 200 mL with water. The dye solution is filtered and stored under refrigeration in an amber glass container. The DCIP concentration is expressed as mg L-ascorbic acid equivalent per 1.0 mL dye solution. The equivalency factor is determined by adding 2 mL of standard L-ascorbic acid (1.0 mg/mL) to 5 mL of the extractant and titrating rapidly with dye solution to a pink color that persists 5 s. This should require approximately 15 mL of the DCIP solution. A blank determination is run by titrating 7 mL of the extractant containing water equal to the average volume of dye required to titrate the ascorbic acid standard. Blanks should approximate 0.1 mL DCIP solution which provides an immediate check on reagent quality.

Notes—

1. The AOAC International *Methods of Analysis*[24] provides specific tests to check for interfering levels of Cu (I), Fe (II) and Sn (II). Application of the SPE clean-up[23] procedure clearly will improve application of AOAC Method 967.21 to complex matrices encountered in processed food, beverages, medical foods, and multivitamins.
2. The AOAC Official Method 985.33, Vitamin C (Reduced Ascorbic Acid) in Ready-to-Feed Milk-Based Infant Formula) (Chapter 50.1.09) is based on the DCIP titration. The method varies from Method 967.21 at the extraction stage of the method. EDTA is added to the metaphosphoric acid-glacial acetic acid extractant to ensure the removal of iron and copper interferences. Iron and copper salts are components of commercial infant formulas.

6.3.2.1.2   Metal Ion Reduction

L-ascorbic acid in biological samples can be measured by redox reactions in which L-ascorbic acid is used to reduce metal ions to produce colored products. Pachla et al.[16] reviewed metal ion redox methods in detail. These methods rely upon the formation of a stable colored complex between the reduced ion and a chelating agent. Reduction of Fe (III) to Fe (II) by L-ascorbic acid is the most common reaction, although many metal ion redox reactions have been utilized for L-ascorbic acid analysis. A chelator is added which complexes with the reduced metal. The reduced metal-chelator complex is then measured by spectroscopic methods. With Fe (II), the most common chelating agents are 2,2'-dipyridine, 2,4,6-tripyridyl-5-triazine and ferrozine.[16]

More recent approaches to metal redox applications for L-ascorbic acid have entailed flow injection techniques, and spectrophotometric methods designed to quantitate ascorbic acid and dehydroascorbic acid. Such techniques are summarized in Table 6.5. A simple flow injection technique developed for pharmaceutical products used Fe (III) and hexacyanoferrate (III) as the chromogenic complexing reagents to produce Prussian Blue.[26]

The reaction sequence is the following:

1. Oxidation of Fe (II)

$$Fe^{2+} + [Fe(CN)_6]^{3-} \rightarrow Fe^{+3} + [Fe(CN)_6]^{4-}$$

2. Formation of hexacyanoferrate (II) ferric complex

$$4Fe^{3+} + 3[Fe(CN)_6]^{4-} \rightarrow Fe_4 [Fe(CN)_6]_3 \text{ Prussian Blue}$$

L-ascorbic acid reduces Fe (III) to Fe (II) resulting in the formation of a deep blue soluble complex. When excess hexacyanoferrate (III) is present, the formation of Prussian Blue is measured at 700 nm. This procedure is detailed in Section 6.4.

6.3.2.2 Derivatization Methods

6.3.2.2.1 o-Phenylenediamine

The o-phenylenediamine (OPD) condensation reaction with dehydroascorbic acid (Figure 6.4) represents one of the most useful derivatization reactions to quantitate total vitamin C. The condensation reaction produces a highly fluorescent quinoxaline product (Ex λ = 350, Em λ = 430). AOAC International Method 967.22 was developed by Deutsch and Weeks[27] for analysis of total vitamin C (L-ascorbic acid + dehydroascorbic acid). This assay improved the scope and specificity of vitamin C methods existing at the time.[9]

AOAC Official Method 967.22, Vitamin C (Total) in Vitamin Preparations, Microfluorometric Method—The AOAC Task Force on Methods for Nutrition Labeling recommended that Method 967.22 be used for most food matrices.[25] The method includes the following steps:

1   Extraction—Samples are extracted with the metaphosphoric acid-glacial acetic acid extractant used with the DCIP assay (Method 967.21). A 100 mL aliquot of the extract is vigorously mixed with 2 g of acid washed Norit. The Norit oxidizes L-ascorbic acid to dehydroascorbic acid. The application of Norit oxidation by Deutsch and Weeks, while simple in approach, greatly improved the accuracy of the methods used to report total vitamin C content of the food supply. Conversion of L-ascorbic acid to dehydroascorbic acid facilitates total vitamin C assay by OPD condensation with formation of the fluorescent quinoxaline and removes potential interfering substances without tedious clean-up steps.

2.   Quinoxaline Fluorescent Derivative Formation—The Norit-treated extract is filtered and 5 mL of the filtrate is added to a 100 mL volumetric flask containing 5 mL sodium acetate solution and 75 mL water. Contents are diluted to 100 mL and 2 mL aliquots are transferred to fluorescence reading tubes. Five milliliters of OPD solution is added to each tube. After mixing, the tubes are incubated for 35 minutes at room temperature in the dark. Fluorescence is determined at Ex λ = 364, Em λ = 440. Standard L-ascorbic acid solution (100 μg/mL) is carried through the procedure.

3   Blank Correction—Blank corrections greatly improve specificity of the assay by accounting for substances other than dehydroascorbic acid that are in the sample extract and reactive with OPD or those that possess native fluorescence that escape Norit treatment.[9] The blank is produced by adding boric acid-sodium acetate buffer to the Norit treated sample and standard solutions. The boric acid complexes with dehydroascorbic acid and prevents condensation with OPD. The fluorescence in the boric acid blank corrects for non-specific fluorescence in the sample extract.

Although few interferences occur in most biological samples, Deutsch and Weeks[27] summarized properties of potential interferences. These include the presence of α-keto groups that react with OPD, fluorescence properties of the dehydroascorbic acid quinoxaline derivative, and presence of adjacent *cis*-hydroxyl groups which react with the boric acid in the blank. The assay is subject to quenching by impurities in the extract. Also, dehydroreductic acid, dehydroreductones, and alloxan interfere by producing fluorescence in the sample solution but not in the blank.[28] Dehydro-reductones are formed by the Maillard reaction (non-enzymatic browning). Therefore, browned foods might be subject to error when assayed for total vitamin C by the procedure.[9] Physical interference results from the extraction of high-starch products such as potatoes, corn, beans, and processed, creamed vegetables.[20,21] The metaphosphoric acid extracts enough starch from these foods to interfere with the fluorescence measurement. Extracts containing starch show a characteristic opalescence which is easily distinguished by trained analysts. The problem can be avoided by diluting the initial extract 1 : 1 with 95% ethanol to precipitate the starch. After removal of the starch, the assay is completed without further modifications. The L-ascorbic acid standard must be treated similarly.

The manual microfluorometric method was modified to semi-automated analysis by use of DCIP[29] and N-bromosuccinimide[30] oxidation in place of Norit oxidation and direct addition of Norit slurry in metaphosphoric acid to the food sample to immediately oxidize L-ascorbic acid to dehydroascorbic acid during the extraction.[31] AOAC International Method 984.26, Vitamin C (Total) in Food, Semiautomated Fluorometric Method (Chapter 45.1.16)[24] was developed by Egberg et al.[31] These investigators added the Norit slurry directly to the metaphosphoric acid-food mixture, allowing adaptation of the method to a Technicon Autoanalyzer system. The semi-automated method gives data comparable to the manual method.[32,33] The modified method provides speed (40 assays per hour) and the same sensitivity and specificity as AOAC International Method 967.22. It has been recommended for possible application to a wide variety of food matrices.[25]

Robotics and flow injection analysis were combined to further automate the general procedure of AOAC Method 967.22.[34,35] Following extraction, the extract is passed through a C_{18} preparative column to remove interferences. The eluent is loaded into autosampler vials and assayed by flow injection analysis. Mercuric chloride is used to oxidize L-ascorbic acid to dehydroascorbic acid and then derivatized with OPD. Results of the automated method compare with results of the manual procedure.

6.3.2.2.2   2,4-Dinitrophenylhydrazine

2,4-Dinitrophenylhydrazine (DNPH) reacts with ketone groups of dehydroascorbic acid under acidic conditions to form a red osazone derivative (Figure 6.4). The method was developed in 1943[36] and several excellent reviews have been written on its application.[10,15,16] DNPH is useful for the analysis of total vitamin C if appreciable quantities of sugars are not present in the product. L-ascorbic acid is oxidized to dehydroascorbic acid by Norit or DCIP. Derivatization is completed with the addition of DNPH and the color is produced upon acidification with sulfuric acid. Maximal absorbance occurs between 500 and 550 nm. Most methods measure the DNPH derivative at 520 nm. Specificity of the reaction for dehydroascorbic acid in complex matrices was attributed to the ability of DNPH to react faster with dehydroascorbic acid compared with other carbohydrates; color is produced more easily with DNPH derivatives of 5- and 6-carbon sugar-like compounds and through the ability to minimize formation of non-ascorbic acid chromogens by carrying out the reaction at low temperatures.[16] Despite the specificity afforded by such factors, DNPH has not been used recently as extensively for food analysis as OPD derivatization. The methods do not compare in simplicity and specificity to the microfluorometric method for total vitamin C assay. DNPH methods for the differential determination of isoascorbic acid are available.[15] Pachla et al.[16] reviewed automated methods based upon DNPH for application to plasma and food analysis.

\   Recently, Wei et al.[37] presented a rapid DNPH based microtiter plate assay for ascorbic acid determination in plasma and leukocytes. The microtiter plate method can be used to assay L-ascorbic acid in a leukocyte-rich fraction prepared from 1 mL of whole blood. The method is capable of high sample throughput, suitable for small sample volumes, and requires smaller amounts of reagents than traditional DNPH methods. Results are similar to standard spectrophotometric methods using DNPH. Because of the potential for use in many different laboratory situations, the microtiter plate assay is summarized in Section 6.4.

6.3.3 ENZYMATIC

Enzyme conversions of L-ascorbic acid to dehydroascorbic acid coupled to a determinative step such as direct spectrophotometric assay following decrease of L-ascorbic acid, OPD, other derivatization reactions, and electrochemical determination of oxygen uptake during the reaction have been used to assay L-ascorbic acid in biological samples. Ascorbate oxidase and ascorbate peroxidase activity represented by the following equations convert the L-ascorbic acid to the dehydro form.[10]

Ascorbate Oxidase—

$$\text{L-ascorbic acid} + \tfrac{1}{2}\, O_2 \rightarrow \text{Dehydroascorbic acid} + H_2O$$

Ascorbate Peroxidase—

$$\text{L-ascorbic acid} + H_2O_2 \rightarrow \text{Dehydroascorbic acid} + 2H_2O$$

A variety of enzyme sources have been used for the enzymatic conversion. Speek et al.[38] used an ascorbate oxidase spatula available from Boehringer-Mannheim to convert L-ascorbic acid and isoascorbic acid to the dehydro forms prior to OPD derivatization and HPLC quantitation of the quinoxaline derivatives. This procedure, summarized in Section 6.4, has been extensively used for quantitation of total vitamin C in foods.[39,40] Total vitamin C and isoascorbic acid can be quantitated at levels as low as 0.2 μg/g. Dehydro forms can be determined individually by omitting the enzymatic oxidation.

Ascorbate peroxidase oxidation of L-ascorbic acid to dehydroascorbic acid has been applied to the spectrophotometric assay of total vitamin C in foods. In more recently published methods quiacol peroxidase from horseradish has been used.[41,42] This peroxidase is commercially available (Sigma Chemical Co.) and catalyzes the oxidation of L-ascorbic acid as well as quiacol. The direct spectrophotometric assay developed by Tsumura et al.[42] was tested on a wide variety of foods and no interferences were apparent. The method was more precise when compared to assays using DCIP and DNPH. The procedure is detailed in Section 6.4.

6.3.4 HIGH PERFORMANCE LIQUID CHROMATOGRAPHY

HPLC methods have been applied to pharmaceuticals and many types of biological samples for analysis of L-ascorbic acid and related compounds. The need to simultaneously assay L-ascorbic acid, dehydroascorbic acid, and isoascorbic acid from food has led to the development of excellent procedures for accurate assay of total vitamin C in the presence of isoascorbic acid. Excellent reviews are available that cover the development of HPLC procedures for vitamin C analysis. In-depth reviews that cover the literature to 1990 are provided by Ball[10] and Parviainen and Nyyssönen.[18] Because of the large number of papers that have been published in the area, we will discuss relatively few but historically important method development papers. Table 6.4 summarizes more pertinent papers. Again, these specific research approaches were selected from quite a large pool of published papers and are not meant to be inclusive.

6.3.4.1 Extraction Procedures for Vitamin C Analysis by HPLC

Most extraction procedures used for biological samples in conjunction with spectrophotometric oxidation-reduction based methods or derivatization procedures are compatible with resolution and detection modes used for HPLC analysis of vitamin C. The analyst must determine extractant compatibility to all components of the LC system. Summaries of recent methodology approaches provided in Table 6.4 show that metaphosphoric acid, mixtures of metaphosphoric acid with glacial acetic acid, trichloroacetic acid, citric acid, mixtures of citric acid and glacial acetic acid, sulfuric acid, and phosphoric acid are usually compatible to LC supports and mobile phases. If the assay requires quantitation of total ascorbic acid, the resolution system must be capable of resolving L-ascorbic acid from dehydroascorbic acid with use of a detection mode capable of detecting both forms of vitamin C. Alternatively, a reducing agent such as dithiothreitol, cysteine, or homocysteine can be added to the extractant to reduce the dehydro form to L-ascorbic acid. Conversely, the L-ascorbic acid can be oxidized to the dehydro form by Norit or enzyme treatment. Total vitamin C assayed as dehydroascorbic acid permits use of OPD derivatization with fluorescence detection to quantitate total vitamin C. Metal chelators, usually EDTA, can be added to the extractant to inhibit metal catalyzed oxidation. Use of metaphosphoric acid as the primary component of the extractant has significant metal chelation properties. Any additions to the extractant must be compatible with the resolution and detection modes of the system. Metaphosphoric acid, with or without glacial acetic acid, has been the most common extractant used to extract vitamin C in HPLC based methods.

6.3.4.2 Chromatography Parameters

6.3.4.2.1 Supports and Mobile Phases

Ball[10] provided an excellent review of the various chromatography systems used for vitamin C analysis. Because of the ionic character of ascorbic acid many different supports have been used. Ball's description of chromatography systems used for resolution of the various compounds of interest in vitamin C analysis included strong anion exchange, weak anion exchange, ion inclusion partition, reversed-phase, ion interaction, cyanopropyl-bonded phase, and hydrophilic gel chromatography. Methods given in Table 6.4 show that reversed-phase systems using C_{18} and macroporous polystyrene divinyl benzene supports are the most commonly applied systems in recently published methods compared to older procedures that relied more on ion-exchange chromatography.

Polymeric styrene divinyl benzene macroporous supports were introduced to food analysis by Lloyd et al.[43,44] The PLRP-S resin has proven to be an advantageous support for HPLC assay of vitamin C. The support is highly stable to chemical and pH extremes that can degrade ODS supports. Polymeric resins were used to overcome support stability problems encountered in method development studies on the HPLC analysis of thiamin (Chapter 7).

Mobile-phase selections suitable for vitamin C analysis are as varied as the supports available for resolution. Selection of the PLRP-S resin leads to relatively simple mobile-phase compositions that effectively resolve L-ascorbic acid, dehydroascorbic acid, isoascorbic acid, and dehydroisoascorbic acid. The Lloyd et al.[43,44] procedure uses isocratic elution with 0.2 M NaH_2PO_4 at pH 2.14. This system has been used effectively to resolve L-ascorbic acid and isoascorbic acid and their dehydro forms in meat products.[45]

TABLE 6.4
Selected HPLC Methods for the Analysis of Ascorbic Acid in Foods, Feed, Pharmaceuticals, and Biologicals

Sample Matrix	Analyte	Sample Preparation	Column	HPLC Parameters Mobile Phase	Detection	Quality Assurance Parameters	References
Food							
1. Cured meats	AA IAA Uric acid	Add 15 mL 5% MPA containing 0.1 mg/mL to 4–10 g sample; Homogenize with and without the addition of AA (IS); Centrifuge; Dilute 10 fold with mobile phase	Altex Ultrasphere ODS 5 µm 25 cm × 4.6 mm	Isocratic 0.04 M NaOAC 0.005 M TBAP 0.2 mg/mL EDTA Adjust to pH 5.25 with HAC 0.4 mL/min or 0.8 mL/min	EC Glassy carbon +0.6 V vs Ag/AgCl	%Recovery 90–94	J. Food Sci., 52, 53, 1987[1]
2–4. Foods, beverages, fruits, vegetables	AA IAA	Blend with 0.3 N TCA containing 0.5 mL octanol per 60 mL; Add NaOAC buffer and ascorbate oxidase; Incubate, 37°C, 5–7 min; Add 0.1% OPD; Incubate, 37°C, 30 min	Spherisorb ODS2 5 µm 12.5 cm × 4 mm	Isocratic 0.08 M KH_2PO_4 : MeOH (80 : 20), pH 7.8 1 mL/min	Fluorescence Ex λ = 365 Em λ = 418	QL (mg/100 g) 1.5–3.4 % Recovery 97.1	J. Food Comp. Anal., 7, 252, 1994[3]; 8, 12, 1995[4]
5–7. Various foods;	A DHAA IAA DHIAA	Blend with 0.1 M citric acid containing 5 mM EDTA plus equal volume of Hex; Centrifuge; Dilute 1 : 1 with mobile phase	Altex ODS 3 columns in series 5 µm 25 cm × 4.6 mm	Isocratic 0.1 M NaH_2PO_4 containing 5 mM EDTA and 5 mM TBAP, pH 5.0 0.5 mL/min	Post-column oxidation with OPD Fluorescence Ex λ = 350 Em λ = 430	DL (ng) On-column 3 % Recovery 90–107	J. Chromatogr. Sci., 22, 485, 1984[5]; J. Micronutr. Anal., 1, 143, 1985[6]; 4, 109, 1988[7]
8. Fruit juice	AA	Dilute with mobile phase; Filter	PLRP-S, 100 Å 5 µm	Isocratic 0.2 M NaH_2PO_4, pH 2.14	220 or 244 nm	DL (µg/mL) 0.02	J. Chromatogr., 437, 447, 1988[8]

No. Sample	Analyte	Sample preparation	Column	Mobile phase / flow	Detection	DL / QL / Recovery	Reference
9. Various foods	AA, DHAA	Solid foods: Homogenize with 10–50 fold excess 20 mM H$_2$SO$_4$; Juices: Homogenize, centrifuge; DHAA: Reduce with DTT	25 cm × 4.6 mm; Sulfonated polystyrene divinyl benzene; 10 cm × 4.6 mm	0. mL/min; 20 mM H$_2$SO$_4$; 0.6 mL/min	EC; Pt electrode +0.6–0.8V vs Ag/AgCl	DL (ng); On-column 0.1; % Recovery 102	J. Assoc. Off. Anal. Chem., 72, 681, 1989[9]
10. Various foods; Animal tissues	AA, DHAA, IAA, DHIAA	Homogenize in MPA : HAC (30 g + 80 mL diluted to 1 L); Vortex with Hex; Centrifuge, filter	PLRP-S; 2 columns in series; 5 µm; 15 cm × 4.6 mm and 25 cm × 4.6 mm	Isocratic; 0.2 M NaH$_2$PO$_4$, pH 2.14; 4°C; 0.5 mL/min	Post-column oxidation with HgCl$_2$ and OPD; Fluorescence Ex λ = 350, Em λ = 430	DL (µg); On-column 1.6	J. Micronutr. Anal., 7, 67, 1990[10]
11. Various foods	AA, DHAA	Homogenize in 17% MPA (0.85% final MPA concentration); Measure before and after conversion of DHAA acid to AA by homocysteine	C$_{18}$; 5 µm; 25 cm × 4.6 mm	Isocratic; 80 mM NaOAC, pH 4.8, containing 1 mM m-octylamine : MeOH : MPA (85 : 15 : 0.00015) pH 4.6, 0.9 mL/min	EC; Glassy carbon + 0.7 V Ag/AgCl; 50 mA	QL (mg/100 g); AA 0.2; DHAA 0.1	J. Food Comp. Anal., 3, 3, 1990[11]
12–13. Various foods	AA, DHAA	Homogenize in 0.1 M citric acid or MPA : HAC (30 g + 80 mL diluted to 1 L)	PLRP-S; 2 columns in series; 5 µm; 15 cm × 4.6 mm and 25 cm × 4.6 mm	Isocratic; 0.2 M NaH$_2$PO$_4$, pH 2.14; 0.5 mL/min	220 nm	QL (mg/100 g); AA—4.0; DHAA—1.3; % Recovery 95–105	Food Chem., 28, 257, 1988[12]
14. Various foods	AA	Homogenize in MPA : HAC (3% MPA in 8% HAC)	µBondapak C$_{18}$; 10 µm; 30 cm × 3.9 mm	MeOH : Water (55 : 45); 1 mL/min	Pre-column oxidation with Norit; OPD derivatization; Fluorescence Ex λ = 350, Em λ = 430	QL (mg/100 g) 0.6; DL (ng/100 µL) 10; % Recovery 90–108	J. Food Comp. Anal., 3, 105, 1990[13]; J. AOAC Int., 75, 887, 1992[14]
15. Diets	AA	Mix with 6% MPA; Filter	Inertsil ODS-2; 5 µm; 25 cm × 4.6 mm	Isocratic; 100 mM KH$_2$PO$_4$ containing 1 mM EDTA-Na, pH 3.0; 0.6 mL/min	EC; 70 mV; Ag/AgCl	QL (mg/100 g) 9.6; % Recovery 97.4–98.4	J. Chromatogr., 606, 277, 1992[15]

TABLE 6.4 Continued

Sample Matrix	Analyte	Sample Preparation	HPLC Parameters			Quality Assurance Parameters	References
			Column	Mobile Phase	Detection		
16–17. Various foods	AA DHAA IAA DHIAA	Homogenize in 17% MPA Centrifuge Filter Reduce with homocysteine to determine AA and IAA	Supelcosil LC-18 DB 3 columns in series 5 μm 25 cm × 4.6 mm	Isocratic 0.08 M NaOAC, pH 5.4, with 5 mM TBAS and 0.15% MPA	EC glassy carbon + 0.6 V Ag/AgCl	DL (ng) On-column 0.5 % Recovery AA—94–107 IAA—94–108	J. Liq. Chromatogr., 15, 753, 1992[16] J. Food Comp. Anal., 7, 158, 1994[17]
18. Various foods	AA DHAA IAA DHIAA	Homogenize in MPA : HAC : EDTA (30 g MPA + 0.5 g EDTA : 80 mL HAC diluted to 1 L) Tissue 10% MPA Add IAA (IS) to all samples prior to blending For processed foods containing IAA, AA can be used as IS if the vitamin is not present in the product.	PLPP-S, 100 Å 5 μm 2 columns in series 15 cm × 4.6 mm and 25 cm × 4.6 mm	Isocratic 0.2 M NaH$_2$PO$_4$, pH 2.14 0.5 mL/min	Post-column derivatization of dehydro-forms with OPD Fluorescence Ex λ = 350 Em λ = 430	DL (ng) On-column 3 % Recovery 80–113	J. Nutr. Biochem., 4, 4, 184, 1993[18]
19. Beer, beverages	AA Sulfites	Add 1.5% MPA (20 mL) to 2 mL sample Flush flask with He Dilute to volume with 1.5% MPA Inject	Ion-exchange Fast Acid 10 cm × 7.8 mm or Aminex HPX 87 H 30 cm × 7.8 mm	Isocratic 0.005 M H$_2$SO$_4$ containing 0.001 M chloride 1 mL/min	EC glassy carbon + 0.6 V Ag/AgCl	QL (mg/L) 0.5 % Recovery 97–100	J. Chromatogr., 640, 271, 1993[19]

Sample	Analytes	Sample preparation	Column	Conditions	Detection	DL/QL/Recovery	Reference
20. Juices	AA DHAA	Dilute to 10 µg/mL with water Filter *Ascorbic acid* Add 10 µL α-methyl-L-DOPA (125 mm/mL) and 800 µL of 2% MPA to 20 µL Inject *Dehydroascorbic acid* To 20 µL of above solution, add 10 µL of α-methyl-L-DOPA and 800 µL L-cysteine in 10 mM phosphate buffer, pH 6.8 (2.5 mg/mL) Inject	Inertsil ODS-2 5 µm 15 cm × 4.6 mm	Isocratic 100 mM KH_2PO_4 (pH 3.0) containing 1 mM EDTA	EC +300 mV vs Ag/AgCl	DL (ng) On-column 0.15 % Recovery AA >90 DHAA 80±	*J. Chromatogr. A,* 654, 215, 1993[20]
21. Fruits, vegetables	AA	Grind with quartz sand Mix macerate with 2% MPA (12 g + 48 mL) Transfer and shake for 10 min Filter	Spherisorb ODS-2 10 µm 25 cm × 4.6 mm	Isocratic 0.01 M KH_2PO_4 : MeOH : 20% TBAH (970 : 30 : 1) Adjust pH to 2.75 with 85% H_3PO_4	PDA 190–340 nm	QL (mg/100 g) DHAA—0.8 AA—1.2	*J. Chromatogr. Sci.,* 32, 481, 1994[21]
22. Food, animal tissue	AA DHAA IAA DHIAA	Homogenize with 17% MPA Centrifuge Filter Mix 500 µL supernatant with 115 mL 45% K_2HPO_4 to final pH of 7.1 Add 0.85% MPA to final volume of 2 µL Dilute 100 µL to 10 mL with mobile phase To second aliquot, mix 45% K_2HPO_4 containing 1% homocysteine to convert DHAA and DHIAA to AA and IAA	PLRP-S 5 µm 25 cm × 4.6 mm Two columns in series	Isocratic 20 mM NaH_2PO_4 containing 0.17% MPA, pH 2.2 *Food* 0.7 mL/min 22°C *Tissue* 0.6 mL/min 5°C	EC glassy carbon vs Ag/AgCl +0.7 V	DL (ng) On-column 0.5 QL (ng/20 µl) 0.5 % Recovery 94–104	*J. Liq. Chromatogr.,* 17, 2445, 1994[22]
23. Infant formula	AA DHAA	Homogenize and dilute 5 g to 100 mL with 1% MPA Centrifuge Filter	Superspher 100 RP-18 5 µm	Isocratic 0.1 M KH_2PO_4, pH 3.5 1 mL/min	254 nm	QL (mg/100 g) 39.7	*Food Chem.,* 52, 99, 1995[23]

TABLE 6.4 CONTINUED

| | | | HPLC Parameters | | | | |
Sample Matrix	Analyte	Sample Preparation	Column	Mobile Phase	Detection	Quality Assurance Parameters	References
24. Fruits	AA	Homogenize 100 g; Dilute 15–25 g with water; Sonicate; Centrifuge; Filter	Supelcosil LC-18; 5 μm; 25 cm × 4.6 mm	Isocratic; 2×10^{-3} M TBAH : MeCN (75 : 25)	254 nm	QL (mg/100 g) 10.2; DL (ng/μL) 1; % Recovery 83.3–100.9	Food Chem., 53, 211, 1995[24]
25. Beverages Apple juice	AA	Neutralize with 0.1 M NaOH; Dilute; Filter	5 C_{18} AR; 25 cm × 4.6 mm	Isocratic; 15 mM NaH_2PO_4-KH_2PO_4, pH 6.5; 0.3 mL/min	Electrochemiluminescence 3 electrode system glassy carbon stainless steel Ag/AgCl + 1.5 V Em λ = 610 nm $Ru(bpy)_3^{2+}$	DL (pmol) On-column 10; % Recovery 94–105	Anal. Sci., 11, 749, 1995[25]
26. Plant materials	AA DHAA	Homogenize 0.2–0.5 g in 5 mL 1.5% MPA containing 1 mM EDTA; Filter; Oxidize to DHAA 700 μL extract, adjust pH to neutrality with 450 mL of 0.2 M Tris; Add OPD	Spherisorb S5-ODS2; 5 μm; 25 cm × 4.6 mm	Isocratic; MeOH : water (1 : 3) containing 1 mM HDTMAB and 0.05% NaH_2PO_4; Adjust pH to 3.6 with 85% H_3PO_4; 1 mL/min	AA 248 nm; OPD derivative of DHAA 348 nm	% Recovery AA— 102.2–103.7; DHAA— 101.6–102.6	Phytochem. Anal., 7, 69, 1996[26]
Feeds 1. Aquatic feed and meals	AA, Ascorbyl-2-sulfate, Ascorbyl-2-polyphosphate	Add 20 mL 1% MPA–0.2% DTT to 1 g, pH 2.16; Vortex for 5–10 min; Homogenize if necessary; Centrifuge; filter consecutively through 0.45 μm and 0.2 μm filters; If ascorbyl-2-polyphosphate is present, digest with phosphatase	Intersil C_4 and C_{18} in series; 5 μm; 15 cm × 4.6 mm	Isocratic; 0.1 M NaOAC containing 174 μL m-octylamine and 200 mg EDTA/L; Adjust pH to 5 with HAC	PDA 255 nm	DL (ppb) 250; % Recovery 97	J. Liq. Chromatogr. Rel. Technol., 19, 3105, 1996[1]

Sample	Analyte	Sample Preparation	Column	Mobile Phase	Detection	QL/DL	Reference
Pharmaceuticals							
1. Fatty pharmaceuticals, cosmetics, butter, margarine	AA Antioxidant Synergists	Mix 10 g product with 5 mL water Heat at 50°C until melted Remove fatty layer and wash twice with 2 mL portions of hot water Add 1 mL sodium γ-hydroxy-butyrate (10 mg/mL) (IS) Centrifuge or extract with water from a Hex dilution	Spherisorb ODS 3 μm 15 cm × 4.6 mm	Isocratic Water acidified with H_2SO_4 pH 1.95 0.7 mL/min	AA 254 nm Antioxidant synergists 210 nm	QL (μg/g) AA 0.6–1.9 % Recovery 95.8–100.7	Chromatographia, 35, 232, 1993[1]
Biologicals							
1. Plasma	AA IAA	Mix plasma with equal volume of 10% MPA Centrifuge Dilute 10 fold with mobile phase	Altex Ultrasphere ODS 5 μm 25 cm × 4.6 mm	Isocratic 0.04 M NaOAC 0.005 M TBAP 0.2 g EDTA/L Adjust pH to 5.25 with HAC	EC glassy carbon + 0.6 V vs Ag/AgCl	DL (ng) On-column 0.25 CV = 2–5.6% % Recovery AA—102–107	J. Liq. Chromatogr., 8, 31, 1985[1]
2. Leukocytes adrenalomedullary chromaffin granules	AA	Suspend 1–2 mg in 1.0 mL TCA/10 mM oxalic acid Store at −70°C Thaw, centrifuge Extract with water-saturated Et_2O Purge with N_2 Add equal volume 40% MeOH : water containing 2 mM EDTA Chromaffin granules were treated with Ag 50W-X 8 cation exchange resin	Axxi-Chrom C$_{18}$ ODS 3 μm 10 cm × 4.6 mm	Isocratic 0.05 M NaH$_2$PO$_4$ 0.05 M NaOAC 180 μM DTMAC 3.66 μM TOAC in 30/70 MeOH/water, pH 4.8 1 mL/min	EC Dual detectors 1. 0.00 V Positive 2. 0.25 V	IAA—92–96 DL (pmol) On-column 3	Anal. Biochem., 181, 276, 1989[2]

Sample	Analyte	Sample preparation	Column	Mobile phase	Detection	DL/Recovery	Reference
3. Plasma	AA DHAA	SPE Apply 1 mL plasma onto 1,2 amino anion exchange column —500 mg resin in 3 mL column Wash with 1 mL 0.05 M NH_4OAC and 0.3 L 0.4 M Na citrate Elute AA with 2 × 0.5 mL of 0.4 M Na citrate Inject	Spherisorb $C_{18\text{-}2}$ 5 µm 25 cm × 4 mm	Isocratic 5 mM NaOAC and 2 mM BAH, pH 2.5 0.5 mL/min	Oxidize AA to DAAA with CuOAC or $CuSO_4$ Post-column derivatization with 1,2-DAB · HCl or 1,2-DA-3,4-DMB · HCl Fluorescence Ex λ = 340 Em λ = 420	DL (ng) On-column AA—16 DHAA—3 % Recovery 97.2–99.2	*Fres. J. Anal. Chem.*, 342, 462, 1992[3]
4. Plasma	AA	Mix 30 µL plasma with 60 mL 90% MeOH in water saturated with EDTA Place on ice for 10-15 min Centrifuge	QC Pak C_{18} 25 cm × 4.5 mm or TSK gel ODS 120 Å 25 cm × 4.5 mm	Isocratic 50 mM Na_2PO_4 50 mM NaOAC 189 µM DTMAC 36.6 µM TOAB 0.2 mM EDTA in MeOH : water (20 : 80), pH 4.8 1 mL/min	EC +350 mV vs Ag/AgCl	DL (ng) On-column 0.1	*J. Nutr. Sci. Vitaminol.*, 40, 73, 1994[4]
5. Plasma	AA DHAA	Mix plasma with 10% MPA Centrifuge Dilute 100 µL with 100 µL 0.125 M Trizma, pH 9.0 Reduce DHAA to AA by adding 100 µL to 50 µL 0.5 M Trizma containing 10 mM DTT	Nova Pak C_{18} 4 µm 7.5 cm × 3.9 mm	Isocratic 0.1 M Na_2HPO_4 2.5 mM EDTA 2.0 mM DTMAC Adjust to pH 3.0 with H_3PO_4	EC +100 mV	DL (fmol) On-column 20	*Anal. Biochem.*, 229, 329, 1995[5]
6. Rat tissue	AA	Mince 0.5 g and homogenize in 50 mM H_3PO_4 containing 0.1 mM EDTA, pH 2.0 Centrifuge	RCM module 8 × 10 Resolve C_{18}	Isocratic 0.2 M KH_2PO_4, pH 3.0 1 mL/min	EC Porous graphite 1. −0.1 V 2. ±0.4 V ± 0.8 V	% Recovery 94	*Biochem J.*, 306, 101, 1995[6]
7. Plasma	AA	Add 25 µL perchloric acid to 500 µL plasma Centrifuge Filter	Supelco C_{18} 5 µm 25 cm × 4.6 mm	Isocratic 80 mM NaOAC, pH 4.6 containing 5% MeOH, 0.5 mM Na_2 EDTA 1 mM NaCl and 1 mM n-octylamine 1.3 mL/min	EC glassy carbon +0.5 V vs Ag/AgCl	DL (pg) On-column 100 % Recovery 100.3	*Eur. J. Pharm. Sci.*, 3, 231, 1995[7]

8. Aqueous humor	AA	*AA* Add 90 µL 0.01 *M* MPA to 10 µL aqueous humor *Total (AA + DHAA)* Add 90 µL 30 µM DTT	CLC-NH$_2$ 15 cm × 6.0 mm	Isocratic *AA* 6 m*M* KH$_2$PO$_4$: 1 *N* HCl : 2 m*M* homocysteine : MeOH : MeCN (66.5 : 1 : 10 : 254 : 70) 0.7 mL/min, 35°C *Total (AA + DHAA)* 6 m*M* KH$_2$PO$_4$: 1 *N* HCl : 0.1 *M* DTT : MeOH : MeCN (66.5 : 1 : 10 : 274 : 70) 0.7 mL/min, 35°C	250 nm	—	*Ophthal. Res*, 27, 347, 1995[8]
9. Biological samples	L-AA D-AA	Add MPA to tissue, store at −70°C Add 40 mL 0.05 *M* KH$_2$PO$_4$ and DTT (1 g/L) to 5 g Add 10 mL MPA (500 g/L), MeCN (20 mL) Centrifuge Remove upper layer	Cap Cell Pak NH$_2$ 40°C	Isocratic 0.68 g KH$_2$PO$_4$ + 200 mL Water +800 mL MeCN + 7.5 mL H$_3$PO$_4$ 1 mL/min	EC +700 mV	—	*J. Chromatog. B*, 690, 25, 1997[9]

6.3.4.2.2 Detection

UV, electrochemical (EC), and fluorescence detection of OPD quinoxaline derivatives of dehydroascorbic acid are the most common detection modes used for quantitation of L-ascorbic acid and its related compounds after HPLC resolution. UV detection of L-ascorbic acid at wavelengths near its absorbance maxima of 245 nm and 265 nm or at 254 nm have frequently been used. UV absorbance due to its lack of specificity is most useful for analysis of high concentration samples such as multivitamins and fruit juices. Absorbance properties of dehydroascorbic acid vary considerably from L-ascorbic acid with maximal absorbance occurring around 223 nm at pH 3.1.[10] The low wavelength often leads to erroneous peaks and solvent interference which complicates the interpretation of the chromatogram.[9] Further, the dehydro form must be present in relatively higher concentrations than L-ascorbic acid due to its weaker UV absorbance characteristic. Investigators are encouraged to use more specific EC or fluorescence derivative techniques to avoid potential sensitivity and specificity problems inherently characteristic to UV detection. Kimoto et al.[46] recently published details of EC detection for ascorbic acid and dehydroascorbic acid.

Summaries of recent HPLC methods (Table 6.4) indicate that EC detection and use of OPD derivatization for fluorescence detection are the most commonly applied detection modes. EC detection relies upon the oxidation of L-ascorbic acid or isoascorbic acid to the dehydro forms. Dehydroascorbic acid is electrochemically inactive. Therefore, EC can be used for total vitamin C only if dehydroascorbic acid is reduced to L-ascorbic acid prior to detection, usually pre-column. The detection limit for EC detection of L-ascorbic acid can be as low as the pmol range. Due to the improvement in available EC detectors, many researchers are now utilizing the sensitivity and selectivity of EC detection.

OPD derivatization is an excellent approach to provide selectivity and sensitivity to vitamin C analysis by HPLC. Derivatization can be by pre-column or post-column since the quinoxaline derivatives can be chromatographically resolved. Well recognized procedures using OPD derivatization are discussed in the following section.

6.3.4.2.3 HPLC Methods Based on OPD Derivatization

6.3.4.2.3.1 Pre-Column Derivatization—Speek et al.[38] developed a highly useful pre-column procedure using OPD derivatization to assay total vitamin C and total isovitamin C in foods. L-ascorbic acid and isoascorbic acid and their dehydro forms were extracted with 0.3 M trichloroacetic acid. Ascorbate oxidase was used to enzymatically oxidize L-ascorbic acid and isoascorbic acid to the dehydro forms. OPD derivatization was completed and the quinoxaline derivatives were isocratically resolved on a reversed-phase system (C_{18}) with 0.08 M KH_2PO_4 containing 20% methanol. By omitting the ascorbate oxidase conversion, dehydro forms can be quantitated. This procedure has been the basis of other OPD methods and has been used extensively in other studies.[39,40] The method is provided in Section 6.4.

Procedural steps based upon the AOAC International Microfluorometric Procedure (Method 967.22) were followed to develop an HPLC procedure with improved sensitivity compared to the manual and semi-automated assays.[47] Complex samples that contained low levels of L-ascorbic acid or produced interferences when assayed by Method 967.22 were successfully assayed by the HPLC procedure. A clarification step was introduced after the Norit oxidation step that consisted of the addition of sodium acetate and methanol to the Norit treated extract. OPD derivatives were formed pre-column in the clarified extract. Some high starch samples like potato chips and canned corn required an additional clean-up step to remove solubilized starch prior to the OPD derivatization. To accomplish the starch removal, an aliquot of the extract was diluted 1 : 1 with 95% ethanol, incubated in an ice bath, and centrifuged. The chromatography system consisted of a μBondapak C_{18} column and mobile phase of methanol : water (55 : 45). Fluorescence detection was at Ex λ = 350 and Em λ = 430. The AOAC Task Force on Methods for Nutrition Labeling recommended the

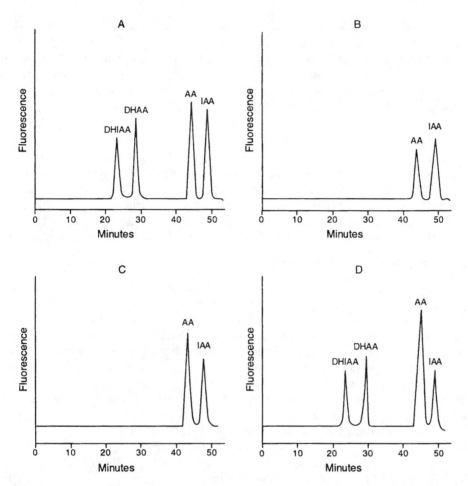

FIGURE 6.5 Chromatograms of L-ascorbic acid and isoascorbic acid in meat products. Either isoascorbic acid or ascorbic acid was used as IS: A—Standards; B—Meat spiked with IAA; C—Hot dog with AA; D—Hot dog spiked with AA. Reprinted with permission from text Reference 49.

method for AOAC collaboration.[25] However, at this time the method has not been collaborated. Procedural steps for the method are provided in Section 6.4.

6.3.4.2.3.2 Post-Column Derivatization—Vanderslice and co-workers published a series of papers that refined LC procedures based on post-column derivatization with OPD.[45,48,49,50] Their final method used an extractant containing 30 g HPO_3 and 0.5 g EDTA dissolved in 500 mL H_2O and 80 mL glacial acetic acid. The solution was diluted to 1 L for extraction of most foods. Animal tissue required an increased HPO_3 concentration to 10% wt/v. The method differs from most vitamin C procedures in that quantitation was based on the use of isoascorbic acid as an internal standard. Chromatography was based on work of Lloyd et al.[43,44] with two PLRP-S columns in series. The basic methodology was used to complete an extensive survey of the vitamin C content in foods in the U.S. diet.[51] Chromatograms are given in Figure 6.5.

6.3.4.2.4 Internal Standards

Internal standards have not been used routinely for HPLC analysis of vitamin C. When derivatives are used to increase sensitivity and selectivity, the internal standard must react similarly to L-ascorbic acid or dehydroascorbic acid. Vanderslice and Higgs[50] showed this problem clearly. They examined 23 different compounds for suitability as an internal standard for post-column OPD derivatization. The derivatives either coeluted or were not sufficiently soluble in the eluting buffer. Many of the compounds gave no detector response under the elution conditions. Vanderslice and Higgs,[50] however, demonstrated the usefulness of using isoascorbic acid as an internal standard in foods to which it has not been added during processing. Also, for many processed meats, L-ascorbic acid can be used as the internal standard for quantitating isoascorbic acid.

6.3.5   CAPILLARY ELECTROPHORESIS

Capillary electrophoresis (CE) represents a newly emerging analytical approach to the analysis of total vitamin C and isoascorbic acid in biological materials. Heiger published an excellent review of CE principles, instrumentation, and modes of operation.[52] Various CE based methods for vitamin C analysis are summarized in Table 6.5. Characteristic of CE methods, the methods are highly efficient, rapid, and versatile, requiring low solvent usage and minimal sample columns. Detection is based on UV absorbance. We have provided a method protocol in Section 6.4 based on the work of Davey et al.[53]

6.3.6   STATUS OF VITAMIN C ANALYSIS

The analyst has a wide selection of accurate methods to choose from that have been applied to many biological matrices. HPLC methods can accurately differentiate between L-ascorbic acid and isoascorbic acid and the dehydro forms of the epimers. However, because of the variability that exists in the application of the methods between laboratories, considerable variation in assayed values can occur when different laboratories assay like samples using proven methods of their choice. This fact was demonstrated by the European Community FLAIR Programme Interlaboratory Assay Method Comparison Study on plasma vitamin C assays.[54] In this study, nine laboratories used DNPH and OPD manual procedures or HPLC procedures based on OPD derivatization and fluorescence detection, UV, or electrochemical detection. The methods were in-house preferred procedures in routine use at the laboratories conducting the study. Samples included spiked plasma samples of known concentration stabilized by addition of an equal volume of 10% metaphosphoric acid. Results of the study from two different plasma samples at three concentrations of L-ascorbic acid showed %CV values ranging from 13 to 87%. Greatest CV% variations occurred at low L-ascorbic acid levels of 4.0 and 4.5 µM. Reasons for the variability summarized in the report included the following:

1. Vitamin C is easily oxidized. Plasma samples must be immediately acidified and frozen. Stabilization was performed in different ways by the participating laboratories.
2. A variety of assay procedures are available that differ in fundamental principle.
3. A biological quality control material does not exist with certified L-ascorbic acid levels for use as an in-house method validation tool.
4. Methods are still in use that measure only the reduced or oxidized forms of vitamin C.
5. Some assay methods are subject to positive or negative interferences by other components in the plasma.

Recommendations coming from the study included:

1. Development of a procedure-calibration protocol with emphasis on low-level spiking of "real samples" to check recoveries at deficiency or borderline concentration ranges.
2. Use of a quality control sample at the borderline concentrations and at two or three higher levels that are stabilized with 5% metaphosphoric acid and stored at −80°C or lower.
3. An urgent need exists for generally available quality control materials with certified vitamin C contents.

The study presents valuable lessons for all involved in micronutrient analysis programs.

TABLE 6.5
Newer Approaches to Vitamin C Analysis—Non-Traditional Methods

Method	Matrix	Analyte	Determinative Parameters	Accuracy/Precision
Flow Injection				
1. *J. Micronutr. Anal.,* 6, 109, 1989	Food	Total AA	Extract with MPA : HAC (Robotic) C_{18} preconditioning clean-up Oxidize AA to DHAA with $HgCl_2$ Derivatize with OPD Fluorescence — Ex λ = 350; Em λ = 430	Results compare to AOAC methods Low recoveries for some samples % Recovery = 69–112
2. *Analyst,* 117, 1635, 1992	Urine Pharmaceuticals	AA	Add 2 mL Na_2H_2EDTA to 15 mL urine and dilute to 25 mL with water Dilute pharmaceuticals with water, filter AA reduction of Co^{III}-EDTA to Co^{II}-EDTA in water-diethylamine solution, pH 12.5 Co^{II}-EDTA detected at 540 nm	RSD = 0.94% DL = 6×10^{-5} mol dm^{-3} QL = 1.2×10^{-4} mol dm^{-3}
3. *Fres. J. Anal. Chem.* 347, 293, 1993	Fruit juices	AA	Juice is dialyzed on line Dialyzed fraction is accepted by Fe (III) reagent 210 µL are injected into a stream of o-phenanthroline and passed through a 100 cm reaction coil Fe (II)/o-phenanthroline complex is monitored at 510 nm	RSD = 0.5% QL = 0.03 g/L
4. *Analyst,* 118, 639, 1993	Fruit juice Pharmaceuticals	AA	Dissolve and dilute with 1% MPA, centrifuge juice Sample is pumped into carrier stream of acidified Fe (III) Luminol is mixed at the reaction coil with the carrier stream Reducing effect of AA on Fe (III) is monitored by measuring Fe (II)-catalyzed light emission from luminol oxidation by H_2O_2	RSD = 1.4% DL = 1×10^{-6} mol L^{-1}

TABLE 6.5 Continued

Method	Matrix	Analyte	Determinative Parameters	Accuracy/Precision
5. *Talanta*, 41, 125, 1994	Drug formulations	AA	Chemiluminescence (CL) is measured with photomutiplier tube and flow-through CL detector Dissolve tablets in water, add H_2SO_4 Inject 110 µL into Fe (III) in 0.05 M H_2SO_4 Merge with 1,10-phenanthroline solution Reduction of Fe (III) by AA monitored by formation of the red tris-1,10, phenanthroline iron (II) complex at 510 nm	RSD = 0.88% % Recovery = +99 QL (ppm) = 100
6. *Talanta*, 42, 779, 1995	Soft drinks Fruit juices Pharmaceuticals	AA	Dissolve in water and/or dilute with carrier solution (6 mg/L 2-mercaptoethanol) Merge with 0.2 M H_2SO_4 Monitor at 245 nm Blank correction for matrix absorbance determined by injecting 0.2 M NaOH and monitoring decrease in absorbance at 245 nm	RSD = 1.2% % Recovery = 101 DL (µg/mL) = 0.2
7. *Anal. Chim. Acta*, 309, 271, 1995	Wine Beer Urine Pharmaceuticals	Total AA	Adjust liquids to pH 6.0 with HCl on NaOH Add 0.1 M EDTA Grind vitamin pills, dilute with 1% oxalic acid Reagent solution of 0.1 M OPD and 0.5 M phosphate buffer, pH 6.0 is merged with sample solution containing 5 mL laccase AA oxidation in the presence of laccase to DHAA is monitored by the formation of quinoxaline derivative Fluorescence, Ex λ = 360; Em λ = 430	RSD = 2.0–4.1% % Recovery = 88–104 QL = 0.025 µg/mL

8. *Anal. Chim. Acta*, 308, 299, 1995	Blood Fruit juice Soft drinks Pharmaceuticals	AA	Dilute or dissolve with water Sample is treated on line with Dowex 50×8^{-200} (Na^+) Sample and toluidine blue solutions are injected simultaneously into two phosphate buffer streams, pH 3.0 Synchronously merged before reaching the irradiated reactor (200 cm $\times$ 0.5 mm), irradiation is by visible light (500 W halogen) The stream is merged downstream with lucigenin The stream is merged with 0.7 M KOH Oxidation of AA in the presence of oxygen Chemiluminescence is measured with a Bio-Orbit luminometer Photosensitized by toluidine blue yield products that react rapidly with lucigenin to yield very strong chemiluminescence	RSD = 1.22% QL = 0.17 mg/mL DL = 2×10^{-10} M
9. *Talanta*, 43, 1275, 1996	Pharmaceuticals	AA	Sample is dissolved in 0.1 M perchloric acid Dilute in 0.1 M phthalate buffer, pH 3.8 Sample is injected into MB^+ carrier stream (MB^+ + 0.1 M phthalate buffer) Stream is irradiated (500 W halogen lamp) Leucomethylene blue is detected amperometrically at 0.05 V using a wall-jet electrode system MB^+ is reduced photochemically to leucomethylene blue two-electron AA oxidation reduction	RSD = 1.3–4.8% DL = 1.9 µg/mL QL = 5.0 µg/mL
10. *Talanta*, 43, 971, 1996	Pharmaceuticals	AA	Dissolve samples in 0.014 M nitric acid Chromogenic reagents 1.0×10^{-3} M Fe^{+3} and 5×10^{-3} M $[Fe(CN)_6]^{-3}$ were merged into the carrier stream of 0.014 M nitric acid Sample stream is merged with chromogenic stream Prussian blue results from the reduction of Fe^{+3} to Fe^{+2} by AA. Deep blue coloration measured at 700 nm	RSD < 1.0%

TABLE 6.5 Continued

Method	Matrix	Analyte	Determinative Parameters	Accuracy/Precision
11. *Analyst*, 122, 115, 1997	Pharmaceuticals Fruit juice Soft drinks	AA	Dissolve sample in water or dilute Inject into manifold with merging lines of 1. 0.5 M phosphate, pH 3.0 2. AA line—5 × 10^{-6} M Thionine Blue Irradiation time—20 sec with a photoreactor length of 200 cm Fluorescence, Ex λ = 340, Em λ = 464 Flow—0.6 mL/min	
Spectrophotometric				
1. *J. Food Sci.*, 58, 619, 1993	Foods	AA	Grind in 2% MPA Centrifuge, filter Mix 0.3 mL sample solution with 2.6 mL phosphate buffer, pH 7.0, containing 1.81 mM EDTA and 0.13 mM 2-mercaptoethanol and 150 μL of quaiacol peroxidase Record absorbance at 265 nm Initiate reaction with 15 μL 50 mM H_2O_2 Record decrease in absorbance at 265 nm Measures oxidation of AA to DHAA	% Recovery = 101.6 (n = 20)
2–3. *Food Chem.*, 53, 397, 1995 *J. Food Sci.*, 60, 360, 1995	Beverages	AA	Dilute with 0.01 M phosphate buffer, pH 7.5 Add riboflavin solution (0.06 g /100 mL) Make volumetric dilution with phosphate buffer Irradiate 20 mg aliquot for 15 min (5500 lux) Measure absorbance at 265 nm before and after irradiation Method measures selective riboflavin-sensitized singlet oxygen oxidation of AA	% Recovery = 97.5–102.3 Data compared favorably to HPLC and indophenol measurements for 9 of 12 beverages

Reference	Analyte	Sample	Procedure	Results
4. *Anal. Biochem.,* 221, 290, 1994	DHAA	Plasma Lymphocytes Mammalian cells	Deproteinize with ice-cold 8% perchloric acid Centrifuge Neutralize with 4 M KOH 700 μL is mixed with 200 μL of MeOH containing 6.25 mM desferrioxamine Add 100 μL of buffer containing 4 M NaH$_2$PO$_4$ and 0.666 M citric acid 1-hydrate, pH 7.9 Follow absorbance changes at 345 nm Stabilization of AA is by desferrioxiamine Method allows direct measurement of DHAA in biologicals	DL < 0.1 μmol/L CV = 3.6–6.8% SD = 0.27–0.55 μM % Recovery = 87.5–105
5. *Talanta,* 42, 1631, 1995	AA	Fruits Vegetables	Homogenize 25 mL juice with 75 mL 3% MPA—8% HAC Centrifuge, filter Determine third order derivative spectra of sample solutions vs extraction solution Determine peak to peak amplitude differences at two wavelengths for each sample matrix Concentration of AA in the sample solution was determined by regression of a calibration graph from the third-order derivative spectra of AA standard vs extraction solution between 190–300 nm	Values compare to those obtained by the 2,6-dichlorophenolindophenol titration RSD = 0.53–2.45% (*n* = 13)
6. *Anal. Sci.,* 11, 853, 1995	AA	Pharmaceuticals	Dissolve in water Add Fe (III) solution (100 μg), 6 μL ferron and 0.1 mL 1 M HCl to sample aliquot Dilute to 10 mL with water Extract green complex with 1% tribenzylamine Dry over sodium sulfate Measure absorbance at 465 nm	RSD = 2.9% % Recovery = 99
7. *Clin. Chem.,* 43, 154, 1997	AA	Plasma	Stabilize 500 μL plasma with MPA/DTT Centrifuge Load 200 μL into Cobas cups of Roche Diagnostics Cobas Fara Centrifugal Analyzer OPD derivatization after AA oxidase treatment Read at 340 nm	% Recovery = 93.8–119 QL = 26.1 μMol/L % CV = 0.51–2.7

TABLE 6.5 Continued

Method	Matrix	Analyte	Determinative Parameters	Accuracy/Precision
Capillary Electrophoresis				
1. *J. Pharm. Biomed. Anal.*, 10, 717, 1992	Fruit juice Pharmaceuticals	AA IAA	Filter juice, 0.2 mM filter Dissolve pharmaceuticals in 0.1 M phosphate buffer, pH 5.0 *CE Parameters* Column—20 cm × 25 µm coated column Buffer—0.1 M phosphate, pH 5.0 Voltage—8 kV Detection—265 nm	RSD < 5% % Recovery-99–101 DL = 0.5 µg/mL
2. *J. Chromatogr.* 633, 245, 1993	Fruit beverages Urine Plasma	AA	Dilute juice and urine with 10% MPA Add 0.1 mL of 100 µg/mL IAA (IS) per 0.1 mL sample; filter (0.45 µm) Mix 0.5 mL serum with 0.5 mL 12% TCA Centrifuge, filter, add 100 µL IAA (IS), 81.5 µg/mL to 0.4 mL filtrate *CE Parameters* Column—30 cm × 75 µm fused-silica capillary Buffer—100 mM tricine, pH 8.8 Voltage—11 kV Detection—254 nm	RSD = 1.9–3.3% Recovery = 98 (plasma) QL = µg/mL
3. *J. Chromatogr.* 645, 197, 1993	Fruits	Total AA AA DHAA	Add 5 mL of 12.5% TCA to 15 g juice Centrifuge, filter Dilute with water, adjust pH to 7.0 Reduce DHAA with 2 mL of 0.8% homocysteine to 0.5 mL extract Assay after 15 min *CE Parameters* Column—40 cm × 1005 µm fused-silica capillary Buffer—20 mM phosphate, pH 7.0 Voltage—6 kV Detection—254 nm	Results agree with HPLC analysis

Reference	Sample	Analyte	Method	Comments
4. *J. Chromatogr. A*, 716, 291, 1995	Foods Beverages	AA Organic acids	Dilute with 2 mM NaOH, pH adjusted to neutrality. Filter (0.2 μm), degas. *CE Parameters* Column—43 cm × 75 μm fused-silica capillary Buffer—5 mM trimellitic acid—1 mM TDTMAB, pH 5.5 or pH 9.0 Voltage—20 kV Detection—on-line PDA, 200–350 nm	RSD = 1–4% DL = $2.0 \times 10^{-6} M$
5. *Anal. Biochem.*, 239, 8, 1996	Plant tissue	AA IAA	Pulverize in liquid N_2 Extract 200 mg (2×) with 2.5 mL 3% MPA/1 mM EDTA; centrifuge Pass 2 mL through C_{18} SPE, keep last 500 μL *CE Parameters* Column—57 cm × 75 μm fused-silica capillary Buffer—200 mM borate, pH 9 Voltage—25 kV Detection—on-line PDA (190–350 nm), quantitation at 260 nm	Compared closely to HPLC analysis DL = 15 pg (84 fmol/injection)
Miscellaneous *Circular Dichroism* 1. *J. Agric. Food Chem.*, 39, 2171, 1991	Fruit juice Apples Peppers Pharmaceuticals	AA Riboflavin Vitamin B_{12}	Blend 20–50 g fruit in $5.5 \times 10^{-5} M$ EDTA dissolved in pH 5.4 buffer Dilute liquids in pH 5.4 buffer Determine differences as a function of wavelength in absorbances between two coincident circularly polarized beams of light that pass simultaneously through the sample. CD Spectral Data for AA Θ_M (deg/M_{cm}) 285 nm -3 251 nm $+105$	—

TABLE 6.5 Continued

Method	Matrix	Analyte	Determinative Parameters	Accuracy/Precision
Stripping Voltammetry				
1. *Food Chem.*, 51, 237, 1994	Fruits Vegetables	AA	Homogenize in 10% HAC, centrifuge Mix extract with Fe (III) and 1,10-phenathroline solutions Dilute with HAC-NaDAC buffer, pH 4.5 Record response curve by scanning the potential from 1.2 V to 0.3 V vs a saturated columel electrode stripping peak at 0.87 V Method follows oxidation of AA with mixture of Fe (III) and 1,10-phenanthroline to form ferroin complex	% Recovery = 102–105 RSD = 5.6%
Chemiluminescence				
1. *J. Biochem. Biophys. Meth.*, 28, 277, 1994	Plasma	AA	Pass plasma through desalting gel filtration column Add 200 µL 0.1 M carbonate buffer containing 0.1 M EDTA and 1 mM luminol, pH 10.5; 400 µL water, and 1800 µL MeOH to 100 µL eluate AA in plasma decreases chemiluminescence of luminol photosynthesized reaction	CV = 2–5%
Isotope Ratio Mass Spectrometry				
1. *J. Agric. Food Chem.*, 43, 2662, 1995	Fruit juice	AA	Centrifuge, filter; flush aliquot with N_2 Add DTT; adjust pH to 5.5 Elute from AG 1 × 8 anion exchange (200–400 mesh, SO_4^{-2}) Lyophilize Redissolve in water (10 mL) Preparatory LC (1 mL) Lyophilize, redissolve in 0.6 mL water Determine carbon isotope ratio	—

Differential Pulse Polarography

1. *Fres., J. Anal. Chem.,* 351, 804, 1995

Asparagus

AA

Cut and grind under N_2
Extract with 1% oxalic acid
Centrifuge
Transfer 1 mL extract to 10 mL phosphate buffer, pH 6.7
   Pulse Amplitude—50 mV
   Drop time—2 s
   Scan rate—2 mV/s

DL = 0.182 µg/mL
RSD = 2.77–4%
% Recovery = 96.9–113.4

Microtiter Plate Assay

1. *Nutr. Biochem.,* 7, 179, 1996

Plasma
Leukocyte

AA

Add 5 mL 10% TCA to 5 mL plasma
Centrifuge
Add DNPH/thiourea/copper to extract (20 µL) to 100 µL extract in microcentrifuge tubes
Incubate at 37°C (2–4h)
Add 150 µL ice-cold 65% H_2SO_4
Vortex, place in dark at ambient temperature for 1 h
Transfer to 96-well microtiter plate
Read with microtiter plate reader at 515 nm and 562 nm

% Recovery = 90

6.4 METHOD PROTOCOLS
Rapid Enzymatic Assay for Ascorbic Acid in Various Foods Using Peroxidase

Principle
- Ascorbic acid was determined by measuring the change in absorbance during oxidation by quaiacol peroxidase.

Chemicals
- Extraction solution—2% metaphosphoric acid
- EDTA
- 2-mercaptoethanol
- USP ascorbic acid

Apparatus
- Spectrophotometer

Procedure

Extraction
- To quartz cuvette, add 2.6 mL $M/30$ phosphate buffer, pH 7.0; 150 μL quaiacol peroxidase (0.5 mg/mL in $M/30$ phosphate buffer, containing 1.81 mM EDTA and 0.13 mM 2-mercaptoethanol)
- Add 0.3 mL sample
- Record initial absorbance at 265 nm
- Initiate reaction with 15 mL of 50 mM H_2O_2
- Record absorbance after 20 min
- Calculate ascorbic acid from calibration plot of ΔA_{265} vs ascorbic acid concentration
- Calibration curve ranges from 0.2 to 1 mg/100 mL

J. Food Sci., 58, 619, 1993

Flow-Injection Spectrophotometric Determination of Ascorbic Acid in Pharmaceutical Products with the Prussian Blue Reaction

Principle
- A deep blue solution forms when Fe^{+3} is reduced to Fe^{+2} by ascorbic acid. The colored complex is monitored at 700 nm.

Chemicals
- Nitric acid
- Fe (III) reagent
  Fe (III) nitrate in 0.014 M nitric acid
    $1.0 \times 10^{-4}, 5.0 \times 10^{-3}, 1.0 \times 10^{-3}, 1.0 \times 10^{-2} M$
- Hexacyanoferrate (III)
    $5.0 \times 10^{-2}, 5.0 \times 10^{-3} M$
- Complexing reagent
  0.5% oxalic acid in 0.1 M NaOH

Apparatus
- Eight channel peristaltic pump
- Spectrophotometer with flow-through cell
- Recorder

Procedure

Extraction

- Dissolve samples in 0.014 M nitric acid

Analysis

- Follow flow-injection procedure schematically shown in Figure 6.6
- Monitor Prussian Blue at 700 nm

Talanta, 43, 971, 1996

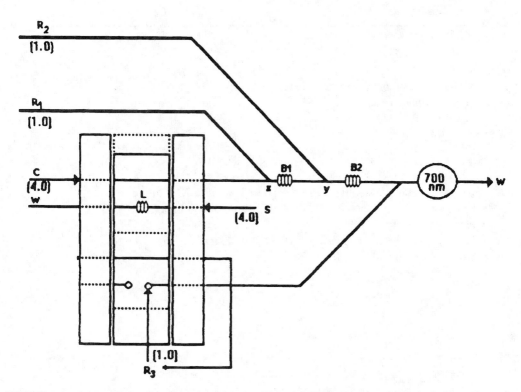

FIGURE 6.6 Schematic for flow-injection analysis of Prussian Blue ascorbic acid analysis. Flow diagram with colorimetric reagents (R_1 and R_2) introduced by confluence (x and y points). B_1 and B_2 are reactors of 150 and 100 cm, respectively. L is a sample loop of 100 cm. C, carrier stream; W, waste; S, sample or reference solution. R_3 is an intermittent flow of an alkaline oxalate solution. Numbers between parentheses represent the flow rates. Reprinted with permission from Reference 10 (Chapter 6, Table 6, Flow-Injection Methods).

Determination of Human Plasma and Leukocyte Ascorbic Acid by Microtiter Plate Assay

Principle
- A microtiter plate technique is used to measure the dinitrophenylhydrazine (DNPH) derivative of ascorbic acid.

Chemicals
- Ascorbic acid standard 0 to 2.0 µg/100 µL
- Trichloroacetic acid (TCA)
- DNPH/thiourea/copper solution (DTC)
- Sulfuric acid

Whole blood fractionation is shown in Figure 6.7.

Apparatus
- 96-well polystyrene microtiter plate
- Microtiter plate reader
- Centrifuge

Procedure

- To 100 µL of TCA-stabilized sample, add 20 µL of DTC solution
- Incubate at 37°C in dark for 2 and 4 h, vortex at 30 min intervals
- Place plates on ice
- Incubate in darkness, 1 h, with vortexing after 30 min
- Read at 515 nm and 562 nm

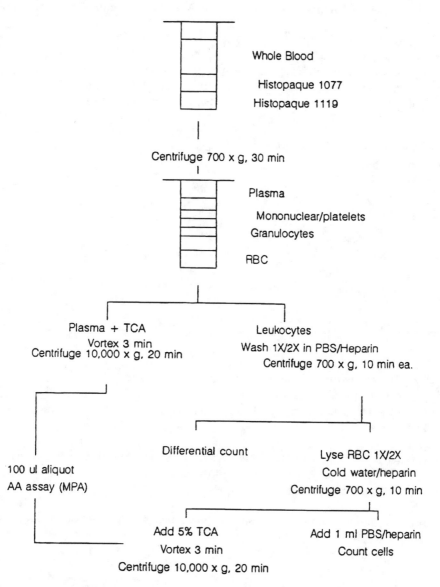

FIGURE 6.7   Isolation of leukocytes from human blood. Reprinted with permission from Reference 1. (Chapter 6, Table 6.5, Microtiter Plate Assay).

Determination of Total Vitamin C in Various Food Matrices by Liquid Chromatography and Fluorescence Detection

Principle

- Food products were extracted with 3% metaphosphoric acid [(MPA)-acetic acid]. Ascorbic acid was oxidized to dehydroascorbic acid with Norite. o-Phenylenediamine fluorescent derivatives were formed pre-column and resolved on μBondapak C_{18}.

Chemicals

- Extraction solution—3% MPA in 8% acetic acid
- USP ascorbic acid
- Sodium acetate
- Acid washed Norit
- Methanol
- o-Phenylenediame (OPD)

Apparatus

- Liquid chromatograph
- Fluorescence detector

Procedure

Extraction

- Homogenize product in food processor
- Weigh sample portion to contain 1.5 to 7.5 mg ascorbic acid
- Mix with 100 mL extraction solution
- Transfer contents to 250 mL g/s flask containing 2 g Norit
- Shake, 30 s
- Filter
- Transfer 20 mL aliquot (300 to 700 μg ascorbic acid) to 100 mL volumetric flask containing 5 mL sodium acetate solution (500 g NaOAC·3H$_2$O per L) and 55 mL methanol
- Dilute to volume with water
- Filter
- Transfer aliquot of filtrate to 100 mL volumetric containing 10 mL of OPD solution (2.5 mg/mL)
- Dilute to volume with mobile phase

Chromatography

Column	30 cm × 3.9 mm
Stationary phase	μBondapak C_{18}
Mobile phase	methanol : water (55 : 45)
Column temperature	Ambient
Flow	1 mL/min
Injection	100 μL
Detector	Fluorescence, Ex λ = 350, Em λ = 430
Calculation	External standard, peak area, linear regression

Note: Some samples require clarification of the extract to remove starch. Extracts were clarified by adding an equal volume of 95% ethanol and filtration before the OPD derivatization.

J. AOAC Int., 75, 887, 1992

Quantitative Determination of Ascorbic, Dehydroascorbic, Isoascorbic and Dehydroisoacscorbic Acids by HPLC in Foods and Other Matrices*

Principle

- Ascorbic acid (AA) and dehydroascorbic acid (DHAA) are extracted with metaphosphoric acid, resolved, and quantitated by isocratic reversed-phase LC with post-column derivatization of DHAA with o-phenylenediamine to give a fluorescent quinoxaline derivative.

Chemicals

- Metaphosphoric acid (MPA)
- Glacial acetic acid
- EDTA (disodium salt)
- *n*-butanol
- hexane

Extraction Solution #1 for Foods

- 30 g MPA, 0.5 g EDTA dissolved in 500 mL H_2O and 80 mL glacial acetic acid and diluted to 1 L

Extraction Solution #2 for Tissue

- 10%, (V/V) MPA
- Standard isoascorbic acid
- DHAA and DHIAA must be prepared and purified using method cited in *J. Assoc. Off. Anal. Chem.*, 48, 1248, 1965

Apparatus

- Waring blender
- Polytron homogenizer
- Centrifuges
- Liquid chromatograph
- Fluorescence detector

Procedure

Extraction of Standards and Samples—Solid Foods

- Prior to blending sample add 10 mL extraction solution #1

a. *For non-fat and low-starch food*

- Transfer 10 mL aliquot to tube and centrifuge at 1200 g at 4°C for 5 min
- Filter (0.45 μm)
- Inject 100 μL onto LC column

b. *For low-starch foods with fat*

- Add 10 mL hexane to 10 mL aliquot
- Vortex 1 min
- Centrifuge at 1200 g
- Filter (0.45 μm) aqueous layer
- Inject 100 μL onto LC column

c. *For high starch foods*

- Add 10 mL *n*-butanol to 10 mL aliquot
- Vortex 1 min
- Centrifuge 48,400 g at 4°C for 10 min
- Filter (0.45 μm) aqueous layer
- Inject 100 μL onto LC column

Chromatography

Column	15.0 cm × 4.6 mm and 25.0 cm × 4.6 mm
Stationary phase	PLRP-S
Mobile phase	0.2 M NaH$_2$PO$_4$ (adjusted to pH 2.14 with H$_3$PO$_4$)
Column temperature	Ambient
Flow	0.8 mL/min
Injection	100 μL
Post-column oxidation and fluorescent derivatization	Oxidant stream = 0.5 mM/L CuCl$_2$
	Reactant stream = 3.1 mM/L o-phenylenediamine
	Reaction coil temperature = 70°C
	Cooling coil temperature = 20°C
Detection	Fluorescence, Ex λ = 350 nm, Em λ = 430 nm
Calculation	Peak area, external standard if both AA and IAA are present

J. Nutr. Biochem., 4, 184, 1993
J. Micronutr. Anal. 4, 109, 1988
J. Food Comp. Anal. 3, 105, 1990

6.5   REFERENCES

Text

1. Olson, R. E., Water-soluble vitamins, in *Principles of Pharmacology,* Munson, P. L., Mueller, R. A. and Breese, G. R., Eds., Chapman and Hall, New York, 1995, chap. 59.
2. Machlin, L. J. and Hüni, J. E. S., *Vitamins Basics,* Hoffmann-LaRoche, Basel, 1994, 24.
3. Gibson, R. S., *Principles of Nutritional Assessment,* Oxford University Press, New York, 1990, chap. 19.
4. National Research Council, *Recommended Dietary Allowances,* 10th ed., National Academy of Sciences, Washington, D.C., 1989, chap. 8.
5. Nutritional Labeling and Education Act of 1990, Fed. Reg., 58, 2070, 1993.
6. Basu, T. K. and Dickerson, J. W., *Vitamins in Human Health and Disease,* CAB International, Wallingford, 1996, chap. 10.
7. Combs, G. R., Jr., *The Vitamins, Fundamental Aspects in Nutrition and Health,* Academic Press, New York, 1992, chap. 9.
8. Moser, U. and Bendich, A., Vitamin C, in *Handbook of Vitamins,* Machlin, L. J., Ed., Marcel Dekker, New York, 1990, chap. 5.
9. Eitenmiller, R. R. and Landen, W. O., Jr., Vitamins, in *Analyzing Food for Nutrition Labeling and Hazardous Contaminants,* Jeon, I. J. and Ikins, W. G., Eds., Marcel Dekker, New York, 1995, chap. 9.
10. Ball, G. F. M., Chemical and biological nature of the water-soluble vitamins, in *Water-Soluble Vitamin Assays in Human Nutrition,* Chapman and Hall, New York, 1994, chap. 2.
11. Tannenbaum, S. R. and Young, V. R., Vitamins and minerals, in *Food Chemistry,* Fennema, O. R., Ed., Marcel Dekker, New York, 1985, 477.
12. Liao, M. L. and Seib, P. A., Selected reactions of L-ascorbic acid related to foods, *Food Tech.,* 41, 104, 1987.
13. Martell, A. E., Chelates of ascorbic acid: formation and catalytic properties, in *Ascorbic Acid: Chemistry, Metabolism and Uses,* Seib, P. A. and Tolbert, Eds., Adv. Chem. Ser. No. 200, American Chemical Society, Washington, D.C., 1982, 153.
14. Sherman, H. C., LaMer, V. K., and Campbell, H. L., The quantitative determination of antiscorbutic vitamin (vitamin C), *J. Am. Chem. Soc.,* 44, 165, 1922.
15. Pelletier, O., Vitamin C, in *Methods of Vitamin Assay,* Augustin, J., Klein, B. P., Becker, D. A., and Venugopal, P. B., Eds., John Wiley and Sons, New York, 1984, chap. 12.

16. Pachla, L. A., Reynolds, D. L., and Kissinger, P. T., Review of ascorbic acid methodology. Analytical methods for determining ascorbic acid in biological samples, food products and pharmaceuticals, *J. Assoc. Off. Anal. Chem.*, 68, 1, 1985.

17. Lumley, I. D., Vitamin analysis in foods, in *The Technology of Vitamins in Food*, Ottaway, P. B., Ed., Chapman and Hall, London, 1993, chap. 8.

18. Parviainen, M. T. and Nyyssönen, K., Ascorbic acid, in *Modern Chromatographic Analysis of Vitamins*, De Leenheer, A. P., Lambert, W. E., and Nelis, H. J., Eds., Marcel Dekker, New York, 1992, chap. 5.

19. Cooke, J. R. and Moxon, R. E. D., The detection and measurement of vitamin C, in *Vitamin C*, Counsell, J. N. and Horning, D. H., Eds., Applied Science Publishers, London, 1985, 303.

20. Remmers, P., The vitamin C level of potato products heated in oil, *Int. J. Vit. Nutr. Res.*, 38, 392, 1968.

21. Pelletier, O., Leduc, N. C., Tremblay, R., and Brassard, R., Vitamin C in potatoes prepared in various ways, *J. Inst. Can. Sci. Technol. Aliment.*, 10, 138, 1977.

22. Tillmans, J., The antiscorbutic vitamin, *Z. Lebensm. Unters.-Forsch*, 60, 34, 1930.

23. Verma, K. K., Jain, A., Sahasrabuddhey, B., Gupta, K., and Mishra, S., Solid-phase extraction clean-up for determining ascorbic acid and dehydroascorbic acid by titration with 2,6-dichlorophenolindophenol, *J. AOAC Int.*, 79, 1236, 1996.

24. AOAC International, *Official Methods of Analysis*, 16th ed., AOAC International, Arlington, VA, 1995.

25. AOAC International, Report on the AOAC International Task Force on Methods for Nutrient Labeling Analyses, *J. AOAC Int.*, 76, 180A, 1993.

26. Nobrega, J. A. and Lopes, G. S., Flow-injection spectrophotometric determination of ascorbic acid in pharmaceutical products with the Prussian Blue reaction, *Talanta*, 43, 971, 1996.

27. Deutsch, M. J. and Weeks, C. E., Microfluorometric assay for vitamin C, *J. Assoc. Off. Anal. Chem.*, 48, 1248, 1965.

28. Bourgeois, C. F. and Mainguy, P. R., Determination of vitamin C (ascorbic acid and dehydroascorbic acid) in foods and feeds, *Int. J. Vit. Nutr. Res.*, 44, 70, 1974.

29. Kirk, J. R. and Ting, N., Fluorometric assay for total vitamin C by continuous flow analysis, *J. Food Sci.*, 40, 463, 1975.

30. Roy, R. B., Conetta, A., and Salpeter, J., Automated fluorometric method for the determination of total vitamin C in food products, *J. Assoc. Off. Anal. Chem.*, 59, 1244, 1976.

31. Egberg, D. C., Potter, R. H., and Heroff, J. C., Semiautomated method for the fluorometric determination of total vitamin C in food products, *J. Assoc. Off. Anal. Chem.*, 60, 126, 1977.

32. DeVries, J. W., Semiautomated fluorometric method for determination of vitamin C in foods: collaborative study, *J. Assoc. Off. Anal. Chem.*, 66, 1371, 1983.

33. Dunmire, D. L., Reese, J. D., Bryan, R., and Seegers, M., Automated fluorometric determination of vitamin C in foods, *J. Assoc. Off. Anal. Chem.*, 62, 648, 1979.

34. Vanderslice, J. T. and Higgs, D. J., Robotic extraction of vitamin C from food samples, *J. Micronutr. Anal.*, 1, 143, 1985.

35. Vanderslice, J. T. and Higgs, D. J., Automated analysis of total vitamin C in foods, *J. Micronutr. Anal.*, 6, 109, 1989.

36. Roe, J. H. and Kuether, C. A., The determination of ascorbic acid in whole blood and urine through the 2,4-dinitrophenylhydrazine derivative of dehydroascorbic acid, *J. Biol. Chem.*, 147, 399, 1943.

37. Wei, Y., Ota, R. B., Bowen, H. T., and Omaye, S. T., Determination of human plasma and leukocyte ascorbic acid by microtiter plate assay, *Nutr. Biochem.*, 7, 179, 1996.

38. Speek, A. J., Schrijver, J., and Schreurs, W. H. P., Fluorometric determination of total vitamin C and total isovitamin C in foodstuffs and beverages by high-performance liquid chromatography with pre-column derivatization, *J. Agric. Food Chem.*, 32, 352, 1984.

39. Hägg, M., Ylikoski, S., and Kumpulainen, J., Vitamin C and α- and β-carotene in vegetables consumed in Finland during 1988–1989 and 1992–1993, *J. Food Comp. Anal.*, 7, 252, 1994.

40. Hägg, M., Ylikoski, S., and Kumpulainen, J., Vitamin C content in fruits and berries consumed in Finland, *Food Comp. Anal.*, 8, 12, 1995.

41. Casella, L., Gullotti, M., Marchesini, A., and Petrarulo, M., Rapid enzymatic method for vitamin C assay in fruits and vegetables using peroxidase, *J. Food Sci.*, 54, 374, 1989.

42. Tsumura, F., Ohsako, Y., Haraguchi, Y., Kumagai, H., Sakurai, H., and Ishii, K., Rapid enzymatic assay for ascorbic acid in various foods using peroxidase, *J. Food Sci.*, 58, 619, 1993.

43. Lloyd, L. L., Warner, F. P., Kennedy, J. F., and White, C. A., Ion suppression reversed phase high performance liquid chromatography method for the separation of L-ascorbic acid in fresh fruit juice, *J. Chromatogr.*, 437, 44, 1988.

44. Lloyd, L. L., Warner, F. P., Kennedy, J. F. and White, C. A., Quantitative analysis of vitamin C (L-ascorbic acid) by ion suppression reversed phase chromatography, *Food Chem.*, 28, 257, 1988.

45. Vanderslice, J. T. and Higgs, D. J., Separation of ascorbic acid, isoascorbic acid, dehydroascorbic acid and dehydoisoascorbic acid in food and animal tissue, *J. Micronutr. Anal.*, 7, 67, 1990.

46. Kimoto, E., Terada, S., and Yamaguchi, T., Analysis of ascorbic acid, dehydroascorbic acid, and transformation products by ion-pairing high performance liquid chromatography with multiwavelength ultraviolet and electrochemical detection, *Meth. Enzymol.*, 279, 3, 1997.

47. Dodson, K. Y., Young, E. R., and Soliman, A. M., Determination of total vitamin C in various food matrices by liquid chromatography and fluorescence detection, *J. AOAC Int.*, 75, 887, 1992.

48. Vanderslice, J. T. and Higgs, D. J., HPLC analysis with fluorometric detection of vitamin C in food samples, *J. Chromatogr. Sci.*, 22, 485, 1984.

49. Vanderslice, J. T. and Higgs, D. J., Quantitative determination of ascorbic, dehydroascorbic, isoascorbic and dehydroisoascorbic acid by HPLC in foods and other matrices, *J. Nutr. Biochem.*, 4, 184, 1985.

50. Vanderslice, J. T. and Higgs, D. J., Chromatographic separation of ascorbic acid, isoascorbic acid, dehydroascorbic acid and dehydroisoascorbic acid and their quantitation in food products, *J. Micronutr. Anal.*, 4, 109, 1988.

51. Vanderslice, J. T., Higgs, D. J., Hayes, J. M., and Block, G., Ascorbic acid and dehydroascorbic acid content of foods as eaten, *J. Food Comp. Anal.*, 3, 105, 1990.

52. Heiger, D. N., *High Performance Capillary Electrophoresis, An Introduction*, Hewlett-Packard GmbH, Waldbronn, Germany, 1992.

53. Davey, M. W., Bauw, G., and Van Montagu, M., Analysis of ascorbate in plant tissue by high performance capillary zone electrophoresis, *Anal. Biochem.*, 239, 8, 1996.

54. Bates, C. J., Plasma vitamin C assays: a European experience, *Int. J. Vit. Nutr. Res.*, 64, 283, 1994.

Table 6.2 Physical Properties of L-Ascorbic Acid and Related Compounds

1. Budavari, S., *The Merck Index*, 12th ed., Merck and Company, Whitehouse Station, NJ, 1996, 139.

2. Friedrich, W., Vitamin C, in *Vitamins*, Walter de Gruyter, Berlin, 1988, chap. 14.

3. Committee on Food Chemicals Codex, Food Chemicals Codex, 4th ed., National Academy of Sciences, Washington, DC, 1996, 33–34.

Table 6.3 Compendium, Regulatory and Handbook Methods of Analysis—Ascorbic Acid (Vitamin C)

1. United States Pharmacopeial Convention, *U.S. Pharmacopoeia National Formulary*, USP 23/NF 18, Nutritional Supplements, Official Monographs, United States Pharmacopoeial Convention, Inc., Rockville, MD, 1995.

2. Scottish Home and Health Department, *British Pharmacopoeia*, 15th ed., British Pharmacopoeic Commission, United Kingdom, 1993.

3. AOAC International, *Official Methods of Analysis*, 16th ed., AOAC International, Arlington, VA, 1995.

4. Deutsch, M.J., Assay for vitamin C: a collaborative study, *J. Assoc. Off. Anal. Chem.*, 50, 798, 1967.

5. Deutsch, M. J. and Weeks, C. E., Microfluorometric assay for vitamin C, *J. Assoc. Off. Anal. Chem.*, 48, 1248, 1965.

6. DeVries, J. W., Semiautomated fluorometric method for determination of vitamin C in foods: collaborative study, *J. Assoc. Off. Anal. Chem.*, 66, 1371, 1983.

7. Tanner, J. T. and Barnett, S. A., Methods of analysis for infant formula: Food and Drug Administration and Infant Formula Council collaborative study, *J. Assoc. Off. Anal. Chem.*, 68, 514, 1985.

8. American Association of Cereal Chemists, *AACC Approved Methods*, 9th ed., vol. 2, American Association of Cereal Chemists, St. Paul, MN, 1966.

9. Robinson, W. B. and Stotz, E., The indophenol-xylene extraction method for ascorbic acid and modifications for interfering substances, *J. Biol. Chem.*, 160, 217, 1945.

10. American Feed Ingredients Association, *Laboratory Methods Compendium,* vol. 1: *Vitamins and Minerals,* American Feed Ingredients Association, West Des Moines, IA, 61, 63.
11. Pongracz, G., Nue potentiometrische bestimmungsmethode für ascorbinsäure and deren verbindungen, *Fresn. Zeits. Anal. Chem.,* 253, 271, 1971.
12. Committee on Food Chemicals Codex, *Food Chemicals Codex,* 4th ed., National Academy of Sciences, Washington, DC, 1996, 33–34.
13. Keller, H. E., *Analytical Methods for Vitamins and Carotenoids,* Hoffmann-LaRoche, Basel, 1988, 20.

Table 6.4 Selected HPLC Methods for the Analysis of Ascorbic Acid Foods, Feeds, Pharmaceuticals, and Biologicals

Foods

1. Kutnink, M. A. and Omaya, S. T., Determination of ascorbic acid, erythorbic acid, and uric acid in cured meats by high-performance liquid chromatography, *J. Food Sci.,* 52, 53, 1987.
2. Speek, A. J., Schrijver, J., and Schreurs, W. H. P., Fluorometric determination of total vitamin C and total isovitamin C in foodstuffs and beverages by high-performance liquid chromatography with pre-column derivatization, *J. Agric. Food Chem.,* 32, 352, 1984.
3. Hägg, M., Ylikoski, S., and Kumpulainen, J., Vitamin C and α- and β-carotene contents in vegetables consumed in Finland during 1988–1989 and 1992–1993, *J. Food Comp. Anal.,* 7, 252, 1994.
4. Hägg, M., Ylikoski, S., and Kumpulainen, J., Vitamin C content in fruits and berries consumed in Finland, *J. Food Comp. Anal.,* 8, 12, 1995.
5. Vanderslice, J. T. and Higgs, D. J., HPLC analysis with fluorometric detection of vitamin C in food samples, *J. Chromatogr. Sci.,* 22, 485, 1984.
6. Vanderslice, J. T. and Higgs, D. J., Robotic extraction of vitamin C from food samples, *J. Micronutr. Anal.,* 1, 143, 1985.
7. Vanderslice, J. T. and Higgs, D. J., Chromatographic separation of ascorbic acid, isoascorbic acid, dehydroascorbic acid and dehydroisoascorbic acid and their quantitation in food products, *J. Micronutr. Anal.,* 4, 109, 1988.
8. Lloyd, L. L., Warner, F. P., Kennedy, J. F., and White, C. A., Ion suppression reversed-phase high-performance liquid chromatography method for the separation of L-ascorbic acid in fresh fruit juice, *J. Chromatogr.,* 437, 447, 1988.
9. Kim, H. J., Determination of total vitamin C by ion exclusion chromatography with electrochemical detection, *J. Assoc. Off. Anal. Chem.,* 72, 681, 1989.
10. Vanderslice, J. T. and Higgs, D. J., Separation of ascorbic acid, isoascorbic acid, dehydroascorbic acid and dehydroisoascorbic acid in food and animal tissues, *J. Micronutr. Anal.,* 7, 67, 1990.
11. Behrens, W. A. and Madère, R., Ascorbic and dehydroascorbic acid contents of canned food and frozen concentrated orange juice, *J. Food Comp. Anal.,* 3, 3, 1990.
12. Lloyd, L. L., Warner, F. P., Kennedy, J. F., and White, C. A., Quantitative analysis of vitamin C (L-ascorbic acid) by ion suppression reversed phase chromatography, *Food Chem.,* 28, 257, 1988.
13. Vanderslice, J. T., Higgs, D. J., Hayes, J. M., and Block, G., Ascorbic acid and dehydroascorbic acid content of foods-as-eaten, *J. Food Comp. Anal.,* 3, 105, 1990.
14. Dodson, K. Y., Young, E. R., and Soliman, A. G. M., Determination of total vitamin C in various food matrices by liquid chromatography and fluorescence detection, *J. AOAC Int.,* 75, 887, 1992.
15. Iwase, H., Determination of ascorbic acid in elemental diet by high-performance liquid chromatography with electrochemical detection, *J. Chromatogr.,* 606, 277, 1992.
16. Behrens, W. A. and Madère, R., Quantitative analysis of ascorbic acid and isoascorbic acid in foods by high-performance liquid chromatography with electrochemical detection, *J. Liq. Chromatogr.,* 15, 753, 1992.
17. Behrens, W. A. and Madère, R., Ascorbic acid, isoascorbic acid, dehydroascorbic acid in selected food products, *J. Food Comp. Anal.,* 7, 158, 1994.
18. Vanderslice, J. T. and Higgs, D. J., Quantitative determination of ascorbic, dehydroascorbic, isoascorbic, and dehydroisoascorbic acid by HPLC in foods and other matrices, *J. Nutr. Biochem.,* 4, 184, 1993.
19. Leubolt, R. and Klein, H., Determination of sulphite and ascorbic acid by high-performance liquid chromatography with electrochemical detection, *J. Chromatogr.,* 640, 271, 1993.

20. Iwase, H. and Ono, I., Determination of ascorbic acid and dehydroascorbic acid in juice by high-performance liquid chromatography with electrochemical detection using L-cysteine as precolumn reductant, *J. Chromatogr. A,* 654, 215, 1993.

21. Daood, H. G., Biacs, P. A., Dakar, M. A., and Hajdu, F., Ion-pair chromatography and photo diode-array detection of vitamin C and organic acids, *J. Chromatogr. Sci.,* 32, 481, 1994.

22. Behrens, W. A. and Madère, R., A procedure for the separation and quantitative analysis of ascorbic acid, dehydroascorbic acid, isoascorbic acid, and dehydroisoascorbic acid in food and animal tissue, *J. Liq. Chromatogr.,* 17, 2445, 1994.

23. Esteve, M. J., Farre, R., Frigola, A., Lopez, J. C., Romera, J. M., Ramirez, M., and Gil, A., Comparison of voltamic and high performance liquid chromatographic methods for ascorbic acid determination in infant formulas, *Food Chem.,* 52, 99, 1995.

24. Vinci, G., Botre, F., Mele, G., and Ruggieri, G., Ascorbic acid in exotic fruits: a liquid chromatographic investigation, *Food Chem.,* 53, 211, 1995.

25. Chen, X. and Sato, M., High performance liquid chromatographic determination of ascorbic acid in soft drinks and apple juice using Tris (2,2'-bipyridine) rutherium (II) electrochemiluminescence, *Anal. Sci.,* 11, 749, 1995.

26. Tausz, M., Kranner, I., and Grill, D., Simultaneous determination of ascorbic acid and dehydroascorbic acid in plant materials by high performance liquid chromatography, *Phytochem. Anal.,* 7, 69, 1996.

Feeds

1. Khaled, M. Y., Simultaneous HPLC analysis of L-ascorbic acid, L-ascorbyl-2-sulfate and L-ascorbyl-2-polyphosphate, *J. Liq. Chromatogr. Rel. Technol.,* 19, 3105, 1996.

Pharmaceuticals

1. Irache, J. M., Ezpeleta, I., and Vega, F. A., HPLC determination of antioxidant synergists and ascorbic acid in some fatty pharmaceuticals, cosmetics and food, *Chromatographia,* 35, 232, 1993.

Biologicals

1. Kutnink, M. A., Skala, J. H., Sauberlich, H. E., and Omaye, S. T., Simultaneous determination of ascorbic acid, isoascorbic acid (erythorbic acid) and uric acid in human plasma by high performance liquid chromatography with amperometric detection, *J. Liq. Chromatogr.,* 8, 31, 1985.

2. Washko, P. W., Hartzell, W. O., and Levine, M., Ascorbic acid analysis using high-performance liquid chromatography with coulometric electrochemical detection, *Anal. Biochem.,* 181, 276, 1989.

3. Capellmann, M. and Bolt, H. M., Simultaneous determination of ascorbic acid and dehydroascorbic acid by HPLC with postcolumn derivatization and fluorometric detection, *Fres. J. Anal. Chem.,* 342, 462, 1992.

4. Umegaki, K., Inoue, K., Takeuchi, N., and Higuchi, M., Improved method for the analysis of ascorbic acid in plasma by high-performance liquid chromatography with electrochemical detection, *J. Nutr. Sci. Vitaminol.,* 40, 73, 1994.

5. Lykkesfeldt, J., Loft, S., and Poulsen, H. E., Determination of ascorbic acid and dehydroascorbic acid in plasma by high-performance liquid chromatography with coulometric detection—are they reliable biomarkers of oxidative stress, *Anal. Biochem.,* 229, 329, 1995.

6. Rose, R. C. and Bode, A. M., Analysis of water-soluble antioxidants by high-pressure liquid chromatography, *Biochem. J.,* 306, 101, 1995.

7. Wang, S., Schram, I. M., and Sund, R. B., Determination of plasma ascorbic acid by HPLC: method and stability studies, *Eur. J. Pharm. Sci.,* 3, 231, 1995.

8. Konomi, N., Hiraki, S., Yano, H., and Hayasaka, S., Intracameral ascorbic acid, glutathione and protein levels in albino and pigmented rabbits, *Ophthal. Res.,* 27, 347, 1995.

9. Margolis, S. A. and Schapira, R. M., Liquid chromatographic measurement of L-ascorbic acid and D-ascorbic acid in biological samples, *J. Chromatogr. B,* 690, 25, 1997.

Table 6.5   Newer Approaches to Vitamin C Analysis—Non-Traditional Methods

Flow Injection

1. Vanderslice, J. T. and Higgs, D. J., Automated analysis of total vitamin C in foods, *J. Micronutr. Anal.,* 6, 109, 1989.
2. Albero, M. I., Garcia, M. S., Sanchez-Pedreño, C., and Rodriguez, J., Determination of ascorbic acid in pharmaceuticals and urine by reverse flow injection, *Analyst,* 117, 1635, 1992.
3. Alamo, J. M., Maquierira, A., Puchades, R., and Sagrado, S., Determination of titratable acidity and ascorbic acid in fruit juices in continuous-flow systems, *Fres. J. Anal. Chem.,* 347, 293, 1993.
4. Alwarthan, A. A., Determination of ascorbic acid by flow injection with chemiluminescence detection, *Analyst,* 118, 639, 1993.
5. Sultan, S. M., Abdennabi, A. M., and Suliman, F. E. O., Flow injection colorimetric method for the assay of vitamin C in drug formulations using tris, 1-10-phenanthroline-iron (III) complex as an oxidant in sulfuric acid media, *Talanta,* 41, 125, 1994.
6. Jain, A., Chaurasia, A., and Verma, K. K., Determination of ascorbic acid in soft drinks, preserved fruit juices and pharmaceuticals by flow injection spectrophotometry: matrix absorbance correction by treatment with sodium hydroxide, *Talanta,* 42, 779, 1995.
7. Huang, H., Cai, R., Du, Y., and Zeng, Y., Flow-injection stopped-flow spectrofluorimetric kinetic determination of total ascorbic acid based on an enzyme-linked coupled reaction, *Anal. Chim. Acta,* 309, 271, 1995.
8. Péréz-Ruíz, T., Martínez-Lozano, C., and Sanz, A., Flow-injection chemiluminometric determination of ascorbic acid based on its sensitized photooxidation, *Anal. Chim. Acta,* 308, 299, 1995.
9. Leon, L. E., Amperometric flow-injection method for the assay of L-ascorbic acid based on the photochemical reduction of Methylene Blue, *Talanta,* 43, 1275, 1996.
10. Nobrega, J. A. and Lopes, G. S., Flow-injection spectrophotometric determination of ascorbic acid in pharmaceutical products with the Prussian Blue reaction, *Talanta,* 43, 971, 1996.
11. Pérez-Ruíz, T., Martínez-Lozano, C., Tomás, V., and Sidrach, C., Flow injection fluorimetric determination of ascorbic acid based on its photooxidation by thionine blue, *Analyst,* 122, 115, 1997.

Spectrophotometric

1. Tsumura, F., Ohsako, Y., Haraguchi, Y., Kumagai, H., Sakurai, H., and Ishii, K., Rapid enzymatic assay for ascorbic acid in various foods using peroxidase, *J. Food Sci.,* 58, 619, 1993.
2. Jung, M. Y., Kim, S. K., and Kim, S. Y., Riboflavin-sensitized photooxidation of ascorbic acid: kinetics and amino acid effects, *Food Chem.,* 53, 397, 1995.
3. Jung, M. Y., Kim, S. K., and Kim, S. Y., Riboflavin-sensitized photodynamic UV spectrophotometry for ascorbic acid assay in beverages, *J. Food Sci.,* 60, 360, 1995.
4. Moeslinger, T., Brunner, M., and Spieckermann, P. G., Spectrophotometric determination of dehydroascorbic acid in biological samples, *Anal. Biochem.,* 221, 290, 1994.
5. Özgür, M. U. and Sungur, S., Third order derivative spectrophotometric determination of ascorbic acid in fruits and vegetables, *Talanta,* 42, 1631, 1995.
6. Arya, S. P. and Mahajan, M., A rapid and sensitive method for the determination of ascorbic acid using Fe (III)—ferronate complex, *Anal. Sci.,* 11, 853, 1995.
7. Lee, W., Roberts, S. M., and Labbe, R. F., Ascorbic acid determination with an automated enzymatic procedure, *Clin. Chem.,* 43, 154, 1997.

Capillary Electrophoresis

1. Lin Ling, B., Baeyens, W. R. G., Van Acker, P., and Dewaele, C., Determination of ascorbic acid and isoascorbic acid by capillary zone electrophoresis: application to fruit juices and to a pharmaceutical formulation, *J. Pharm. Biomed. Anal.,* 10, 717, 1992.
2. Koh, G. V., Bissell, M. G., and Ito, R. K., Measurement of vitamin C by capillary electrophoresis in biological fluids and fruit beverages using a stereoisomer as an internal standard, *J. Chromatogr.,* 633, 245, 1993.
3. Chiari, M., Nesi, M., Carrea, G., and Righetti, P. G., Determination of total vitamin C in fruits by capillary zone electrophoresis, *J. Chromatogr.,* 645, 197, 1993.

4. Wu, C. H., Lo, Y. S., Lee, Y. H., and Lin, T. I., Capillary electrophoretic determination of organic acids with indirect detection, *J. Chromatogr. A,* 716, 291, 1995.
5. Davey, M. W., Bauw, G., and Van Montagu, M., Analysis of ascorbate in plant tissues by high performance capillary zone electrophoresis, *Anal. Biochem.,* 239, 8, 1996.

Miscellaneous

Circular Dichroism—
1. Purdie, N. and Swallows, K. A., Direct determination of water-soluble vitamins by circular dichroism, *J. Agric. Food Chem.,* 39, 2171, 1991.

Stripping Voltammetry—
1. Guanghan, L., Yu, W., Leiming, Y., and Shuanglong, H., Determination of ascorbic acid in fruits and vegetables by stripping voltammetry on a glassy carbon electrode, *Food Chem.,* 51, 237, 1994.

Chemiluminescence—
1. Lewin, G. and Popov, I., Photochemiluminescent detection of antiradical activity; III: a simple assay of ascorbate in blood plasma, *J. Biochem. Biophys. Meth.,* 28, 277, 1994.

Isotope Ratio—
1. Gensler, M., Rossmann, A., and Schmidt, H. J., Detection of added L-ascorbic acid in fruit juices by isotope ratio mass spectrometry, *J. Agric. Food Chem.,* 43, 2662, 1995.

Differential Pulse Polarography—
1. Esteve, M. J., Farre, R., and Frigola, A., Determination of ascorbic acid in asparagus by differential pulse polarography, *Fres. J. Anal. Chem.,* 351, 804, 1995.

Microtiter plate—
1. Wei, Y., Ota, R. B., Bowen, H. T., and Omaye, S. T., Determination of human plasma and leukocyte ascorbic acid by microtiter plate assay, *Nutr. Biochem.,* 7, 179, 1996.

7 Thiamin

7.1 REVIEW

Thiamin was isolated and characterized in 1926. It was the first of the water-soluble vitamins structurally characterized and was formally given the designation vitamin B_1 in 1927 by the British Medical Research Council. Descriptions of beriberi, the principle form of thiamin deficiency, were recorded centuries earlier, and associations of the deficiency to diets high in polished rice were made before the 20th century. Beriberi was epidemic in populations consuming polished rice as a dietary staple until rice fortification became a common practice. Thiamin deficiency occurs as a marginal deficiency and in the more extreme states of beriberi and Wernicke-Korsakoff's syndrome. Marginal deficiency is characterized by fatigue, irritability, and lack of concentration. Beriberi, resulting from prolonged, low dietary intake, includes dry beriberi (muscle wasting with heart involvement, hypotension, sodium retention, tachycardia and pulmonary edema), and wet beriberi (edema, anorexia, muscle weakness, ataxia, and peripheral paralysis). Infantile beriberi which can be quickly fatal is characterized by vomiting, convulsions, abdominal distention, and anorexia. Infantile beriberi can result in heart failure.[1] Wernicke-Korsakoff syndrome is a severe deficiency state characterized by mental disorder, including confusion, hallucinosis, psychosis, and coma. It is frequently seen in alcoholics after long periods of alcohol intake without food intake. Clinically, thiamin status is indicated by measurement of urinary excretion of thiamin and erythrocyte transketolase activity. Transketolase requires thiamin pyrophosphate (TPP) and is a highly reliable measure of thiamin status. Serum, erythrocyte, and blood thiamin levels are insensitive thiamin status indices.[2]

Dietary sources considered to be primary sources to the human include unrefined cereal grains, legumes, nuts, and pork which is higher in thiamin content than most muscle foods. In developed countries, severe thiamin deficiency is rare; however, marginal deficiency is documented more frequently. Situations that can lead to marginal deficiency include pregnancy and lactation, heavy physical work, regular heavy alcohol intake, high carbohydrate intake, and various disease states.[2] Recommended Dietary Allowances (RDAs) for thiamin are based upon a calorie intake relationship of 0.5 mg/1000 kcal and a minimum intake of 1.0 mg/day for individuals consuming low calorie diets containing less than 2000 kcal/day.[1] RDAs range from 1.0 to 1.1 mg for women and 1.2 to 1.5 mg for men. The RDA for infants less than six months old is 0.3 mg. RDAs are increased to 1.5 mg for pregnant women and to 1.6 mg for lactating women. The Nutritional Labeling and Education Act of 1990 (NLEA) specifies a Reference Daily Intake (RDI) of 1.5 mg for use in nutritional labeling.[3]

Thiamin exists naturally as free thiamin and phosphorylated as thiamin monophosphate (TMP), thiamin diphosphate or thiamin pyrophosphate (TPP), and thiamin triphosphate (TTP). All forms exist in animal and plant tissue although plant tissue contains higher levels of the free vitamin than found in animal tissue. TPP is one of the principle cofactors for decarboxylation of α-keto acids characterized by the pyruvate dehydrogenase complex's role in synthesis of acetyl-CoA from pyruvate in the TCA cycle. TPP also functions as the cofactor for the transketolase reaction in the pentose phosphate pathway. The transketolase reaction transfers a two-carbon fragment from xylulose-5-phosphate to ribose-5-phosphate, forming glyceraldehyde-3-phosphate and the seven-carbon sugar, sedoheptulose-7-phosphate. TPP plays a central role in metabolism and is essential to normal carbohydrate, nucleic acid, and amino acid metabolism. TPP and other thiamin phosphorylated esters function in nerve impulse transmission. The exact role of thiamin in neurotransmission is unknown; however, TPP is involved in synthesis of acetyl choline, a primary neurotransmitter.

7.2 PROPERTIES

7.2.1 CHEMISTRY

7.2.1.1 General Properties

The structure of thiamin in the free base form is given in Figure 7.1. The vitamin is characterized by a pyrimidine ring (4' amino-2'-methylpyrimidinyl-5'-ylmethyl) linked by a methylene bridge to the 3-nitrogen atom in a substituted thiazole (5-(2-hydroxyethyl)-4-methyl-thiazole). Conversion of thiamin to TMP, TPP, and TTP is shown in Figure 7.2. Thiamin hydrochloride ($C_{12}H_{18}ON_4SCl_2$) and thiamin mononitrate ($C_{12}H_{17}O_4N_5S$) are the commercially available forms used in pharmaceuticals and for food fortification (Figure 7.2). Thiamin hydrochloride is the USP reference standard. Physical properties of the thiamin salt and naturally occurring phosphorylated forms are given in Table 7.1. Thiamin hydrochloride is a white crystalline powder with a yeast-like odor and salty, nut-like taste.[4] The most distinguishing difference between the hydrochloride salt and the mononitrate is water-solubility. The hydrochloride is soluble in water (1 g/mL) and the mononitrate is only slightly water-soluble (0.027 g/mL). This solubility difference leads to differentiation in industrial uses for the two thiamin forms. The hydrochloride salt is used in injectable and parenteral pharmaceuticals and for fortification of foods requiring solubility. The lower hydroscopicity of the mononitrate makes it ideal for use in dry blends, multivitamins, and dry products such as enriched flour.[5] Thiamin hydrochloride is nearly insoluble in methanol, ethanol, and glycerol. It is insoluble in ether, acetone, benzene, hexane, and chloroform.

7.2.1.2 Spectral Properties

Thiamin hydrochloride absorbs in the region of 200 to 300 nm. Absorption maxima vary with the pH of the solution. At pH 2.9, a single maxima is present at 246 nm. At pH levels above 5 but below neutrality, two absorption maxima exist at 234 nm and 264 nm, representing the pyrimidine and thiazole rings, respectively.[6] Characteristic absorption spectra are given in Figure 7.3.I. The $E_{1cm}^{1\%}$ values in phosphate buffer at 246 nm (pH 2.9), 234 nm (pH 5.5), and 264 nm (pH 5.5) are 425, 345, and 255, respectively (Table 7.1).

Oxidation of thiamin or its phosphate esters with alkaline potassium ferricyanide or cyanogen bromide quantitatively forms thiochrome (Thc), thiochrome monophosphate (ThcMP), thiochrome pyrophosphate (ThcPP), and thiochrome triphosphate (ThcTP) (Figure 7.4). At alkaline pH above 8.0, thiochrome products have excitation maxima at 375 nm and emission maxima at 432 to 435 nm

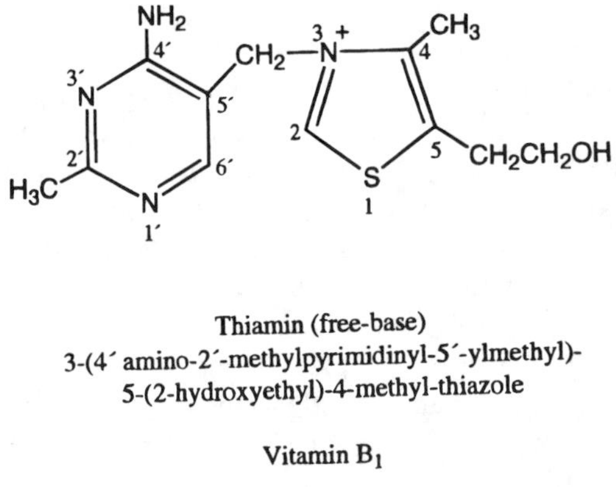

Thiamin (free-base)
3-(4´ amino-2´-methylpyrimidinyl-5´-ylmethyl)-
5-(2-hydroxyethyl)-4-methyl-thiazole

Vitamin B$_1$

FIGURE 7.1   Structure of thiamin.

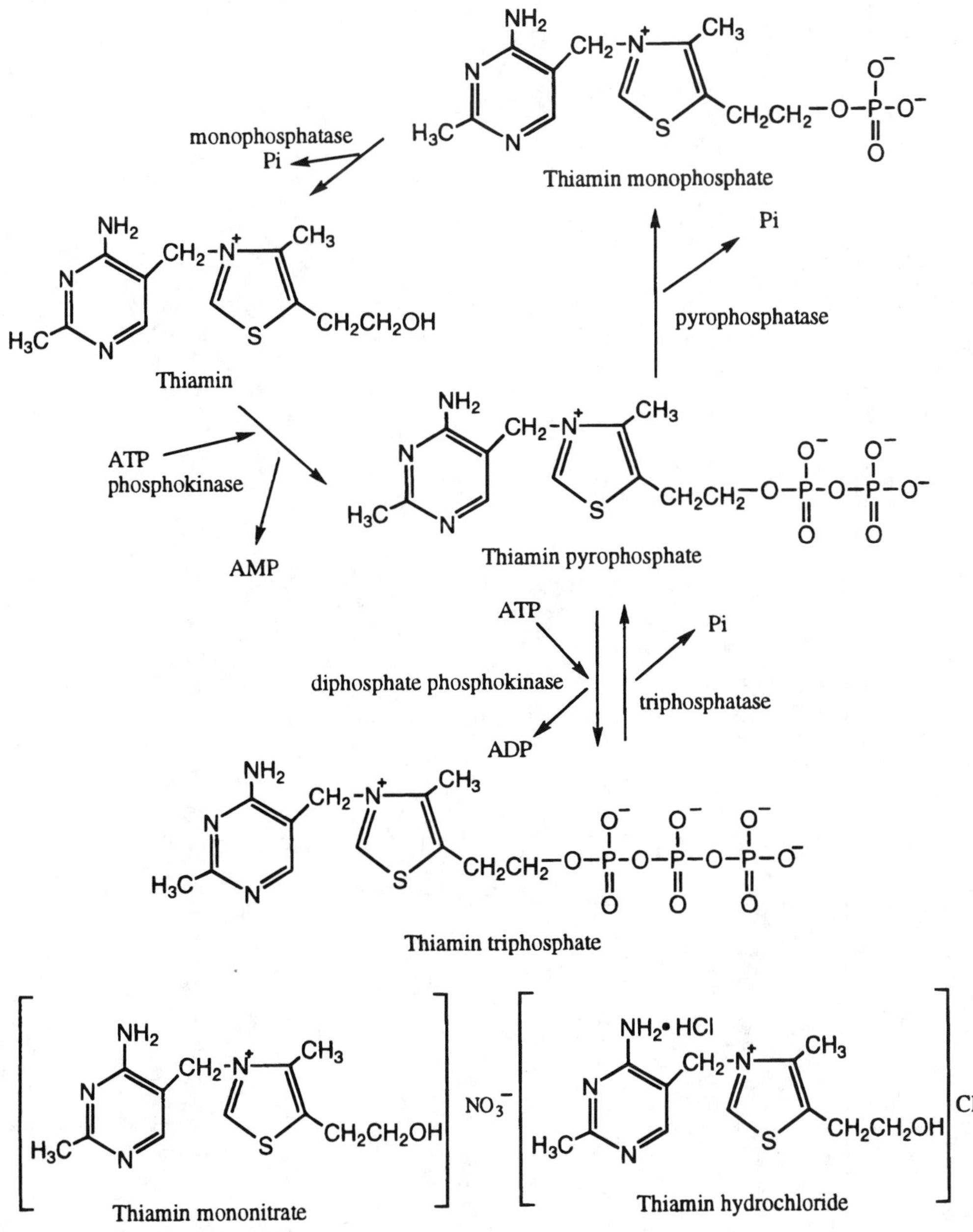

FIGURE 7.2   Structures of thiamin and related compounds.

(strong blue fluorescence) (Figure 7.3.II).[7,8] These highly fluorescent oxidation products are the basis of the thiochrome procedure for thiamin quantitation.[4] Thiochrome analysis has been used to develop most of the analytical data available on the thiamin content of the food supply.[9] Since thiamin does not fluoresce, development of the thiochrome analysis in the 1930s provided a highly specific method for thiamin quantitation from most matrices.

TABLE 7.1
Physical Properties of Thiamin Salts

Substance[a]	Molar Mass	Formula	Solubility	Crystal Form	Melting Point °C	λ max nm	Absorbance[b] $E_{1\,cm}^{1\%}$	$\epsilon \times 10^{-3}$
Thiamin hydrochloride CAS No. 67-03-5 **9430**	337.26	$C_{12}H_{17}ClN_4OS \cdot HCl$	Water—1.0 g/mL Ethanol (95%)— 1.0 g/100 mL Ethanol (100%)— 0.3 g/100 mL Glycerol—5 g/100 mL Insol. in ether, benzene, hexane, chloroform	White crystalline powder, colorless, monoclinic, needles	246–250 (dec.)	246[c] 234[d] 264[d]	425 345 255	[14.3] [11.6] [8.6]
Thiamin mononitrate CAS No. 532-43-4 **9430**	327.37	$C_{12}H_{17}N_5O_4S$	Water—2.7 g/100 mL	White to yellow, white crystals	196–200 (dec.)			
Thiamin monophosphate CAS No. 532-40-1 **9431**	344.33	$C_{12}H_{17}N_4O_4PS$						
Thiamin pyrophosphate CAS No. 157-87-0 **9431**	424.31	$C_{12}H_{18}N_4O_7P_2S$			(Tetrahydrate form) 220–222 (dec.)			
Thiamin triphosphate CAS No. 3475-65-8	504.29	$C_{12}H_{19}N_4O_{10}P_3S$			(Hydrochloride form) 228–232 (dec.)			

[a] Common or generic name; CAS No.–Chemical Abstract Service number, bold print designates the Merck Index monograph number.
[b] Values in brackets are calculated from corresponding $E_{1\,cm}^{1\%}$ values.
[c] In 0.1 M phosphate buffer, pH 2.9.
[d] In 0.1 M phosphate buffer, pH 5.5.

Ball, G. F. M., Water-Soluble Vitamin Assays in Human Nutrition.[1]
Budavari, S. The Merck Index.[2]
Ellefson, W. C., Methods of Vitamin Assay.[3]

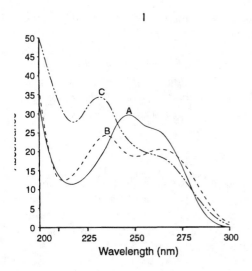

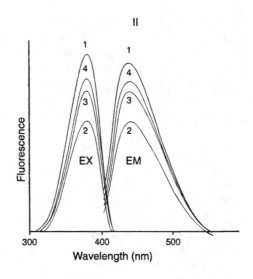

FIGURE 7.3.I Absorption spectra of thiamin at pH 10.6 (broken line), thiamin hydrochloride at pH 2.9 (solid line), and pH 5.5 (dashed line). Spectra reproduced with permission from References 4 and 6; λ max, A = 246 nm; B and C = 234 nm.

FIGURE 7.3.II Fluorescence excitation and emission spectra of Thc (1), ThcMP (2), ThcPP (3) and ThcTP (4). Modified from Reference 8.

7.2.2 STABILITY

Thiamin is one of the least stable of the water-soluble vitamins when the pH of the matrix approaches neutrality. Maximum stability in solution is between pH 2.0 to 4.0. Therefore, in low-acid foods, the vitamin is highly susceptible to losses during thermal processing.[9] Thiamin is highly unstable at alkaline pH. Stability is dependent upon the extent of heating and on the food matrix characteristics. Thermal degradation occurs even under slightly acid conditions. Dwivedi and Arnold[10] found that thermal degradation was primarily due to scission of the methylene bridge yielding pyrimidine and thiazole. Further destruction of thiazole liberates hydrogen sulfide. Both reactions are influenced by oxidation–reduction, inorganic bases (sulfites and bisulfites), metal complexes, radiation, and thiaminases with pH being the controlling factor. Ball[6] reported that alkaline pH during cooking or processing leads to extensive thiamin losses. Use of baking powder in cake mixes was mentioned as an example where 50% or higher loss can occur. Thiamin is destroyed in chocolate, baked products.

Thiochrome Reaction

$$CH_3-C \overset{N}{\underset{N}{\underset{\overset{|}{C}}{\cdots}}} C-NH_2 \quad HC \overset{S}{\underset{C-CH_2-N}{\cdots}} C-C_2H_4OH \quad \xrightarrow[\substack{CNBr \\ OH}]{\substack{Fe(CN)_6^{\equiv} \\ HgCl_2 \\ or}} \quad CH_3 \cdots C \overset{N}{\underset{N}{\cdots}} \overset{N}{\underset{\overset{|}{C}}{\cdots}} \overset{S}{\underset{C-CH_2-N}{\cdots}} C-C_2H_4OH$$

Thiamin   Thiochrome

FIGURE 7.4 Thiochrome reaction.

Thiaminase is present in unprocessed foods of plant and animal origin. Thiamin degradation occurs either by nucleophilic displacement of the methylene of the pyrimidine or by hydrolysis of thiamin into thiazole and pyrimidine.[11] Thiaminase reactions are initiated by bruising, blending or homogenization, or other processes that break tissue structure. Sulfhydryl groups and other reducing agents usually protect thiamin from thiaminase action. Degradation of thiamin in the presence of sulfite proceeds through cleavage of the methylene bridge similar to degradation at alkaline pH. Use of sulfite as a food processing aid to inhibit browning reactions can lead to extensive losses.

7.3 METHODS

Current methods for thiamin analysis include the classic thiochrome methods, microbiological analysis, and HPLC procedures. The following section provides pertinent information on each of these approaches. Reviews available on thiamin assay procedures include Ellfeson,[4] Kawasaki,[8] Ottaway,[5] Eitenmiller and Landen,[9] and Fayol.[12] Many of the standard procedures are available in various compendiums and handbooks. These methods are summarized in Table 7.2.

7.3.1 CHEMICAL

The thiochrome reaction (Figure 7.4) has been used since its development in 1935[11] for analysis of thiamin from biological matrices. In the absence of other fluorescent compounds that can interfere with the assay, the fluorescence intensity of thiochrome is proportional to the total thiamin in the sample.[4] Thiochrome is used as the determinative step in USP methods for pharmaceuticals,[13] AOAC International Official Methods,[14] American Association of Cereal Chemists Approved Methods,[15] and as suggested methods for feeds and premixes.[16] Procedural descriptions of AOAC International Methods, because of their world-wide influence, are given below.

AOAC Official Method 942.23, Thiamin (Vitamin B$_1$) in Foods, Fluorometric Method, *AOAC Official Methods of Analysis*, 45.1.05

The method includes the following steps:

1. Acid Hydrolysis

Samples are hydrolyzed with 0.1 N HCl for 30 min at 95 to 100°C or autoclaved at 121°C for 30 min. Most thiamin procedures use HCl hydrolysis because the vitamin is stable under the acidic environment. The hydrolysis breaks protein complexes and effectively liberates thiamin from cellular material in most sample matrices.

2. Enzyme Hydrolysis

An aliquot of the acid hydrolysate is adjusted to pH 4.0 to 4.5 with 2 N sodium acetate. Phosphorylated thiamin esters are converted to free thiamin using takadiastase, Mylase 100 (U.S. Biochemical Corporation), or α-amylase. The digest is incubated at 45 to 50°C for three hours.

The products of the phosphate esters are insoluble in isobutanol used in the subsequent extraction step and complete conversion must be assured.[4] Proper selection of the phosphatase source, therefore, is a significant but often slighted part of the procedure. Studies by Hasselmann et al.[17] found that a mixture of β-amylase and takadiastase was satisfactory for thiamin hydrolysis. β-amylase, alone, did not produce complete dephosphorylation. Suitability of the enzyme for hydrolysis of thiamin phosphate esters can be determined by digesting a thiamin phosphate standard and comparing the digest to a thiamin reference standard.[4] A 3 h incubation period is considered sufficient for total hydrolysis when the enzyme has high, documented phosphatase activity.[18]

3. Extract Clean Up

The digest is adjusted to pH 3.5, filtered, and an aliquot containing approximately 5 mg thiamin is passed through an absorption column filled with a 100 mm bed of Bio-Rex 70 (Hydrogen form) (Bio Rad Laboratories) to remove possible interfering compounds. Decalso® was formally used as the support, but became unavailable in the 1970s. Bio-Rex 70 was chosen as the replacement. Reversed-phase C_{18} open-column chromatography was reported to be equivalent to Bio-Rex 70 for extract clean up.[19] The C_{18} clean up requires elution with cold 3% KCl-methanol (70 : 30) which is easier to work with than the boiling acid-KCl solution required for elution from Bio-Rex 70.

4. Thiochrome Formation

An aliquot of the purified extract is oxidized with 1% potassium ferricyanide in 15% sodium hydroxide. Thiochrome is extracted with isobutanol and quantitated fluorometrically. The blank in the manual thiochrome procedure is produced by eliminating the oxidation step. This blank does not account for fluorescence developed during the oxidation.[20] Several studies have been completed to improve the blank determination. Leveille[21] used benzenesulfonyl chloride (BSC) to inhibit thiochrome formation in the presence of potassium ferricyanide. His procedure for urine analysis eliminated the column chromatography and isobutanol extraction by use of a BSC-treated sample to correct for blank fluorescence. Soliman[20] adapted the BSC technique to food analysis using a semi-automated technique. The method has been used by the Atlanta Center for Nutrient Analysis, FDA, for a large variety of sample matrices.

AOAC Official Method 953.17, Thiamin (Vitamin B₁) in Grain Products, Fluorometric (Rapid Method), *AOAC Official Methods of Analysis,* 45.1.06

Method 953.17 is used for enriched products where natural ester forms of thiamin make up a negligible amount of the total thiamin. It is only applicable to enriched grain products since the enzyme digestion and Bio-Rex 70 purification steps are eliminated. The method should not be used until the amount of phosphorylated forms are verified to be negligible when compared to the amount of thiamin hydrochloride added through enrichment.[9] For flour, a non-enriched product can be used for comparative assays.

AOAC Official Method 957.17, Thiamin (Vitamin B₁) in Bread, Fluorometric Method, *AOAC Official Methods of Analysis,* 45.1.07

Method 957.17 was originally designated for the analysis of air-dried bread. All steps are essentially the same as Method 957.17. The AOAC Task Force on Methods for Nutrition Labeling recommended the method for assay of beverages, juices, fruits, dairy products, fish, and shellfish.[22] The AOAC Official Methods of Analysis, 16th ed. (1995)[14] states that the method is applicable to all foods.

AOAC Official Method 986.27, Thiamin (Vitamin B₁) in Milk-Based Infant Formula, Fluorometric Method, *AOAC Official Methods of Analysis,* 50.1.08

Method 986.27 is identical to Method 942.23. The AOAC Task Force on Methods for Nutrient Labeling recommended the method for assay of all foods.[22]

7.3.2 MICROBIOLOGICAL

Microbiological analysis provided some of the earliest methods to assay thiamin from biological matrices. *Lactobacillus fermenti* was originally used, but problems with specificity limited its

TABLE 7.2
Compendium, Regulatory, and Handbook Methods for the Analysis of Thiamin

Source	Form	Methods and Application	Approach	Most Current Cross-Reference
U.S. Pharmacopeia *National Formulary*, 1995, USP 23/NF 18, Nutritional Supplements Official Monographs[1]				
1. pages 2143, 2146, 2148, 2153	Thiamin Thiamin hydrochloride	Thiamin in oil- and water-soluble vitamin capsules/tablets w/wo minerals	HPLC 280 m	None
2. pages 2162, 2168, 2170, 2172	Thiamin Thiamin hydrochloride	Thiamin in water-soluble vitamin capsules/tablets w/wo minerals	HPLC 280 nm	None
3. page 1530	Thiamin Thiamin hydrochloride	Thiamin hydrochloride (NLT 98.0%, NMT 102.0%)	HPLC 254 nm	None
4. pages 1530–1531	Thiamin Thiamin hydrochloride	Thiamin hydrochloride Elixir/injection	HPLC 254 nm	None
5. pages 1531, 1571	Thiamin Thiamin hydrochloride	Thiamin hydrochloride tablets	Thiochrome Fluorometric Ex λ = 365 Em λ = 435	None
6. page 1532	Thiamin mononitrate	Thiamin mononitrate (NLT 98.0%, NMT 102.0%);	HPLC 254 nm	None
7. page 1532	Thiamin mononitrate	Thiamin mononitrate elixir	HPLC 254 nm	None
British Pharmacopoeia, 15th ed., 1993[2]				
vol. 1, pages 664–665	Thiamin hydrochloride	Thiamin hydrochloride	Potentiometric	None
vol. 1, page 665	Thiamin mononitrate	Thiamin nitrate	Titration	None
vol. 2, page 1128	Thiamin hydrochloride	Thiamin injection	HPLC 244 nm	None

AOAC Official Methods of Analysis, 16th ed., 1995[3]				
1. 45.1.05	Thiamin Thiamin hydrochloride	AOAC Official Method 942.23, Thiamin (Vitamin B_1) in Foods	Thiochrome Fluorescence Ex λ = 365 Em λ = 435	*J. Assoc. Off. Anal. Chem.*, 64, 1336, 1981[4]
2. 45.1.06	Thiamin Thiamin hydrochloride	AOAC Official Method 953.17, Thiamin (Vitamin B_1) in Grain Products	Thiochrome Fluorescence Ex λ = 365 Em λ = 435	*J. Assoc. Off. Anal. Chem.*, 36, 837, 1953[5]; 37, 122, 1954[6]; 37, 154, 1954[7]; 38, 722, 1955[8]
3. 45.1.07	Thiamin Thiamin hydrochloride	AOAC Official Method 957.17, Thiamin (Vitamin B_1) in Bread	Thiochrome Fluorescence Ex λ = 365 Em λ = 435	*J. Assoc. Off. Anal. Chem.*, 40, 843, 1957[9]; 41, 603, 1958[10]; 43, 47, 1960[11]
4. 50.1.08	Thiamin Thiamin hydrochloride	AOAC Official Method 986.27, Thiamin (Vitamin B_1) in Milk-Based Infant Formula	Thiochrome Fluorescence Ex λ = 365 Em λ = 435	*J. Assoc. Off. Anal. Chem.*, 69, 777, 1986[12]
American Association of Cereal Chemists, 1996, *Approved Methods*, vol. 2[13]				
AACC 86–80	Thiamin Thiamin hydrochloride	Thiamin in complete feeds (> 0.4 mg/kg)	Thiochrome Fluorescence Ex λ = 370 Em λ = 430	*AOAC Official Methods of Analysis*, 16th ed., 1995[3]
American Feed Ingredients Association, *Laboratory Methods Compendium*, vol. 1, 1991[14] pages 145–148	Thiamin Thiamin hydrochloride	Thiamin in bread, wheat, rice, corn grits, corn meal, puffed cereal, farina and flour	Thiochrome Fluorescence Ex λ = 365 Em λ = 435	*Cereal Chem.*, 35, 1, 1958[15]

TABLE 7.2 Continued

Source	Form	Methods and Application	Approach	Most Current Cross-Reference
Food Chemicals Codex, 4th ed., 1996[16]				
1. pages 411–412	Thiamin hydrochloride	Thiamin hydrochloride (NLT 98.0%, NMT 102.0%)	HPLC 254 nm	None
2. page 412	Thiamin mononitrate	Thiamin mononitrate (NLT 98.0%, NMT 102.0%)	HPLC 254 nm	None
Hoffmann-LaRoche, *Analytical Methods for Vitamins and Carotenoids in Feed*, 1988[17]				
1. pages 23–26	Thiamin and its phosphate esters	Determination of vitamin B$_1$ in complete feeds (< 4 mg/kg)	Thiochrome Fluorescence Ex λ = 370 Em λ = 430	*Handbuch der Lebensmittel-Chemie*, vol. 2, part 2, Springer Verlag, Berlin, 1967, 721[18]
2. pages 27–29	Thiamin and its phosphate esters	Determination of vitamin B$_1$ in complete feeds and premixes	Thiochrome Fluorescence Ex λ = 378 Em λ = 430	
Methods for the Determination of Vitamins in Foods, COST 91, 1985[19]	Thiamin and its phosphate esters	Thiamin in foods	Thiochrome Ex λ = 378 Em λ = 430	*J. Assoc. Off. Anal. Chem.*, 64, 616, 1981[20]

use. The organism is susceptible to both stimulatory and inhibitory matrix effects. Responses are reported for pentoses, reducing agents, fructose, maltose, calcium, and glucose heat degradation products.[17, 23] Deibel et al.[24] introduced *Lactobacillus viridescens* (ATCC 12706) as an improved assay for thiamin. *L. viridescens* is much more specific for thiamin, requiring intact thiamin for growth. The organism is not as subject to matrix effects as *L. fermenti*. Table 7.3 summarizes responses of several bacteria and protozoans used in the past for thiamin assay. Analytical data obtained from the *L. viridescens* assay corresponds closely to properly run thiochrome assays. The organism is widely accepted for food analysis.[9] AOAC International does not provide an official microbiological assay for thiamin. The *L. viridescens* assay was recommended for collaboration,[22] but, at the present, the collaborative study has not been completed.

Extraction procedures for the microbiological analysis of thiamin generally follow the thiochrome analysis procedures (AOAC International Method 942.23). Enzyme hydrolysis of the phosphate esters is necessary to avoid differential growth response to TMP, TPP, and TTP.

7.3.3   High Performance Liquid Chromatography

For the past 25 years, HPLC has been commonly used for the analysis of thiamin. Reviews on HPLC methodology include those given in Section 7.3. Table 7.4 provides details on selected papers that provide a historical perspective of method development and recent research approaches. Because thiamin and riboflavin can be conveniently assayed concurrently or simultaneously, many methods are available to assay the two vitamins from the same extract. These procedures are discussed in Chapter 8.

7.3.3.1   Extraction Procedures for Thiamin by HPLC

Extraction protocols depend on the investigator's need to quantitate total thiamin or thiamin and the phosphate esters. To assay total thiamin, the extraction must liberate thiamin from the sample matrix and hydrolyze the esters. Such extractions use acid and enzyme hydrolysis that closely follow AOAC International Method 942.23. Recently, two multilaboratory studies were conducted that gave extraction parameters for the concurrent extraction of thiamin and riboflavin. In a French study conducted by the Commission Generale d'Unification des Methods d'Analysis,[25] a procedure originally reported by Hasselmann et al.[17] was used. Hydrolysis with 0.1 N HCl was followed by enzyme digestion with a combination of β-amylase and takadiastase. The method gave high recoveries except for chocolate powder which required an increase in HCl concentration to 0.5 N to obtain reliable results.

The European Union Measurement and Testing Program recently published details of an optimal extraction procedure developed from earlier studies.[26] Steps in the extraction were the following:

1. Autoclave a 0.2 to 5 g sample in 0.1 N HCl for 30 min at 121°C. Sample size and volume were chosen by laboratories in the study.

TABLE 7.3
Responses Induced by Thiamin and Related Compounds Relative to thiamin[a]

Organism	Thiamin	Pyrimidine	Thiazole	TPP
Lactobacillus viridescens	1.0	0	0	1.0
Saccharomyces cerevisiae	1.0	0	0	0.7
Ochromonas malhamensis	1.0	0	0	1.0
Lactobacillus fermenti	1.0	0[b]	0[b]	0.3

[a]Table adapted from Reference 23.
[b]Response after long incubation periods.

TABLE 7.4

HPLC Methods for the Analysis of Thiamin in Foods, Feed, Pharmaceuticals, and Biologicals

		Sample Preparation			HPLC Parameters			
Sample Matrix	Analyte	Sample Extraction	Clean Up	Column	Mobile Phase	Detection	Quality Assurance Parameters	References
Foods								
1. Cereals, urine	Thiamin	Add 0.1 N HCl 1 g sample/100 mL Autoclave, 30 min Centrifuge	C_{18} disposable columns Elute thiamin with 5 mM NH$_4$H$_2$O$_4$, pH 2.8 : MeCN : H3PO$_4$ (3.9 : 1 : 0.1) Inject eluate	MicroPak AX-5 5 μm 30 cm × 4.6 mm	Isocratic 5 mM NH$_4$H$_2$PO$_4$, pH 2.85 0.5 mL/min, 30°C	245 nm	—	*J. Chromatogr.*, 231, 433, 1982[1]
2. Rice flour	Thiamin	Takadiastase digestion Centrifuge	—	Nucleosil C_{18} 5 μm 15 cm × 4 mm	Isocratic 0.01 M NaH$_2$PO$_4$ and 0.15 Na perchlorate, pH 2.2, 0.6 mL/min	Thiochrome Post-column Fluorescence Ex λ = 375 Em λ = 435	—	*J. Chromatogr.*, 284, 281, 1984[2]
3. Various foods	Thiamin, TMP, TPP, TTP	Add amprolium (IS) Homogenize with 5% sulfosalicylic acid Centrifuge Filter water layer	AG2-X8 Anion exchange	Perkin Elmer C_{18} 3 μm 30 cm × 3 mm	Gradient 0.1 M Na$_3$PO$_4$, pH 5.5 6.0 min 0.1 M Na$_3$PO$_4$, pH 2.6 19 min	Thiochrome Post-column Fluorescence Ex λ = 339 Em λ = 432	—	*J. Micronutr. Anal.*, 2, 189, 1986[3]
4. Infant formula, various foods	Thiamin, non-phosphorylated	Adjust pH to 1.7–2.0 with 6 N HCl Adjust pH to 4.0–4.2 withNaOH Filter Inject filtrate	—	μBondapak C_{18} 10 μm 30 cm × 4.6 mm	Isocratic EDTA (2 g) + sodium hexane sulfonate (3 g) + acetic acid (15 mL) + MeOH (400 mL) Dilute to 2 L with water 2.5 mL/min, 50°C	248 nm	—	*J. Assoc. Off. Anal. Chem.*, 73, 792, 1990[4]

		Sample preparation	Cleanup	Column	Mobile phase	Detection	DL	Reference
5. Various foods	Thiamin	Hydrolyze with 0.1 M HCl (30 mL) and 6 M HCl (0.1 mL) 121°C for 1 min Adjust pH to 4.0–4.5 Digest with takadiastase, 48°C, 3 h	Amberlite CG-50 C$_{18}$ Sep-Pak	μBondapak C$_{18}$ 10 μm 30 cm × 3.9 mm	Isocratic MeOH : HAC : sodium hexane sulfonate various 1.0 mL/min	254 nm	DL (ng) On-column 0.5	Z. Lebensm. Unters.-Forsch., 191, 313, 1990[5]
6. Chicken breast	Thiamin, TMP	Blend 80 g meat with 160 mL water under N$_2$ Add 8 mL 1 N HCl to 80 g slurry. To 16.3 g, add 15 g water, 1.5 mL 1/N HCl Dilute to 35 mL Heat at 100°C for 30 min Adjust pH to 4.5–4.7 Add α-amylase Digest overnight at 37.5°C Centrifuge	Bio-Rex 70	Shodex DM-614 or Hypersil APS	Isocratic 0.5 M citrate, pH 4.5	Thiochrome Pre-column Fluorescence Ex λ = 365 Em λ = 425	—	J. AOAC Int., 75, 346, 1992[6]
7. Various foods	Thiamin	Add 0.25 N H$_2$SO$_4$ (10 mL) to 2 g sample Autoclave, 30 min Adjust pH to 4.6 with NaOH : HAC mixture Digest with takadiastase, 40–45°C, 25 min Digest with papain, 40–45°C, 2 h Add TCA, heat at 50–60°C, 5 min Centrifuge	—	Mercksorb Si60 10 μm 25 cm × 4.5 mm	Isocratic Phosphate buffer pH 5.6 : EtOH (100 : 12) 1 mL/min	Thiochrome Post-column Fluorescence Ex λ = 366 Em λ = 464	—	Food Chem, 43, 393, 1992[7]
8. Various foods	Thiamin	Add 0.1 N HCl 5 g sample/65 mL Autoclave 30 min Adjust pH to 4.5 Digest with takadiastase Add TCA Dilute and filter	Form thiochrome derivative and pass through Baker C$_{18}$ SPE column or other C$_{18}$ SPE columns	Novapak C$_{18}$ 4 μm 15 cm × 3.9 mm	Isocratic MeOH : 50 mM phosphate, pH 7.0 (30 : 70) 1 mL/min	Thiochrome Pre-column Fluorescence Ex λ = 366 Em λ = 436	DL (pg) On-column 10	J. Food Comp. Anal., 6, 152, 1993[8]

TABLE 7.4 Continued

| Sample Matrix | Analyte | Sample Preparation | | HPLC Parameters | | | | |
		Sample Extraction	Clean Up	Column	Mobile Phase	Detection	Quality Assurance Parameters	References
9. Dried yeast	Thiamin	Add 1 mL of 10% HCl and 80 mL water to 1 g sample Incubate at 80–85°C, 30 min Add NaOAC buffer, pH 4.5 Digest with diastase, 45–50°C, 3 h	Extract with isobutanol Add p-chloroaniline (IS)	CAPCELL PAK C₁₈ 6 μm 15 cm × 4.6 mm	Isocratic 0.05 M acetate, pH 3.5 : MeCN (80 : 15) with 0.15% sodium 1-octane sulfonate	254 nm	—	Chromatographia, 39, 91, 1994[9]
10. Various foods	Thiamin	Add HCl (concentration unknown) Digest, 100°C for 30 min Adjust pH to 4–4.5 Digest with takadiastase 47°C, 3 h	Weak anion exchange column	Lichrosphere 100 RP-18 5 μm 12.5 cm × 4 mm	Isocratic H_3PO_4/KH_2PO_4, 10^{-2} M, pH 2.8 : MeOH (85 : 15) with 5 μM hexane sulfonic acid and 0.1% triethylamine	254 nm	—	J. Liq. Chrom. Rel. Technol., 19, 2155, 1996[10]
11. Dried yeast	Thiamin	Add 1 mL of 10% HCl and 80 mL water to 1 g sample Incubate at 80–85°C 30 min Add NaOAC buffer Digest with takadiastase, 45–50°C, 3 h	CM-Cellulose column Add phenacetin (IS) to eluate	Nucleosil C₁₈ 5 μm or CAPCELL-PAK C₁₈ 5 μm 15 cm × 4.6 mm	Isocratic 0.02 M phosphate buffer, pH 3.5, containing 0.2% sodium 1-octane sulfonate : MeCN (4 : 1) 40°C 1 mL/min	254 nm	—	J. Chromatogr. A, 726, 237, 1996[11]
Feed								
1. Rodent feed	Thiamin	Add 0.1 N HCl (20 mL) to 1 g sample Heat at 100°C, 30 min Centrifuge Adjust aliquot to pH 4.0 with HAC	—	SynChropak SCD-100 25 cm × 4.6 mm	Isocratic MeOH : water (40 : 60) containing 0.05 M	Thiochrome Post-column Fluorescence	DL (pg) On-column 5	J. AOAC Int., 78, 307, 1995[1]

Sample	Analyte	Sample preparation	Column	Mobile phase	Detection		Reference
				pentane sulfonate Adjust to pH 4.0 with HAC 0.5 mL/min	Ex λ = 370 Em λ = 430		
Pharmaceuticals							
1. Multivitamins	Thiamin	Dissolve in 0.1 M NaOH Shake for 15 min Centrifuge Dilute with mobile phase	Polymeric RP Jones Chromatography 5 µm 25 cm × 4.6 mm	Isocratic MeCN : 0.02 M Phosphate buffer pH 11.0 (20 : 80) 2 mL/min	EC Wall-jet amperometric Glassy carbon working electrode Gold counter electrode Ag/AgCl reference + 0.7 vs Ag/AgCl	—	Analyst, 120, 1059, 1995[1]
Biologicals							
1-3. Blood, erythrocytes, plasma	Thiamin, TMP, TPP, TTP	Add 0.1 mL TCA (100 g/L) to 0.2 mL vortex, centrifuge	ISA-07/S$_{25}$O$_4$ Shimadzu 25 cm × 0.4 mm	Isocratic 0.7 M NaOAC 0.5 mL/min 25°C	Thiochrome Post-column Fluorescence Ex λ = 375 Em λ = 450, 435	—	J. Chromatogr., 188, 417, 1980[1]; 245, 141, 1982[2] Clin. Chem., 29, 2073, 1983[3]
4. Blood, milk, cerebrospinal fluid	Thiamin, TMP, TPP	Blood Add perchloric acid Hold at 0°C for 15 min Centrifuge Add salicylamide (IS) with phosphatase overnight, 37°C	C$_{18}$	Isocratic MeOH : 0.05 M citrate buffer, pH 4.0 (45 : 55) containing 10 mmol/L sodium l-octane-sulfonate	Thiochrome Post-column Fluorescence Ex λ = 367 Em λ = 435	—	J. Chromatogr., 277, 145, 1983[4]
5. Excitable tissues	Thiamin, TMP, TPP, TTP	Homogenize in 5% TCA Centrifuge Extract supernatant with water saturated E$_2$0 Water phase reacted to form thiochrome	Ultrasphere-ODS 5 µm 15 cm or 25 cm × 4.6 mm	Gradient 25 mM phosphate buffer, pH 8.4 : 10% MeOH for 1 min to 100% MeOH in 3 min	Thiochrome Pre-column Fluorescence Ex λ = 390 Em λ = 475	—	J. Chromatogr., 307, 283, 1984[5]

TABLE 7.4 Continued

| Sample Matrix | Analyte | Sample Preparation | | HPLC Parameters | | | | |
		Sample Extraction	Clean Up	Column	Mobile Phase	Detection	Quality Assurance Parameters	References
6. Standards	Thiamin, TMP, TPP, TTP	—	—	PRP-1 25 cm × 4.1 mm	Isocratic 25 mM phosphate buffer, pH 8.4	Thiochrome Post-column Fluorescence Ex λ = 375–400 filter Em λ = 460–600 filter	—	J. Chromatogr. 295, 486, 1984[6]
7. Erythrocytes	TPP	Add 4 mL MeOH to 2 mL cell hemolysate Shake, centrifuge Form thiochrome fluorophore	—	Spherisorb-NH₂ 5 μm 15 cm × 4.6 mm	Isocratic MeOH : 0.1 M K₃PO₄ buffer, pH 7.5 (60 : 40) 2 mL/min	Thiochrome Pre-column Fluorescence Ex λ = 340 Em λ = 437	—	Clin. Chim. Acta 153, 43, 1985[7]
8. Serum	Thiamin, TMP, TPP, TTP	Add 0.1 mL TCA to 0.5 mL serum Centrifuge Extract with water-saturated Et₂O	—	PRP-1 10 μM 25 cm × 4.1 mm	Isocratic 15 mM sodium phosphate buffer, pH 8.5, containing 10% MeOH for esters or 10% THF for thiamin 0.5 mL/min	Thiochrome Pre-column Fluorescence Ex λ = 365 Em λ = 433	—	J. Chromatogr. 382, 297, 1986[8]
9. Animal tissue	Thiamin, TMP, TPP, TTP	Homogenize with 10% TCA; Centrifuge Extract with water-saturated Et₂O Lyophilize	—	CLC-ODS 15 cm × 6 mm	Isocratic 100 μM phosphate buffer, pH 2.5 : MeOH (92 : 8) 0.5 mL/min	Thiochrome Post-column Fluorescence Parameters not reported	—	J. Chromatogr. 450, 317, 1988[9]
10. Blood, tissue	Thiamin	Blood and tissue Add 0.19 M HCl (blood) or 0.1 M HCl (tissue) Hold at 100°C, 1 h Cool to 37°C Hydrolyze with papain	—	Lichrosorb Li60 5 μm 25 cm × 4 mm	Isocratic CHCl₃ : MeOH (80 : 20) 2 mL/min	Thiochrome Pre-column Fluorescence Ex λ = 375 Em λ = 430	—	J. Micronutr. Anal. 7, 147, 1990[10]

No. Sample	Analytes	Sample preparation	Column	Mobile phase	Detection	Performance	Reference
11–12. Blood, serum	Thiamin, TMP, TPP, TTP	and takadiastase Form thiochrome fluorophores / Add 0.25 mL of 2.44 M TCA to 2 mL / Allow to stand 1 h in dark, centrifuge / Extract with water-saturated Et_2O / Form thiochrome fluorophores	Supelcosil NH_2 25 cm × 4.6 mm	Step-wise MeCN: 85 mM phosphate buffer, pH 7.5 (90:10) for thiamin and (60:40) for phosphate esters 1.5 mL/min	Thiochrome Pre-column Fluorescence Ex λ = 375 Em λ = 450	—	J. Chromatogr., 564, 127, 1991[11], Meth. Enzymol., 279, 67, 1997[12]
13. Blood, serum	Thiamin, TMP, TPP, TTP	Add 0.2 mL 10% perchloric acid to 0.2 mL sample / Hold at 4°C, 15 min / Dilute with 1.8 M NaOAC in 0.6 M NaOH / Filter with Costar centrifuge filter unit	Partisphere C_{18} 5 μm 11 cm × 4.7 mm	Gradient A. 15 mM citric acid, pH 4.2 / B. 0.1 M formic acid containing 4% diethylamine, pH 3.2 / 0–25 min / 90% A, 10% B / 2.5 min 50% A, 50% B / 3.0–6.0 min / 5% A, 95% B / 7.0–10 min / 95% A, 5% B	Thiochrome Post-column Fluorescence Ex λ = 365 Em λ = 435	—	J. Chromatogr., 567, 71, 1991[13]
14. Neurons, astrocytes	Thiamin, TMP, TPP, TTP	Collect cells, disrupt with 60% TCA / Extract with Et_2O / Derivatize to thiochrome	PRP-1 5 μm 15 cm × 4.1 mm	Isocratic 50 mM phosphate containing 25 mM TBAHS and 4% THF 0.5 mL/min	Thiochrome Pre-column Fluorescence Ex λ = 365 Em λ = 433	DL (TTP) 50 fmol; —	Anal. Biochem., 198, 52, 1991[14]
15–16. Erythrocytes	Thiamin, TMP, TPP, TTP	Deproteinize with 10% TCA, 0.5 mL TCA + 0.5 mL hemolysate / Centrifuge / Extract with Et_2O	μBondapak C_{18} 10 μm 30 cm × 3.9 mm	Isocratic 0.15 mM citric acid adjusted to pH 4.2 with ammonia : 0.4% diethylamine in 0.1 M formic acid (90:10)	Thiochrome Post-column Fluorescence Ex λ = 365 Em λ = 435	DL (ng) 1 nmol; CV% 2.6–11.5; % Recovery 95–110	J. Chromatogr. B, 653, 217, 1994[15], Clin. Chim. Acta, 234, 91, 1995[16]
17. Whole blood	Thiamin, TMP, TPP,	To 1 mL blood, add 1 mL 7.2% perchloric	Microsphere C_{18} 3 μm	Gradient A. 31.9 g $K_2HPO_4 \cdot 3H_2O$	Thiochrome Pre-column	% Recovery Thiamin—90	Meth. Enzymol., 279, 74, 1997[17]

TABLE 7.4 Continued

| Sample Matrix | Analyte | Sample Preparation | | | HPLC Parameters | | | |
		Sample Extraction	Clean Up	Column	Mobile Phase	Detection	Quality Assurance Parameters	References
	TTP	acid in 0.25 M NaOH and 0.1 mL water Mix, place on ice Centrifuge Derivatize		10 cm × 4.6 mm	in 800 mL water + 120 mL MeOH + 0.6 mL 0.5 M TBAH + 15 mL DMF Adjust to pH 7.0 Make to 1 L with water B. 70% MeOH Linear Gradient 0 min 100% A 2–6 min 80% A, 20% B 6–7 min To 100% A 1 mL/min	Fluorescence Ex λ = 367 Em λ = 435	TMP—102 TPP—99 TTP—101 % CV Recovery 2.4–8.3 Intraassay 0.6–16	
18. Plasma	Thiamin, TMP, TPP, TTP as thiamin	Mix 1 mL plasma with 0.15 mL 3 M perchloric acid Vortex, centrifuge Add 0.3 mL 1 M NaOAC/HAC buffer, pH 4.6 containing 2.4 g NaOH per 100 mL to supernatant. Digest with acid phosphatase, 16 h, 40°C Add 0.15 mL 3 M perchloric acid and centrifuge	—	Nucleosil 120 5 C_{18} 12.5 cm × 4 mm	Isocratic MeCN : (10 mM perchloric acid : 100 mM octane sulfonic acid) (25 : 75) 2 mL/min	Thiochrome Post-column Fluorescence Ex λ = 365 Em λ = 435	Precision %CV 0.9–4.3 Reproducibility %CV 1.8–4.3	*Meth. Enzymol.*, 279, 83, 1997[18]

Complete reference information follows the main reference section at the end of the chapter and is listed by table.

2. Adjust an aliquot to pH 4.0 with 4.0 *M* sodium acetate buffer (pH 6.1).
3. Add 100 mg takadiastase per g sample.
4. Incubate at 37 to 45°C for 4 h for thiamin (18 h for riboflavin).
5. Cool, filter, or centrifuge.

At this point, the extract was ready for either microbiological or HPLC analysis. This extraction procedure uses a high ratio of enzyme to sample which could produce high enzyme blanks.

Quantitation of free thiamin and the individual phosphate esters requires conditions that do not hydrolyze the ester bonds. Sample extraction is limited to acid hydrolysis to free matrix-bound thiamin.[27] Enzyme digestion common to thiochrome and microbiological assay is eliminated. Sulfosalicylic acid has been successfully used for extraction of free thiamin, TMP, TPP, and TTP from foods.[27] Further extract clean up by solid-phase extraction, solvent partitioning, and protein precipitation is common. For blood, serum, urine, and other biological fluids, acid hydrolysis is not necessary. For these matrices, the sample is deproteinized with trichloroacetic acid (TCA) or perchloric acid. If TCA is used, the extract is treated with water-saturated diethyl ether to remove excess TCA. Tissue samples are often digested with protease to aid liberation of thiamin.

7.3.3.2 Chromatography Parameters

7.3.3.2.1 Supports and Mobile Phases

Reversed-phase chromatography on C_{18} support with an isocratic mobile phase works efficiently for the resolution of thiamin, TMP, TPP, and TTP. While C_{18} has been the most common support for thiamin chromatography, polystyrene resin provides advantages when pre-column thiochrome procedures are used. Various investigators have used PRP-1 (polystyrene-divinyl-benzene beads) for chromatography of the thiochromes. Bontemps et al.[28] observed that silica based C_{18} supports quickly degraded at pH 8.4 and that poly(styrene-divinylbenzene) resins could be used for reversed-phase resolution of thiochrome products of thiamin and the phosphate esters at higher mobile phase pH levels. These authors subsequently reported that 10 μm PRP-1 was useful for the chromatography at pH 8.4 which was sufficiently close to the fluorescence optima of the thiochromes to provide excellent sensitivity.[29]

Application of silica based C_{18} supports for pre-column thiochrome procedures was facilitated with the use of an acid mobile phase of 100 m*M* NaH_2PO_4-H_3PO_4 buffer, pH 2.5—8% methanol.[30] To provide for maximal fluorescence of the thiochrome products, 0.2 *M* NaOH—70% methanol was pumped into the column effluent to raise the pH to 8.6. The procedure developed by Iwata et al.[30] is given in detail in Section 7.4.

Mobile-phase components of published reversed-phase systems suitable for thiamin resolution include methanol-water, methanol-buffers (phosphate and acetate), acetonitrile-buffers, and buffers of various concentrations. Ion-pair reagents, usually heptane or hexane sulfonates, are often added to the mobile phase to improve resolution. Gradients, while not necessary, have been successfully used for the chromatography. Mobile phases for the methods outlined in Table 7.4 indicate the variability in chromatography systems that have been efficiently used for HPLC resolution of thiamin and its esters from complex sample digests.

7.3.3.2.2 Detection

UV detection at 245 to 254 nm can be used for high potency samples such as pharmaceuticals or enriched foods. However, lack of sensitivity and selectivity precludes its use for most HPLC separations. Recent studies on dried yeast and foods relied on UV detection at 254 nm.[31, 32] UV detection is not sensitive enough for naturally occurring levels of thiamin, TMP, TPP, and TTP in foods and most biological samples. Further, extensive extract clean up is required to allow UV detection.

The utility of thiochrome as a specific and highly fluorescent product of thiamin oxidation has led to the routine use of pre-column and post-column thiochrome procedures for fluorescence quantitation of thiamin and its esters. Thiochrome formed pre-column refers to procedures that form the thiochromes directly in the sample extract. The thiochrome products are chromatographically resolved. Pre-column thiochrome procedures are simpler to set up compared to post-column systems. To maximize fluorescence (Ex λ 365 to 375, Em λ 425 to 435), pH of the mobile phase must be kept above 8.0.[8] C_{18} reversed-phase columns are quickly degraded under the high pH environment. As discussed in Section 7.3.3.2.1, polystyrene-divinylbenzene supports help to overcome this obstacle.

Post-column procedures are based on the conversion of thiamin compounds to their respective thiochromes after chromatographic resolution of the thiamin forms. Post-column oxidation requires an additional pumping system to deliver the oxidizing agent which is usually 0.01% potassium ferricyanide in 15% sodium hydroxide. The oxidizing agent is pumped into the column effluent and sent through a mixing coil ahead of the fluorescence detector. Post-column methods provide resolution and sensitivity in the fentomole range equivalent to pre-column methods.

7.3.3.2.3   Internal Standards

The general consensus of researchers involved in the development of HPLC methods for thiamin analysis is that adequate internal standards are not available. Salicylamide, sodium salicylate, and anthracene fluoresce similarly to thiochrome and have been used for injection volume correction.[8] Amprolium was reported to be a usable internal standard to carry through the thiochrome reaction[27]; however, Ollilainin et al.[33] found that amprolium produced an unknown compound during oxidation to form thiochrome products with a K′ value over 60. Band broadening of the amprolium thiochrome product also occurred. These investigators concluded that amprolium could not be used reliably as an internal standard for thiochrome. Recently, phenacetin was applied to the UV detection of thiamin; however, the compound was added immediately before injection and was not a true internal standard.[34]

7.4   METHOD PROTOCOLS

Improved High-Performance Liquid Chromatographic Determination of Thiamin and Its Phosphate Esters in Animal Tissues

Principle

- Thiamin, TMP, TDP, and TTP were converted into thiochrome fluorophores by pre-column alkaline oxidation with cyanogen bromide. Thiochromes were resolved by reversed-phase chromatography on ODS using an acidic mobile phase. Alkaline methanol was mixed with the column effluent prior to the fluorescent detector.

Chemicals

- Trichloroacetic acid (TCA)
- Diethyl ether
- Cyanogen bromide
- Sodium hydroxide
- Hydrochloric acid
- Thiamin monophosphate
- Thiamin diphosphate
- Thiamin triphosphate

Apparatus

- Liquid chromatograph
- Fluorescent detector
- Proportioning pump

Procedure

Animal Tissue Extraction

- Homogenize with cold TCA
- Centrifuge (16,000 × g), 15 min
- Extract TCA with water-saturated diethyl ether
- Lyophilize, store at −20°C

Thiochrome Formation

- Divide extract into two fractions, A + B
- A:
  - To 200 μL A, add 25 μL 0.3 M CNBr
  - Vortex 1 min
  - Add 25 μL 1 M NaOH
  - Vortex 1 min
  - Neutralize with 3 M HCl
- B:
  - To 200 μL B, add 25 μL 1 M NaOH
  - Vortex 1 min
  - Add 25 μL 0.3 M CNBr
  - Vortex 1 min
  - Neutralize with 3 M NaOH

Note: B serves as the blank. Addition of the NaOH destroys thiamin compounds. Chromatography of the blank will indicate possible non-thiochrome fluorescent compounds that are not resolved from the thiamin derivatives.

Chromatography

Mobile phase	100 mM sodium dihydrogen phosphate-phosphoric acid buffer, pH 2.5, 8% methanol
Column	15 cm × 6 mm
Stationary phase	Shimpak CLC-ODS
Column temperature	50°C
Flow	0.5 mL/min
Injection volume	20–40 μL
Alkali delivery	0.2 M NaOH + Methanol (30 : 70) at 0.5 mL/min, CRB-IB incubator box at 50°C
Detection	Fluorescence, excitation and emission at wavelengths suitable for thiochrome
Calculation	External standard, peak area, linear regression

J. Chromatogr., 450, 317, 1988

Determination of Thiamin and Riboflavin in Meat and Meat Products by High-Performance Liquid Chromatography

Principle

- Extract thiamin and riboflavin by autoclaving in 0.1 *N* HCl and digestion with papain and Takadiastase. Convert thiamin to thiochrome and quantitate by isocratic elution from silica with fluorescence detection. Convert riboflavin to lumiflavin by UV irradiation and quantitate by isocratic elution from silica with fluorescence detection.

Chemicals

- Hydrochloric acid
- Sodium acetate
- Thiamin HCl (USP)
- Riboflavin (USP)
- Chloroform
- Trichloroacetic acid (TCA)
- Glacial acetic acid
- Potassium ferricyanide
- Sodium sulfate
- Isobutyl alcohol
- Methanol

Enzymes

- Papain
- Takadiastase

Apparatus

- HPLC
- Fluorescence detector
- Chromato-VUE cabinet, model C-5 with long- and short-wavelength UV lamps
- Autoclave

Procedure

Sample Extraction

- Weigh 5 g sample
- Add 60 mL 0.1 *N* HCl, autoclave, 121°C, 30 min
- Adjust pH to 4.0–4.5 with 2 *M* sodium acetate
- Digest with papain and Takadiastase, 3 h, 42-45°C
- Precipitate protein with 2 mL of 50% TCA
- Steambath, 5 min
- Dilute to 100 mL with water

Thiochrome Formation

- Oxidize 10 mL filtrate with 5 mL 1% alkaline potassium ferricyanide
- Extract thiochrome with 10 mL isocutyl alcohol
- Treat standard in same manner to generate standard curve

Riboflavin Conversion to Lumiflavin

- Adjust pH of 10 mL of filtrate to 10–12 with 15% NaOH
- Irradiate for 30 min
- Add 1 mL glacial acetic acid
- Extract with 10 mL chloroform
- Dry extract with anhydrous sodium sulfate
- Treat standards in same manner to generate standard curve

Chromatography

Column	50 cm × 2.1 mm
Stationary phase	Spherisorb silica, 20 μ
Mobile phase	Chloroform : methanol (90 : 10)
Flow	Thiochrome—1.0 mL/min
	Lumiflavin—0.8 mL/min
Column temperature	Ambient
Detection	Fluorescence
	Thiochrome Ex λ = 367, Em λ = 418
	Lumiflavin Ex λ = 270, Em λ = 418
Calculation	Internal standard, peak area, linear regression

J. Agric. Food Chem., 28, 483, 1980

7.5   REFERENCES

TEXT

1. National Research Council, *Recommended Dietary Allowances,* 10th ed., National Academy of Sciences, Washington, D.C., 1989, chap. 8.
2. Machlin, L. J. and Huni, J. E. S., *Vitamins Basics,* Hoffmann-LaRoche, Basel, 1994, 26.
3. *Nutritional Labeling and Education Act of 1990,* Fed. Reg., 58, 2070, 1993.
4. Ellefson, W. C., Thiamin, in *Methods of Vitamin Assay,* 4th ed., Augustin, J., Klein, B. P., Becker, D. A., and Venugopal, P. B., Eds., John Wiley and Sons, New York, 1985, chap. 13.
5. Ottaway, P. B., Stability of vitamins in foods, in *The Technology of Vitamins in Food,* Chapman and Hall, London, 1993, chap. 5.
6. Ball, G. F. M., Chemical and biological nature of the water-soluble vitamins, in *Water-Soluble Vitamin Assays in Human Nutrition,* Chapman and Hall, New York, 1994, chap. 2.
7. Ishii, K., Sarai, K., Sanemori, H., and Kawasaki, T., Analysis of thiamin and its phosphate esters by high-performance liquid chromatography, *Anal. Biochem.,* 97, 191, 1979.
8. Kawasaki, T., Vitamin B_1: Thiamin, in *Modern Chromatographic Analysis of Vitamins,* 2nd ed., De Leenheer, A. P., Lambert, W. E., and Nelis, H. J., Eds,. Marcel Dekker, New York, 1992, chap. 8.
9. Eitenmiller, R. and Landen, W. O., Vitamins, in *Analyzing Food for Nutrition Labeling and Hazardous Contaminants,* Jeon, I. G. and Ikins, W. G., Eds., Marcel Dekker, New York, 1995, chap. 9.
10. Dwivedi, B. K. and Arnold, R. G., Chemistry of thiamin degradation in food products and model systems. A review, *J. Agric. Food Chem.,* 21, 54, 1973.
11. Barger, G., Bergel, F., and Todd, R. A., Über das thiochrom aus vitamin B_1 (Antineuria), *Chem. Ber.,* 68, 257, 1935.
12. Fayol, V., High-performance liquid chromatography determination of total thiamin in biological and food products, *Meth. Enzymol.,* 279, 57, 1997.
13. United States Pharmacopeial Convention, *U.S. Pharmacopeia National Formulary,* USP 23/NF18, Nutritional Supplements Official Monographs, 1995.
14. AOAC International, *Official Methods of Analysis,* 16th ed., AOAC International, Arlington, VA, 1995.

15. American Association of Cereal Chemists, *Approved Methods,* vol. 2, 1996.
16. American Feed Ingredients Association, *Laboratory Methods Compendium, Vitamins and Minerals,* vol. 1, American Feed Ingredients Association, Des Moines, IA, 1991, 145.
17. Hasselmann, C., Franck, D., Grimm, P., Diop, P. A., and Soules, C., High-performance liquid chromatographic analysis of thiamin and riboflavin in dietetic foods, *J. Micronutr. Anal.,* 5, 269, 1989.
18. Lumley, I. D., Vitamin analysis in food, in *The Technology of Vitamins in Food,* Ottaway, P. B., Ed., Chapman and Hall, London, 1993, chap. 8.
19. Alyabis, A. M. and Simpson, K. L., Comparison of reverse-phase C_{18} open-column with the Bio-Rex 70 column in the determination of thiamin, *J. Food Comp. Anal.,* 6, 166, 1993.
20. Soliman, A. M., Comparison of manual and benzenesulfonyl chloride-semiautomated thiochrome method for the determination of thiamin in food, *J. Assoc. Off. Anal. Chem.,* 64, 616, 1981.
21. Leveille, G. A., Modified thiochrome procedure for the determination of urinary thiamin, *Am. J. Clin. Nutr.,* 25, 273, 1972.
22. AOAC International, Report on the AOAC International Task Force on Methods for Nutrient Labeling Analyses, *J. AOAC Int.,* 76, 180A, 1993.
23. Voigt, M. N. and Eitenmiller, R. R., Comparative review of the thiochrome, microbial and protozoan analysis of B-vitamins, *J. Food Prot.,* 41, 730, 1978.
24. Deibel, R. H., Evans, J. B., and Niven, C. F., Jr., Microbiological assay for thiamin using *Lactobacillus viridescens, J. Bacteriol.,* 74, 818, 1957.
25. Arella, F., Lahely, S., Bourguignon, J. B., and Hasselmann, C., Liquid chromatographic determination of vitamins B_1 and B_2 in foods. A collaborative study, *Food Chem.,* 56, 81, 1996.
26. van den Berg, H., von Schaik, F., Finglas, P. M., and de Froidmont-Gortz, I., Third EUMAT intercomparison on methods for the determination of vitamins B_1, B_2, and B_6 in foods, *Food Chem.,* 57, 101, 1996.
27. Vanderslice, J. T. and Huang, M. H. A., Liquid chromatographic analysis of thiamin and its phosphates in food products using amprolium as an internal standard, *J. Micronutr. Anal.,* 2, 189, 1986.
28. Bontemps, J., Phillippe, P., Bettendorff, L., Lombet, J., Dandrifosse, G., Schoffeniels, E., and Crommen, J., Determination of thiamin phosphates in excitable tissues as thiochrome derivatives by reversed-phase high performance liquid chromatography on octadecyl silica, *J. Chromatogr.,* 307, 283, 1984.
29. Bontemps, J., Bettendorff, L., Lombet, J., Grandfils, C., Dandrifosse, G., Schoffeniels, E., Nevejans, F. and Crommen, J., Poly (styrene-divinylbenzene) as reversed-phase adsorbent for the high-performance liquid chromatographic analysis of thiochrome derivatives of thiamin and phosphorylated esters, *J. Chromatogr.,* 295, 486, 1984.
30. Iwata, H., Matsuda, T., and Tonomura, H., Improved high-performance liquid chromatographic determination of thiamin and its phosphate esters in animal tissues, *J. Chromatogr.,* 450, 317, 1988.
31. Yamanaka, K., Matsuoka, M. and Banno, K., Determination of thiamin in dried yeast by high-performance liquid chromatography using a clean-up column of CM-cellulose, *J. Chromatogr.,* 726, 237, 1996.
32. Blanco, D., Llaneza, M. B., and Gutierrez, M. D., A paired ion liquid chromatographic method for thiamin determination in selected foods, *J. Liq. Chrom. Rel. Technol.,* 19, 2155, 1996.
33. Ollilainen, V., Vahteristo, L., Uusi-Rauva, A., Varo, P., Koivistoinen, P., and Huttunen, J., The HPLC determination of total thiamin (vitamin B_1) in foods, *J. Food Comp. Anal.,* 6, 152, 1993.
34. Yamanaka, K., Horimoto, S., Matsuoka, M., and Banno, K., Analysis of thiamin in dried yeast by high-performance liquid chromatography and high-performance liquid chromatography/atmospheric pressure chemical ionization-mass spectrometry, *Chromatographia,* 39, 91, 1994.

TABLE 7.1   Physical Properties of Thiamin Salts

1. Ball, G. F. M., Chemical and biological nature of the water-soluble vitamins, in *Water-Soluble Vitamin Assays in Human Nutrition,* Chapman and Hall, New York, chap. 2.
2. Budavari, S., *The Merck Index,* 12th ed., Merck and Company, Whitehouse Station, NJ, 1996, 1586.
3. Ellefson, W. C., Thiamin, in *Methods of Vitamin Assay,* 4th ed., Augustin, J., Klein, B. P., Becker, D. A., and Venugopal, P. B., Eds., John Wiley and Sons, New York, 1985, chap. 13.

TABLE 7.2   Compendium, Regulatory, and Handbook Methods for the
Analysis of Thiamin

1. United States Pharmacopeial Convention, *U.S. Pharmacopeia National Formulary,* USP 23/ NF 18, Nutritional Supplements, Official Monographs, United States Pharmacopeial Convention, Rockville, MD, 1995.
2. Scottish Home and Health Department, *British Pharmacopoeia,* 15th ed., British Pharmacopoeic Commission, United Kingdom, 1993.
3. AOAC International, *Official Methods of Analysis,* 16th ed., AOAC International, Arlington, VA, 1995.
4. Ellefson, W. L., Richter, E., Adams, M., and Baillies, N. T., Evaluation of ion exchange resins and various enzymes in thiamin analysis, *J. Assoc. Off. Anal. Chem.,* 64, 1336, 1981.
5. McRoberts, L. H., Report on the determination of thiamine in enriched flour: comparison of acid hydrolysis and fluorometric methods, *J. Assoc. Off. Anal. Chem.,* 36, 837, 1953.
6. Association Official Agricultural Chemists, Nutritional adjuncts (vitamins), *J. Assoc. Off. Agric. Chem.,* 37, 122, 1954.
7. Schoenherr, W. H., Identification of insect fragments in cereal products, *J. Assoc. Off. Anal. Chem.,* 37, 154, 1954.
8. McRoberts, L. H., Report on the determination of thiamine in enriched flour, *J. Assoc. Off. Anal. Chem.,* 38, 722, 1955.
9. McRoberts, L. H., Report on thiamine in enriched cereal and bakery products, *J. Assoc. Off. Anal. Chem.,* 40, 843, 1957.
10. McRoberts, L. H., Report on the determination of thiamine in enriched cereal and bakery products, *J. Assoc. Off. Anal. Chem.,* 41, 603, 1958.
11. McRoberts, L. H., Determination of thiamine in enriched cereal and bakery products, *J. Assoc. Off. Anal. Chem.,* 43, 47, 1960.
12. Tanner, J. T. and Barnett, S. A., Methods of analysis for infant formula in Food and Drug Administration and infant formula collaborative study, phase III, *J. Assoc. Off. Anal. Chem.,* 69, 777, 1986.
13. American Association of Cereal Chemists, *AACC Approved Methods,* 9th ed., vol. 2, American Association of Cereal Chemists, St. Paul, MN, 1996.
14. American Feed Ingredients Association, *Laboratory Methods Compendium,* vol. 1: *Vitamins and Minerals,* American Feed Ingredients Association, West Des Moines, IA, 1991, 145.
15. Bechtel, W. G. and Hollenbeck, C. M., A revised thiochrome procedure for the determination of thiamin in cereal products, *Cereal Chem.,* 35, 1, 1958.
16. Committee on Food Chemicals Codex, *Food Chemicals Codex,* 4th ed., National Academy of Sciences, Washington, D.C., 1996, 411, 412.
17. Keller, H. E., *Analytical Methods for Vitamins and Carotenoids,* Hoffmann-LaRoche, Basel, 1988, 23, 27.
18. Von Acker, H., *Handbuch der Lebensmittel-Chemie,* vol. 2, Springer Verlag, Berlin, 1967, 721.
19. Brubacher, G., Müller-Mulot, W., and Southgate, D. A. T., *Methods for the Determination of Vitamins in Food, Recommended by COST 91,* Elsevier Applied Science Publishers, New York, 1985, chap. 4.
20. Soliman, A. G. M., Comparison of manual and benzenesulfonyl chloride semiautomated thiochrome methods for determination of thiamin in foods, *J. Assoc. Off. Anal. Chem.,* 64, 616, 1981.

TABLE 7.4   HPLC Methods for the Analysis of Thiamin in Food, Feed,
Pharmaceuticals, and Biologicals

Food

1. Hilker, D. M. and Clifford, A. J., Thiamin analysis and separation of thiamin phosphate esters by high-performance liquid chromatography, *J. Chromatogr.,* 231, 433, 1982.
2. Ohta, H., Baba, T., Suzuki, Y., and Okada, E., High-performance liquid chromatographic analysis of thiamine in rice flour with fluorimetric post-column derivatization, *J. Chromatogr.,* 284, 281, 1984.
3. Vanderslice, J. T. and Huang, M. H. A., Liquid chromatographic analysis of thiamin and its phosphates in food products using amprolium as an internal standard, *J. Micronutr. Anal.,* 2, 189, 1986.

4. Nicolas, E. C. and Pfender, K. A., Fast and simple liquid chromatographic determination of nonphosphorylated thiamine in infant formula, milk, and other foods, *J. Assoc. Off. Anal. Chem.,* 73, 792, 1990.
5. Vidal-Valverde, C. and Reche, A., An improved high performance liquid chromatographic method for thiamin analysis in foods, *Z. Lebensm. Unters. Forsch.,* 191, 313, 1990.
6. Fox, J. B., Ackerman, S. A., and Thayer, D. W., Fluorometric determination of thiamin vitamers in chicken, *J. AOAC Int.,* 75, 346, 1992.
7. Abdel-Kader, Z. M., Comparison of AOAC and high-performance liquid chromatographic methods for thiamin determination in foods, *Food Chem.,* 43, 393, 1992.
8. Ollilainen, V., Vahteristo, V., Uusi-Rauva, L. A., Varo, P., Koivistoinen, P., and Huttunen, J., The HPLC determination of total thiamin (vitamin B_1) in foods, *J. Food Comp. Anal.,* 6, 152, 1993.
9. Yamanaka, K., Horimoto, S., Matsuoka, M., and Banno, K., Analysis of thiamine and dried yeast by high-performance liquid chromatography and high-performance liquid chromatography/atmospheric pressure chemical ionization-mass spectrometry, *Chromatographia,* 39, 91, 1994.
10. Blanco, D., Llaneza, M. B., and Gutierrez, M. D., A paired ion liquid chromatographic method for thiamine determination in selected foods, *J. Liq. Chrom. Rel. Technol.,* 19, 2155, 1996.
11. Yamanaka, K., Matsuoka, M., and Banno, K., Determination of thiamine in dried yeast by high-performance liquid chromatography using a clean-up column of CM-cellulose, *J. Chromatogr.,* 726, 237, 1996.

Feed

1. Gehring, T. A., Cooper, W. M., Holder, C. L., and Thompson, H. C., Jr., Liquid chromatographic determination of thiamine in rodent feed by post-column derivatization and fluorescence detection, *J. AOAC Int.,* 78, 307, 1995.

Pharmaceuticals

1. Hart, J. P., Norman, M. D., and Tsang, S., Voltammetric behaviours of vitamin B_1 (thiamine) at a glassy carbon electrode and its determination in multivitamin tablets using anion-exchange liquid chromatography with amperometric detection under basic conditions, *Analyst,* 120, 1059, 1995.

Biologicals

1. Kimura, M., Fujita, T., Nishida, S., and Itokawa, Y., Differential fluorometric determination of picogram levels of thiamin, thiamin monophosphate, diphosphate, triphosphate using high performance liquid chromatography, *J. Chromatogr.,* 188, 417, 1980.
2. Kimura, M., Panijpan, B., and Itokawa, Y., Separation and determination of thiamin and its phosphate esters by reversed-phase high-performance liquid chromatography, *J. Chromatogr.,* 245, 141, 1982.
3. Kimura, M. and Itokawa, Y., Determination of thiamin and thiamin phosphate esters in blood by liquid chromatography with post-column derivatization, *Clin. Chem.,* 29, 2073, 1983.
4. Weilders, J. P. M. and Mink, C. J. K., Quantitative analysis of total thiamine in human blood, milk, and cerebrospinal fluid by reversed-phase ion-pair high-performance liquid chromatography, *J. Chromatogr.,* 277, 145, 1983.
5. Bontemps, J., Philippe, P., Bettendorff, L., Lombet, J., Dandrifosse, G., and Schoffeniels, E., Determination of thiamine phosphates in excitable tissues as thiochrome derivatives by reversed-phase high-performance liquid chromatography on octadecyl silica, *J. Chromatogr.,* 307, 283, 1984.
6. Bontemps, J., Bettendorff, L., Lombet, J., Grandfils, C., Nevejans, F., and Crommen, J., Poly (styrene-divinylbenzene) as reversed-phase adsorbent for the high-performance liquid chromatographic analysis of thiochrome derivatives of thiamin and phosphorylated esters, *J. Chromatogr.,* 295, 486, 1984.
7. Baines, M., Improved high performance liquid chromatographic determination of thiamin diphosphate in erythrocytes, *Clin. Chim. Acta,* 153, 43, 1985.
8. Bettendorff, L., Grandfils, C., DeRycker, C., and Schoffeniels, E., Determination of thiamine and its phosphate esters in human blood serum at fentomole levels, *J. Chromatogr.,* 382, 297, 1986.
9. Iwata, H., Matsuda, T., and Tonomura, H., Improved high-performance liquid chromatographic determination of thiamine and its phosphate esters in animal tissues, *J. Chromatogr.,* 450, 317, 1988.

10. Bailey, A. L. and Finglas, P. M., A normal phase high performance liquid chromatographic method for the determination of thiamin in blood and tissue samples, *J. Micronutr. Anal.,* 7, 147, 1990.
11. Tallaksen, C. M. E., Bohmer, T., and Bell, H., Concomitant determination of thiamin and its phosphate esters in human blood and serum by high-performance liquid chromatography, *J. Chromatogr.* 564, 127, 1991.
12. Tallaksen, C. M. E., Bohmer, T., Karlsen, J., and Bell, H., Determination of thiamin and its phosphate esters in human blood, plasma, and urine, *Meth. Enzymol.,* 279, 67, 1997.
13. Lee, B. L., Ong, H. Y., and Ong, C. N., Determination of thiamine and its phosphate esters by gradient elution high-performance liquid chromatography, *J. Chromatogr.,* 567, 71, 1991.
14. Bettendorff, L., Peeters, M., Jouan, C., Wins, P., and Schoffeniels, E., Determination of thiamin and its phosphate esters in cultured neurons and astrocytes using an ion-pair reversed-phase high-performance liquid chromatographic method, *Anal. Biochem.,* 198, 52, 1991.
15. Herve, C., Beyne, P., and Delacoux, E., Determination of thiamine and its phosphate esters in human erythrocytes by high-performance liquid chromatography with isocratic elution, *J. Chromatogr. B,* 653, 217, 1994.
16. Herve, P., Beyne, P., Lettiron, Ph., and Delacoux, E., Comparison of erythrocyte transketolase activity with thiamine and thiamine phosphate ester levels in chronic alcoholic patients, *Clin. Chim. Acta,* 234, 91, 1995.
17. Gerrits, J., Eidhof, H., Brunnekreeft, J. W. I., and Hessels, J., Determination of thiamin and thiamin phosphates in whole blood by reversed-phase liquid chromatography with precolumn derivatization, *Meth. Enzymol.,* 279, 74, 197.
18. Mascher, H. J. and Kikuta, C., High-performance liquid chromatography determination of total thiamin in human plasma, *Meth. Enzymol.,* 279, 83, 1997.

8 Riboflavin

8.1 REVIEW

Riboflavin (Vitamin B_2) was isolated in 1932 from Brewer's yeast as a yellow enzyme thought to function in cell respiration. From 1933 to 1935, the structure was determined and riboflavin was synthesized. The coenzymes, flavin mononucleotide (FMN) and flavin adenine dinucleotide (FAD) were characterized from 1934 to 1938. Riboflavin deficiency or ariboflavinosis usually occurs along with other water-soluble vitamin deficiencies. The close relationship of riboflavin metabolism with the metabolism of vitamin B-6, folic acid, and niacin leads to deficiency symptoms that are often interrelated or the result of improper functioning of metabolic systems requiring other nutrients.[1] Generalized symptoms result from the involvement of FMN and FAD in many aspects of energy, protein, and lipid metabolism. A characteristic symptom of riboflavin deficiency is oral-buccal cavity lesions including angular stomatitis (characteristic fissures at the corners of the mouth). Other symptoms include seborrheic dermatitis, scrotal and vulvar skin changes, and mono-cystic anemia.[1]

Biochemical status tests are usually required to substantiate riboflavin deficiency. Subclinical deficiency is assessed by measurement of erythrocyte glutathione reductase (EGR) which requires FAD as the cofactor. The enzyme catalyzes the conversion of glutathione to reduced glutathione with the participation of NADPH. The assay follows the *in vitro* stimulation of EGR activity through the addition of FAD. The assay results are converted to an activity coefficient which rises in subjects to a riboflavin intake level of 0.5 mg/1000 kcal.[2] Riboflavin levels in urine based on 24 h urine collections can be used to confirm EGR observations. As noted for thiamin, riboflavin in blood, serum, and erythrocytes are not dependable measures of status.

Good dietary sources of riboflavin include most animal products. Milk and other dairy foods are excellent natural sources. Cereals, unless fortified, are low but consistent sources. Green vegetables are generally higher in riboflavin compared with fruits which contain lower amounts of the vitamin. Cooking can result in large losses through leaching of riboflavin into the cooking medium. Additionally, light exposure can lead to significant losses during storage. Recommended Dietary Allowances (RDAs) are based upon clinical observations that an intake of 0.6 mg/1000 kcal will prevent deficiency.[1] RDAs range from 0.4 mg/day for the 0- to 6-month-old infant to 1.8 mg/day for the 15- to 18-year-old male and the lactating female (first 6 months). A minimum intake of 1.2 mg/day is recommended for the adult consuming 2000 kcal/day. The Reference Daily Intake (RDI) used for the nutritional label declaration is 1.7 mg.[3]

The principle form of riboflavin in biological materials is FAD.[4] FAD and FMN occur as protein bound flavoproteins in tissue and primarily bound to albumin in serum. The flavoprotein enzymes function in one- or two-electron oxidation-reduction reactions. Flavin enzymes that act aerobically are oxidases and those that function anaerobically are dehydrogenases. Notable reactions involving the flavins include electron transfer between NADH and the cytochromes, amino acid oxidase reactions, glutathione reductase, succinate and fumarate dehydrogenase, conversion of tryptophan to niacin, pyridine-linked dehydrogenases, acyl-CoA dehydrogenases, and many other reactions involving oxidation–reduction.

8.2   PROPERTIES

8.2.1   CHEMISTRY

8.2.1.1   General Properties

Riboflavin is 7,8-dimethyl-10-(1′-D-ribity)isoalloxazine (Figure 8.1). The isoalloxazine ring is commonly known as the flavin ring. The flavin ring is methylated at the 7 and 8 positions. The vitamin is substituted on the 10 position with a D-ribityl side chain. Phosphorylation at the 5′ position of the ribityl side chain produces FMN. Addition of adenosine-5′-monophosphate yields FAD. Structural relationships of riboflavin, FMN, and FAD are shown in Figure 8.2. The carbon-nitrogen bond linking the ribityl side chain to the isoalloxazine is stable to acid hydrolysis; whereas, FMN and FAD are easily converted to riboflavin below pH 5.0.[4] For this reason, analytical procedures often incorporate acid hydrolysis as the first step with subsequent quantitation of total riboflavin. Conversely, acid conditions must be avoided in the quantitation of the co-enzyme forms.

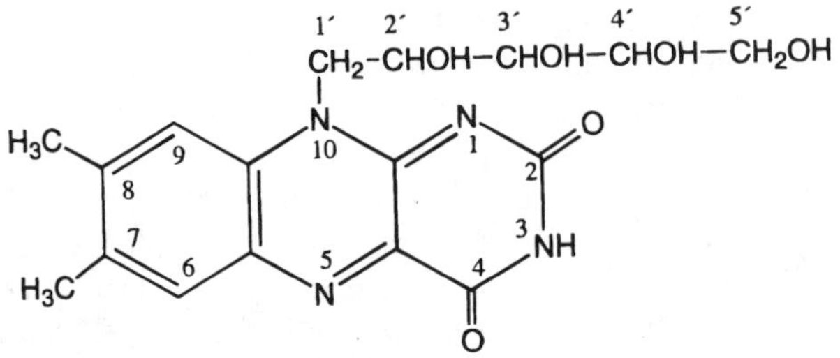

Riboflavin
7,8-dimethyl-10-(1′-D-ribityl)isoalloxazine
Vitamin B$_2$

FIGURE 8.1   Structure of riboflavin.

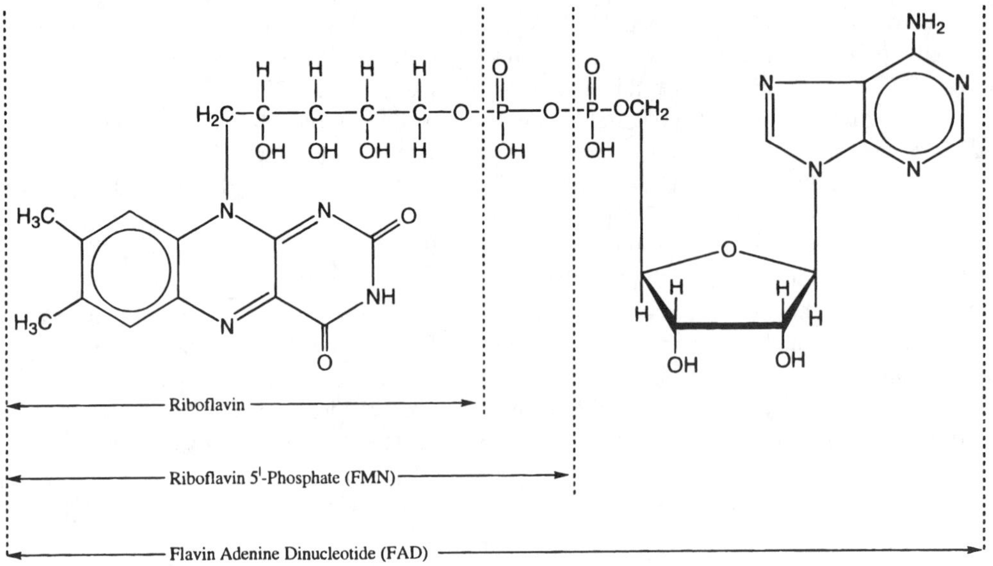

FIGURE 8.2   Structures of riboflavin and the flavin co-enzymes.

Physical properties of riboflavin ($C_{17}H_{20}N_4O_6$), FMN ($C_{17}H_{21}N_4O_9P$) which is known commercially as riboflavin monophosphate or riboflavin 5'-phosphate, and FAD ($C_{27}H_{33}N_9O_{15}P_2$) are given in Table 8.1. Riboflavin is available as the USP standard. The vitamin is a yellow-green, fluorescent compound which produces yellow-orange needle shaped crystals.[5] Riboflavin, FMN, and FAD are slightly soluble in alcohol and insoluble in ether, acetone, benzene, and chloroform. Water-solubility of riboflavin and riboflavin 5'-phosphate differ with riboflavin having only slight solubility in water (0.10 to 0.13 g/L) compared to high water-solubility of riboflavin 5'-phosphate (30 g/L).[6] Water-solubility limits the use of riboflavin to products that do not require rehydration. Riboflavin in high concentrations is bitter. Fat enrobed forms are available commercially for use in products where off-flavors due to riboflavin addition is problematic.

8.2.1.2 Spectral Properties

The characteristic spectral properties of riboflavin, FMN, and FAD provide the basis of chemical assays and the sensitivity and specificity for HPLC analysis.[7] In aqueous solutions, riboflavin shows absorption maxima of 223, 266, 373, and 445 nm (Fig. 8.3.I).[8] In the oxidized state, flavins and flavoproteins have absorption maxima at 370 and 450 nm.[6] The maxima shown around 370 nm for riboflavin and the co-enzymes is affected by the solvent environment and shifts to lower wavelengths as the polarity of the solvent decreases.[5] Absorption maxima are quite similar for riboflavin and FMN with slight variations being apparent in the spectrum of FAD.[8] Reduction of the flavins and flavoproteins produces atypical and variable absorption spectra above 300 nm that make interpretation of spectroscopic data difficult.[9] Strong absorbance with the characteristic maxima is absent in the reduced states. $E_{1cm}^{1\%}$ values for riboflavin determined in 0.1 M phosphate buffer, pH 7.0, at 260, 375, and 450 nm are 736, 282, and 324, respectively (Table 8.1).

The UV-visible spectral properties have been used for riboflavin analysis; however, most chemical and HPLC methods capitalize on the strong native fluorescence of the flavins (Ex λ : 440 to 500, Em λ : 520 to 530).[7] Riboflavin and FMN fluoresce similarly and FAD less strongly. FAD has 10 to 20% of the fluorescent intensity on an equimolar basis compared to riboflavin and FMN.[6,10] Interaction of the adenine with the isoalloxazine ring leads to quenching of the fluorescence producing a quantum yield that is approximately ten times less than the quantum yield of riboflavin or FMN.[6] Fluorescence excitation and emission spectra of riboflavin in water is shown in Fig. 8.3.II.

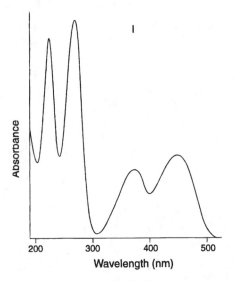

FIGURE 8.3.I Absorption spectrum of riboflavin dissolved in water. Adapted from Reference 8.

TABLE 8.1
Physical Properties of Riboflavin, FMN, and FAD

Substance[a]	Molar Mass	Formula	Solubility	Crystal Form	λ max nm[b]	Spectral Properties $E^{1\%}_{1cm}$	$\epsilon \times 10^{-3}$	Fluorescence Ex: nm	Em: nm
Riboflavin Vitamin B$_2$ CAS No. 83-88-5 **8367**	376.37	C$_{17}$H$_{20}$N$_4$O$_6$	Soluble but unstable in dilute alkali; Slightly soluble in water, 0.10–0.13 g/L; Slightly soluble in alcohol, phenol; Insoluble in CHCl$_3$, acetone, benzene, ether	Fine yellow-orange needles M.P. 278–282°C (dec.)	260 / 375 / 450	[736] / [282] / [324]	27.7 / 10.6 / 12.2	360, 465; pH 3.5–7.5	521
Riboflavin-5′-phosphate CAS No. 130-40-5 **8368**	456.35	C$_{17}$H$_{21}$N$_4$O$_9$P	Soluble in water, 30 g/L (Na salt); Insoluble in acetone, benzene, ether	Fine, yellow-orange crystalline powder M.P. 280–290°C (dec.)	260 / 375 / 450	[594] / [228] / [267]	27.1 / 10.4 / 12.2	440–500; pH 3.5–7.5	530
Flavin-adenine dinucleotide FAD CAS No. 146-14-5 **4131**	785.56	C$_{27}$H$_{33}$N$_9$O$_{15}$P$_2$	Soluble in water; Insoluble in CHCl$_3$, acetone, benzene, ether		260 / 375 / 450	[471] / [118] / [144]	37.0 / 9.3 / 11.3	440–500; pH 2.7–3.1	530

[a] Common or generic name; CAS No.—Chemical Abstract Service number, Merck Index Monograph number in bold.
[b] Values in brackets are calculated from corresponding ε values, 0.1 M phosphate buffer.

Ball, G. F. M., *Water-Soluble Vitamin Assays in Human Nutrition*.[1]
Budavari, S., *The Merck Index*.[2]
Nielsen, P., *Modern Chromatographic Analysis of Vitamins*.[3]
Food Chemicals Codex.[4]

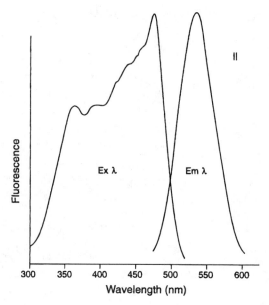

FIGURE 8.3.II Fluorescence excitation and emission spectra of riboflavin dissolved in water. Reproduced with permission from Reference 8.

Fluorescence intensity is not affected at intermediate pH levels. Reduced forms of the flavins do not fluoresce.[8]

8.2.2 STABILITY

Riboflavin is stable to heat and oxidation if protected from light; thus, most food processing operations have little effect on riboflavin content. Physical loss can be quite extensive through leaching effects, but little chemical degradation is likely to occur. Stability increases as acidity increases. Maximal stability to heat degradation is between pH 2.0 to 5.0. Destruction of the isoalloxazine ring occurs above pH 7.0,[8] and FMN and FAD are converted to riboflavin below pH 5.0.[4]

Riboflavin, FMN, and FAD are easily degraded by UV and visible light with the range of 420 to 560 nm causing the greatest effect.[7,11] Photochemical degradation proceeds through reduction of the isoalloxazine ring by electrons donated by the ribityl side chain.[10,12] The pH of the solution controls the route of degradation. In acidic or neutral solutions, the ribityl side chain is cleaved, forming lumichrome (Figure 8.4). Under alkaline pH, UV light exposure forms lumiflavin through cleavage at the deoxy-end carbon of the ribityl side chain.[13] The lumiflavin reaction is an important analytical tool to enhance flavin detection in chromatographic analysis, since it fluoresces more strongly than the native riboflavin.[14,15]

The high sensitivity of flavins to light degradation is a significant factor influencing food packaging. The light induced loss of riboflavin in fluid milk packaged in glass containers and subjected to sunlight was one of the first nutrient losses in food products documented by scientific study. More recent studies have documented riboflavin loss in translucent containers in refrigerated dairy cases leading to the use of light barriers in blow-molded polyethylene containers.[16] Even in dry products, light exposure can lead to riboflavin loss. Enriched pasta lost up to 80% of the riboflavin within 12 weeks under fluorescent light.[17] The extreme lability under even dim light conditions dictates that the analyst protect riboflavin preparations under all phases of analysis. Darkness and use of red light and low-actinic glassware can minimize riboflavin loss during analysis.

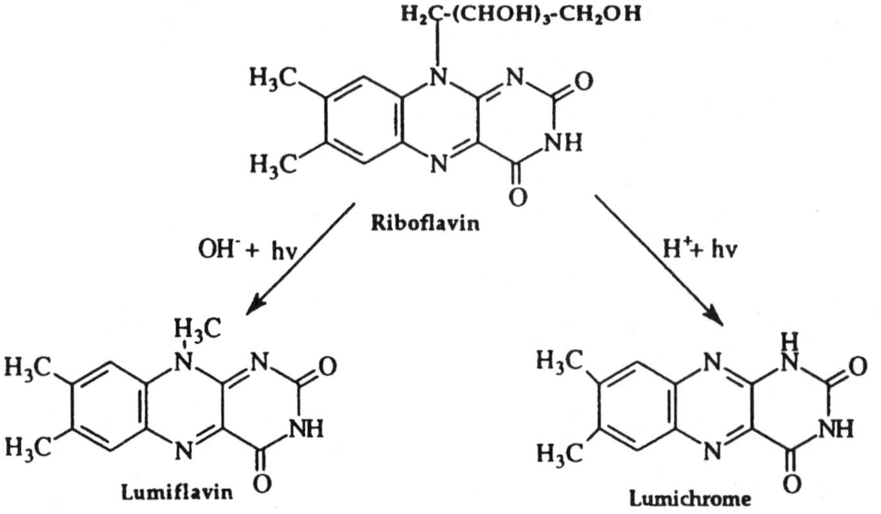

FIGURE 8.4   Conversion of riboflavin to lumiflavin and lumichrome.

8.3   METHODS

Rat and chick assays were developed for the analysis of riboflavin in the early 1930s. The animal assays were mostly replaced in the next decade by microbiological and fluorometric procedures followed by HPLC techniques in the 1970s. Recent reviews on methodology for riboflavin assay include Shah,[5] Nielsen,[6] Russell and Vanderslice,[10] Ottaway,[11] Ball[8] and Eitenmiller and Landen.[7] Compendium, handbook, and other standard methods are summarized in Table 8.2.

8.3.1   CHEMICAL

8.3.1.1   Direct Fluorometry

AOAC International methods[18] are based on the measurement of the native fluorescence of riboflavin. These methods include:

1. AOAC Official Method 970.65,
   Riboflavin (Vitamin B_2) in Foods and Vitamin Preparations—
   Fluorometric Method,
   AOAC Official Methods of Analysis, 45.1.07.
2. AOAC Official Method 981.15,
   Riboflavin in Foods and Vitamin Preparations—
   Automated Method,
   AOAC Official Methods of Analysis, 45.1.09.
3. AOAC Official Method 985.31,
   Riboflavin in Ready-to-Feed Milk-Based Infant Formula—
   Fluorometric Method,
   AOAC Official Methods of Analysis, 50.1.07.

These methods are closely related in principle and will be discussed to explain the chemistry, method development, and application aspects.

8.3.1.1.1   *Manual Procedure*

AOAC Official Method 970.65 has been the primary method used to determine published riboflavin content of the food supply. It remains an important procedure for analysis of riboflavin.[19] The

TABLE 8.2
Compendium, Regulatory, and Handbook Methods for the Analysis of Riboflavin

Source	Form	Method and Application	Approach	Most Current Cross-Reference
U.S. Pharmacopeia National Formulary, USP23/NF18 1995, Nutritional Supplements, Official Monograph[1]				
1. pages 2143, 2146, 2148, 2153	Riboflavin	Riboflavin in oil and water-soluble capsules/tablets w/wo minerals	HPLC 280 mm	None
2. pages 2162, 2168, 2170, 2172	Riboflavin	Riboflavin in water-soluble capsules/tablets w/wo minerals	HPLC 280 mm	None
3. page 1379	Riboflavin	Riboflavin (NLT 98.0%, NMT 102.0%)	Fluorescence Ex λ = 444 Em λ = 530	None
4. page 1379	Riboflavin	Riboflavin tablets/injection	Fluorescence Ex λ = 440 Em λ = 530	None
5. page 1380	Riboflavin 5′-phosphate sodium and other phosphate esters	Riboflavin 5′-phosphate sodium	HPLC Fluorescence Ex λ = 440 Em λ = 530	None
British Pharmacopeia, 15th Ed., 1993[2]				
1. vol. 1, page 558	Riboflavin	Riboflavin	Spectrophotometric 444 nm	None
2. vol. 1, page 559	Riboflavin 5′-phosphate sodium salt	Riboflavin sodium phosphate	Spectrophotometric 444 nm	None
AOAC International Official Methods of Analysis, 16 Ed., 1995[3]				
1. 45.2.01	Riboflavin	AOAC Official Method 960.46 Riboflavin, Microbiological Assays	Microbiological	*J. Assoc. Off. Anal. Chem.*, 42, 529, 1959[4]

TABLE 8.2 Continued

Source	Form	Method and Application	Approach	Most Current Cross-Reference
2. 45.1.08	Riboflavin	AOAC Official Method 970.65 Riboflavin in Foods and Vitamin Preparations	Fluorescence Ex λ = 440 Em λ = 565	J. Assoc. Off. Anal. Chem., 53, 542, 1970[5]
3. 50.1.07	Riboflavin	AOAC Official Method 985.31 Riboflavin in Ready-To-Feed Milk-Based Infant Formulas	Fluorescence Ex λ = 440 Em λ = 565	J. Assoc. Off. Anal. Chem., 68, 514, 1985[6]
4. 45.2.06	Riboflavin	AOAC Official Method 940.33 Riboflavin in Vitamin Preparations	Microbiological	J. Assoc. Off. Anal. Chem., 42, 529, 1959[4]
American Association of Cereal Chemists, Approved Methods, vol. 2, 1996[7]				
1. AACC 86–70	Riboflavin	Riboflavin in whole-grain, grits, meal, and puffed cereal, farina and bread	Fluorescence Automated Ex λ = 436 Em λ = 570	Cereal Sci. Today, 7 198, 1962[8] Anal. Chem., 19, 243, 1947[9]
2. AACC 86–72	Riboflavin	Riboflavin in whole-grain, grits, meal, flaked and puffed cereal, farina and bread	Microbiological	Ind. Eng. Chem., 14, 271, 1942[10]; 17, 176, 1945[11]
3. AACC 86–73	Riboflavin	Riboflavin in whole-grain, grits, meal, flaked and puffed cereal, farina and bread	Fluorescence Automated Ex λ = 436 Em λ =570	J. Agric. Food Chem., 23, 815, 1975[12]
American Feed Ingredients Association, Laboratory Methods Compendium, vol. 1, 1991[13]				
page 153	Riboflavin	Determination of vitamin B_2 in complete feeds and premixes with HPLC (> 0.5 mg/kg)	HPLC Fluorescence Ex λ = 453 Em λ = 521	None
Food Chemicals Codex, 4th Ed.,1996[14]				
1. pages 338–339	Riboflavin	Riboflavin (NLT 98.0%, NMT 102.0%)	Fluorescence Ex λ = 440 Em λ = 530	None

2. pages 339–341	Riboflavin 5´-phosphate sodium	Riboflavin 5´-phosphate sodium (NLT equivalent of 73.0% of Riboflavin, NMT equivalent of 79.0% of Riboflavin)	Fluorescence Ex λ = 440 Em λ = 530	None
Hoffmann-LaRoche, Analytical Methods for Vitamins and Carotenoids, 1988[15]				
1. pages 30–32	Riboflavin and co-enzyme forms	Determination of B_2 in complete feeds and premixes with HPLC (> 0.5 mg/kg)	HPLC Fluorescence Ex λ = 453 Em λ = 521	None
Methods for Determination of Vitamins in Foods Recommended by COST 91[16]	Riboflavin	Tentative method, foods	HPLC Fluorescence Ex λ = 453 Em λ = 521	*Anal. Chem.* 130, 359, 1983[17]

Atlanta Center for Nutrient Analysis, Food and Drug Administration uses this method for routine nutritional label compliance analysis. Method 970.65 measures total riboflavin after acid hydrolysis of FMN and FAD to free riboflavin. Hydrolysis is completed by autoclaving in 0.1 N HCl for 30 min. Specific parameters are provided in the *AOAC Official Methods of Analysis*[18] for preparation of dry and semi-dry samples, those containing basic materials, liquids, concentrates, premixes, and multivitamins. Proteins are removed by adjusting the pH to 4.5 and filtering or centrifuging to clarify the extract. pH is sequentially increased to 6.8 to check that no further precipitation occurs.

Interfering fluorescent substances are destroyed by acidifying the extract with glacial acetic acid and oxidation with potassium permanganate. After 2 min of oxidation, excess permanganate is destroyed with the addition of hydrogen peroxide. Hydrogen peroxide decolorizes the solution. If MnO_2 precipitate is noted at this point, the solution should be filtered or centrifuged. The oxidation step does not affect riboflavin, but is essential to limiting fluorescence as much as possible to riboflavin. A long standing criticism of the general procedure is that an overestimation of the true riboflavin content can occur through non-specific fluorescence.

Fluorescence measurements (Em λ = 440, Ex λ = 565) include sample solutions containing added riboflavin as an internal standard (spike) and on sample solutions containing water in place of the spike solution. After initial measurement of the sample fluorescence, sodium hydrosulfite is added to sample tubes and fluorescence is measured. The sodium hydrosulfite converts riboflavin to the non-fluorescent, reduced leuco form to provide a blank to correct for remaining fluorescence (not from riboflavin) after the addition of permanganate oxidation. The AOAC International procedure notes that addition of sodium hydrosulfite in excess of 20 mg per tube can reduce interfering fluorescing materials, leading to inaccuracies in the assay.

8.3.1.1.2   Modifications of AOAC International Method 970.65

Method 970.65 was modified for flow injection analysis to reduce manual error and increase laboratory output. AOAC Method 981.15 is a semi-automated procedure based on Method 970.65. Original studies were completed by Egberg and Potter[20] and Egberg.[21] The procedure used the Technicon AutoAnalyzer II system. Modifications to the manual method include the use of sodium bisulfite to reduce excess permanganate in place of hydrogen peroxide to eliminate oxygen bubble formation within the system. Blanks are run by replacing the sodium acetate diluent added in front of the fluorometer with sodium hydrosulfite solution. The samples are then pumped through the system a second time for the blank determination. To prevent precipitation and build up of MnO_2 in the coil where the excess permanganate is reduced, metaphosphoric acid is introduced as a manganese sequestering ligand. Egberg and Potter[20] obtained a correlation coefficient of 0.9869 with an overall standard error of 0.23 mg/100 g when the manual and semi-automated methods were compared on 61 different foods. Method 981.15 gives comparable results to the microbiological assay by *Lactobacillus rhamnosus*.[5]

Semi-automated procedures based on the Technicon Auto Analyzer were modified to a simpler flow injection analysis system.[19] Lack of a true internal standard for the AOAC International Methods is a recognized deficiency of the methods. Further, lack of defatting steps in the AOAC International Methods led to low recoveries for some matrices. This study also showed that raw liver could rapidly decrease spiked riboflavin if the addition was completed prior to autoclaving. Indigenous enzymes were, therefore, indicated to act rapidly to degrade riboflavin. The authors concluded that AOAC International Methods were not suitable for samples containing active enzyme systems.[19] This, again, draws attention to the need for the analyst to pay particular attention to stability factors early in the extraction stage for the analysis of all vitamins.

8.3.1.2   Indirect Fluorometry

Excellent discussions exist in the older literature on the use of lumiflavin for the indirect quantitation of riboflavin.[22,23] Riboflavin is converted to lumiflavin when irradiated under alkaline conditions (Figure 8.4). The reaction adds specificity since other fluorescing compounds in the sample extract are not converted to lumiflavin. Further specificity is added by extraction of the lumichrome into chloroform. Lumiflavin increases sensitivity since it fluoresces more strongly than native riboflavin (Ex λ = 450, Em λ = 513). Chloroform extraction of lumiflavin eliminates naturally occurring fluorescent materials from the sample extract which are not soluble in chloroform. Even though these advantages exist for the lumiflavin procedure, the method has seen little use.[8] The strong fluorescence and specificity of lumiflavin can be applied to HPLC methodology, eliminating the need for extract clean up. Lumiflavin was used for the HPLC analysis of riboflavin in meat and meat products with detection limits as low as 0.05 ng per injection.[15] Addition of riboflavin standard to the sample as an internal reference standard is recommended to compensate for possible intensity differences in irradiation of the sample extract and the reference riboflavin solution.[22] Extractions of natural products might require amylase or protease treatment to obtain optimal extraction efficiency.

8.3.2 MICROBIOLOGICAL

Lactobacillus rhamnosis (formerly *L. casei*) ATCC 7469 is considered to be the best and most often used microorganism for riboflavin assay. Since the *L. rhamnosis* response to FMN and FAD differs from the growth promotion by riboflavin, all methods based on *L. rhamnosis* are for total riboflavin. Procedures incorporate an acid hydrolysis step to convert FMN and FAD to free riboflavin. Other microorganisms including *Leuconostoc mesenteroides*,[23] *Tetrahymena pyriformis*,[24] and *Enterococcus faecalis*[8,25] have riboflavin growth requirements but have not been extensively used. *L. rhamnosis* growth is affected by common biological sample constituents including starch, protein degradation products, and free fatty acids. Free fatty acids can stimulate or inhibit the growth response, and fat should be extracted with ether or hexane prior to the acid hydrolysis step. The fat extraction step should be considered routine unless the analyst verifies that the fat content of the sample is inconsequential to the assay results. Proteins are removed through precipitation at pH 4.5. Ball[8] points out that *E. faecalis* is not affected as extensively by matrix effects compared to *L. rhamnosis,* and that it could be used in place of *L. rhamnosis*. However, lack of commercial media for the *E. faecalis* assay makes its use more difficult.

AOAC International Method 940.33, "Riboflavin (Vitamin B₂) in Vitamin Preparations, Microbiological Methods (960.46)," Chapter 45.2.06, is approved only for vitamin preparations. However, because of the broad application of *L. rhamnosis* to food analysis, the AOAC Task Force on Methods for Nutrient Labeling recommended collaboration of the assay for all food matrices.[26] At this time, the procedure has not been collaborated. In the procedure, FMN and FAD are converted to free riboflavin by hydrolysis with 0.1 N HCl (121°C for 30 min). The hydrolyzed extracts are adjusted to pH 4.5, precipitated protein is filtered or centrifuged from the extract and the pH is adjusted to 6.8. Digestion with amylolytic or proteolytic enzymes are not required in Method 940.33. However, enzyme digestions can be highly beneficial for efficient extraction of riboflavin from high starch or high protein matrices as well as ensuring the complete conversion of FMN and FAD to riboflavin.

Combined extractions for thiamin and riboflavin analysis have been commonly used for food analysis.[27,28] Recently, the European Measurement and Testing Program reported an optimal combined extraction procedure for thiamin and riboflavin suitable for either microbiological or HPLC analysis.[29] Details of this extraction are given in Chapter 7, Thiamin.

8.3.3 HIGH PERFORMANCE LIQUID CHROMATOGRAPHY

Reviews on HPLC methods for analysis of riboflavin, FMN, and FAD include Finglas and Faulks,[30] Van Niekerk,[31] Russell and Vanderslice,[10] Nielsen,[6] Ottaway,[11] and Ball.[8] Russell and Vanderslice[10] categorized HPLC methods for riboflavin and its coenzymes as follows:

1. Total riboflavin analysis using C_{18} columns and fluorescence detection.
2. Total riboflavin analysis using C_{18} columns and UV detection.
3. Total riboflavin analysis using silica and amino columns with either fluorescence or UV detection.
4. Individual flavin analysis excluding the simultaneous determination of riboflavin, FMN, and FAD.
5. Simultaneous analysis of riboflavin, FMN and FAD.

To broaden this classification, HPLC methods for the concurrent or simultaneous analysis of other water-soluble vitamins in addition to total riboflavin should be added. In more recent published methods for food analysis, thiamin and riboflavin are frequently analyzed together. We define concurrent methods as those that utilize the same sample extract with different chromatography systems; whereas, simultaneous procedures quantitate the two vitamins from the same LC injection. HPLC methods are summarized in Table 8.3 (total riboflavin), Table 8.4 (concurrent methods for riboflavin and thiamin), and Table 8.5 (simultaneous methods for riboflavin and thiamin and occasionally other water-soluble vitamins).

8.3.3.1   Extraction Procedures for Riboflavin Analysis by HPLC

Summaries of extraction procedures for riboflavin are provided in Tables 8.3, 8.4, and 8.5. Total riboflavin analysis is initiated with acid hydrolysis by HCl or H_2SO_4 to convert co-enzyme forms into free riboflavin. These procedures either duplicate or closely follow procedures recommended for the chemical or microbiological assay procedures. Solid phase clean-up procedures are often used prior to injection. Supports for extract clean up include C_{18} or Florisil. Extraction procedures for urine and serum commonly start with the addition of trichloroacetic acid (TCA), ammonium sulfate, or metaphosphoric acid to the sample for deproteinization. When TCA is used, excess TCA must be removed with water-saturated diethyl ether. These procedures do not incorporate acid hydrolysis and, therefore, allow quantitation of FAD and FMN in addition to free riboflavin. Lopez-Anaya and Mayersohn[32] precipitated proteins in urine with acetonitrile followed by shaking with chloroform and injected the extract directly for analysis of riboflavin, FMN, and FAD in urine and plasma.

Specific methods for quantitation of riboflavin and its co-enzymes in foods include those by Russell and Vanderslice[4] and Bilic and Sieber.[33] Russell and Vanderslice extracted the flavins with methanol and dichloromethane followed by partitioning with 100 mM citrate phosphate buffer, pH 5.5. Bilic and Sieber[33] extracted dairy products with 6% formic acid containing 2 M urea followed by C_{18} solid phase clean up. Both procedures used internal standards and proved useful for accurate quantitation of the native riboflavin forms in foods.

Usually, acid digestion with autoclaving completely liberates riboflavin from bound forms. However, difficult matrices such as those high in starch or protein can be more effectively extracted through use of amylolytic or proteolytic enzymes.[10] Enzyme digestion can benefit analyte recovery, ensure conversion of FMN and FAD, and aid in sample clean up. For certain foods such as milk, dairy products, and eggs where the predominant form is free riboflavin or loosely-bound forms (not FMN or FAD), acid and enzyme conversion is not always necessary for accurate riboflavin assay.[8] Russell and Vanderslice[4] reported that approximately 85% of the riboflavin in pasteurized whole milk was riboflavin with the remainder as FMN and FAD. No detectable co-enzyme forms were present in raw and cooked whole egg or raw egg yolk. Various studies have used simple extraction procedures for the analysis of riboflavin in milk and dairy products.[16,34,35] Munoz et al.[35] deproteinized the sample with 10% lead acetate solution acidified to pH 3.2 with glacial acetic acid followed by filtration to prepare milk extracts for LC injection. For foods containing appreciable amounts of FMN and FAD, efficient conversion of the co-enzymes to free riboflavin must be assured. Recommendations include the routine application of enzymatic hydrolysis

TABLE 8.3

HPLC Methods for the Analysis of Riboflavin in Foods, Feed, Pharmaceuticals and Biologicals

Sample Matrix	Analyte	Sample Preparation		HPLC Parameters				
		Sample Extraction	Clean Up	Column	Mobile Phase	Detection	Quality Assurance Parameters	References
Foods								
1. Eggs, dairy products	Riboflavin	Milk Acidify to pH 3.0 with HAC Centrifuge Dairy products and eggs Suspend in water : MeOH (2 : 1) Homogenize Acidify to pH 3.0 Centrifuge	—	μBondapak C$_{18}$ 30 cm × 3.9 mm	Isocratic Water : MeOH : HAC (65 : 35 : 0.1) 1 mL /min	270 nm	DL (ng) On-column 10 % CV 0.98–8.6 % Recovery 91.3–109	J. Food Sci., 48, 92, 1983[1]
2. Milk, dairy products	Riboflavin	Milk Pass through C$_{18}$ Sep-Pak Elute riboflavin with 0.02 M acetate buffer, pH 4.0 : MeOH (1 : 1) Dairy products Blend with 0.02 M acetate buffer, pH 4.0 Pass through C$_{18}$ Sep-Pak	—	Bio-Sil ODS—5S C$_{18}$ 25 cm × 4 mm	Isocratic Water : MeOH : HAC (65 : 35 : 0.1) 1 mL/min	270 nm	DL (ng) On-column 10 % CV 1.6–5.4 % Recovery 94.5–100.7	J. Assoc. Off. Anal Chem., 68, 693, 1985[2]

TABLE 8.3 Continued

Sample Matrix	Sample Preparation			HPLC Parameters				
	Analyte	Sample Extraction	Clean Up	Column	Mobile Phase	Detection	Quality Assurance Parameters	References
3. Cheese	Riboflavin	Homogenize in water : MeOH (2 : 1) Acidify with HAC Centrifuge	—	LiChrosorb RP$_{18}$ 5 μm 25 cm × 4 mm	Isocratic MeCN : water (20 : 80) 1 mL/min	446 nm	DL (ng) On-column 2.5 % CV 2.1–6.5 % Recovery 90.2	J. Food Sci., 51, 857, 1986[3]
4. Milk	Riboflavin	Mix with 10% TCA Dilute and filter	—	Spherisorb ODS 5 μm 25 cm × 4.5 mm	Isocratic MeCN : water (20 : 80) 1.5 mL/min	Fluorescence Ex λ = 453 Ex λ = 580	DL (ng) On-column 0.5 % CV 6.5–8 % Recovery 93–98	Die Nahr, 31, 77, 1987[4]
5. Milk	Riboflavin	Mix 2 mL of 10% lead acetate with 20 mL milk. Filter	—	LiChrosorb C$_{18}$ 10 μm 25 cm × 4.6 mm	Isocratic water : MeOH : HAC (50 : 49 : 1) 1.5mL/min	Fluorescence Filter fluorometer	—	J. Food Sci., 53, 436, 1988[5]
6. Various foods	Riboflavin	Add 0.1 N HCl Autoclave, 30 min Adjust pH to 4.5 Dilute, filter	—	LiChrosorb C$_{18}$ 10 μm 25 cm × 4 mm	Isocratic 0.005 M 1-Hex sulfonic acid : MeOH (60 : 40) 1.0 mL/min	Fluorescence Ex λ = 440 Ex λ = 565	QL (mg/100g) 0.02 % CV 2.7 % Recovery 86–99	J. Assoc. Off. Anal. Chem., 71, 16, 1988[6]

7. Various foods	Riboflavin	Homogenize Add 0.2 M H_2SO_4 Autoclave, 20 min Adjust pH to 4.5 with 2.5 M acetate buffer Digest with Claradiastase or Takadiastase, 45° C Dilute, filter	Sep-Pak C_{18}	Spherisorb S5 ODS2 5 µm 25 cm × 4.6 mm	Isocratic MeOH : water (35 : 65) 1 mL/min	Fluorescence Ex λ = 445 Ex λ = 525	DL (pg) On-column 20 % CV 3.4–6.2 % Recovery 93–108	*J. Micronutr. Anal.*, 8, 199, 1990[7]
8. Various foods	Riboflavin	Add 0.1 N HCl (30 mL) and 6 N HCl (1 mL) to 5–10 g sample Autoclave, 15 min Adjust pH to 4.0–4.5 Digest with Takadiastase, 48° C, 3 h Filter and dilute	Florisil followed by Sep-Pak C_{18}	µBondapak C_{18} 10 µm 30 cm × 3.9 mm	Isocratic MeOH : water : HAC (32 : 67 : 1) containing 5mM Na Hexsulfonate or MeOH : water : HAC (31 : 68 : 0.5) containing 5 mM Na heptane sulfonate and 5 mM hexsulfonate (25 : 75)	254 nm	DL (ng) On-column 0.4 % Recovery 98	*J. Liq. Chromatogr.*, 13, 2089, 1990[8]
9. Dairy Products	Riboflavin, FMN, FAD	Add formic acid-urea (6% formic acid containing 2 M urea) Homogenize or mix Centrifuge to remove fat Add sorboflavin (IS)	Silica gel C_{18}	Supelco LC$_{18}$ 3 µm 7.5 cm × 4.6 mm	Isocratic MeCN : 00 mM KH_2PO_4 (14 : 86), pH 2.9	Fluorescence Ex λ = 450 Em λ = 530	DL (nmol/L) FMN = 2.5 B_2 = 2.5 FAD = 3 % CV 6.7 % Recovery 95–101	*J. Chromatogr.*, 511, 359, 1990[9]

TABLE 8.3 Continued

Sample Matrix	Analyte	Sample Preparation — Sample Extraction	Clean Up	HPLC Parameters — Column	Mobile Phase	Detection	Quality Assurance Parameters	References
10. Various foods	Riboflavin, FMN, FAD	AddMeOH (9.0 mL) and CH_2Cl_2 (10 mL) per 0.5–4.0 g sample Add 7-ethyl-8-methyl-riboflavin (IS) Homogenize Add 100 mM citrate-phosphate buffer, pH 5.5 containing sodium azide Homogenize Centrifuge, filter	—	2 PLRP-S 100 Å in series 5 μm 25 cm × 4.6 mm 15 cm × 4.6 mm	Gradient MeCN : 0.1% sodium azide in 10 mM citrate-phosphate buffer, pH 5.5 0 min (3 : 97) linear gradient to (6 : 94) at 43 min Isocratic at (14 : 86) to 70 min linear gradient to (3 : 97) to 80 min Isocratic at (3 : 97) to 90 min	Fluorescence Ex λ = 450 Em λ = 522	% Recovery 96–113	Food Chem., 43, 151, 1992[10]
11. Milk, non-dairy imitation milk	Riboflavin	Add 10 lead acetate, pH 3.2 Filter	—	Spherisorb ODS 5 μm 15 cm × 3.9 mm 1 L water 0.6 mL/min	Isocratic water-acetic acid : MeOH (70 : 30) Add 1.5 mL HAC to 1 L water 0.6 mL/min	270 nm	% Recovery 92.2± 1.2	Food Chem., 49, 203, 1994[11]
12. Casein	Riboflavin	To 1 g, add 50 mg pepsin, 7 mL 0.1 M HCl Incubate, 37° C, 18 or 24 h Add 1.0 mL 0.35 M NaOAC, pH 5.5 Add 0.1 g Tatadiastase Incubate, 45° C, 2 or 18 h Dilute to 10mL Filter	—	Spherisorb ODS 5 μm 25 cm × 4.6 mm	Isocratic 0.05 M NaOAC in MeOH : water (35 : 65)	Fluorescence Ex λ = 447 Em λ = 517	QL (ng/kg) 0.1 RSD = 3%	Analyst, 121, 1671, 1996[12]

Biologicals

Sample	Analytes	Sample preparation	Cleanup	Column	Conditions	Detection	Performance	Reference
1. Blood	Riboflavin, FMN, FAD	Add 10% TCA Hold at 4° C, 30 min Add NaOAC buffer Centrifuge	—	Hypersil ODS 5 µm 15 cm × 4.6 mm	Isocratic 0.3 M KH$_2$PO$_4$: MeOH (83.3 : 16.7) pH 2.9 2 mL/min	Fluorescence Ex λ = 470 Em λ = 525	DL (nmol/L) B$_2$ = 10 FAD = 20 FMN = 15 QL (nmol/L) FAD = 240 % Recovery 94	J. Chromatogr., 228, 311, 1982[1]
2. Fish serum	Riboflavin, FMN, FAD	Add 10% TCA Hold at 0° C, 30 min Add NaOAC buffer Centrifuge	—	Zorbax–NH$_2$ 5 µm 15 cm × 4.6 mm	Isocratic MeOH : 0.2 M NAH$_2$PO$_4$, pH 3.0 (90 : 10) 1.3 mL/min 50° C	Fluorescence Ex λ = 328 Em λ = 526	DL (ng/mL) B$_1$ = 4.9 FMN = 9.1 FAD = 73.1 CV 11–13% % Recovery 92–97	Analyst, 110, 1505, 1985[2]
3. Serum, urine	Riboflavin	Add isoriboflavin (IS) Add TCA (100g/L) Centrifuge	Sep-Pak C$_{18}$ for serum	ROSIL C$_{18}$HL 5 µm 15 cm × 3.2 mm	Isocratic MeOH : water : HAC (36.7 : 63.7 : 0.1) 0.75 mL/min	Fluorescence Ex λ = 450 Em λ = 530	DL (µg/L) 10 (serum) % CV 2.2–4.9	Clin. Chem., 318, 1371, 1985[3]
4-6. Urine	Riboflavin	Add HAC and toluene Saturate with (NH$_4$)$_2$SO$_4$ Centrifuge Add 80% aqueous phenol Centrifuge Add water, extract with water saturated Et$_2$O	—	µBondaPak C$_{18}$	Gradient 5 mM NH$_4$OAC buffer, pH 6.0 for 2 min Linear gradient To 21% MeOH in 2 min To 50% MeOH in 17 min to 70% MeOH in 2 min	Fluorescence Ex λ = 305–365 Em λ = 475–650	—	J. Nutr. 115, 496, 1985[4]; 117, 468, 1987[5] Am. J. Clin. Nutr., 46, 830, 1987[6]

TABLE 8.3 Continued

		Sample Preparation		HPLC Parameters				
Sample Matrix	Analyte	Sample Extraction	Clean Up	Column	Mobile Phase	Detection	Quality Assurance Parameters	References
7. Urine	Riboflavin FMN, FAD 7α-OH-riboflavin Lumiflavin	Add 5% metaphosphoric acid containing 5% β-thiodiglycol Centrifuge Filter	—	AsahiPak-G5 320H Hydrophilic gel 25 cm × 7.5 mm	Isocratic 148 g propionic acid and 32 g NaOH in 2 L water, pH 4.4 55° C	Fluorescence Ex λ = 450 Em λ = 525	% Recovery 98.7 ± 2.5	*J. Chromatogr.*, 385, 283, 1987[7]
8. Plasma, urine	Riboflavin FMN, FAD, degradation products	Plasma Add MeCN to plasma (1 : 1) Centrifuge Extract with $CHCl_3$ Assay aqueous phase Urine Inject directly or dilute with water	—	PRP-1 10 μm 25 cm × 4.6 mm	Isocratic MeCN : water : 10% trifluoroacetic acid : (14 : 84 : 1.5 : 0.09) pH 1.8	Fluorescence Ex λ = 470 Em λ = 525	DL (ng/mL) 1–5 % Recovery >84	*J. Chromatogr.*, 423, 105, 1987[8]
9. Tissues	FAD	Add TCA : 0.6 M Et_2O to 200–300 mg sample Homogenize (Polytron) Extract with 4 mL TCA : water (10 : 90) Centrifuge Extract supernatant with Et_2O Filter	—	Hypersil APS-NH_2 5 μm 15 cm × 4.6 mm	Isocratic MeCN : 0.1 M NaH_2PO_4, pH 3.05 (30 : 70) 0.8 mL/min	Electrochemical glassy carbon Ag/AgCl reference 280mV	DL (pmol) On-column FAD = 1.25 % Recovery 95	*J. Chromatogr.*, 442, 441, 1988[9]

					Isocratic	Fluorescence	% Recovery	
10–11. Retina	Riboflavin, FMN, FAD	Homogenize Add TCA to 4% final concentration Centrifuge, 4°C Add 5% NH_4Cl in 10 mM NaH_2PO_4 pH 5.5 Filter	—	Sepralyte CH 5 µm 15 cm × 4.0 mm	2% $(NH_4)_2PO_4$: MeCN (90 : 10) 2 mL/min	Ex λ = 447 Em λ = 530	~100	Anal. Biochem., 188, 164, 1990[10] Exp. Eye Res., 54, 605, 1992[11]

TABLE 8.4
HPLC Methods for the Concurrent Analysis of Riboflavin and Thiamin in Foods, Feed, Pharmaceuticals, and Biologicals

| Sample Matrix | Analyte | Sample Preparation | | HPLC Parameters | | | |
		Sample Extraction	Clean Up	Column	Mobile Phase	Detection	Quality Assurance Parameters	References
1. Meat, meat products	Thiamin, riboflavin	Add 0.1 N HCl (60 mL) to 5 g sample Autoclave, 30 min Adjust pH to 4.0–4.5 Digest with Takadiastase and papain Add 2 mL of 10% TCA Heat on steam bath, 5 min Dilute, filter Convert thiamin to thiochrome and riboflavin to lumiflavin	—	Spherisorb Silica 20 μm 50 cm × 2.1 mm	Isocratic CHC_3 : MeOH (90 : 10) 1 mL/min—thiamin 0.8 mL/min—riboflavin	Thiochrome Pre-column Fluorescence Ex λ = 367 Em λ = 418 Lumiflavin Pre-column Fluorescence Ex λ = 270 Em λ = 418	DL (mg) B_1 = 0.05 Lumiflavin = 0.02 % Recovery 84–100	*J. Agric. Food Chem.,* 28, 483, 1980[1]
2. Potatoes	Thiamin, riboflavin	Add 0.1 N HCl to 25 g sample Reflux for 30 min Cool, adjust pH to 4.5 through addition of 16mL of Takadiastase solution in 1 M acetate buffer, pH 4.6 Digest at 45–50° C, 2h Dilute, filter	—	μBondapak C_{18} 25 cm × 4.6 mm	Isocratic water : MeOH (70 : 30) 2 mL/min	Thiochrome Pre-column Fluorescence Ex λ = 365 Em λ = 435 Riboflavin Fluorescence Ex λ = 450 Em λ = 510	DL (ng) On-column B_1 = 0.5 B_2 = 0.1 % CV B_1 = 7.4 B_2 = 7.9 % Recovery B_1 = 95.2 ± 1.2 B_2 = 94.3 ± 2.9	*Food Chem.,* 15, 37, 1984[2]

3. Meats	Thiamin Riboflavin Niacin	Add 0.1 N HCl (60 mL) and 6 N HCl (2mL) to 5 g sample Autoclave, 121° C, 60 min Adjust pH with 2 N NaOAC Digest with Takadiastase and papain 40–45° C, 2.5–3.0 h Add 50% TCA (2 mL) Heat at 100° C, 10 min Dilute, filter	Extract thiochrome reaction mixture with isobutyl alcohol	Alltech C$_{10}$ 10 μm	Isocratic 0.02 M phosphate buffer : MeOH (70 : 30) pH 7.0 1 mL/min	Thiochrome Pre-column Fluorescence Ex λ = 378 Em λ = 430 Riboflavin Fluorescence Ex λ = 378 Em λ = 430 Niacin 254 Riboflavin and Niacin assayed simultaneously with detectors in series	% Recovery B$_1$ = 98.1 B$_2$ = 96.3 Niacin= 97.5	*J. Agric. Food Chem.,* 36, 1176, 1988[3]
4. Dietetic foods	Thiamin Riboflavin	Add 0.1 M HCl (65 mL) to 5 g sample Heat at 100° C, 30 min Adjust pH to 4.5 with 2.5 M NaOAC Digest overnight with mixture of β-amylase and Takadiastase Dilute, filter	Sep-Pak C$_{18}$ to remove excess oxidizing reagent from thiochrome reaction	μBondapak C$_{18}$	Isocratic MeOH : 0.05 M NaOAC, pH 4.5 (60 : 40) 1 mL/min	Thiochrome Pre-column Fluorescence Ex λ = 366 Em λ = 435 Riboflavin Fluorescence Ex λ = 422 Em λ = 522	QL (mg/100g) B$_1$ = 0.02 B$_2$ = 0.02 % Recovery 95–100	*J. Micronutr. Anal.,* 5, 269, 1989[4]
5. Soybeans, tofu	Thiamin Riboflavin	Soak in water at 4°C for 10 h Heat at 90°C for 30 min Adjust to pH 2.0 Autoclave, 15 min Adjust pH to 4.5 Filter Dilute	—	Ultrasphere C$_{18}$ 5 μm 15 cm × 4.6 mm	Isocratic MeCN : 0.01 acetate buffer, pH 5.5 (13 : 87) 1.2 mL/min	Thiochrome Pre-column Fluorescence Ex λ = 362 Em λ = 436 Riboflavin Fluorescence Ex λ = 436 Em λ = 535	% Recovery B$_1$ = 84 B$_2$ = 95	*J. Agric. Food Chem.,* 38, 163, 1990[5]

TABLE 8.4 Continued

| Sample Matrix | Analyte | Sample Preparation | | HPLC Parameters | | | | |
		Sample Extraction	Clean Up	Column	Mobile Phase	Detection	Quality Assurance Parameters	References
6–8. Cereals, various foods	Thiamin Riboflavin	Add 0.1 N HCl (30mL) to 5 g sample Autoclave, 125°C 15 min Adjust to pH 4.0–4.5 with 2 N NaOAC Digest with Claradiastase, 50°C, 3h Add 1 mL of 50% TCA Heat at 90°C, 15 min Adjust pH to 3.5 with 2 N NaOAC Dilute, filter	—	μBondapak C_{18} RCM 8 × 10	Isocratic MeOH : 0.005 M phosphate buffer, pH 7.0 (35 : 65) 0.8 mL/min	Thiochrome Pre-column Fluorescence Ex λ = 360 Em λ = 425 Riboflavin Fluorescence Ex λ = 440 Em λ = 520	% CV B_1 = 5.5 B_2 = 10 % Recovery B_1 = 85–94 B_2 = 80–96	*J. Food Comp. Anal.,* 6, 299, 1993[6] *J. AOAC Int.,* 77 681, 1994[7] *J. Food Comp. Anal.,* 7, 94, 1994[8]
9. Meat, liver	Thiamin Riboflavin	Add 0.01 M HCl (35 mL) to 5 g minced sample Autoclave, 121°C 30 min Add 2 mL Takadiastase in 2.5 M NaOAC buffer Add 2 mL Claradiastase and 2 mL papain (in water) Adjust pH to 4.5 Digest 16–18 h at 37°C Filter, adjust pH to 6.0 Filter, dilute	Nucleosil C_{18} Centrifuge	Nucleosil C_{18} 3 μm 15 cm × 4.6 mm	Isocratic 0.01 M KH_2PO_4 pH 3.0 : MeCN (84 : 16) meat or (85 : 15) liver containing 5 mM sodium hexsulfonate	254	DL (μg/mL) B_1 = 0.1 B_2 = 0.03 QL (μg/mL) B_1 = 50 B_2 = 16 % CV B_1 = 8 B_2 = 5 % Recovery B_1 = 83 B_2 = 89	*J. Chromatogr. A.* 668, 359, 1994[9]

| 10. Various foods | Thiamin
Riboflavin | Add 0.1 M HCl (65 mL) to 5 g sample
Heat at 100°C, 30 min
Adjust pH to 4.5 with 2.5 M NaOAC
Digest with β-amylase and Takadiastase,
37°C, 18 h
Dilute, filter | Sep-Pak C$_{18}$ for thiochrome | C$_{18}$
10 μm
25 cm × 4 mm | Isocratic
MeOH : 0.05 M NaOAC (30 : 70)
1 mL/min | Thiochrome
Pre-column
Fluorescence
Ex λ = 366
Em λ = 435
Riboflavin
Fluorescence
Ex λ = 422
Em λ = 522 | % CV
B$_1$ = 13–21
B$_2$ = 5–13
% Recovery
89 | *Food Chem.*, 56, 81, 1996[10] |

TABLE 8.5
HPLC Methods for the Simultaneous Analysis of Riboflavin and Thiamin in Foods, Feed, Pharmaceuticals, and Biologicals

| Sample Matrix | Analyte | Sample Preparation | | HPLC Parameters | | | |
		Sample Extraction	Clean Up	Column	Mobile Phase	Detection	Quality Assurance Parameters	References
1. Various foods	Thiamin Riboflavin	Add 0.1 N HCl (30 mL) and 6 N HCl (1 mL) to 1 g sample Autoclave, 121° C 15 min Adjust pH to 4.0–4.5 with 2 N NaOAC Digest with Takadiastase, 48° C, 3 h Add 50% TCA (2 mL) Heat on steam bath, 15 min Adjust pH to 3.5 Dilute, filter	Sep-Pak C$_{18}$ after thiochrome formation	Radial-Pak C$_{18}$ 10 cm × 18 mm	Isocratic MeOH : 0.01 M phosphate buffer, pH 7.0 (37 : 63) 1.5 or 3.0 mL/min	Thiochrome Pre-column Fluorescence Ex λ = 360 Em λ = 415 Riboflavin Fluorescence Ex λ = 360, 450 Em λ = 415, 530	DL (ng) On-column B$_1$ = 0.5 B$_2$ = 1.0 % Recovery B$_1$ = 99.5–110 B$_2$ = 85.6–104	J. Food Sci., 47, 2048, 1982[1]
2. Various foods	Thiamin Riboflavin	See J. Food Sci., 47, 2048, 1982[1]	See J. Food Sci., 47, 2048, 1982[1]	Ultrasphere ODS 5 μm 25 cm × 4.6 mm	Isocratic MeOH : water (20 : 80) pH 7.0, containing 0.005 M tetrabutyl ammonium phosphate	Thiochrome Pre-column Fluorescence Ex λ = 360 Em λ = 415 Riboflavin Fluorescence Ex λ = 450 Em λ = 530	DL (ng) On-column B$_1$ = 0.5 B$_2$ = 1.0	J. Assoc. Off. Anal. Chem. 67, 1012, 1984[2]

No. Sample	Analytes	Extraction	Cleanup	Column	Mobile Phase	Detection	Performance	Reference
3–4. Fortified cereal	Thiamin Riboflavin Pyridoxine	Add 0.1 N H_2SO_4 (35 mL) to 2 g sample Heat at 100°C, 30 min Add Clarase in 5 mL 2.5 M NaOAC Digest, 55°C, 60 min Centrifuge	—	μBondapak C$_{18}$ 30 cm × 4.1 mm	Isocratic MeOH : water (36:64) containing 1% HAC and 0.005 M hexsulfonic acid 1 mL/min	Thiochrome Post-column Fluorescence Ex λ = 360 Em λ = 460 Riboflavin Pyridoxine Fluorescence Ex λ = 288 Em λ = 418	QL (μg/g) B$_1$ = 1 B$_2$ = 1 B$_6$ = 2 % CV B$_1$ = 2.1 B$_2$ = 1.5 B$_6$ = 1.7 % Recovery B$_1$ = 92 B$_2$ = 91 B$_6$ = 90	J. Agric. Food Chem., 32, 1326, 1984[3] J. Chromatogr., 299, 281, 1984[4]
5–6. Various foods	Thiamin Riboflavin	AOAC extraction	—	μBondapak C$_{18}$ Radial Pak 10 μm	Isocratic MeOH : water (40:60) containing 5 mM PicB$_6$, 1.5 mL/min	Thiochrome Post-column Fluorescence Ex λ = 360 Em λ = 425 Riboflavin Fluorescence Ex λ = 360 Em λ = 500	DL (μg) On-column B$_1$ = 0.002 B$_2$ = 0.003 % Recovery B$_1$ = 98.7 ± 1.8 B$_2$ = 98.6 ± 1.5	J. Micronutr. Anal., 1, 23, 1985[5] J. Chromatogr., 318, 412, 1985[6]
7. Goat milk	Thiamin Riboflavin Ascorbic acid	Acid digestion, autoclave, 125°C, 15 min Digest with takadiastase	Sep-Pak C$_{18}$	Nova-Pak C$_{18}$ Cartridge RCM-100 5 μm	Isocratic water : MeOH (70:30) containing 0.0005 M hexsulfonate 2 mL/min	Diode array 214 nm 200 to 400 nm	% CV B$_1$ = 5.9 B$_2$ = 8.0 % Recovery B$_1$ = 92.1 B$_2$ = 89.0	J. Chromatogr., 410, 201, 1987[7]

TABLE 8.5 Continued

	Sample Preparation		HPLC Parameters				
Sample Matrix	Analyte	Sample Extraction	Clean Up	Column	Mobile Phase	Detection	Quality Assurance Parameters	References
8–9. Infant formula, medical foods	Thiamin Riboflavin Pyridoxine	Weigh sample equivalent of 120–180 µg of each vitamin Add water to 60 mL Add 2 mL perchloric acid, stir for 30 min Add 6 M KOH dropwise to pH 3.2 ± 0.4 Transfer to 200 mL volumetric, dilute with mobile phase Refrigerate overnight Filter	—	Pico Tag 30 cm × 3.9 mm	Isocratic Hexsulfonic acid (0.95 M) in 1 L water containing 9.5 mL MeCN and 0.5 mL NH$_4$OH, pH 3.6 Dilute 930 mL to 1 L	Thiochrome Post-column Fluorescence Ex λ = 360 Em λ = 435 Riboflavin Fluorescence Ex λ = 440 Em λ = 565 Pyridoxine Fluorescence Ex λ = 295 Em λ = 395	Medical Foods DL (µg/mL) B$_1$ = 0.05 B$_2$ = 0.05 B$_6$ = 0.01 % CV B$_1$ = 5.9 B$_2$ = 6.0 B$_6$ = 10.7 % Recovery B$_1$ = 111 B$_2$ = 96.3 B$_6$ = 113	J. AOAC Int., 75, 561, 1992[8] 76, 276, 1993[9]
10. Various foods	Thiamin Riboflavin	Add 0.1 N HCl (50 mL) to sample weight containing 30–40 µg of each vitamin Autoclave, 121° C, 30 min Adjust pH to 4.5 with 2 M NaOAC Dilute, filter	Sep-Pak C$_{18}$	µBondapak C$_{18}$ 30 cm × 3.9 mm	0.005 M NH$_4$OAC, pH 5.0 : MeOH (72 : 28) 1.5 mL/min	Thiochrome Post-column Fluorescence Ex λ = 370 Em λ = 435 Riboflavin Fluorescence Ex λ = 370	DL (ng) On-column B$_1$ = 0.05 B$_2$ = 0.05 % CV B$_1$ = 1.9 B$_2$ = 1.6	J. AOAC Int., 76, 1156, 1993[10]

by an enzyme preparation containing phosphatase activity to convert any remaining phosphorylated forms remaining after acid hydrolysis to free riboflavin[8,30] Extraction procedures provided by the French Commission Générale d'Unification des Méthods d'Analyse[36] and the Standards, Measurement, and Testing Program (EUMAT)[29] provide excellent proven protocols for riboflavin extraction. The French procedure is summarized in Section 8.4. An indication of inadequate hydrolysis is the presence of phosphorylated riboflavin peaks in the chromatogram. For this reason, the quality control program for the analysis should include chromatographic characterization of FMN.

8.3.3.2 Chromatography Parameters

8.3.3.2.1 Supports and Mobile Phases

Various supports have been used for riboflavin chromatography. C_{18} stationary phases are most commonly used for total riboflavin analysis in foods and biologicals (Tables 8.3 to 8.5). Other supports such as C_{10}, -NH_2, hydrophilic gel, and normal-phase chromatography on silica have been less frequently, although successfully, applied. Mobile phases consist of mixtures of methanol or acetonitrile with water or buffers. Ion-pair chromatography with heptane or hexane sulfonate or triethyl- or tetrabutyl ammonium phosphate can improve resolution, but ion-pairs have not been needed in most published resolution systems. Methods that simultaneously determine riboflavin and thiamin as thiochrome (Table 8.5) more frequently utilize ion-pair chromatography.

Methods for the quantitation of riboflavin, FMN, and FAD use polymer-based columns (PLRP-5, Polymer Laboratories) of polystyrene/divinylbenzene resin to avoid stability problems noted for silica based supports under the column conditions required for FMN and FAD stability. PLRP-5 was used by Russell and Vanderslice[4] with gradient elution by acetonitrile/0.1% sodium azide : 10 mM citrate-phosphate buffer, pH 5.5 (3 : 97 to 6 : 94 to 14 : 86) to effectively resolve riboflavin, FMN, FAD, and 7-ethyl-8-methyl-riboflavin (internal standard) in various food extracts. Lopez-Anaya and Mayersohn[32] used a macroporous co-polymer support (PRP-1, Hamilton) to isocratically resolve riboflavin, FMN, and FAD in plasma and urine with acetonitrile : water : 10% trifluoroacetic acid : phosphoric acid (14 : 84 : 1.5 : 0.09), pH 1.8.

Tables 8.3 to 8.5 show a small but selective segment of the many successful chromatography systems available in the literature for riboflavin chromatography. The efficient coupling of riboflavin analysis and analysis of other water-soluble vitamins, primarily thiamin, into simultaneous assays requiring a single LC injection are summarized in Table 8.5. Reliable methods developed by Chase et al.,[37,38] and Sims and Shoemaker[39] for simultaneous analysis of riboflavin, thiamin, and vitamin B_6 are provided in Section 8.4.

8.3.3.2.2 Detection

Fluorescence detection (Ex λ = 440—450, Em λ = 530) is sensitive and specific for riboflavin quantitation after LC resolution. Detection limits for riboflavin by fluorescence is <1 pmol (0.38 ng) compared to 30 pmol (11 ng) by UV detection at 254 nm.[6] UV detection is adequate for pharmaceuticals and enriched foods. However, its use for samples with lower, naturally occurring vitamin levels most likely will require concentration and clean up of the extract prior to chromatography. Vidal-Valverde and Reche[40] treated acid and enzyme hydrolysates of foods by Florisil and C_{18} Sep-Pak chromatography to allow use of UV detection at 254 nm.

Conversion of riboflavin to lumiflavin was effectively used to increase the sensitivity of fluorescence detection of riboflavin at low levels in meat and meat products (Section 8.4).[15] Riboflavin in extracts prepared by autoclaving in 0.1 N HCl, digestion by papain and takadiastase, and TCA precipitation of protein was converted to lumiflavin by UV irradiation at pH 10 to 12. The lumiflavin was extracted with chloroform. The chloroform extract was injected into the LC system with fluorescence detection at Ex λ = 270, Em λ = 418. The detection limit was 0.02 ng per injection.

Advantages of sensitivity and selectivity make fluorescence detection of the flavins a clear choice over UV detection. Added sensitivity and reliability of newer, dedicated fluorescent detectors plus the convenience of wavelength programmability adds to the utility of fluorescence detection as the preferred mode for flavin analysis.

8.3.2.2.3   Internal Standards

Internal standards for riboflavin and flavin co-enzyme analysis are not generally available. Compounds used in past research include 2,2′diphenic acid, nicotinamide, p-hydroxy-benzoic acid, acetosalicyclic acid, theobromine, isoriboflavin, sorboflavin, and 7-ethyl-8-methyl riboflavin. All of these compounds have different structural properties compared to riboflavin except the riboflavin analogs isoriboflavin (8-demethyl-6-methyl riboflavin),[41] sorboflavin (glucityl side chain on the ribityl chain),[33] and 7-ethyl-8-methyl-riboflavin.[4] They are not commercially available, but Bilic and Sieber[33] provides detailed synthesis instructions for sorboflavin.

8.4   METHOD PROTOCOLS
Simultaneous Liquid Chromatographic Determination of Thiamin and Riboflavin in Selected Foods

Principle
- Extract sample containing 30 to 40 μg thiamin and riboflavin by autoclaving at 121°C for 30 min. Complete thiochrome formation and clean reaction mixture by Sep-Pak C_{18} SPE. Thiochrome and riboflavin are chromatographed on C_{18} with fluorescence detection.

Chemicals
- Thiamin-HCl (USP)
- Riboflavin (USP)
- Hydrochloric acid
- Sodium acetate
- Potassium ferricyanide
- Sodium hydroxide
- Methanol
- Acetic acid
- Ammonium acetate

Apparatus
- HPLC
- Fluorescence detector, programmable
- Sep-Pak C_{18} cartridge
- Autoclave

Procedure

Sample Extraction
- Weigh sample containing 30 to 40 μg of thiamin and riboflavin
- Add 50 mL 0.1 N HCl, autoclave, 12°C, 30 min
- Cool, adjust pH to 4.5 with 2 N sodium acetate
- Dilute to 100 mL with water, filter
- Pipet 4.0 mL filtrate into test tube

Thiochrome Formation
- To 4 mL filtrate, add 3.0 mL 1% potassium ferricyanide in 15% NaOH, vortex 30 s
- Allow 1 min for oxidation, add 3.0 mL 3.75 N HCl, vortex

Sep-Pak Clean-Up
- Condition C_{18} cartridge with 5.0 mL methanol, followed by 0.005 M ammonium nitrate, pH 5.0
- Load 5.0 mL of reacted filtrate
- Rinse cartridge with 5 mL 0.005 M ammonium acetate, pH 5.0
- Elute vitamins with 4.0 mL methanol : 0.005 M ammonium acetate, pH 5.0 (60 : 40)
- Filter, 0.45 μm

Chromatography

Column	30 cm × 3.9 mm
Stationary phase	μBondapak C_{18}
Mobile phase	0.005 M NH_4OAC; pH 5.0 : methanol (72 : 8)
Flow	1.5 mL/min
Column temperature	Ambient
Detection	Fluorescence
	Thiochrome—Ex λ = 370, Em λ = 435
	Riboflavin—Ex λ = 370, Em λ = 520
Calculation*	External standards, linear regression, peak area

Note: Thiamin is calculated as thiamin-HCl.

J. AOAC Int., 76, 1156, 1993

Thiamin, Riboflavin and Pyridoxine in Supplements, Infant Formulas and Medical Foods

Principle

Multivitamin supplements
- Extracted with weak acid, sonicated, filtered and diluted with mobile phase prior to injection and quantitation by reversed-phase LC with fluorescence detection.

Infant formulas and medical foods
- Extracted with a perchloric acid solution, pH adjusted, filtered and diluted with mobile phase and quantitated by reversed-phase LC with fluorescence detection.

Chemicals
- Water
- Hexane sulfonic acid, sodium salt
- Perchloric acid (69 to 72%)
- Acetonitrile
- Sodium hydroxide
- Ammonium hydroxide
- Phosphoric acid
- Potassium hydroxide
- Hydrochloric acid

- Potassium ferricyanide
- Thiamin standard (USP)
- Riboflavin standard (USP)
- Pyridoxine HCl standard (USP)
- Derivatizing solution—1 g potassium ferricyanide in 100 mL water. Dilute a 60 mL aliquot to 100 mL with 15% NaOH.

Fluorescence
- HPLC
- Fluorescence detector—programmable
- Reaction coil
- Post-column reactant pump
- pH meter
- Filter paper—32 cm grade 588 pre-pleated
- Eldex pump

Procedure

Multivitamin Supplements
- Weigh portion in 100 mL volumetric flask
- Dilute to volume with 0.1 N HCl
- Sonicate 30 min
- Filter
- Transfer aliquot to 100 mL volumetric flask
- Dilute to volume with mobile phase

Infant Formulas and Medical Foods
- Weigh portion into a 250 mL beaker
- Add 50 mL water, mix to dissolve
- Add 2mL perchloric acid
- Stir 30 min
- Add 6 m KOH dropwise to pH 3.3
- Transfer solution to 200 mL volumetric flask
- Dilute to volume with mobile phase
- Refrigerate overnight
- Filter
- Inject 125 μL for riboflavin and pyridoxine analysis
- Repeat injection for thiochrome analysis

Chromatography

Mobile phase	0.95 g hexane sulfonic acid dissolved in 1 L H_2O containing 9.5% acetonitrile and 0.5 mL ammonium hydroxide. Adjust to pH 3.6 with phosphoric acid. Dilute 930 mL to 1 L with water.
Column	30.0 cm $\times$ 3.9 mm
Stationary phase	C_{18} Novapak
Column temperature	29°C
Flow	1 mL/min
Derivative reactant	For B_1 deliver reactant at 0.3 mL/min
Reactioncoil temperature	55°C
Retention time	B_1 = 19 min; B_2 = 14 min; B_6 = 7.5 min (approximate)
Programmable	

Fluorescence detection	Time	B_2 and B_6
	0	Ex λ = 295 nm, Em λ = 395 nm
	11	Ex λ = 440 nm, Em λ = 565 nm
	27	Ex λ = 295 nm, Em λ = 395 nm
		(B_1)
		Ex λ = 360 nm, Em λ = 435 nm
Calculation		External standard, peak area, standard curve, 0.2, 0.4, 0.8, and 1.0 μg/mL
		Linear regression

J. AOAC Int., 75, 561, 1992; *J. AOAC Int.*, 76, 1276, 1993; *J. Micronutrient Analysis*, 71, 15, 1990

Liquid Chromatographic Determination of Vitamins B_1 and B_2 in Foods: A Collaborative Study

Principle
- Extract thiamin and riboflavin with 0.1 N HCl (100°C), β-amylase and Takadiastase digestion. Quantitate riboflavin directly from the extract by isocratic reversed-phase chromatography with fluorescence detection. Convert thiamin pre-column into thiochrome. Isolate thiochrome from the reaction mixture by Sep-Pak C_{18} chromatography and quantitate by reversed-phase liquid chromatography with fluorescence detection.

Chemicals
- Acetic acid
- Hydrochloric acid
- Sodium acetate
- Sodium hydroxide
- Potassium ferricyanide
- Methanol

Enzymes
- β-amylase (from barley)
- Takadiastase *(Aspergillus orizae)*

Apparatus
- HPLC
- Fluorescence detector
- Cellulose acetate filtration unit

Procedure

Sample Extraction
- Weigh 5 g of finely ground sample
- Add 65 mL of 0.1 M HCl
- Digest at 100°C, 30 min
- Adjust pH to 4.5 with 2.5 M sodium acetate
- Digest with β-amylase and Takadiastase, 18 h, 37°C
- Filter through filter paper and cellulose acetate (0.1 μm)
- Inject for riboflavin analysis

Thiochrome Formation
- To 1mL of filtrate add 3 mL potassium ferricyanide solution and 24 mL of 3.75 M NaOH
- Mix, allow to stand 1 min

- Pass through Sep-Pak C_{18} cartridge
- Wash cartridge with 10 mL 0.05 M sodium acetate
- Elute thiochrome with 8 mL methanol : water (70 : 30)
- Dilute eluent to 10 mL, filter through cellulose acetate (0.1 μm)
- Inject

Chromatography

Column	25 cm $\times$ 4 mm, 10μm
Stationary phase	C_{18}
Mobile phase	Methanol : 0.5 M sodium acetate (30 : 70)
Column temperature	Ambient
Flow	1 mL/min
Detection	Riboflavin: Fluorescence, Ex λ = 366, Em λ = 435
	Thiochrome: Fluorescence, Ex λ = 422, Em λ = 522
Calculation	External standard, peak area

Food Chem., 56, 81, 1996

Non-Degradative Extraction and Simultaneous Quantitation of Riboflavin, Flavin Mononucleotide, and Flavin Adenine Dinucleotide in Foods by HPLC

Principle

- Extract flavins by homogenization in methanol and methylene chloride. Flavins are stabilized in McIlvaine buffer (100 mM citrate-phosphate, pH 5.5) containing 0.1% sodium azide. Quantitate by gradient elution from two PLRP-S columns in series, fluorescence detection, and 7-ethyl-8-methyl-riboflavin as an internal standard.

Chemicals

- Methanol
- Methylene chloride
- 7-Ethyl-8-methyl-riboflavin (IS)
- Citrate-phosphate buffer, 100 mM, pH 5.5
- Sodium azide

Apparatus

- HPLC
- Fluorescence detector
- Centrifuge
- Polytron® homogenizer

Procedure

Sample Extraction

- Weigh 0.5 to 4.0 g ground sample
- Add 9.0 mL methanol and 100 mL methylene chloride
- Add 2 mL IS
- Homogenize, 75 s at 50% full speed
- Add 9.0 mL citrate-phosphate buffer containing 0.1% sodium azide

- Homogenize, 30 s
- Centrifuge
- Decant aqueous phase, filter
- Inject

Chromatography

Column	25 cm × 4.6 mm and 15 cm × 4.6 mm in series
Stationary phase	PLRP-S, 100 Å
Mobile phase	Acetonitrile / 0.1% sodium azide in 10 mM citrate-phosphate buffer, pH 5.5, 6 step gradient
Column temperature	40°C
Flow	1.0 to 1.2 mL/min
Detection	Fluorescence, Ex λ = 450, Em λ = 522
Calculation	Internal standard

Food Chem., 43, 151, 1992

Determination of Thiamin and Riboflavin in Meat and Meat Products by High-Pressure Liquid Chromatography

Principle

- Extract thiamin and riboflavin by autoclaving in 0.1 N HCl and digestion with papain and takadiastase. Convert thiamin to thiochrome and quantitate by isocratic elution from silica with fluorescence detection. Convert riboflavin to lumiflavin by UV irradiation and quantitate by isocratic elution from silica with fluorescence detection.

Chemicals

- Hydrochloric acid
- Sodium acetate
- Thiamin HCl (USP)
- Riboflavin (USP)
- Chloroform
- Trichloroacetic acid (TCA)
- Glacial acetic acid
- Potassium ferricyanide
- Sodium sulfate
- Isobutyl alcohol
- Methanol

Enzymes

- Papain
- Takadiastase

Apparatus

- HPLC
- Fluorescence detector
- Chromato-VUE cabinet, model C-5 with long- and short-wavelength UV lamps
- Autoclave

Procedure

Sample Extraction
- Weigh 5 g sample
- Add 60 mL 0.1 N HCl, autoclave, 121°C, 30 min
- Adjust pH to 4.0 to 4.5 with 2 M sodium acetate
- Digest with papain and Takadiastase, 3 h, 42 to 45°C
- Precipitate protein with 2 mL of 50% TCA
- Steambath, 5 min
- Dilute to 100 mL with water

Thiochrome Formation
- Oxidize 10 mL filtrate with 5 mL 1% alkaline potassium ferricyanide
- Extract thiochrome with 10 mL isocutyl alcohol
- Treat standard in same manner to generate standard curve

Riboflavin Conversion to Lumiflavin
- Adjust pH of 10 mL of filtrate to 10 to 12 with 15% NaOH
- Irradiate for 30 min
- Add 1 mL glacial acetic acid
- Extract with 10 mL chloroform
- Dry extract with anhydrous sodium sulfate
- Treat standards in same manner to generate standard curve

Chromatography

Column	50 cm × 2.1 mm
Stationary phase	Spherisorb silica, 20 μm
Mobile phase	Chloroform : methanol (90 : 10)
Flow	Thiochrome—1.0 mL/min
	Lumiflavin — 0.8 mL/min
Column temperature	Ambient
Detection	Fluorescence
	Thiochrome: Ex λ = 367, Em λ = 418
	Lumiflavin: Ex λ = 270, Em λ = 418
Calculation	Internal standard, peak area, linear regression

J. Agric. Food Chem., 28, 483, 1980

8.5   REFERENCES

Text

1. National Research Council, *Recommended Dietary Allowances*, 10th ed., National Academy of Sciences, Washington, D.C., 1989, chap. 8.
2. Gibson, R. S., *Principles of Nutritional Assessment*, Oxford University Press, New York, 1990, chap. 20.
3. *Nutritional Labeling and Education Act of 1990*, Fed. Reg., 58, 2070, 1993.
4. Russell, L. F. and Vanderslice, J. T., Non-degradative extraction and simultaneous quantitation of riboflavin, flavin mononucleotide and flavin adenine dinucleotide in foods by HPLC, *Food Chem.,* 43, 151, 1992.
5. Shah, J. J., Riboflavin, in *Methods of Vitamin Assay*, Augustin, J., Klein, B. P., Becker, D. A. and Venugopal, P. B., Eds., John Wiley and Sons, New York, 1985, chap. 14.
6. Nielsen, P., Flavins, in *Modern Chromatographic Analysis of Vitamins*, De Leenheer, A. P., Lambert, W. E. and Nelis, H. J., Eds., Marcel Dekker, New York, 1992, chap. 9.

7. Eitenmiller, R. R. and Landen, W. O., Jr., Vitamins, in *Analyzing Food for Nutrition Labeling and Hazardous Contaminants*, Jeon, I. J. and Ikins, W. G., Eds., Marcel Dekker, New York, 1995, chap. 9.

8. Ball, G. F. M., Chemical and biological nature of the water-soluble vitamins, in *Water-Soluble Vitamin Assays in Human Nutrition*, Chapman and Hall, New York, 1994, chap. 2.

9. Friedrich, W., Vitamin B_2: Riboflavin and its bioactive variants, in *Vitamins*, Walter de Gruyter, New York, 1988, chap. 7.

10. Russell, L. F. and Vanderslice, J. T., A comprehensive review of vitamin B_2 analytical methodology, *J. Micronutr. Anal.,* 8, 257, 1990.

11. Ottaway, P. B., Stability of vitamins in food, in *The Technology of Vitamins in Food*, Chapman and Hall, London, 1993, chap. 5.

12. Cairns, W. L. and Metzler, D. E., Photochemical degradation of flavins. VI. A new photoproduct and its use in studying the photolytic mechanism, *J. Am. Chem. Soc.,* 93, 2772, 1971.

13. Woodcock, E. A., Warthesen, J. J. and Labuza, T. P., Riboflavin photochemical degradation in pasta measured by high performance liquid chromatography, *J. Food Sci.,* 47, 545, 1982.

14. Wagner-Jauregg, T., in *The Vitamins*, vol. V., Sebrell, W. H. and Harris, R. S., Eds., Academic Press, New York, 1972, chap. 14.

15. Ang, C. Y. and Moseley, F. A., Determination of thiamin and riboflavin in meat and meat products by high pressure liquid chromatography, *J. Agric. Food Chem.,* 28, 483, 1980.

16. Palanuk, S. L., Warthesen, J. J. and Smith, D. E., Effect of agitation, sampling and protective films on light-induced riboflavin loss in skim milk, *J. Food Sci.,* 53, 436, 1988.

17. Furuya, E. M. and Warthesen, J. J., Influence of initial riboflavin content on retention in pasta during photodegradation and cooking, *J. Food Sci.,* 49, 986, 1984.

18. AOAC International, *AOAC Official Methods of Analysis*, 16th ed., AOAC International, Arlington, VA, 1995.

19. Russell, L. F. and Vanderslice, J. T., Comments on the standard fluorometric determination of riboflavin in foods and biological tissues, *Food Chem.,* 42, 79, 1991.

20. Egberg, D. C. and Potter, R. H., An improved automated determination of riboflavin in food products, *J. Agric. Food Chem.,* 23, 815, 1975.

21. Egberg, D. C., Semiautomated method for riboflavin in food products: collaborative study, *J. Assoc. Off. Anal. Chem.,* 62, 1041, 1979.

22. Strohecker, R. and Henning, H. M., *Vitamin Assay Tested Methods*, Verlag Chemie, Darmstadt, 1965, 110.

23. Pearson, W. N., Bliss, C. I. and Gyorgy, P., Riboflavin, in *The Vitamins*, vol. 2, Gyorgy, P. and Pearson, W. N., Eds., Academic Press, New York, 1968, 99.

24. Baker, H. and Frank, O., *Clinical Vitaminology, Methods and Interpretation*, Interscience Publishers, New York, 1968, chap. 5.

25. Kornberg, H. A., Langdon, R. S. and Cheldelin, V. H., Microbiological assay for riboflavin, *Anal. Chem.,* 20, 81, 1948.

26. AOAC International, Report of the AOAC International Task Force on Methods for Nutrient Labeling Analyses, *J. AOAC Int.,* 76, 180A, 1993.

27. Saarivirta, M., The content of B-vitamins in the milk of cows fed purified or low-protein feed, with urea as the sole or main nitrogen source, and evaluation of the microbiological assay methods, *Anal. Acad. Sci. Fenn., II, Chem.,* 147, 7, 1969.

28. Eitenmiller, R. R., Johnson, C. D., Bryan, W. D., Warren, D. B. and Gebhardt, S. E., Nutrient composition of cantaloupe and honeydew melons, *J. Food Sci.,* 50, 136, 1985.

29. van den Berg, H., van Schaik, F., Finglas, D. M. and de Froidmont-Gortz, I., Third EUMAT intercomparison for the determination of vitamins B_1, B_2 and B_6 in food, *Food Chem.,* 57, 101, 1996.

30. Finglas, P. M. and Faulks, R. M., Critical review of HPLC methods for the determination of thiamin, riboflavin and niacin in food, *J. Micronutr. Anal.,* 3, 251, 1987.

31. Van Niekerk, P. J., Determination of vitamins, in *HPLC in Food Analysis*, 2nd ed., MaCrae, R., Ed., Academic Press, New York, chap. 9.

32. Lopez-Anaya, A. and Mayersohn, M., Quantification of riboflavin, riboflavin 5'-phosphate and flavin adenine dinucleotide in plasma and urine by high-performance liquid chromatography, *J. Chromatogr.,* 423, 105, 1987.

33. Bilic, N. and Sieber, R., Determination of flavins in dairy products by high performance liquid chromatography using sorboflavin as internal standard, *J. Chromatogr.,* 511, 359, 1990.

34. Rashid, I. and Potts, D., Riboflavin determination in milk, *J. Food Sci.,* 45, 744, 1980.

35. Munoz, A., Ortiz, R. and Murcia, M. A., Determination by HPLC of changes in riboflavin levels in milk and nondairy imitation milk during refrigerated storage, *Food Chem.,* 49, 203, 1994.

36. Arella, F., Lahely, S., Bourguignon, J. B. and Hasselmann, C., Liquid chromatographic determination of vitamins B₁ and B₂ in foods—a collaborative study, *Food Chem.,* 56, 81, 1996.

37. Chase, G. W., Jr., Landen, W. O., Jr., Eitenmiller, R. R., and Soliman, A. G. M., Liquid chromatographic determination of thiamine, riboflavin, and pyridoxine in infant formula, *J. AOAC Int.,* 75, 561, 1992.

38. Chase, G. W., Landen, W. O., Jr., Soliman, A.G.M., and Eitenmiller, R. R., Method modification for liquid chromatographic determination of thiamine, riboflavin and pyridoxine in medical foods, *J. AOAC Int.,* 76, 1276, 1993.

39. Sims, A. and Shoemaker, D., Simultaneous liquid chromatographic determination of thiamine and riboflavin in selected foods, *J. AOAC Int.,* 76, 1156, 1993.

40. Vidal-Valverde, C. and Reche, A., Reliable system for the analysis of riboflavin in foods by high performance liquid chromatography and UV detection, *J. Liq. Chromatogr.,* 13, 2089, 1990.

41. Lambert, W. E., Cammaert, P. M. and De Leenheer, A. P., Liquid chromatographic measurement of riboflavin in serum and urine with isoriboflavin as internal standard, *Clin. Chem.,* 31, 1371, 1985.

Table 8.1   Physical Properties of Riboflavin, FMN, and FAD

1. Ball, G. F. M., Chemical and biological nature of the water-soluble vitamins, in *Water-Soluble Vitamin Assays in Human Nutrition,* Chapman and Hall, New York, 1994, chap. 2.

2. Budavari, S., *The Merck Index,* 12th Ed., Merck and Company, Whitehouse Station, NJ, 1996, 1410.

3. Nielsen, P., Flavins, in *Modern Chromatographic Analysis of Vitamins,* De Leenheer, A. P., Lambert, W. E. and Nelis, H. J., Eds., Marcel Dekker, New York, 1992, chap. 9.

4. National Academy of Sciences, *Food Chemicals Codex,* National Academy of Science, Washington, D.C., 1996, 339.

Table 8.2   Compendium, Regulatory and Handbook Methods for the Analysis of Riboflavin

1. The United States Pharmacopeial Convention, Inc., *U.S. Pharmacopeia National Formulary,* USP23/NF18, Nutritional Supplements, Official Monographs, United States Pharmacopeial Convention, Inc., Rockville, MD, 1995.

2. Scottish Home and Health Department, *British Pharmacopoeia,* 15th ed., British Pharmacopoeia Commission, United Kingdom, 1993.

3. AOAC International, *Official Methods of Analysis,* 16th ed., AOAC International, Arlington, VA, 1995.

4. Lay, H. W., Report on revision of microbiological methods for the B vitamins, *J. Assoc. Off. Anal. Chem.,* 42, 529, 1959.

5. DeRitter, G., Collaborative study of extraction methods for fluorometric assay of riboflavin, *J. Assoc. Off. Anal. Chem.,* 53, 542, 1970.

6. Tanner, J. T. and Barnett, S. A., Methods of analysis for infant formula: Food and Drug Administration and Infant Formula Council: collaborative study, *J. Assoc. Off. Anal. Chem.,* 68, 514, 1985.

7. American Association of Cereal Chemists, *AACC Approved Methods,* 9th ed., vol. 2, American Association of Cereal Chemists, St. Paul, MN, 1996.

8. Bechtel, W. G., Fluorometric procedure for riboflavin in cereals and cereal products, *Cereal Sci. Today,* 7, 198, 1962.

9. DeRitter, E. and Rubin, S. H., Determination of thiamine and riboflavin in the presence of reduced iron, *Anal. Chem.,* 19, 243, 1947.

10. Andrews, J. S., Boyd, H. M. and Terry, D. E., Riboflavin analysis of cereals, *Ind. Eng. Chem.,* 14, 271, 1942.

11. Rubin, S. H., DeRitter, E., Schurman, R. L. and Bauernfeind, J. C., Determination of riboflavin in low-potency foods and feeds, *Ind. Eng. Chem.,* 17, 136, 1945.

12. Egberg, D. C. and Potter, R. H., An improved automated determination of riboflavine in food products, *J. Agric. Food Chem.,* 23, 815, 1975.

13. American Feed Ingredients Association, *Laboratory Methods Compendium, vol. 1: Vitamins and Minerals,* American Feed Ingredients Association, West Des Moines, 1A, 1991, 153.

14. Committee on Food Chemicals Codex, *Food Chemicals Codex*, 4th ed., National Academy of Sciences, Washington, D.C., 1996, 338.

15. Keller, H. E., *Analytical Methods for Vitamins and Carotenoids*, Hoffman-LaRoche, Basel, 1988, 30.

16. Brubacher, G., Müller-Mulot, W. and Southgate, D. A. T., *Methods for the Determination of Vitamins in Foods Recommended by COST 91*, Elsevier Applied Science Publishers, New York, 1985, chap. 10.

17. Nielsen, P., Reuschenbach, P. and Bacher, A., *Anal. Biochem.*, 130, 359, 1983. Phosphates of riboflavin and riboflavin assays: a reinvestigation by high performance liquid chromatography.

Table 8.3   HPLC Methods for the Analysis of Riboflavin in Foods, Feed, Pharmaceuticals, and Biologicals

Food

1. Ashoor, S. H., Seperich, G. J., Monte, W. C. and Welty, J., HPLC determination of riboflavin in eggs and dairy products, *J. Food Sci.*, 48, 92, 1983.

2. Ashoor, S. H., Knox, M. J., Olsen, J. R. and Deger, D. A., Improved liquid chromatographic determination of riboflavin in milk and dairy products, *J. Assoc. Off. Anal. Chem.*, 68, 693, 1985.

3. Stancher, B. and Zonta, F., High performance liquid chromatographic analysis of riboflavin (vitamin B_2) with visible absorbance detection in Italian cheese, *J. Food Sci.*, 51, 857, 1986.

4. Ribarova, F., Shishkov, S., Obretenova, N. and Metchkneva, L., Comparative determination of riboflavin in milk by HPLC and lumiflavin methods, *Die Nahr.*, 31, 77, 1987.

5. Palanuk, S. L., Warthesen, J. J. and Smith, D. E., Effect of agitation, sampling location and protective films on light-induced riboflavin loss in skim milk, *J. Food Sci.*, 53, 436, 1988.

6. Reyes, G. S. P., Norris, K. M., Taylor, C. and Potts, D., Comparison of paired-ion liquid chromatographic method with AOAC fluorometric and microbiological methods for riboflavin determination in selected foods, *J. Assoc. Off. Anal. Chem.*, 71, 16, 1988.

7. Ollilainen, V., Matilla, P., Vara, P., Koivistoinen, P. and Huttunen, J., The HPLC determination of total riboflavin in foods, *J. Micronutr. Anal.*, 8, 199, 1990.

8. Vidal-Valverde, C. and Reche, A., Reliable system for the analysis of riboflavin in foods by high performance liquid chromatography and UV detection, *J. Liq. Chromatogr.*, 13, 2089, 1990.

9. Bilic, N. and Sieber, R., Determination of flavins in dairy products by high performance liquid chromatography using sorboflavin as internal standard, *J. Chromatogr.*, 511, 359, 1990.

10. Russell, L. F. and Vanderslice, J. T., Non-degradative extraction and simultaneous quantitation of riboflavin, flavin, mononucleotide, and flavin adenine dinucleotide in foods by HPLC, *Food Chem.*, 43, 151, 1992.

11. Muñoz, A., Ortiz, R. and Murcia, M. A., Determination by HPLC of changes in riboflavin levels in milk and nondairy imitation milk during refrigerated storage, *Food Chem.*, 49, 203, 1994.

12. Hewavitharna, A. K., Method for the extraction of riboflavin for high performance liquid chromatography and application to casein, *Analyst*, 121, 1671, 1996.

Biologicals

1. Speek, A. J., Van Schaik, F., Schrijver, J. and Schruers, W. H. P., Determination of the B_2 vitamer flavin-adenine dinucleotide in whole blood by high-performance liquid chromatography with fluorometric detection, *J. Chromatogr.*, 228, 311, 1982.

2. Ichinose, N., Adachi, K. and Schwedt, G., Determination of B_2 vitamers in serum of fish using high-performance liquid chromatography with fluorescence detection, *Analyst*, 110, 1505, 1985.

3. Lambert, W. E., Cammaert, P. M. and De Leenheer, A. P., Liquid-chromatographic measurement of riboflavin in serum and urine with isoriboflavin as internal standard, *Clin, Chem.*, 318, 1371, 1985.

4. Oka, M. and McCormick, D. B., Urinary lumichrome-level catabolites of riboflavin are due to microbial and photochemical events and not rat tissue enzymatic cleavage of the ribityl chain, *J. Nutr.*, 115, 496, 1985.

5. Chastain, J. L. and McCormick, D. B., Clarification and quantitation of primary (tissue) and secondary (microbial) catabolites of riboflavin that are excreted in mammalian (rat) urine, *J. Nutr.*, 117, 468, 1987.

6. Chastain, J. L. and McCormick, D. B., Flavin catabolites: Identification and quantitation in human urine, *Am. J. Clin. Nutr.*, 46, 830, 1987.

7. Seki, T., Noguchi, K. and Yanagihara, Y., Determination of riboflavine in human urine by the use of a hydrophilic gel column, *J. Chromatogr.*, 385, 283, 1987.

8. Lopez-Anaya, A. and Mayersohn, M., Quantification of riboflavin, riboflavin-5-phosphate and flavin adenine dinucleotide in plasma and urine by high performance liquid chromatography, *J. Chromatogr.*, 423, 105, 1987.

9. Cann-Moisan, C., Caroff, J. and Girin, F., Determination of flavin adenine dinucleotide in biological tissues by high-performance liquid chromatography with electrochemical detection, *J. Chromatogr.*, 442, 441, 1988.

10. Batey, D. W. and Eckhart, C. D., Identification of FAD, FMN, and riboflavin in the retina by microextraction and high-performance liquid chromatography, *Anal. Biochem.*, 188, 164, 1990.

11. Batey, D. W., Daneshgar, K. K. and Eckhert, C. D., Flavin levels in rat retina, *Exp. Eye Res.*, 54, 605, 1992.

Table 8.4   HPLC Methods for the Concurrent Analysis of Riboflavin and Thiamin in Foods, Feed, Pharmaceuticals, and Biologicals

1. Ang, C. Y. W. and Moseley, F. A., Determination of thiamin and riboflavin in meat and meat products by high-pressure liquid chromatography, *J. Agric. Food Chem.*, 28, 483, 1980.

2. Finglas, P. M. and Faulks, R. M., The HPLC analysis of thiamin and riboflavin in potatoes, *Food Chem.*, 15, 37, 1984.

3. Dawson, K. R., Unklesbay, N. F. and Hedrick, H. B., HPLC determination of riboflavin, niacin, and thiamin in beef, pork, and lamb after alternate heat-processing methods, *J. Agric. Food Chem.*, 36, 1176, 1988.

4. Hasselmann, C., Franck, D., Grimm, P., Diop, P. A. and Soules, C., High performance liquid chromatographic analysis of thiamin and riboflavin in dietetic foods, *J. Micronutr. Anal*, 5, 269, 1989.

5. Fernando, S. M. and Murphy, P. A., HPLC determination of thiamin and riboflavin in soybeans and tofu, *J. Agric. Food Chem.*, 38, 163, 1990.

6. Hägg, M. and Kumpulainen, J., Thiamine and riboflavin contents in domestic and imported cereal products in Finland, *J. Food Comp. Anal.*, 6, 299, 1993.

7. Hägg, M., Effect of various commercially available enzymes in the liquid chromatographic determination with external standardization of thiamin and riboflavin in food, *J. AOAC Int.*, 77, 681, 1994.

8. Hägg, M. and Kumpulainen, J., Thiamine and riboflavin contents of Finnish breads and their corresponding flours, *J. Food Comp. Anal.*, 7, 94, 1994.

9. Barna, E. and Dworschak, E., Determination of thiamine (vitamin B_1) and riboflavin (vitamin B_2) in meat and liver by high-performance liquid chromatography, *J. Chromatogr. A*, 668, 359, 1994.

10. Arella, F., Lahély, S., Bourguignon, J. B. and Hasselmann, C., Liquid chromatographic determination of vitamins B_1 and B_2 in foods. A collaborative study, *Food Chem.*, 56, 81, 1996.

Table 8.5   HPLC Methods for the Simultaneous Analysis of Riboflavin and Thiamin in Foods, Feed, Pharmaceuticals, and Biologicals

1. Fellman, J. K., Artz, W. E., Tassinari, P. D., Cole, C. L., and Augustin, J., Simultaneous determination of thiamin and riboflavin in selected foods by high-performance liquid chromatography, *J. Food Sci.*, 47, 2048, 1982.

2. Augustin, J., Simultaneous determination of thiamine and riboflavin in foods by liquid chromatography, *J. Assoc. Off. Anal. Chem.*, 67, 1012, 1984.

3. Wehling, R. L. and Wetzel, D. L., Simultaneous determination of pyridoxine, riboflavin, and thiamin in fortified cereal products by high-performance liquid chromatography, *J. Agric. Food Chem.*, 32, 1326, 1984.

4. Mauro, B. J. and Wetzel, D. L., Simultaneous determination of thiamine and riboflavin in enriched cereal based products by high-performance liquid chromatography using selective detection, *J. Chromatogr.*, 299, 281, 1984.

5. Wills, R. B. H., Wimalasiri, P. and Greenfield, H., Comparative determination of thiamin and riboflavin in foods by high-performance liquid chromatography and fluorometric methods, *J. Micronutr. Anal.*, 1, 23, 1985.

6. Wimalasiri, P. and Wills, R. B. H., Simultaneous analysis of thiamin and riboflavin in foods by high-performance liquid chromatography, *J. Chromatogr.,* 318, 412, 1985.
7. Lavigne, C., Zee, J. A., Simard, R. E. and Gosselin, C., High-performance liquid chromatographic-diode-array determination of ascorbic acid, thiamine and riboflavin in goats' milk, *J. Chromatogr.,* 410, 201, 1987.
8. Chase, G. W., Jr., Landen, W. O., Jr., Eitenmiller, R. R. and Soliman, A. G. M., Liquid chromatographic determination of thiamine, riboflavin, and pyridoxine in infant formula, *J. AOAC Int.,* 75, 561, 1992.
9. Chase, G. W., Landen, W. O., Jr., Soliman, A. G. M. and Eitenmiller, R. R., Method modification for liquid chromatographic determination of thiamine, riboflavin and pyridoxine in medical foods, *J. AOAC Int.,* 767, 1276, 1993.
10. Sims, A. and Shoemaker, D., Simultaneous liquid chromatographic determination of thiamine and riboflavin in selected foods, *J. AOAC Int.,* 76, 1156, 1993.

9 Niacin

9.1 REVIEW

Niacin deficiency "Pellagra" was described by Casel in Spain in 1735 and by Pugati in Italy in 1755. Pellagra is derived from the Italian term "pelle agra" for rough skin. Recognition of the disease as a dietary deficiency did not occur until Goldberger (1920) showed that pellagra was not an infectious disease and could be induced by the lack of a nutritional factor in corn. The factor was called the "pellagra preventive factor."[1] Goldberger's studies led to the recognition of black tongue disease in dogs fed diets that caused pellagra in humans. Consequently, in 1937, nicotinic acid was recognized as a curative factor for black tongue in dogs[2] and for pellagra.[3]

Although corn consumption as a dietary staple was linked to pellagra incidence for centuries, the etiology was not clearly defined until the relationship between dietary tryptophan and its conversion to niacin was understood. Krehl et al.[4] showed that tryptophan could replace nicotinic acid and prevent pellagra-like symptoms in rats. Later work showed that tryptophan is a precursor for the biosynthesis of nicotinic acid.[5] Studies conducted from 1961 to 1980 designed to determine the contribution of dietary tryptophan to the niacin requirement led to the accepted interconversion factor of 60 to 1.[6] Sixty mg of dietary tryptophan is considered equivalent to 1 mg of niacin. The concept of niacin equivalents (NE) was introduced by Horwitt et al.[7] One NE is equal to 1 mg of niacin and 60 mg of dietary tryptophan. RDAs are reported as NEs to include the impact of metabolic conversion of tryptophan to our niacin requirements. The historically significant role of corn diets in pellagra incidence is explained by the low levels and poor bioavailability of both tryptophan and nicotinic acid in corn. Clear relationships of other micronutrients to the onset of pellagra are not available.

Marginal niacin deficiency shows multiple symptoms including insomnia, loss of appetite, weight and strength loss, soreness of the tongue and mouth, indigestion, abdominal pain, burning sensation in various parts of the body, vertigo, headache, numbness, nervousness, distractibility, apprehension, mental confusion and forgetfulness.[8] Pellagra or frank niacin deficiency includes symptoms of dermatosis, dementia, and diarrhea (Three-D Disease). In developed countries, alcoholics are at risk of developing pellagra. Pellagra continues to be problematic in dietary deficient areas where corn and other cereals are major dietary staples. Clinical status tests include the measurement of the niacin metabolites N'-methylnicotinamide (NMN) and N'-methyl-2-pyridone-5-carboxamide (2-pyridone) in the urine. The test centers around the observed ratio of 2-pyridone to NMN in healthy adults of 1.3 to 4.0. Values below 1.0 indicate niacin deficiency.[9] Blood levels of niacin or its co-factors and metabolites are not used as status indicators owing to inconsistent results or unsatisfactory methodology. Levels in plasma respond rapidly to dietary intake and do not provide an accurate index of tissue stores.[9]

Owing to the contribution of dietary tryptophan to NE intake, foods containing balanced protein are important dietary sources. Milk, eggs, and meats can be good dietary sources even though the actual niacin content might be quite low. Niacin is widely distributed in the food supply; however, bioavailability (Section 9.2.3) might be quite low. Niacin is bioavailable and in good concentration in meats. Fortified cereal grain products are important dietary sources in countries where fortification is used. In the United States, calculated NE intakes are 27 for women and 41 for men.[6] Recommended Dietary Allowances (RDAs) are based on an intake of 6.6 NE/1000 kcal and not less than 13 NE at a caloric intake less than 2000 kcal/day. RDAs range from 13 for the 51+ year-old female to 20 for the 15 to 18 year-old male and pregnant and lactating female.[6] The Reference Daily Intake (RDI) is 20 NE.[10]

Few foods, unless fortified, contain free niacin in appreciable quantities. In unprocessed foods, naturally occurring niacin is present mostly in the pyridine co-enzymes nicotinamide adenine dinucleotide (NAD) and nicotinamide adenine dinucleotide phosphate (NADP). Nicotinic acid and nicotinamide serve as precursors for the synthesis of NAD and NADP. The dietary forms (NAD and NADP) are hydrolyzed in the intestinal mucosa, and nicotinic acid is converted to nicotinamide during co-enzyme biosynthesis. The metabolically active form in the co-enzymes is nicotinamide, the primary circulating form of niacin.[11] NAD and NADP function in oxidation-reduction reactions. Nicotinamide acts as an electron acceptor or hydrogen donor. Jacob and Swendseid[11] summarized the function of NAD as an electron carrier for intracellular respiration and a co-dehydrogenase involved in the oxidation of fuel molecules such as glyceraldehyde 3-phosphate, pyruvate and lactate. NADP functions as a hydrogen donor in reductive processes for biosynthesis of fatty acids and steroids and as a co-dehydrogenase for oxidation of glucose 6-phosphate to ribose 5-phosphate in the pentose phosphate pathway.[11] Niacin metabolism is summarized in Figure 9.1. NAD and NADP enzyme dependent reactions are summarized in Table 9.1.[12]

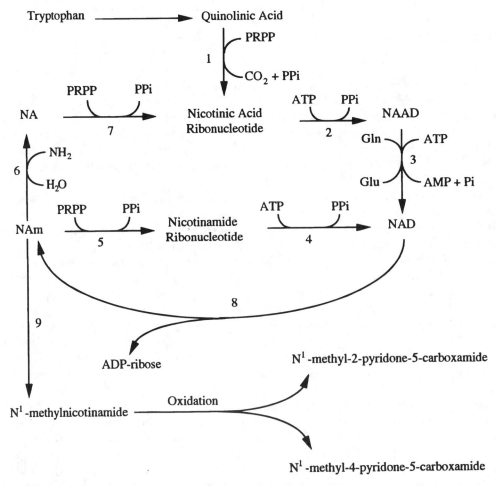

FIGURE 9.1   Pathways of niacin metabolism. NA, nicotinic acid; NAm, nicotinamide; NAAD, nicotinic acid adenine dinucleotide; PRPP, phosphoribosyl pyrophosphate. Enzymes: 1, quinolinate phosphoribosyltransferase; 2 and 4, adenyltransferase; 3, NAD synthetase; 5, nicotinamide phosphoribosyltransferase; 6, nicotinamide deamidase; 7, nicotinate phosphoribosyltransferase; 8, poly (ADP-ribose) synthetase or NAD glycohydrolase; 9, N'-methyltransferase. Reproduced with permission from Reference 11.

TABLE 9.1
NAD and NADP Dependent Enzymes[a]

Enzyme	Pyridine Nucleotide
Carbohydrate Metabolism	
3-phosphoglyceraldehyde dehydrogenase	NAD(H)
glucose-6-phosphate dehydrogenase	NADP(H)
6-phosphogluconate dehydrogenase	NADP(H)
lactate dehydrogenase	NAD(H)
alcohol dehydrogenase	NAD(H)
Lipid Metabolism	
α-glycerophosphate dehydrogenase	NAD(H)
β-hydroacyl CoA dehydrogenase	NAD(H)
3-ketoacyl ACP reductase	NADP(H)
enoyl-ACP-reductase	NADP(H)
3-hydroxy-3-methylglutaryl-CoA reductase	NADP(H)
Amino Acid Metabolism	
glutamate dehydrogenase	NAD(H)/NADP(H)
Other	
glutathione reductase	NADP(H)
dihydrofolate reductase	NADP(H)
thioredoxin-NADP reductase	NADP(H)
4-hydroxybenzoate hydroxylase	NADP(H)
NADH dehydrogenase/NADH-ubiquinone reductase complex	NAD(H)
NADPH-cytochrome P[450] reductase	NADP(H)

[a]Table adapted from Reference 12.

9.2 PROPERTIES

9.2.1 CHEMISTRY

Niacin refers to nicotinic acid ($C_6H_5O_2N$) and nicotinamide ($C_6H_6ON_2$) which have equal biological activity. Structures are given in Figure 9.2. Nicotinic acid is, chemically, pyridine 3-carboxylic acid and nicotinamide is pyridine 3-carboxylic acid amide. The acid and amide forms are readily interconvertible (Figure 9.1) and nicotinic acid is converted to the amide in formation of NAD and NADP. Structures of the co-enzyme, are given in Figure 9.3.

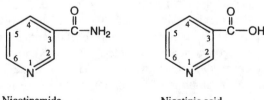

Nicotinamide
pyridine-3-carboxylic
acid amide

Nicotinic acid
pyridine-3-carboxylic
acid

FIGURE 9.2 Structures of nicotinic acid and nicotinamide.

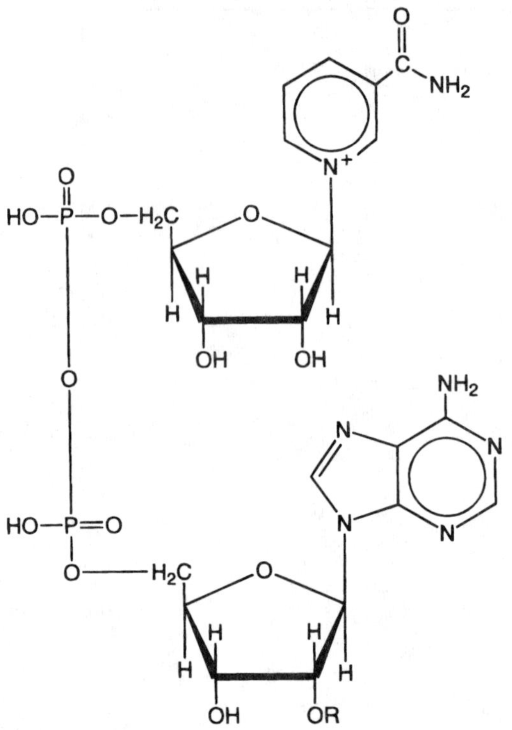

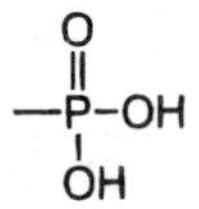

FIGURE 9.3   Structures of nicotinamide adenine dinucleotide (NAD) and nicotinamide adenine dinucleotide phosphate (NADP).

9.2.1.1   General Properties

Physical properties of nicotinic acid, nicotinamide and the co-enzymes are given in Table 9.2. Nicotinic acid is the USP reference standard. Both compounds are white needle-shaped crystals. Nicotinamide is more water-soluble (100 g/100 mL) than nicotinic acid (1.67 g/100 mL).[13] The compounds are odor free. Nicotinamide exhibits a bitter flavor which can be detected at higher levels in fortified foods. Both free niacin forms are bases and form quaternary ammonium salts when dissolved in acid solutions.[14] Nicotinic acid is amphoteric and forms carboxylic acid salts in basic solution.[14] Both compounds are available for fortification and supplementation. Nicotinamide is used in dry and liquid products, and nicotinic acid is used in products in which its lower solubility does not pose problems.[14] Bitterness of nicotinamide can be masked by enrobing techniques. Analysts or production workers must handle nicotinic acid carefully. It is a powerful vasodilator leading to a rapid flushing through inhalation of the dust. Oral dosages designed to lower serum cholesterol are great enough to cause the flushing response in such patients.[15]

TABLE 9.2
Physical Properties of Nicotinic Acid and Nicotinamide

Substance[a]	Molar Mass	Formula	Solubility	Melting Point °C	Crystal Form	λ max nm	Absorbance[b]		
							$E_{1\,cm}^{1\%}$	$\epsilon \times 10^{-3}$	Solvent
Nicotinic acid CAS No. 58-67-6 **6612**	123.11	$C_6H_5NO_2$	Water 1.67 g/100 mL Ethyl alcohol 0.73 g/100 mL Soluble in alkali hydroxides and carbonates, propylene glycol Insoluble in ether	236.6	Needles	260	[227]	2.8	50 mM potassium phosphate buffer, pH 7.0
Nicotinamide CAS No. 68-92-0 **6574**	122.13	$C_6H_6N_2O$	Water 100 g/100 mL Ethyl alcohol 66.6 g/100 mL Soluble in glycerol	128–131	Needles	261	478	[5.8]	0.1 $N\,H_2SO_4$

[a] Common or generic name; CAS No. — Chemical Abstract Service number, bold print designates the Merck Index monograph number.
[b] Values in brackets are calculated from corresponding ϵ or $E_{1\,cm}^{1\%}$ values.

Ball, G.F.M., *Water-Soluble Vitamin Assays in Human Nutrition*, [1]
Budavari, S. *The Merck Index*, [2]
Shibata, K., and Shimono, T., *Modern Chromatographic Analysis of Vitamins*, [3]
Eitenmiller, R.R., and DeSouza, S., *Methods of Vitamin Assay*, [4]

9.2.1.2 Spectral Properties

Nicotinic acid and nicotinamide show similar absorption properties with an absorption maxima near 260 nm. Absorption intensity is pH dependent. Spectra at pH 7.0 and 2.0 are shown in Figure 9.4. The free forms of the vitamin do not fluoresce. Co-enzymes show two UV maxima at 260 nm (nicotinamide ring) and 340 nm (adenine ring).[1] The co-enzymes fluoresce at 470 nm (Em λ) when excited at 260 nm or 340 nm.[1] The lack of fluorescence of nicotinic acid and nicotinamide and relatively low specificity of UV detection is problematic for LC analysis of niacin in biological materials. Most extraction procedures require time consuming clean-up steps to produce interference free chromatograms (Section 9.3.3).

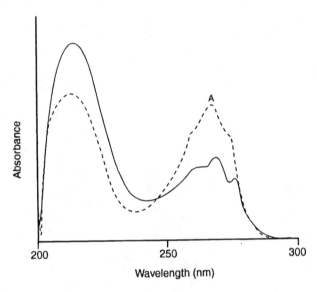

FIGURE 9.4 Absorption spectra of nicotinic acid in 0.1 M phosphate buffer at pH 7.0 (solid line) and pH 2.0 (broken line), A = 261 nm. Reproduced with permission from Reference 14.

9.2.2 STABILITY

Niacin is the most stable water-soluble vitamin.[16] Biological activity is not affected by thermal processing, light, acid, alkali, or oxidation. Owing to its stability, acid or alkali hydrolysis can be used for extraction from biological samples. Such conditions free the niacin from co-enzyme structures and destroy the sample matrix. From a food processing standpoint, processing and cooking procedures do not inactivate niacin. Leaching is usually the primary route for loss during food preparation.[16] Dairy processing operations do not affect niacin content.[14]

9.2.3 BIOAVAILABILITY

Bioavailability of niacin in unfortified foods is often low. Significant proportions of total niacin can exist in bound forms that are not absorbed by the human or can not be utilized if absorbed. Without specific processing, such as alkali treatment of corn, the bound vitamin is partially unavailable. As much as 50% of the total niacin in unenriched wheat and wheat products is unavailable.[17] Other cereals are assumed to contain significant amounts of bound "unavailable" niacin. Koetz et al.[18] identified 3-0-nicotinyl-O-glucose as an acid hydrolysis product of wheat bran, thus establishing that the ester linkage between nicotinic acid and the 3-position of glucose as one mechanism for formation of unavailable niacin in the plant kingdom. Unavailable forms of niacin in foods have never been fully characterized. Other complexed forms include amide linkages between amino groups of proteins and peptide and the carboxyl group of nicotinic acid. Protein bound nicotinic acid and glucose esters are thought to be partially available to the human.[19,20] The methylated derivative of nicotinic acid, 1-methylnicotinic acid, or trigonelline, is not biologically active. However, it is converted to nicotinic acid by thermal processing.[12] Treatment of corn with alkali liberates bound niacin and improves the bioavailability to humans.[21] Alkali processing of tortilla flour largely prevents pellagra in Central and South America where corn is the primary staple cereal.[16]

Of significance to accurate assessment of niacin intake, extraction methods that use acid hydrolysis do not hydrolyze most bound forms found in cereals. Such methods do not overestimate available niacin. Extraction by alkaline hydrolysis will liberate nicotinic acid from the macromolecules. Alkali hydrolysis, therefore, measures total niacin, but overestimates the amount naturally available from the food.[22]

9.3 METHODS

Several time tested methods based on chemical and microbiological assays are still routinely used. HPLC methods are available; however, LC methods rely on UV detection, and sensitivity and selectivity remains a problem. Some gas chromatography procedures are available, but these methods have seen little use. Regulatory methods use chemical procedures based on the classical König reaction. Other AOAC International[23] methods are based on microbiological assay by *Lactobacillus plantarum* ATCC No. 8014. The following section discusses chemical, microbiological and HPLC procedures. Methodology reviews include Eitenmiller and DeSouza,[13] Ball,[14] Shibata and Shimono,[15] Eitenmiller and Landen,[16] and Lumley.[22] Various handbook and compendium methods are summarized in Table 9.3.

9.3.1 CHEMICAL

The colorimetric determination of niacin is based upon the König reaction in which nicotinic acid and nicotinamide react with cyanogen bromide, yielding a pyridinium compound (Figure 9.5). Rearrangement produces derivatives that couple with aromatic amines to form colored compounds in the polymethine dye family with absorption maxima at 436 nm.[13,24] Under properly controlled conditions, color produced is proportional to the niacin content. Factors that must be controlled

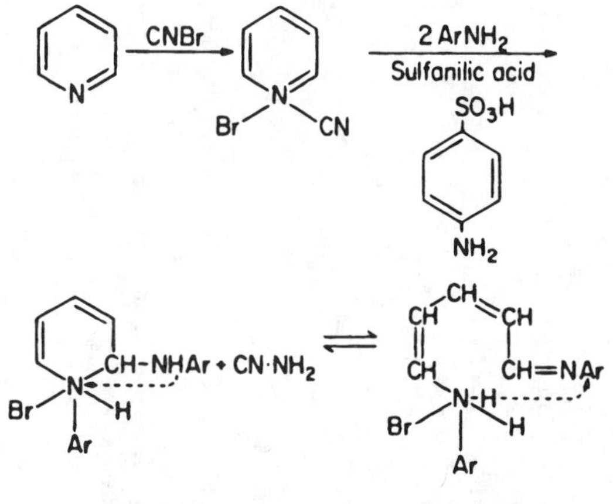

FIGURE 9.5 Colorimetric reaction for niacin determination. Reproduced with permission from Reference 13.

TABLE 9.3
Compendium, Regulatory, and Handbook Methods of Analysis for Niacin, Nicotinic Acid, and Nicotinamide

Source	Form	Methods and Application	Approach	Most Current Cross-Reference
U.S. Pharmacopeia National Formulary, 1995, USP 23/NF 18, Nutritional Supplements Official Monographs[1]				
1. pages 2143, 2146, 2148, 2153	Nicotinic acid Nicotinamide	Niacin/niacinamide in oil- and water-soluble vitamin capsules/tablets w/wo minerals	HPLC 280 nm	None
2. pages 2162, 2168, 2170, 2172	Nicotinic acid Nicotinamide	Niacin/niacinamide in water-soluble vitamin capsules/tablets w/wo minerals	HPLC 280 nm	None
3. page 1080	Nicotinic acid	Niacin (NLT 99.0%, NMT 101.0%)	Spectrophotometric 262 nm	None
4. page 1081	Nicotinic acid	Niacin in tablets	HPLC 262 nm	None
5. page 1081	Nicotinic acid	Niacin in injection	Colorimetric 450 nm	None
6. page 1082	Nicotinamide	Niacinamide in injection/tablets	Colorimetric 450 nm	None
7. page 1082	Nicotinamide	Niacinamide (NLT 98.5%, NMT 101.5%)	HPLC 254 nm	None
British Pharmacopoeia, 15th ed., 1993[2]				
1. vol. I, page 447	Nicotinic acid	Nicotinic acid	Titration	None
2. vol. II, pages 1025-1026	Nicotinamide	Nicotinamide tablets	Spectrophotometric 262 nm	None
AOAC Official Methods of Analysis, 16th ed., 1995[3]				
1. 45.2.04	Nicotinic acid Nicotinamide	AOAC Official Method 944.13, Niacin and Niacinamide in Vitamin Preparations	Microbiological	*J. Assoc. Off. Anal. Chem.*, 42, 529, 1959[4]
2. 45.1.10	Nicotinic acid Nicotinamide	AOAC Official Method 961.14, Niacin and Niacinamide in Drugs, Food and Feeds	Colorimetric 470 nm	*J. Assoc. Off. Anal. Chem.*, 58, 799, 1975[5]
3. 45.1.11	Nicotinic acid Nicotinamide	AOAC Official Method 975.41, Niacin and Niacinamide in Cereal Products	Automated Colorimetric 470 nm	*J. Assoc. Off. Anal. Chem.*, 58, 799, 1975[5]
4. 45.1.12	Nicotinic acid	AOAC Official Method 981.16, Niacin	Automated	*J. Assoc. Off. Anal.*

	Analyte	Description	Method	Reference
5. 45.1.13	Nicotinamide Nicotinamide	and Niacinamide in Foods, Drugs and Feed AOAC Official Method 968.32, Niacinamide in Multivitamin Preparations	Colorimetric 470 nm Spectrophotometric 550 nm	Chem., 62, 1027, 1979[6] J. Assoc. Off. Anal. Chem., 51, 828, 1968[7]
6. 50.1.19	Nicotinic acid Nicotinamide	AOAC Official Method 985.34, Niacin and Niacinamide in Ready-To-Feed Milk-Based Infant Formula	Microbiological	J. Assoc. Off. Anal. Chem., 68, 514, 1985[8]
American Feed Ingredients Association, *Laboratory Methods Compendium*, vol. 1, 1991[9]				
1. pages 99–101	Nicotinamide	Niacinamide in compound feed (5–100 ppm)	HPLC 264 nm	J. Chromatogr., 502, 79, 1990[10]
2. pages 103–105	Nicotinic acid Nicotinamide	Nicotinamide and nicotinic acid in multivitamin preparations and vitamin premixes	HPLC 264 nm	None
3. pages 107–110	Nicotinic acid	Nicotinic acid in complete feeds and premixes	Colorimetric 420 nm	Handbuch der Lebensmittle-Chemie, vol. 2, 1967, 738[11]
4. pages 111–114	Nicotinic acid Nicotinamide	Nicotinic acid, nicotinamide, pyridoxine, folic acid, riboflavin and thiamin in liquid and solid vitamin mixtures (>50 mg/kg)	HPLC 263 nm	None
American Association of Cereal Chemists, *Approved Methods*, 1996, vol. 2[12]				
1. AACC 86–49	Nicotinic acid	Niacin in enriched concentrates	Colorimetric	AOAC Int. 16th ed., 45.1.10, (1995)[3]
2. AACC 86–50	Nicotinic acid Nicotinamide	Niacin and nicotinamide in cereal products	Colorimetric 470 nm	J. Assoc. Off. Anal. Chem., 45, 449, 1962[13]
	Nicotinamide		400 nm	AOAC Int. 16th ed., 45.2.04, (1995)[3]
3. AACC 86–51	Nicotinic acid Nicotinamide	Niacin in cereal products	Microbiological	Cereal Chem. 19, 553, 1982[14]

TABLE 9.3 Continued

Source	Form	Methods and Application	Approach	Most Current Cross-Reference
4. AACC 86-52	Nicotinic acid Nicotinamide	Niacin and niacinamide automated determination in cereal products	Automated Colorimetric 470 nm	*J. Agric. Food Chem.,* 22, 323, 1974[15] AOAC Int., 16th ed., 45.1.12, (1995)[3]
Hoffmann-LaRoche, Analytical Methods for Vitamins and, Carotenoids in Feed, 1988[16]				
1. pages 39–41	Nicotinic acid Nicotinamide	Determination of nicotinic acid in complete feeds and premixes (>1 mg/kg)	Colorimetri 420 nm	*Handbuch der Lebensmittle-Chemie,* vol. 2, 1967, 738[11]
				American Feed Ingredients Association, *Laboratory Methods Compendium,* vol. 1, 107[9]
Food Chemicals Codex, 4th ed., 1996[17]				
1. page 264	Nicotinic acid	Niacin (NLT 99.5%, NMT 101.0%)	Titration, NaOH	None
2. pages 264–265	Nicotinamide	Niacinamide (NLT 98.5%, NMT 101.0%)	Titration, perchloric acid	None
3. page 265	Niacinamide ascorbate	Niacinamide ascorbate (NLT 73.5% Ascorbic Acid) (NLT 24.5% Niacinamide)	Titration, perchloric acid	None

include reaction temperature, pH, the choice of an aromatic amine for maximum color development, and the preparation of a proper blank for background correction.[25]

Current AOAC International[23] colorimetric methods use the König reaction. The methodology was developed by Pelletier and Campbell.[26]

AOAC Official Method 961.14, Niacin and Niacinamide in Drugs, Foods, and Feeds, Colorimetric Method *AOAC Official Methods of Analysis of AOAC International,* 45.1.10

Method 961.14 is the manual AOAC International Method. Procedural steps include the following as summarized by Eitenmiller and DeSouza.[13]

9.3.1.1 Sample Preparation

1. *Pharmaceuticals.* Prepare sample containing at least five tablets or capsules by dispersing in small volume of water with heating. Tablets may be ground. Cool and transfer to volumetric flask and dilute to volume so that final solution contains 50 to 200 μg niacin per mL. Pipette 10 mL aliquot into 250 mL Erlenmeyer flask and add 10 mL concentrated HCl. Evaporate on hot plate to approximately 2 mL, cool, and add 25 to 50 mL of water. Adjust pH to 2.5 to 4.5 with 40% NaOH or KOH. Adjust volume with water so that final volume contains approximately 4 μg niacin per mL. If cloudy, filter or centrifuge.

2. *Noncereal foods and feeds.* Weigh approximately one ounce (25 to 30 g) of sample into 1000 mL Erlenmeyer flask and disperse with 200 mL of 1 N H_2SO_4. Autoclave for 30 minutes at 15 psi, cool, and adjust pH to 4.5 with 10 N NaOH. Dilute to 250 mL with water and filter. Weigh 17 g of $(NH_4)_2SO_4$ into 50 mL volumetric flask and pipette in 40 mL of sample solution. Dilute to volume with water and shake vigorously. Clarify by filtration or centrifugation, and use 1 mL for niacin quantitation.

3. *Cereal products.* Add 1.5 g $Ca(OH)_2$ to each of six 250 mL Erlenmeyer flasks. Add 0, 5, 10, 15, 20, and 25 mL of 10 μg niacin per mL standard solution to each flask for standard curve preparation. Weigh approximately 2.5 g sample into another flask containing 1.5 g $Ca(OH)_2$. Add water to each flask so that volume is approximately 90 mL, mix, and autoclave at 15 psi for 2 hours. Mix while hot, cool to 40°C, and transfer to 100 mL volumetric flask. Dilute to volume with water. Extracts can be stored, refrigerated, at this point.

Transfer approximately 50 mL from each flask to centrifuge tubes and place in ice bath for 15 min or in refrigerator for at least 2 h. Centrifuge and pipette 20 mL of supernatant from each tube into separate centrifuge tubes containing 8 g of $(NH_4)_2SO_4$ and 2 mL phosphate buffer, pH 8.0. Dissolve by shaking and warm to 55 to 60°C. Clarify by centrifugation or filtration.

Determinative steps of the König reaction are provided in Part C of Method 961.14.[23]

Note: The König reaction involves the use of 10% cyanogen bromide solution. All determinative steps should be completed under an approved hood. Do not breathe vapors, and, if solution comes into contact with skin, wash immediately with water.

AOAC Official Method 975.41, Niacin and Niacinamide in Cereal Products, Automated Method, *Official Methods of Analysis of AOAC International,* 45.1.11

Method 961.14 was automated for the determination of niacin in cereals.[27] The automated method uses in-line dialysis for the last clarification step, replacing $(NH_4)_2SO_4$ precipitation. One drop of

Brij-35 is added to 100 mL of the diluted extract to avoid bubble formation in the autoanalyzer tubing. The method was based on the Technicon AutoAnalyzer II system.

AOAC Official Method 981.16, Niacin and Niacinamide in Foods, Drugs, and Feeds, Automated Method *Official Methods of Analysis of AOAC International*, 45.1.12, American Association of Cereal Chemists Method 86-52

Method 961.14 was further modified and collaborated for all products other than cereals.[28] Collaborative studies showed that Method 975.41 and Method 981.16 are more precise than the manual procedure (Method 961.14). Also, labor and analysis time are decreased owing to greater sample throughout.

AOAC Official Method 968.32, Niacinamide in Multivitamin Preparations, Spectrophotometric Method, *Official Methods of Analysis of AOAC International*, 45.1.13

Method 968.32 uses the König reaction to quantitate nicotinamide. Nicotinic acid does not interfere unless present at much higher concentrations than nicotinamide.

Note: Collaborated AOAC International Methods using colorimetric procedures provide data that closely compare to microbiological analysis by *Lactobacillus plantarum*.

9.3.2   MICROBIOLOGICAL

Microbiological assay of the niacin content in biological samples continues to be an important method world wide. This, in part, is owing to selectivity and sensitivity problems still influencing the use of LC methods for niacin assay of complex matrices. Additionally, microbiological assay of niacin is a well-accepted assay that is quite simple to conduct in the vitamin analysis laboratory.

Lactobacillus plantarum, Lactobacillus mesenteroides, and the protozoan, *Tetrahymena thermophila* (pyriformis) have been used for niacin analysis. *L. plantarum* is the primary assay organism. It responds equally on a molar basis to nicotinic acid, nicotinamide and NAD. *L. plantarum* assay is a reliable measure of the total niacin in biologicals and pharmaceuticals. *L. mesenteroides* responds only to nicotinic acid.[29] *T. thermophila* responds equally to nicotinic acid and nicotinamide; however, studies have shown non-additive responses for the two niacin forms.[30] For analysis of NMN in urine, only *L. plantarum* has growth response. Drift (growth stimulation or inhibition) is seldom encountered with the use of *L. plantarum*. The bacteria is not affected by free fatty acids in the growth media.[31]

AOAC International microbiological methods for niacin use *L. plantarum* ATCC No. 8014. Summaries of the regulatory methods were provided by Eitenmiller and DeSouza[13] and Ball.[14]

AOAC Official Method 944.13, Niacin and Niacinamide (Nicotinic Acid and Nicotinamide) in Vitamin Preparations, Microbiological Method, *Official Methods of Analysis of AOAC International*, 45.2.04

Method 944.13 was recommended for application to all foods by the AOAC Task Force on Methods for Nutrition Labeling.[32] Samples are extracted by autoclaving for 30 min in 1.0 N H_2SO_4. After autoclaving, proteins are removed by precipitation at pH 4.5. AOAC International also provides Method 985.34 (Chapter 50.1.9) "Niacin and Niacinamide (Nicotinic Acid and Nicotinamide) in Ready-To-Feed Milk-Based Infant Formula." Method 985.34 is similar to Method 944.13.

Use of 1 N H_2SO_4 hydrolysis for extraction of niacin from cereals should be approached with caution. Method 985.34 is stated to be applicable to cereals; however, it is generally accepted that alkaline hydrolysis must be used to free niacin from the documented bound forms in cereals (Section 9.2.3). The $Ca(OH)_2$ procedure given in AOAC Method 961.41 provides suitable extracts for microbiological analysis. Other, more simple, alkaline digestions are available that have been used in conjunction with LC analysis.[33,34,35] These methods are summarized in Table 9.4 (Table 9.4, References 1, 2, and 6—Foods).

Modified microbiological methods, as opposed to the use of traditional microassay techniques, are available. Guilarte and Pravlik[36] used *Kloeckera apiculata* (brevis) ATCC No. 9774 and radiometric techniques to assay niacin in blood and food. The yeast responded equally to nicotinic acid and nicotinamide, but did not respond to nicotinuric acid, trigonelline, NMN, 2-pyridone, picolinic acid, and quinolinic acid. The method consisted of growing the yeast in media containing L-[1-^{14}C] methionine as substrate with measurement of $^{14}CO_2$. The assay was precise and specific, but the method has not been used by other investigators.

A highly automated microplate method was developed by Solve et al.[37] with *L. plantarum*. The procedure was conducted using 48- and 96-well microplates, video digital-image processing, and an ELISA reader. The method reduced material and time expenditures compared to conventional microbiological assay. Digital imaging was an efficient approach to turbidity measurement. Coefficients of variation ranged from 3.7 to 4.8% for the 48-well and from 16.7 and 25.8% for the 96-well plate assay. The detection limit was 0.5 ng niacin per well. The authors concluded that the 48-well microplate assay had advantages of automation, speed, and minimum reagent costs. Results compared favorably to conventional approaches.

9.3.3 HIGH PERFORMANCE LIQUID CHROMATOGRAPHY

Use of LC methods for the measurement of niacin in biological samples has been hindered somewhat by the necessity to use UV detection. While UV detection is suitable for high concentration vitamin premixes and concentrates and for some fortified foods, it lacks specificity and often produces chromatograms with unresolved interferences. Methods for biological samples based on UV detection include clean-up procedures to remove interfering compounds. Useful reviews of LC methodology include Ball,[14] Shibata and Shimono,[15] Eitenmiller and Landen,[16] and Lumley.[22] Other, more general, but useful reviews include Finglas and Faulks[38] and Rizzolo and Polesello.[39] LC methods for the analysis of niacin in food and biological samples are summarized in Table 9.4.

9.3.3.1 Extraction Procedures for Niacin Analysis by HPLC

Both acid and alkaline hydrolysis are used as the initial step in niacin extraction procedures. HCl and H_2SO_4 and NaOH or $Ca(OH)_2$ are the common acids or bases. Details of acid and alkaline hydrolysis procedures are detailed in Table 9.4. Acid hydrolysis will not completely liberate bound niacin forms (Section 9.2.3), and is often used to assay "available" niacin. Alkaline hydrolysis liberates most bound forms and provides a measure of total niacin. Choice of extraction parameters depends on the following factors:

1. If total niacin is to be determined in cereals, alkaline hydrolysis must be used.
2. Fortified forms of niacin can be extracted by acid, water, or ethanol extractions, usually without autoclaving. Hydrolysis is necessary for extraction of complex food and clinical samples.
3. Blood, serum, and urine do not require hydrolysis for efficient niacin extraction.
4. Acid hydrolysis can produce partial conversion of nicotinamide to nicotinic acid.[40]
5. Alkaline hydrolysis converts nicotinamide to nicotinic acid, resulting in simpler chromatography of fortified foods that might contain both forms.
6. Biological samples usually require extract purification following initial extractions. Clean up is necessary owing to a lack of specificity of UV detection.

TABLE 9. 4
HPLC Methods for the Analysis of Niacin in Food, Feeds, Pharmaceuticals, and Biologicals

Sample Matrix	Analyte	Sample Preparation		HPLC Parameters				
		Sample Extraction	Clean Up	Column	Mobile Phase	Detection	Quality Assurance Parameters	References
Food								
1. Cereal	Niacin	Weigh sample equivalent to 0.2 mg niacin	AGI-X8 anion-exchange KMnO$_4$ oxidation	µBondapak C$_{18}$	Isocratic MeOH : water (5 : 95) containing 0.005 TBAP 2.0 mL/min	254 nm	—	*J. Liq. Chromatogr.*, 3, 269, 1980[1]
		Add 80 mL water and 10 mL Ca(OH)$_2$ suspension (50 g/ 500 mL water)						
		Heat, steambath, 30 min						
		Autoclave, 30 min Cool, add water to 200 mL						
		Refrigerate, overnight Centrifuge						
2. Various foods	Niacin	*Acid Hydrolysis* Autoclave 1–5 g in 60 mL 0.1M H$_2$SO$_4$, 1 h	—	Nucleosil 5 C$_{18}$ 15 cm × 4.6 mm and Nucleosil SB anion-exchange Column switching	Column switching A. 5.7 mL HAC+ 800 mL water, to pH 3.0 with NaOH Adjust to 100 mL	254 nm Also, assayed microbiologically	QL 0.5 mg/100 g % CV 6.6 % Recovery 100	*J. Agric. Food Chem.*, 32, 304, 1984[2]
		Cool, digest with Diastase®, 45°C, 3 h			B. A : MeOH (5 : 95)			
		Alkaline Hydrolysis Add 80 mL water and 10 mL Ca(OH)$_2$ suspension (1 g/10 mL water)			C. 22.8 mL HAC + 800 mL water, adjust pH to 3.0 with NaOH, dilute to 1000 mL with water			
		Heat, steambath, 30 min						

Sample	Analyte	Sample preparation	Cleanup	Column	Mobile phase	Detection	Performance	Reference
3. Instant coffee	Nicotinic acid	Autoclave 30 min Dilute to 100 mL with water Refrigerate, overnight Centrifuge Dissolve 1 g in hot water (30 mL at 80°C) Cool, dilute to 50 mL Filter, 0.45 µm	Sep-Pak C_{18}	Spherisorb ODS-2 15 cm × 5 mm	Column switching A to B to C to A over 55 min Isocratic 8% MeOH with 0.005M TBAH, pH 7.0 1.5 mL/min	254 nm	% CV 2.8 % Recovery 102.5	J. Micronutr. Anal., 1, 55, 1985[3]
4. Beef, pork	Nicotinic acid Nicotinamide	Blend Add 30 mL water to 10 g sample Homogenize (Biotron) Dilute to 100 mL with water Centrifuge Transfer 20 mL to 25 mL volumetric Add 1 mL saturated $ZnSO_4$ and 0.5 L 1 N NaOH (deproteinization) Dilute to volume Allow to stand at ambient temperature, 30 min Filter	—	µBondapak C_{18} 30 cm × 3.9 mm or Radial-Pak 2 module	Isocratic *Nicotinic acid* MeOH : water (1 : 9) with 5 mm PIC-A, pH 3.5, 1 mL/min *Nicotinamide* 2 PIC-B7 vials in 1000 mL water 1 mL/min	263 nm	QL 1 ng/100 g % CV 105 % Recovery 96–105	J. Assoc. Off. Anal. Chem., 70, 698, 1987[4]
5. Meats	Nicotinic acid Nicotinamide	Add 30 mL water to 5 g sample Homogenize, Polytron® Boil, 10 min Cool, dilute to 50 mL Filter, 0.45 µm	—	Partisil SCX 10 µm 25 cm × 4.6 mm cation-exchange	Isocratic 50 mM phosphate buffer, pH 3.0 1 mL/min 25°C	260 nm	DL (ng) On-column nicotinic acid 2 nicotinamide 4 % Recovery 98–100	J. Chromatogr., 457, 403, 1988[5]

TABLE 9. 4 Continued

Sample Matrix	Analyte	Sample Preparation		HPLC Parameters				References
		Sample Extraction	Clean Up	Column	Mobile Phase	Detection	Quality Assurance Parameters	
6. Beef, semolina, cottage cheese	Total niacin as nicotinic acid	Weigh sample to contain ≥ 0.04 mg niacin or greater sample weight for representative sample; Add 200 g-sample weight of water; Add 10 g Ca(OH)$_2$ Blend; Autoclave, 15 min; Cool, filter, Whatman 2V; Add 300–320 mg oxalic acid to 100 mL aliquot; Mix, adjust pH to 6.5–7.0; Filter, Whatman 42	Sep-Pak plus C$_{18}$	Supelco LC-18–08; 5 μm; 15 cm × 4.6 mm	Isocratic; MeCN : H$_3$PO$_4$ (23 + 0.1) containing 0.1% SDS; 1.5 mL/min	254 nm	QL 0.05 mg/100 g; % CV 1.0–10.0; % Recovery 99.5	J. Assoc. Off. Anal. Chem., 73, 467, 1990[6]
7. Feeds	Nicotinamide	Add 10 mL 0.2 M HCl to 2 g sample; Stir, 10 min; Centrifuge, filter, 0.5 μm	—	A. RP-18 5 μm 25 cm × 4.6 mm and B. Nucleosil 5 SA anion-exchange 25 cm × 4.6 mm Column switching	Column switching; Eluent A 0.01M KH$_2$PO$_4$; Eluent B 0.01M KH$_2$PO$_4$: MeCN (60 : 40); A. 0–17 min B. 17–20 min A at 20 min Column switching	264 nm	DL 0.5 ppm; QL 2 ppm	J. Chromatogr., 502, 79, 1990[7]
8. Various foods	Nicotinic acid	Add 4 mL of 40% NaOH to 5–10 g sample; Add 4 mL water	AGI-X8 anion-exchange and IC-SPM cation-	Asahipak NH 2 P-50 5 μm	MeCN : water (60 : 40) containing 0.075M NaOAC	261 nm	% Recovery 91–94	J. Chromatogr., 588, 171, 1991[8]

Food	Form	Sample preparation	Cleanup	Column	Mobile phase / flow	Detection	Performance	Reference
		Heat, steambath, 30 min / Neutralize with 25% HCl / Add same volume of MeOH / Filter / Rinse residue with 50% MeOH / Dilute to 100 mL with 50% MeOH / Evaporate 30 mL aliquot to dryness / Dissolve in 20 mL water	exchange	25 cm × 4.6 mm	0.5 mL/min			
9. Legumes, meat	Nicotinic acid	Add 30 mL 0.1 N HCl to 1–10 g sample plus 1 mL 6 N HCl / Autoclave, 15 min / Adjust pH to 4.0–4.5 with 2 N NaOAC / Add 5 mL of 6% Takadiastase® / Digest at 48°C, 3 h / Filter, dilute to 100 mL with water	Dowex 1-X8	μBondapak C$_{18}$ 10 μm 30 cm × 3.9 mm or Spherisorb ODS2 10 μm 30 cm × 3.9 mm	Isocratic 0.005M TBAB in MeOH : 0.01M NaOAC (1 : 9), pH 4.72 1.5 mL/min	254 nm	—	J. Agric. Food Chem., 39, 116, 1991[9]
10. Fortified foods	Nicotinic acid	Weigh sample containing 100 mg niacin into 500 mL Phillips beaker / Add 50 mL water / Add 6 mL H$_2$SO$_4$ (1 : 1) / Mix / Autoclave, 45 min / Cool, adjust pH to 6.0–6.5 with 7.5 N NaOH / Dilute to 100 mL with water	Florisil	PRP-X100 25 cm × 4.1 mm	Isocratic 20 mL HAC diluted to 1 L with water	254 nm	QL 0.11 μg/mL / CV % 2.4–2.9 / % Recovery 99.8	J. AOAC Int., 76, 390, 1993[10]

TABLE 9. 4 Continued

| Sample Matrix | Analyte | Sample Preparation | | HPLC Parameters | | | | |
		Sample Extraction	Clean Up	Column	Mobile Phase	Detection	Quality Assurance Parameters	References
		Filter, Whatman 40 Adjust 20 mL aliquot to pH 0.5–1.0 with H_2SO_4 (1 : 1)						
Biologicals								
1. Plasma, urine	Nicotinamide	*Plasma* Mix 1 mL with 10 µL isonicotinamide (IS), 400 mg/L Add 10 µL water Vortex *Urine* Mix 1 mL with 10 mL isonicotinamide (IS), 5000 mg/L Add 10 µL water Vortex	Sep-Pak C_{18}	µBondapak C_{18} 30 cm × 4 mm or LiChrosorb RP-18 10 µm 25 cm × 4 mm	Isocratic Dissolve 4.446 g sodium dioctyl-sulfosuccinate in 1450 mL water Adjust pH to 2.5 with formic acid Add 1050 mL MeOH 2.0 mL/min	254 nm	QL (mg/L) 0.1 (plasma) 1.0 (urine) % Recovery 91.8–92.4	*J. Chromatogr.,* 221, 161, 1980[1]
2. Urine	Nicotinamide Metabolites	To 1 mL urine, add 1.2 g K_2CO_3 Add isonicotinamide (IS) Cool on ice Add 5 mL Et_2O, mix Centrifuge Remove Et_2O layer (3×) Dissolve residue in water Filter	—	7-ODS-L 7 µm 25 cm × 4.6 mm	Isocratic 10 mM KH_2PO_4 : MeCN (96 : 4), pH 3.0 1 mL/min	260 nm	DL (pg) On-column 304–1220 % Recovery 97.9	*J. Chromatogr.,* 424, 23, 1988[2]

3. Urine	Nicotinic acid Nicotinuric acid	Dilute urine (300 μL) with 600 μL water Add 6-methyl nictonic acid (IS) (20 μg/mL)	Bond Elut SCX	Invertisil ODS-2 5 μm 25 cm × 4.6 mm	Isocratic 10 mM K_2HPO_4 containing 5 μM TBAP, pH 7.0 : MeCN (90 : 10) 1 mL/min 35°C	254 nm	QL 5 μg/mL % CV 8.1–8.8	J. Chromatogr. B, 661, 154, 1994[3]
4. Biological samples	Nicotinic acid Nicotinamide	Homogenize in saline Add 18 mL acetone to 3 mL, homogenate Centrifuge Mix with 14 mL $CHCl_3$ Centrifuge Filter 500 mL of upper aqueous phase, 0.45 μm Add [³H] nicotinic acid for recovery study	—	Hypersil ODS 5 μm 25 cm × 4.6 mm	Gradient A. 100% MeOH B. 5 mM TBAP, pH 7.0 0–10 min A : B (90 : 10) To (30 : 70) 1.2 mL/min	Post-column derivatization using König reaction 410 nm	DL (Pmol) On-column 12–21 RSD% <5 % Recovery 92.4	J. Chromatogr. B, 665, 71, 1995[4]

The most common extract purification approaches use ion-exchange chromatography with anion-exchange resin and solid phase C_{18} extraction columns. Chase et al.[41] used Florisil open-column chromatography to successfully purify H_2SO_4 extracts of fortified foods. Detection at 254 nm following chromatography on PRP-X100 anion exchange resin gave interference free chromatograms. The Chase et al.[41] procedure is detailed in Section 9.4.

9.3.3.2.   Chromatography Parameters

9.3.3.2.1   Supports and Mobile Phases

Supports and mobile phases used in recently developed methods for niacin analysis are given in Table 9.4. Poor resolution of niacin because of the necessity to use UV detection has led investigators to develop quite complex chromatographic systems in addition to the use of extensive extract purification methods. Most methods capable of resolving niacin use anion- and cation-exchange resins or reversed-phase chromatography on C_{18}. van Niekerk et al.[34] introduced a complex column switching technique to resolve niacin from eluting UV absorbing intereferences. The method used C_{18} reversed-phase and anion-exchange chromatography on Nucleosil 5-SB support. Mobile phases used with the system were based upon glacial acetic acid : water combinations and the cycle was completed in 55 min. Other investigators have used column switching on C_{18} and anion-exchange columns effectively.[42] Ion-pair chromatography can improve resolution of niacin from interfering peaks, but ion-pairing reagents have not been universally used. Commonly used ion-pair reagents include tert-butylammonium hydroxide (TBAH), tetrabutylammonium phosphate (TBAP), sodium dodecylsulfate (SDS), tetrabutylamminoum bromide (TBAB), and sodium dioctylsulfosuccinate.

9.3.3.2.2   Detection

UV detection presents a convenient, although non-specific, detection mode for niacin. Most studies to date utilized absorbance at 254 to 264 nm. A newer approach to niacin detection after LC resolution uses the chromaphore developed by the König reaction with KCN.[43] The post-column derivatization provided extremely clean chromatograms with high specificity for nicotinic acid and nicotinamide. The method is summarized in Section 9.4 and deserves investigation for its general application to biological samples. Use of KCN remains an obstacle, but the reagent can be safely handled.

9.3.3.2.3   Internal Standards

Internal standards have not been routinely used in LC quantitation of niacin. Isonicotinamide was the internal standard in methods developed for plasma and urine.[44,45]

9.3.4   CAPILLARY ELECTROPHORESIS

Capillary electrophoresis (CE) offers another highly promising approach for quantitating total niacin in biological samples. Ward and colleagues[46,47] recently published methodology using CE for analysis of a wide variety of foods. After alkali extraction, the extract was purified and concentrated by solid-phase extraction on Sep-Pak C_{18} and SCX cation exchange columns connected in series. CE used a 75 μm uncoated fused silica capillary column (50 cm) with acetonitrile : phosphate buffer, pH 7.0 (15 : 85). Detection was at 254 nm. The CE procedure and HPLC determinations gave comparable values. The CV for the method was 0.9% and provided cleaner chromatograms, more speed, and lower sample cost compared to the HPLC method. Because of the potential for this approach to niacin analysis for all types of sample matrices, the procedural details are given in Section 9.4.

9.4   METHOD PROTOCOLS

Liquid Chromatographic Analysis of Niacin in Fortified Food Products

Principle

- After initial extraction by autoclaving with H_2SO_4 (1 + 1), the extracts were purified using Florisil open column chromatography. The amount of niacin was determined by LC and UV detection at 254 nm.

Chemicals

- Florisil
- H_2SO_4
- Methanol

Apparatus

- Liquid chromatograph
- UV detector
- Glass columns, 300 × 10.5 mm for open-column chromatography

Procedure

Extraction of Standards and Samples

- Weigh sample to contain 100 μg niacin
- Add 150 mL water and 6 M H_2SO_4 (1 + 1)
- Mix well to break up clumps
- Autoclave at 121°C to 123°C for 45 min
- Adjust pH to 6.0 to 6.5 with 7.5 N NaOH
- Adjust pH to 4.5 with H_2SO_4 (1 + 1)
- Dilute extract to 100 mL with water
- Filter, Whatman No. 40
- Adjust 20.00 mL aliquot of filtrate to pH 0.5 to 1.0 with H_2SO_4 (1 + 1)

Open-column Clean Up

Preparation of Florisil Column
- Add 4 g Florisil to column
- Top with small pledglet of glass wool
- Prewash column with 30 mL methanol, followed by two 15 mL portions of 0.5 N H_2SO_4

Sample Extract
- Transfer extract to Florisil column
- Wash column with two 15 mL portions of 0.5 N H_2SO_4
- Discard effluent
- Elute niacin with 25 mL 0.5 N NaOH into a 50 mL volumetric flask containing 1.0 mL glacial acetic acid
- Dilute to volume with water
- Filter (0.45 μm filter)

Chromatography*

Column	25.0×4.1 mm
Stationary phase	PRP* X100
Mobile phase	glacial acetic acid + water (20 + 980)
Column temperature	Ambient
Flow	1.5 mL/min
Retention time	8 min
Detection	UV, 254 nm
Calculation	External standard, linear regression: 0.25, 0.48, 0.64, and 0.80 μg/mL

*Figures 9.6.I and 9.6.II.

J. AOAC International, 76, 390, 1993

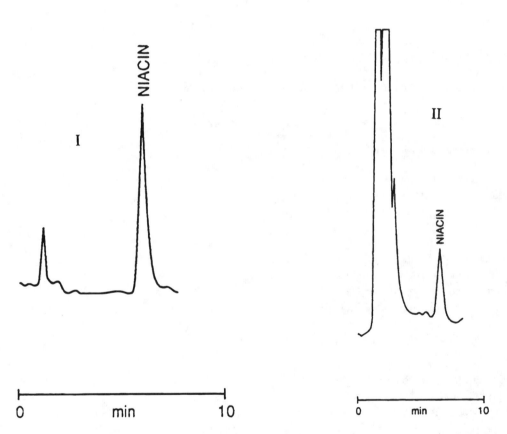

FIGURE 9.6.I Chromatogram of a niacin standard solution. Reproduced with permission from Reference 41.

FIGURE 9.6.II Chromatogram of nicotinic acid in a milk-based infant formula. Reproduced with permission from Reference 41.

High-Performance Liquid Chromatographic Determination of Nicotinic Acid and Nicotinamide in Biological Samples Applying Post-column Derivatization Resulting in Bathmochrome Absorption Shifts

Principle

- Tissue was homogenized in saline. After addition of acetone, the extract was centrifuged. After chloroform addition, the extract was recentrifuged. The aqueous layer was filtered and injected. LC analysis used C_{18} support and a linear gradient of tetrabutylammonium phosphate (TBAP) and methanol. Post-column derivatization with KCN (König reaction) yielded clean chromatograms at 410 nm.

Chemicals

- Nicotinic acid, nicotinamide
- Chloramin T
- Tris
- Methanol
- Acetone
- Chloroform
- TBAP
- Potassium cyanide

Apparatus

- HPLC, gradient controller
- Visible detector
- Centrifuge
- Solvent metering pump
- Water bath

Procedure

Sample Extraction

- Homogenize tissue in saline
- Add acetone, centrifuge
- Add chloroform to supernatant
- Centrifuge
- Filter aqueous layer

Chromatography*

Column	25 cm × 4.6 mm
Stationary phase	ODS Hypersil, 5 μm
Mobile phase	Linear gradient of 100% methanol and 5 mM TBAP, pH 7.0
Column temperature	Ambient
Flow	1.2 mL/min
Detector	410 nm
Post-column derivatization	KCN (Figure 9-7-I), 60°C
Calculation	External calibration, peak area, regression

* See Figures 9.7.I and 9.7.II.

J. Chromatogr. B, 665, 71, 1995

I

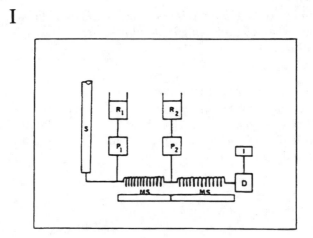

FIGURE 9.7.I   Schematic for the chromatography system and post-column derivatization of niacin by KCN. 1 to 2% chloramine T, P_1-pump, R_2-0.25% KCN, 25 mM Tris, 40 mM HCl, P_2-pump, D-detector, I-integrator. Reaction coils are 2 m PTFE, 0.5 mm ID after R_1 delivery and 8 m PTFE, 0.5 mm ID after R_2 delivery. Coils are immersed in a 60°C water bath. Flow rate equals 0.5 mL/min. Reproduced with permission from Reference 43.

II

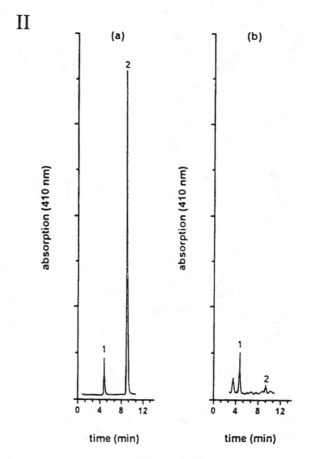

FIGURE 9.7.II   Chromatograms of nicotinic acid and nicotinamide after post-column derivatization. $a =$ standards, $b =$ rat intestinal tissue, Peak 1 = nicotinic acid, Peak 2 = nicotinamide. Reproduced with permission from Reference 43.

The Determination of Niacin in Cereals, Meat, and Selected Foods by Capillary Electrophoresis and High Performance Liquid Chromatography

Principle

- Total niacin is extracted by alkaline hydrolysis and concentration and purification on C_{18} and SCX cation exchange columns in series. Capillary electrophoresis on fused silica resolved niacin with detection at 254 nm.

Chemicals

- Niacin
- Saccharin (IS)
- Disodium hydrogen orthophosphate
- Oxalic acid
- Methanol
- Ammonium hydroxide
- Acetonitrile

Apparatus

- Capillary electrophoresis unit with UV detector
- Sep-Pak C_{18} Vac cartridge
- SCX column (500 mg)
- Cellulose acetate filter assembly (0.8 μm)

Procedure

Extraction

- To 1 g of sample, add 0.75 g calcium hydroxide and 20 mL deionized water
- Autoclave, 2 h at 121°C
- Cool, dilute to 50 mL with water
- Centrifuge
- To 15 mL aliquot of supernatant, adjust pH to 7.0 with 10% solution of oxalic acid
- Dilute to 25 mL with water, centrifuge at 0°C

SPE Clean-Up and Concentration

- Condition Sep-Pak Vac C_{18} and SCX columns connected in series with 10 mL methanol followed by 10 mL deionized water
- Load 10 mL extract onto the C_{18} column
- Wash columns with 5 mL water
- Discard C_{18} column
- Wash SCX column with 5 mL methanol
- Elute niacin with 5 mL of freshly prepared 2% solution of ammonium hydroxide in methanol
- Evaporate eluate under nitrogen
- Dissolve residue in 1 mL of aqueous saccharin (40 μg/mL)
- Filter, 0.8 μm cellulose acetate

Capillary Electrophoresis*

Column	75 cm × 75 μm uncoated fused silica
Effective length	50 cm to detection
Buffer	15% acetonitrile and 85% of a 1 : 1 mixture of 0.02 *M* potassium ihydrogen orthophosphate and 0.02 *M* disodium hydrogen orthophosphate, pH 7.0

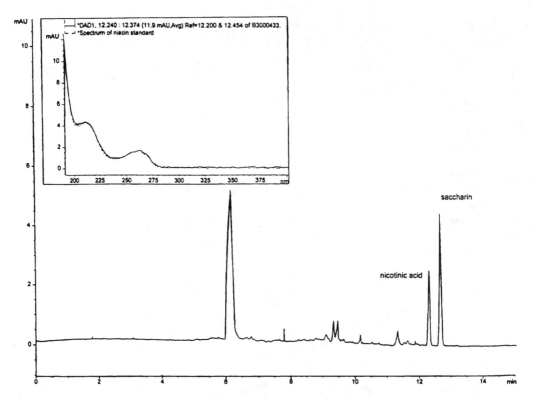

FIGURE 9.8 Capillary electrophoretic resolution of nicotinic acid and saccharin (IS) from cereal containing 6.4 mg nicotinic acid/100 g. Reproduced with permission from Reference 47.

Voltage	+ 20 kV
Temperature	30°C
Detection	254 nm
Load	Under vacuum

* See Figure 9.8.

Food Chem., 60, 667, 1997

9.5   REFERENCES

Text

1. Friedrich, W. F., Niacin: nicotinic acid, nicotinamide, NAD(P), in *Vitamins*, Walter de Gruyter, Berlin, 1988, chap. 8.
2. Elvehjem, C. A., Madden, R. J., Strong, R. M., and Woolby, D.W., Relation of nicotinic acid and nicotinic acid amide to canine black tongue, *J. Am. Chem. Soc.,* 59, 1767, 1937.
3. Spies, T. D., Cooper, C., and Blankenhorn, M. A., The use of nicotinic acid in the treatment of pellagra, *JAMA,* 110, 622, 1938.
4. Krehl, W. A., Tepley, L. J., Sarma, P. S., and Elvehjem, C. A., Growth retarding effects of corn in nicotinic acid-low rations and its counteraction by tryptophane, *Science,* 101, 489, 1945.
5. Heidelberger, C., Morgan, G., and Lefkovsky, F., Tryptophan metabolism, *J. Biol. Chem.,* 179, 151, 1948.
6. National Research Council, *Recommended Dietary Allowances,* 10th ed., National Academy of Sciences, Washington, D.C., 1989, chap. 8.

7. Horwitt, M. K., Harper, A. E., and Henderson, L. M., Niacin-tryptophan relationships for evaluating niacin equivalents, *Am. J. Clin. Nutr.*, 34, 423, 1981.
8. Machlin, L. J. and Hüni, J. E. S., *Vitamin Basics*, Hoffmann-LaRoche, Basel, 1994, 42.
9. Gibson, R. S., *Principles of Nutritional Assessment*, Oxford University Press, New York, 1990, 440.
10. *Nutritional Labeling and Education Act of 1990*, Fed. Reg., 58, 2070, 1993.
11. Jacob, R. A. and Swendseid, M. E., Niacin, in *Present Knowledge in Nutrition*, 7th ed., Ziegler, E. E. and Flier, L. J., Jr., Eds., ILSI Press, Washington, D.C., 1996, chap. 19.
12. Combs, G. F., Jr., *The Vitamins, Fundamental Aspects in Nutrition and Health*, Academic Press, New York, 1992, chap. 12.
13. Eitenmiller, R. R. and DeSouza, S., Niacin, in *Methods of Vitamin Assay*, 4th ed., Augustin, J., Klein, B. P., Becker, D. A., and Venugopal, P. B., Eds., John Wiley and Sons, New York, 1985, chap. 15.
14. Ball, G. F. M., Chemical and biological nature of the water-soluble vitamins, in *Water-Soluble Vitamin Assays in Human Nutrition*, Chapman and Hall, New York, 1994, chap. 2.
15. Shibata, K. and Shimono, T., Nicotinic acid and nicotinamide in *Modern Chromatographic Analysis of Vitamins*, 2nd ed., De Leenheer, A. P., Lambert, W. E., and Nelis, H. J., Eds., Marcel Dekker, New York, 1992, chap. 7.
16. Eitenmiller, R. and Landen, W. O., Jr., Vitamins, in *Analyzing Food for Nutrition Labeling and Hazardous Contaminants*, Jeon, I. J. and Ikins, W. G., Eds., Marcel Dekker, New York, 1995, chap. 9.
17. Hepburn, F. N., Nutrient composition of selected wheats and wheat products, VII. Total and free niacin, *Cereal Chem.*, 48, 369, 1971.
18. Koetz, R., Armado, R., and Neukom, H., Nature of bound nicotinic acid in wheat bran, *Lebensm., Wiss. Technol*, 12, 346, 1979.
19. Carter, E. G. A. and Carpenter, K. J., The bioavailability for humans of bound niacin from wheat bran, *Am. J. Clin. Nutr.*, 36, 855, 1982.
20. Carter, E. G. A. and Carpenter, K. J., The available niacin values of foods for rats and their relation to analytical values, *J. Nutr.*, 112, 2091, 1982.
21. Kodicek, E., Braudi, R., Kon, S. K., and Mitchell, K. G., The availability to pigs of nicotinic acid in tortilla baked from maize treated with lime-water, *Br. J. Nutr.*, 13, 363, 1959.
22. Lumley, I. D., Vitamin analysis in food, in *The Technology of Vitamins in Food*, Ottaway, P.B., Ed., Chapman and Hall, New York, 1993, chap. 8.
23. AOAC International, *Official Methods of Analysis*, 16th ed., AOAC International, Arlington, VA, 1995.
24. Strohecker, R. and Henning, H., *Vitamin Assay Tested Methods*, Verlag Chemie, Darmstadt, 1965, 198.
25. Goldsmith, G. A. and Miller, D. N., Niacin, in *The Vitamins*, Gyorgy, P. and Pearson, Eds., Academic Press, New York, 1967, 137.
26. Pelletier, O. and Campbell, J. A., A modified procedure for the determination of niacin in cereal products, *J. Assoc. Off. Anal. Chem.*, 42, 625, 1959.
27. Gross, A.F., Automated method for the determination of niacin and niacinamide in cereal products: collaborative study, *J. Assoc. Off. Anal. Chem.*, 58, 799, 1975.
28. Egberg, D., Automated method for niacin and niacinamide in food products: Collaborative study, *J. Assoc. Off. Anal. Chem.*, 62, 1027, 1979.
29. Voigt, M. N. and Eitenmiller, R. R., Comparative review of the thiochrome, microbial and protozoan analyses of B-vitamins, *J. Food Prot.*, 41, 730, 1978.
30. Baker, H. and Frank, O., *Clinical Microbiology*, Interscience Publishers, New York, 1968, 31.
31. Kodicek, E. and Pepper, C. R., A critical study of factors influencing the microbiological assay of nicotinic acid, *J. Gen. Microbiol.*, 2, 292, 1948.
32. AOAC International, Report of the AOAC International Task Force on Methods for Nutrient Labeling Analyses, *J. AOAC Int.*, 76, 180A, 1993.
33. Tyler, T. A., Shrago, R. R., and Shuster, H. V., Determination of niacin in cereal samples by HPLC, *J. Liq. Chromatogr.*, 3, 269, 1980.
34. van Niekerk, P. J., Smit, S. C. C., Strydom, E. S. P. and Armbruster, G., Comparison of a high-performance liquid chromatographic and microbiological method for the determination of niacin in foods, *J. Agric. Food Chem.*, 32, 304, 1984.
35. Tyler, T. A. and Genzale, J. A., Liquid chromatographic determination of total niacin in beef, semolina and cottage cheese, *J. Assoc. Off. Anal. Chem.*, 73, 467, 1990.

36. Guilarte, T. R. and Pravlik, K., Radiometric-microbiological assay of niacin using *Klocckera brevis*: analysis of human blood and food, *J. Nutr.,* 13, 2587, 1983.

37. Solve, M., Eriksen, H., and Brogren, C. H., Automated microbiological assay for quantitation of niacin performed in culture microplates read by digital image processing, *Food Chem.,* 49, 419, 1994.

38. Finglas, P. M. and Faulks, R. M., Critical review of HPLC methods for the determination of thiamin, riboflavin and niacin in food, *J. Micronutr. Anal.,* 3, 251, 1987.

39. Rizzolo, A. and Polesello, S., Chromatographic determination of vitamins in foods, *J. Chromatogr.,* 624, 103, 1992.

40. Rees, D. I., Determination of nicotinamide and pyridoxine in fortified food products by HPLC, *J. Micronutr. Anal.,* 5, 53, 1989.

41. Chase, G. W., Jr., Landen, W. O., Jr., Soliman, A. M., and Eitenmiller, R. R., Liquid chromatographic analysis of niacin in fortified food products, *J. AOAC Int.,* 76, 390, 1993.

42. Balschukat, D. and Kress, E., Use of column switching for the determination of niacinamide in compound feed, *J. Chromatogr.,* 502, 79, 1990.

43. Stein, J., Hahn, A., and Rehner, G., High-performance liquid chromatographic determination of nicotinic acid and nicotinamide in biological samples applying post-column derivatization resulting in bathmochrome absorption shifts, *J. Chromatogr. B,* 665, 71, 1995.

44. DeVries, J., Günthert, W., and Ding, R., Determination of nicotinamide in human plasma and urine by ion-pair reversed-phase high-performance liquid chromatography, *J. Chromatogr.,* 221, 161, 1980.

45. Shibata, K., Kawada, T., and Iwai, K., Simultaneous microdetermination of nicotinamide and its major metabolites, N′-methyl-2-pyridone-5-carboxamide and N′-methyl-4-pyridone-3-carboxamide, by high-performance liquid chromatography, *J. Chromatogr.,* 424, 23, 1988.

46. Ward, C., Trenerry, V. C., and Pant, I., The application of capillary electrophoresis to the determination of total niacin in concentrated yeast spreads, *Food Chem.,* 58, 185, 1996.

47. Ward, C. M. and Trenerry, V. C., The determination of niacin in cereals, meat, and selected foods by capillary electrophoresis and high performance liquid chromatography, *Food Chem.,* 60, 667, 1997.

Table 9.2   Physical Properties of Nicotinic Acid and Nicotinamide

1. Ball, G. F. M., Chemical and biological nature of the water-soluble vitamins, in *Water-Soluble Vitamin Assays in Human Nutrition*, Chapman and Hall, New York, 1994, chap. 2.

2. Budavari, S., *The Merck Index*, 12th ed., Merck and Company, Whitehouse Station, NJ, 1996, 1114, 1130.

3. Shibata, K. and Shimono, T., Nicotinic acid and nicotinamide, in *Modern Chromatographic Analysis of Vitamins*, 2nd ed., De Leenheer, A. P., Lambert, W. E. and Nelis, H. J., Eds., Mercel Dekker, New York, 1992, chap. 7.

4. Eitenmiller, R. R. and DeSouza, S., Niacin, in *Methods of Vitamin Assay*, 4th ed., Augustin, J., Klein, B. P., Decker, D. A. and Venugopal, P. B., Eds., John Wiley & Sons, New York, 1985, chap. 15.

Table 9.3   Compendium, Regulatory and Handbook Methods of Analysis for Niacin

1. The United States Pharmacopeial Convention, *U.S. Pharmacopeia National Formulary*, USP23/NF18, Nutritional Supplements Official Monographs, United States Pharmacopeial Convention, Rockville, MD, 1995.

2. Scottish Home and Health Department, *British Pharmacopoeia*, 15th ed., British Pharmacopoeial Commission, United Kingdom, 1993.

3. AOAC International, *Official Methods of Analysis*, 16th ed., AOAC International, Arlington, VA, 1995.

4. Loy, H. W., Report on revision of microbiological methods for the B vitamins, *J. Assoc. Off. Anal. Chem.,* 42, 529, 1959.

5. Gross, A. F., Automated method for the determination of niacin and niacinamide in cereal products: collaborative study, *J. Assoc. Off. Anal. Chem.,* 58, 799, 1975.

6. Egberg, D. C., Automated method for niacin and niacinamide in food products: collaborative study, *J. Assoc. Off. Anal. Chem.,* 62, 1027, 1979.

7. Pelletier, O., Chemical determination of niacinamide in multivitamin preparations, *J. Assoc. Off. Anal. Chem.,* 51, 828, 1968.

8. Tanner, J. T. and Barnett, S. A., Methods of analysis for infant formula: Food and Drug Administration and Infant Formula Council: collaborative study, *J. Assoc. Off. Anal. Chem.,* 68, 514, 1985.

9. American Feed Ingredients Association, *Laboratory Methods Compendium,* vol. 1: *Vitamins and Minerals,* American Feed Ingredients Association, West Des Moines, IA, 1991, 99.
10. Balschukat, D. and Kress, G., Use of column switching for the determination of niacinamide in compound feed, *J. Chromatogr.,* 502, 79, 1990.
11. *Handbuch der Lebensmittel-Chemie,* vol. 2, Springer-Verlag, Berlin, 1967, 738.
12. American Association of Cereal Chemists (AACC), *Approved Methods,* 9th ed., vol. 2, American Association of Cereal Chemists, St. Paul, MN, 1996.
13. Campbell, J. A. and Pelletier, O., Determination of niacin (niacinamide) in cereal products, *J. Assoc. Off. Anal. Chem.,* 45, 449, 1962.
14. Dexter, J.E., Matsuo, R.R. and Morgan, B.C., Effects of processing conditions and cooking time on riboflavin, thiamine and niacin levels in enriched spaghetti, *Cereal Chem.,* 19, 553, 1982.
15. Egberg, D. C., Potter, R. H. and Honold, G. R., The semiautomated determination of niacin and niacinamide in food products, *J. Agric. Food Chem.,* 22, 323, 1974.
16. Keller, H. E., *Analytical Methods for Vitamins and Carotenoids,* Hoffmann-LaRoche, Basel, 1988, 39.
17. Committee on Food Chemicals Codex, *Food Chemicals Codex,* 4th ed., National Academy of Sciences, Washington, D.C., 1996, 264.

Table 9.4 HPLC Methods for the Analysis of Niacin in Foods, Feeds, Pharmaceuticals, and Biologicals

Food

1. Tyler, T. A., Shrago, R. R. and Shuster, H. V., Determination of niacin in cereal samples by HPLC, *J. Liq. Chromatogr.,* 3, 269, 1980.
2. van Niekerk, P. J., Smit, S. C. C., Strydom, E. S. P. and Armbruster, G., Comparison of a high-performance liquid chromatographic and microbiological method for the determination of niacin in foods, *J. Agric. Food Chem.,* 32, 304, 1984.
3. Trugo, L. C., Macrae, R. and Trugo, N.M.F., Determination of nicotinic acid in instant coffee using HPLC, *J. Micronutr. Anal.,* 1, 55, 1985.
4. Takatsuki, K., Suzuki, S., Sato, M., Sakai, K. and Ushizawa, I., Liquid chromatographic determination of free and added niacin and niacinamide in beef and pork, *J. Assoc. Off. Anal. Chem.,* 70, 698, 1987.
5. Hamano, T., Mitsuhashi, Y., Aoki, N., Yamamoto, S. and Oji, Y., Simultaneous determination of niacin and niacinamide in meats by high-performance liquid chromatography, *J. Chromatogr.,* 457, 403, 1988.
6. Tyler, T. A. and Genzale, J. A., Liquid chromatographic determination of total niacin in beef, semolina and cottage cheese, *J. Assoc. Off. Anal. Chem.,* 73, 467, 1990.
7. Balschukat, D. and Kress, E., Use of column switching for the determination of niacinamide in compound feed, *J. Chromatogr.,* 502, 79, 1990.
8. Hirayama, S. and Maruyama, M., Determination of a small amount of niacin in foodstuffs by high-performance liquid chromatography, *J. Chromatogr.,* 588, 171, 1991.
9. Vidal-Valverde, C. and Reche, A., Determination of available niacin in legumes and meat by high-performance liquid chromatography, *J. Agric. Food Chem.,* 39, 116, 1991.
10. Chase, G. W., Jr., Landen, W. O., Jr., Soliman, A. M. and Eitenmiller, R. R., Liquid chromatographic analysis of niacin in fortified food products, *J. AOAC Int.,* 76, 390, 1993.

Biologicals

1. de Vries, J. X., Günthert, W. and Ding, R., Determination of nicotinamide in human plasma and urine by ion-pair reversed-phase high-performance liquid chromatography, *J. Chromatogr.,* 221, 161, 1980.
2. Shibata, K., Kawada, T. and Iwai, K., Simultaneous microdetermination of nicotinamide and its major metabolites, n-methyl-2-pyridone-5-carboxamide and N'-methyl-4-pyridone-3-carboxamide, by high-performance liquid chromatography, *J. Chromatogr.,* 424, 23, 1988.
3. Iwaki, M., Ogiso, T., Hayashi, H., Lin, E. T. and Benet, L. Z., Simultaneous measurement of nicotinic acid and its major metabolite, nicotinuric acid in urine using high-performance liquid chromatography: application of solid-liquid extraction, *J. Chromatogr. B,* 661, 154, 1994.
4. Stein, J., Hahn, A. and Rehner, G., High-performance liquid chromatographic determination of nicotinic acid and nicotinamide in biological samples applying post-column derivatization resulting in bathmochrome absorption shifts, *J. Chromatogr. B,* 665, 71, 1995.

10 Vitamin B-6

10.1 REVIEW

In 1934, Gyorgy identified vitamin B-6 as a curative factor for a characteristic dermatitis in rats. The vitamin was isolated in the pure crystalline state in 1938 by several researchers. Gyorgy named the vitamin pyridoxine which was structurally characterized and synthesized in 1939. The complexity of the vitamin B-6 group was not understood until Snell[1] identified the existence of pyridoxal and pyridoxamine in some of the early historically significant growth studies on the lactic acid bacteria. Human deficiency symptoms were first observed in 1950 by Mueller and Vilter.[2] Marginal vitamin B-6 deficiency is usually associated with other nutritional deficiencies. General symptoms include weakness, sleeplessness, nervous disorders, appetite and growth depression, and various dermatologic disorders. Table 10.1 summarizes deficiency symptoms as presented by Combs.[3] Genetic

TABLE 10.1
Symptoms of Vitamin B-6 Deficiency*

System	Signs
General	
Appetite	Decrease
Growth	Decrease
Dermatologic	Acrodynia, cheilosis, stomatitis, glossitis
Muscular	Weakness
Skeletal	Dental caries
Organs	Hepatic steatosis
Vascular	
Vessels	Arteriosclerosis
Erythrocytes	Anemia
Nervous	Paralysis, convulsions, peripheral neuropathy
Reproductive	Decreased egg production
Fetal	Malformations, death
Congenital Disorders	
Homocysteinuria cystathione β-synthetase deficiency	Thrombosis, skeletal and connective tissue malformation, mental retardation
Cystathionuria cystathione g-lyase deficiency	Mental retardation
γ-Amino butyric acid (GABA) deficiency Glutamic decarboxylase deficiency	Neuropathies
Sideroblastic anemia δ-aminolevulinate synthase deficiency	Anemia, cystathionuria, xanthuremic aciduria

* Adapted from Reference 3.

defects involving vitamin B-6 dependent enzymes, while not diet dependent, produce symptoms that mimic deficiency.[4] Individuals with congenital enzyme deficiencies sometimes respond to high doses of vitamin B-6.

The metabolically active form is pyridoxal-5'-phosphate (PLP). PLP acts as a co-factor in a large number of amino acid transformations, most notable of which is transamination. In general, PLP enzymes act through Schiff base aldimine intermediates with the formation of a resonance stabilized carbanion. Vitamin B-6 dependent enzymes are categorized in Table 10.2. The primary route for PLP catabolism is through oxidation to 4-pyridoxic acid (4-PA) which is excreted in the urine. Pyridoxal (PL) and 4-PA are the primary urinary excretion forms. Clinical status tests for the human include plasma PLP quantitation and urinary measurements of PL expressed as mg per g creatinine, and 4-PA. LC methods for analysis of PLP, PL, and 4-PA are discussed in Section 10.3. Since PLP is the co-enzyme for kynureninase and kynurenine aminotransferase in the kynurenine stage of the conversion of tryptophan to niacin, decreased activity of these enzymes during vitamin B-6 deficiency leads to increased urinary excretion of kynurenine and 3-hydroxykynurenine. Excretion levels are increased by oral loading of tryptophan, hence, the status test is known as the tryptophan load test. Plasma PLP levels and the tryptophan load test when completed concurrently provide excellent biochemical confirmation of vitamin B-6 status. Plasma PLP levels correlate with tissue concentrations.[5]

Because of its major role in amino acid metabolism, vitamin B-6 is widely dispersed throughout the plant and animal kingdoms. Foods considered as excellent sources include meats, cereal grains, vegetables, and nuts. However, bioavailability, discussed in Section 10.2, is highly variable and

---

TABLE 10.2
PLP-Dependent Enzymes*

Reaction	Enzyme
Decarboxylations	Aspartate 1-decarboxylase
	Glutamine decarboxylase
	Ornithine decarboxylase
	Aromatic amino acid decarboxylase
	Histidine decarboxylase
R-group interconversions	Serine hydroxymethyltransferase
	d-Aminolevulinic acid synthase
Transaminations	Aspartate aminotransferase
	Alanine aminotransferase
	γ-Aminobutyrate aminotransferase
	Cysteine aminotransferase
	Tyrosine aminotransferase
	Leucine aminotransferase
	Ornithine aminotransferase
	Glutamine aminotransferase
	Branched-chain amino acid aminotransferase
	Serine-pyruvate amino transferase
	Aromatic amino acid transferase
	Histidine aminotransferase
Racemization	Cystathione β-synthase
α,β-Elimination	Serine dehydratase
γ-Elimination	Cystathione γ-lyase
	Kynureninase

* Adapted from Reference 3.

poorly documented. Vitamin B-6 intake of 0.016 mg/g protein provides adequate status for the normal individual. The RDA set in the 1989 Recommended Dietary Allowances[6] was established using upper boundary levels of acceptable protein intake (126 g/day for men and 100 g/day for women). The RDA for vitamin B-6 is 2.0 mg for men and 1.6 mg for women. RDAs are increased by 0.6 mg during pregnancy and by 0.5 mg during lactation. The Reference Daily Intake (RDI) set by the NLEA is 2.0 mg.[7]

10.2 PROPERTIES

10.2.1 CHEMISTRY

10.2.1.1 General Properties

Vitamin B-6 refers to all 2-methyl-3-hydroxy-5-hydroxy methyl pyridine compounds that possess the biological activity of pyridoxine (PN) (2-methyl-3-hydroxy-4,5-bis (hydroxymethyl)-pyridine in rats). PN, substituted at the 4-position with a hydroxymethyl group, has been commonly referred to as pyridoxol; however, the preferred name is pyridoxine. Other vitamin B-6 forms distributed throughout nature include pyridoxal (PL) and pyridoxamine (PM) with an aldehyde (-CHO) and aminoethyl ($-CH_2NH_2$) substituted at the 4-position of the pyridine ring, respectively. The structure and accepted ring numbering system for PN is given in Figure 10.1. Pyridoxal kinase phosphorylates PN, PL, and PM to the 5′-phosphates (PNP, PLP, and PMP). The metabolically active form is PLP. PNP and PMP are oxidized to PLP by PM (PN) 5′-phosphate oxidase.[8] PN, PL, and PM are metabolically interconvertible and considered to be biologically active equivalents. Since each of the six vitamers are found in food, analytical techniques must be capable of quantification of each, to accurately assess vitamin B-6. Resolution and quantitation of the phosphorylated forms and 4-PA, the catabolized form excreted in urine, are often required. LC methods, as discussed in Section 10.3, are well suited to these analytical demands. Structures of the six metabolically active vitamers 4-PA, and pyridoxine-glucoside (PN-glucoside) are given in Figure 10.2.

Physical characteristics of vitamin B-6 are summarized in Table 10.3. Pyridoxine hydrochloride ($C_8H_{12}ClNO_3$, M wt 205.64) is the commonly available commercial form. The PN · HCl salt is a white, odorless crystalline powder with a slightly salty taste. It presents few problems from a food fortification standpoint. The PN · HCl is readily soluble in water (22 g/100 mL), alcohol, and propylene glycol. It is sparingly soluble in acetone and practically insoluble in ethyl ether and chloroform. PN is more stable than PL and PM, providing a highly usable form for food fortification and formulation of pharmaceuticals. PN · HCl is the USP reference standard.

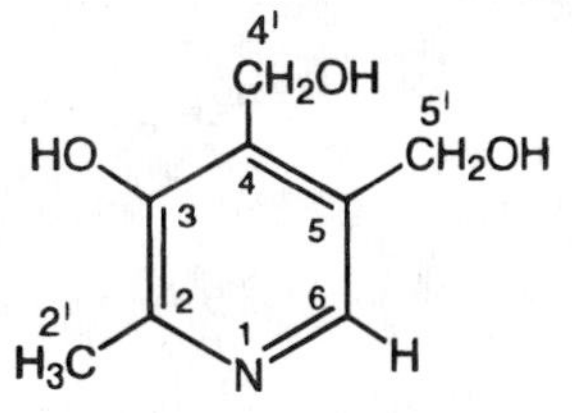

Pyridoxine
2-methyl-3-hydroxy-4,5-bis (hydroxymethyl)-pyridine
Pyridoxol
Vitamin B_6
PN

FIGURE 10.1   Structure of pyridoxine (PN).

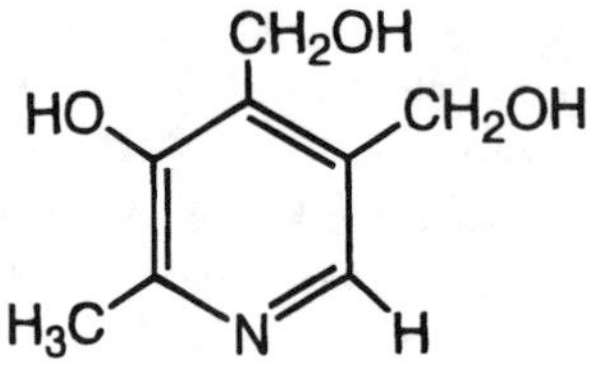

Pyridoxine
PN

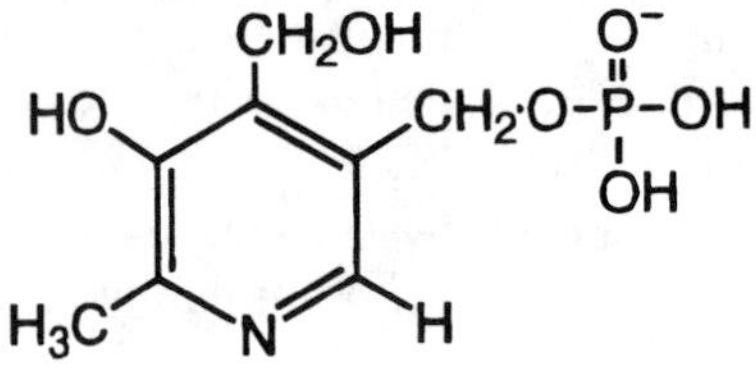

Pyridoxine 5'-phosphate
PNP

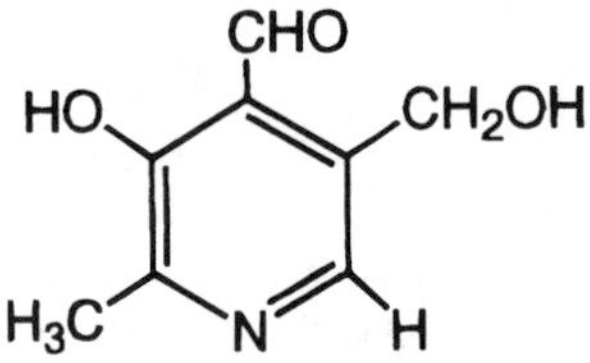

Pyridoxal
PL

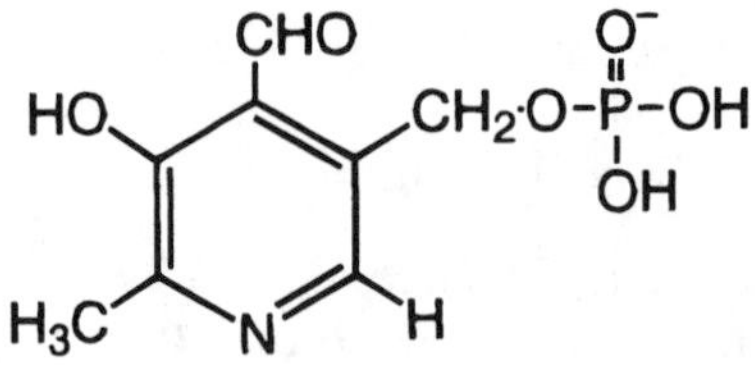

Pyridoxal 5'-phosphate
PLP

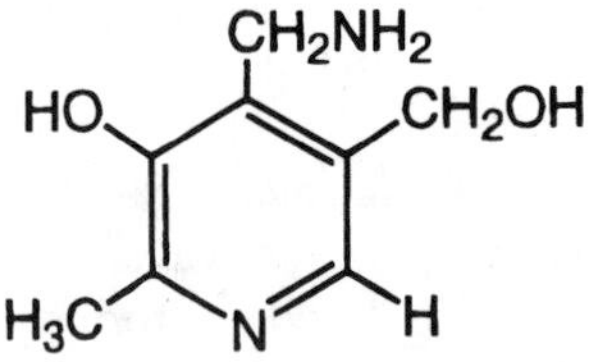

Pyridoxamine
PM

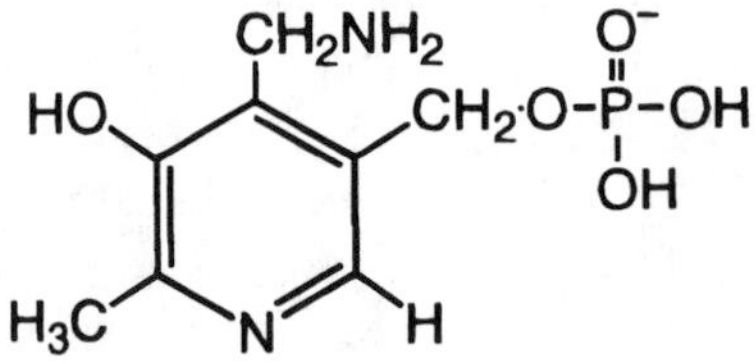

Pyridoxamine 5'-phosphate
PMP

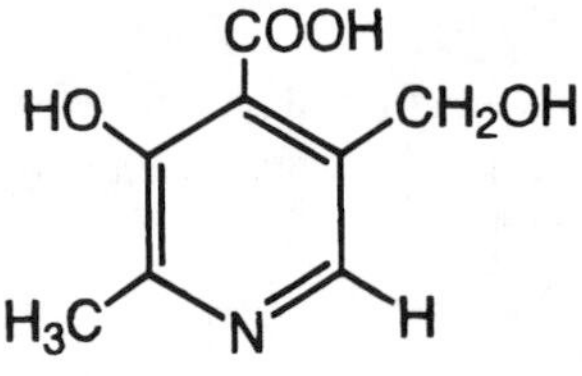

4-Pyridoxic Acid
4-PA

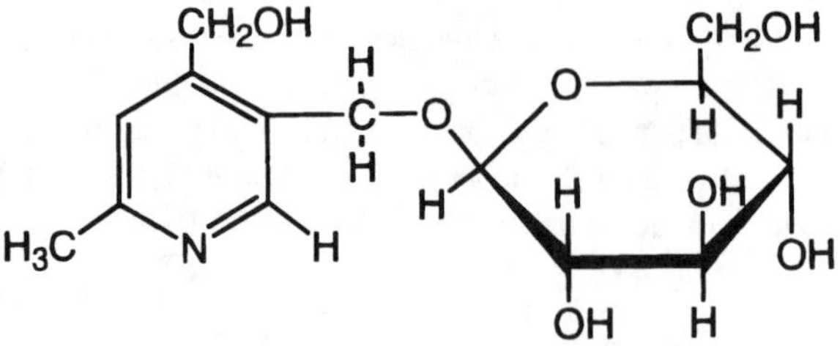

5'-O-(β-D-glucopyranosyl) pyridoxine
PN-Glucoside

FIGURE 10.2 Structures of pyridoxine and related compounds.

10.2.1.2 Spectral Properties

Spectral properties of vitamin B-6 compounds and other hydroxypyridines were presented by Bridges et al.[9] Ball[10] and Ubbink[8] recently summarized UV and fluorescence properties of the vitamin B-6 group. For specifics of the spectral properties, the reader is referred to the excellent study provided by Bridges et al.[9] PN, PL, PM, and the 5′-phosphates show absorption maxima at 290 nm when dissolved in 0.1 *M* HCl.[8,9] At pH 7.0, PL and PLP show maximum absorbance at 390 nm;

TABLE 10.3
Physical Properties of Vitamin B-6

Substance[a]	Molar Mass	Formula	Solubility	Melting Point°C	Absorbance[b] λ max mm	Absorbance[b] $E^{1\%}_{1cm}$	Absorbance[b] ε	Solvent	Fluorescence Maxima Ex nm	Fluorescence Maxima Em nm	Fluorescence Maxima pH Range
Pyridoxal HCl CAS No. 65-22-5 **8162**	203.63	$C_8H_9NO_3 \cdot HCl$	Soluble in water, 95% ethanol	165 (dec.)	390	[9.8]	200	Water	330	382	6.0
					318	[399]	8128	Water	310	365	12.0
Pyridoxine HCl CAS No. 58-56-0 **8166**	205.64	$C_8H_{12}ClNO_3$	Soluble in water, alcohol, propylene glycol, sparingly soluble in acetone Insoluble in ether, $CHCl_3$	206–208 Sublimes	292	[375]	7720	Methanol			
					290	[408]	8400	0.1 N HCl			
					253	[180]	3700	Phosphate buffer, pH 7.0			
					325	[345]	7100	Phosphate buffer, pH 7.0			
Pyridoxine CAS No. 65-23-6 **8166**	169.18	$C_8H_{11}NO_3$	Soluble in water Weakly soluble in alcohol, acetone Insoluble in ether, $CHCl_3$	160	324	[428]	7244	pH 6.8	332	400	6.5–7.5
					254	[23]	3891	pH 6.8	320	380	12.0–14.0
Pyridoxamine Dihydrochloride CAS No. 524-36-7 **8164**	241.12	$C_8H_{12}N_2O_2 \cdot 2HCl$	Soluble in water, 95% alcohol	226–227 (dec.)	328	322	7763	Water	337	400	4.0–5.5
					253	[190]	4571	Water	320	370	14
Pyridoxal 5′-phosphate CAS No. 54-47-7 **8163**	247.14	$C_8H_{10}NO_6P$			330	[101]	2500	Phosphate buffer, pH 7.0	365	423	2.5–4.8
									360	430	8.7–13.0
					388	[198]	4900	Phosphate buffer, pH 7.0	330	410	6.0

[a] Common or generic name; CAS No. — Chemical Abstract Service number, bold print designates the Merck Index monograph number.
[b] Values in brackets are calculated from corresponding ε values.
Budavari, S., *The Merck Index*.[1]
Friedrich, W., *Vitamins*.[2]
Ubbink, J.B., *Modern Chromatographic Analysis of Vitamins*.[3]
Ball, G.F.M., *Water-soluble Vitamin Assays in Human Nutrition*.[4]

whereas, the other vitamers maximally absorb at 253 and 325 nm.[8,9] UV spectra of PN·HCl at pH 1.8, 4.5, and 7.0 are shown in Figure 10.3.I).

Fluorescence properties are given in Table 10.3. Excitation and emission maxima are those originally provided by Bridges et al.[9] The non-phosphorylated vitamers fluoresce strongly from slightly acidic to strongly alkaline pH.[8] PLP fluoresces weakly compared to PMP and PNP which fluoresce similarly to the respective non-phosphorylated forms. Structurally, PL exists in solution as the hemiacetal which provides for its strong fluorescence intensity. The low intensity fluorescence of PLP is the result of the phosphate ester on the 5-position of the pyridine ring prohibiting hemiacetal formation.[8,9] Several approaches are available to enhance fluorescence of PLP for effective detection after LC resolution (Section 10.3). Fluorescence excitation and emission spectra for PN·HCl are shown in Figure 10.3.II. Fluorescence provides a highly sensitive and specific detection mode for the analysis of all vitamin B-6 forms commonly encountered in food and other biological samples.

10.2.2   STABILITY

Model system studies with PN, PL, and PM hydrochloride salts have clearly demonstrated the significance of pH and light to the stability of the different vitamin B-6 forms. Stability characteristics can be summarized as follows:

1. All forms are quite stable in acidic solutions if protected from light.
2. Laboratory light conditions or exposure of foods to light during storage, marketing, or preparation can significantly affect vitamin B-6 retention.
3. PN is more stable than PL and PM. PM is the least stable.
4. Light exposure can degrade all forms even at acidic pH values. Stability greatly decreases as pH increases to levels above neutrality.[11,12]
5. Near-UV and UV radiation are the most damaging wavelengths.[13]

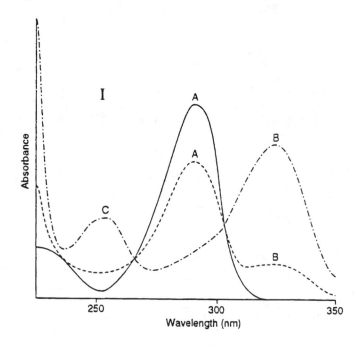

FIGURE 10.3.I   UV spectra of PN · HCl. Solid line—0.1 M phosphate buffer, pH 1.8. Broken line—0.1 M phosphate buffer, pH 4.5. Discontinuous line—0.1 M phosphate buffer, 7.0. λ max—A, 290 nm; B, 324 nm; C, 253 nm. Reproduced with permission from Reference 10.

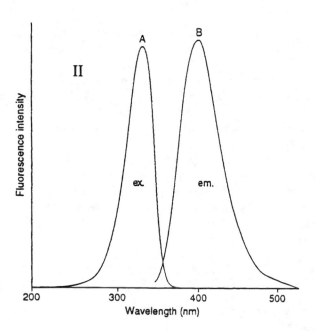

FIGURE 10.3.II Fluorescence excitation and emission spectra of PN · HCl in 0.1 M phosphate buffer, pH 7.0. λ max—A, 327 nm; B, 393 nm. Reproduced with permission from Reference 10.

6. Use of low actinic glassware[9] and yellow or golden fluorescent light are essential for the analytical laboratory.[11]
7. Processing and cooking conditions cause variable losses. Heat degradation increases as pH increases. PN is more heat stable than PL and PM.
8. Processing losses of vitamin B-6 in vegetables can be large and variable due to physical loss from leaching. Heat degradation plays a greater role in animal products, since PN is the primary vitamer in plants and PL and PM are more predominant in animal tissues and milk.
9. Interconversion of the vitamin B-6 forms occurs during heat processing of food and during preparation of biological samples. Relative concentrations of the vitamers can dramatically change during processing.[14,15]
10. Bioavailability can be significantly affected by food processing (Section 10.2.3).

10.2.3 BIOAVAILABILITY

Excellent research studies during the last two decades provided in-depth knowledge on the bioavailability of vitamin B-6. It has been recognized for many years that vitamin B-6 exists in nature in protein and non-protein bound forms. Extraction procedures designed for biological samples have a primary role to free such bound forms to ensure complete analysis of the vitamin. It is now understood that unique bound forms of vitamin B-6 can affect bioavailability to the animal or human and that interpretation of analytical values for certain foods should be based upon the forms naturally present in the food. A general point is that animal products contain more bioavailable forms of vitamin B-6 compared to plant food sources.

In plants, PN can exist in quite significant amounts as a β-glucoside. The glucoside was identified as 5′-0-(β-D-gluco-pyranosyl) pyridoxine (PN-glucoside, Figure 10.2) as a constituent of rice bran.[16,17] Kabir et al. [18] called attention to the bioavailability question of PN-glucoside for humans by showing an inverse relationship between the glycosylated vitamin B-6 content of food and its bioavailability to humans. Differential assays were developed based upon varying extraction procedures (Section 10.3.2.1) to differentiate PN and PN-glucoside in foods.[16,19] The first highly descriptive paper on PN-glucoside in common plant foods was provided by Kabir et al.[19] Table 10.4 data clearly show that the levels of PN-glucoside is quite variable in plant products and non-existent in animal products. In broccoli, cauliflower, carrots, and cooked soybeans greater than 50% of the vitamin B-6 was in the PN-glucoside form. In a later study, PN-glucoside was identified in potatoes and shown to increase during storage.[20] More recently, 5'-0-[6-0-((+))-5-hydroxy-dioxindole-3-acetyl)-β-cellobiosyl] pyridoxal was identified in rice bran, representing another confirmed, conjugated form of vitamin B-6.[21]

Studies of PN-glucoside were advanced with the development of an LC procedure for its quantitation.[22] The method, developed by Gregory and Ink,[22] is provided in Section 10.4. Work by Gregory and colleagues[23,24,25] on the bioavailability of PN-glucoside proved that the substance is poorly available to humans and animals as a source of vitamin B-6. The bioavailability studies conducted by Gregory's group represent some of the most in-depth studies completed on the bioavailability of a water-soluble vitamin form from the food supply.

TABLE 10.4
Vitamin B-6 and Glycosylated Vitamin B-6 Content of Different Foods*

Food	Total Vitamin B-6[a] μg/100g	Nonconjugated Vitamin B-6[a] μg/100g	%[b]	Glycosylated Vitamin B-6[a] μg/100g	%	Sum[e]
Vegetables						
Broccoli, raw	168 ± 0.8[c]	140 ± 4	84	n.d.[d]	—	84
Broccoli, frozen	119 ± 13	48 ± 2	23	78 ± 10	65	88
Cauliflower, raw	156 ± 0.8	148 ± 0.2	95	9 ± 0.5	5	100
Cauliflower, frozen	84 ± 7	20 ± 4	23	69 ± 8	82	105
Green beans, raw	60	51	85	6	10	95
Green beans, canned	28 ± 2	16 ± 0.1	56	8 ± 0.1	28	84
Carrots, raw	170	75	44	87	51	95
Fruits						
Bananas	313 ± 6	308 ± 31	98	10 ± 14	3	101
Avocados, fresh	443 ± 4	221 ± 1	50	15 ± 6	3	53
Orange juice, fresh	43 ± 0.1	18 ± 0.5	42	16 ± 0.6	37	79
Orange juice, concentrate	165 ± 2	54 ± 1	33	78 ± 0.8	47	80
Peaches, canned	9 ± 0.3	7 ± 0.5	71	2 ± 0.1	21	92
Nuts						
Filberts, raw	587 ± 15	707 ± 16	120	26 ± 29	4	124
Almonds, raw	86	69	81	n.d.	0	81
Grains						
Corn, frozen	88 ± 14	38 ± 9	44	6 ± 1	6	50
Rice (white) cooked	138 ± 2	50 ± 2	37	19 ± 1	14	51
Rice bran	3515 ± 84	600 ± 6	17	153 ± 30	4	21
Whole wheat bread	169 ± 2	69 ± 1	40	29 ± 3	17	57
Wheat bran	903 ± 1	117 ± 3	13	236 ± 17	36	49
Whole wheat flour	265	129	48	19	11	59
Legumes						
Navy beans, cooked	381 ± 35	143 ± 6	37	159 ± 9	42	79

Peanut butter	302 ± 21	49 ± 5	16	54 ± 11	18	34
Soybeans, cooked	627 ± 11	130 ± 4	21	357 ± 4	57	78
Animal Products						
Beef, ground, cooked	263	83	31	n.d.	—	31
Tuna, canned	316	158	50	n.d.	—	50
Chicken						
Breast, raw	700	454	65	n.d.	—	65
Breast, cooked	684	316	46	n.d.		46
Leg, raw	388	176	45	n.d.		45
Leg, cooked	306	150	49	n.d.		49
Milk, skim	5 ± 1	4 ± 0.3	79	n.d.		79

[a]Total vitamin B-6 refers to the amount of vitamin B-6 measured microbiologically after acid hydrolysis. Nonconjugated vitamin B-6 is the amount measured in a sample that was mixed with 0.1 M phosphate buffer for 2 h. Glycosylated vitamin B-6 refers to the difference between the enzyme treated value and the free vitamin B-6 value. All values are as pyridoxine equivalents per 100 g of food.

[b]The percent of non-conjugated and glycosylated forms was calculated by dividing the amount of free or glycosylated forms by the total vitamin B-6 content of each corresponding food.

[c]The values listed are means ± standard deviation for duplicate samples. Values without a standard deviation are based on a single analysis.

[d]n.d. = not detected by the enzyme treatment.

[e]Sum of the % non-conjugated and glycosylated vitamin B-6 as a percentage of the total vitamin B-6.

*Reproduced with permission from Reference 19.

10.3 METHODS

For many reasons, HPLC analysis is the preferred method for vitamin B-6 assay. Food analysis can be accurately completed microbiologically and blood analysis by enzymatic and immunological procedures, but the sensitivity and specificity provided by current LC based methods make them the clear choice for use in the modern nutrient analysis laboratory. Our discussion is limited to microassay, because of its still common usage, and to LC analysis of vitamin B-6. Helpful reviews available on vitamin B-6 assay methods include Polansky et al.,[26] Ubbink,[8] Lumley,[27] Gregory,[28] Ball,[10] and Eitenmiller and Landen.[29] Handbook and compendium procedures are summarized in Table 10.5.

10.3.1 MICROBIOLOGICAL

Several different microorganisms have been used to assay vitamin B-6. None are without problems. Strohecker and Henning[30] in their early text on vitamin assay provided methodology based on *Saccharomycus carlsbergensis (S. uvarum)*, *Streptococces faecalis (Enterococcus faecalis)*, and *Lactobacillus helviticus*. Other organisms used in the past include *Lactobacillus casei, Neurospora sitophila, Saccharomyces cerevisiae,* and the protozoan, *Tetrahymenia pyriformis.* Of these, the most commonly used and preferred organism is *S. uvarum* (ATCC 9080). The assay was introduced in 1943,[31] and refined for food analysis at the Beltsville Human Nutrition Research Center, United States Department of Agriculture. Studies by Parrish et al.[32,33] showed that *S. uvarum* responded unequally to the three vitamin B-6 vitamers. Response to PN and PL were similar, but growth response to PM was less. The differential growth response to the vitamers led to the development of chromatographic procedures to separate PN, PL, and PM, and then to assay them individually by *S. uvarum*. This procedure forms the basis of AOAC Method 961.15. The chromatographic method as developed by MacArthur and Lehmann,[34] Toepfer and Lehmann,[35] and Toepfer and Polansky[36] is shown in Figure 10.4. Cation-exchange chromatography on Dowex AG50W-X8 resin resolves the vitamers and allows their subsequent individual quantitation.

TABLE 10.5
Compendium, Regulatory, and Handbook Methods for Analysis of Pyridoxine Hydrochloride, Pyridoxine, Pyridoxal, and Pyridoxamine

Source	Form	Methods and Application	Approach	Most Current Cross-Reference
U.S. Pharmacopeia National Formulary, 1995, USP 23/NF 18, Nutritional Supplements Official Monographs[1]				
1. pages 2143, 2146, 2148, 2153	Pyridoxine Hydrochloride	Pyridoxine hydrochloride in oil- and water-soluble vitamin capsules/tablets w/wo minerals	HPLC 280 nm	None
2. pages 2162, 2168, 2170, 2172	Pyridoxine Hydrochloride	Pyridoxine hydrochloride in water-soluble vitamin capsules/tablets w/wo minerals	HPLC 280 nm	None
3. page 1347	Pyridoxine Hydrochloride	Pyridoxine hydrochloride (NLT 98.0%, NMT 102.0%)	Colorimetric 650 nm	None
4. pages 1347–1349	Pyridoxine Hydrochloride	Pyridoxine hydrochloride injection/tablets	Colorimetric 650 nm	None
British Pharmacopoeia, 15th ed., 1993[2]				
1. vol. 1, page 565	Pyridoxine Hydrochloride	Pyridoxine hydrochloride	Titration	None
2. vol. 2, page 1087	Pyridoxine Hydrochloride	Pyridoxine tablets	Spectrophotometric 290 nm	None
AOAC Official Methods of Analysis, 16th ed., 1995[3]				
1. 45.2.08	Pyridoxine Pyridoxal	AOAC Official Method 961.15, Vitamin B-6 (Pyridoxine, Pyridoxal, Pyridoxamine) in Food Extracts	Microbiological	*J. Assoc. Off. Anal. Chem.*, 44, 426, 1961[4]; 47, 750, 1964[5]; 53, 546, 1970[6]
2. 50.1.18	Pyridoxine Pyridoxal Pyridoxamine	AOAC Official Method 985.32, Vitamin B-6 (Pyridoxine, Pyridoxal, Pyridoxamine) in Ready-To-Feed Milk Based Infant Formula	Microbiological	*J. Assoc. Off. Anal. Chem.*, 68, 514, 1985[7]

American Feed Ingredients Association, *Laboratory Methods Compendium*, vol. 1, 1991[8]

1. pages 157–158	Vitamin B-6 (pyridoxine hydrochloride) in concentrates and premixes	Pyridoxine Hydrochloride	HPLC 280 nm	*J. Chromatogr. Sci.*, 15, 262, 1977[9]
2. pages 159–161	Vitamin B-6 in complete feeds and premixes	Pyridoxine Pyridoxal Pyridoxamine	Microbiological	*Methods in Vitamin B-6 Nutrition, Analysis and Status*, Plenum Press, 1981, 21[10] Hoffmann-LaRoche, *Analytical Methods for Vitamins and Carotenoids in Feed*, 1988, 23[11]

American Association of Cereal Chemists, *Approved Methods*, vol. 2, 1996[12]

1. AACC 86-31	Vitamin B-6 complete in cereal products	Pyridoxine Pyridoxal Pyridoxamine	Microbiological	Official Methods of Analysis, AOAC Int., 16th ed.[3]

Food Chemicals Codex, 4th ed., 1996[13]

1. page 334	Pyridoxine hydrochloride (NTL 98%, NMT 100.5%	Pyridoxine Hydrochloride	Titration, perchloric acid	None

Hoffmann-LaRoche, *Analytical Methods for Vitamins and Carotenoids in Feed*, 1988[11]

1. pages 33–35	Microbiological assay of vitamin B-6 in complete feeds and premixes	Pyridoxine Pyridoxal Pyridoxamine	Microbiological	*Methods in Vitamin B-6 Nutrition*, Plenum Press, 1981, 21[10]
Methods for the Determination of Vitamins in Foods, COST 9 1[14]	HPLC assay of Vitamin B-6 fresh and processed foods	Pyridoxine Pyridoxal Pyridoxamine Phosphate esters	HPLC	5 related references

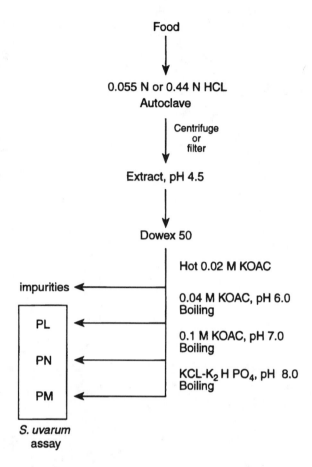

FIGURE 10.4   Open-column fractionation of PN, PL, and PM for assay by *S. uvarum*. Adapted from Reference 37.

It is generally accepted that *S. uvarum* gives differential response to PN, PL, and PM. Also, the lower response to PM can be slight or quite significant depending on individual cultures and the laboratory culture procedures in use. Polansky[37] pointed out that when studies are completed with *S. uvarum*, the effects of the differential growth response can be eliminated by use of the chromatographic separation prior to microbiological assay. The tedious nature of the procedure has led to the use of rapid and precise LC procedures capable of resolution of the 3 vitamers and their phosphate esters. The work at the USDA on the vitamin B-6 assay by *S. uvarum* represents an important era in vitamin B-6 analysis.

Various researchers[38,39] have suggested that *Kloeckera apiculata* (ATCC 9774) replace *S. uvarum* for vitamin B-6 assay. Observations by Barton-Wright[38] and, later, by Guilarte et al.[39] indicated essentially equal growth response by *K. apiculata* to PL, PN, and PM. However, other investigators showed a lower growth response to *K. apiculata* to PM, similar to the growth response of *S. uvarum*, compared to the response to PL and PN.[37,40] *K. apiculata* has not seen wide usage for food analysis. However, Guilarte et al.[41] used *K. apiculata* to develop a radiometric assay for B-6 analysis. Radiometric procedures for vitamin B-6 and other water-soluble vitamin assays have not been widely applied.

AOAC International[42] provides two methods based upon microbiological assay with *S. uvarum* (ATCC 9080).

AOAC Official Method 961.15, Vitamin B-6 (Pyridoxine, Pyridoxal, Pyridoxamine) in Food Extracts, Microbiological Method, *AOAC Official Methods of Analysis,* 45.2.08

Method 961.15 and most other applications of *S. uvarum* rely on early studies[43,44] that established acid extraction procedures suitable for efficient extraction of vitamin B-6 from most food matrices. It was shown that optimal extraction of vitamin B-6 from plant tissues can be achieved by autoclaving the tissue in 0.44 *N* HCl for 2 h at 121°C. Animal products and tissues are hydrolyzed with 0.055 *N* HCl by autoclaving at 121°C for 5 h. These extraction procedures have not been modified to any great extent over the years. Following digestion, the hydrolyzates are cooled, adjusted to pH 4.5 with 6 *N* KOH, and diluted with water. The digests are filtered and chromatographed on Dowex AG 50W-X8 according to procedures established by Toepfer and Lehmann[35] and Toepfer and Polansky.[36] The procedure is tedious, cumbersome, and generally disliked by nutritional analysts. Hot 0.02 *M* potassium acetate, pH 5.5 is used to elute impurities. Boiling 0.04 *M* potassium acetate, pH 6.0, is used to elute PL, followed by boiling 0.1 *M* potassium acetate, pH 7.0, for PN and boiling $KCl-K_2HPO_4$, pH 8.0, for elution of PM. Each vitamer is individually quantitated and summed to obtain total vitamin B-6 (Figure 10.4). Polansky[37] detailed the historical development and application of the procedure.

AOAC Official Method 985.32, Vitamin B-6 (Pyridoxine, Pyridoxal, Pyridoxamine), in Ready-To-Feed Milk-Based Infant Formula, Microbiological Method, *AOAC Official Methods of Analysis,* 50.1.18

Method 985.32 has been approved only for milk-based infant formula. The method does not require the chromatography step since the primary form of vitamin B-6 is PN added during manufacture of the formula. Vitamin B-6 is extracted with 0.05 *M* HCl and autoclaved for 5 h. The procedure was provided as a collaborative study in 1985.[45]

The U.S. Food and Drug Administration, Atlanta Center for Nutrient Analysis (ACNA) uses *S. uvarum* to quantitate vitamin B-6 in Total Diet Program marketbasket food samples. The procedure follows Method 961.15; however, the chromatographic separation of PN, PL, and PM is not included in the analysis. An SOP for the procedure is available and is provided in Section 10.4.

10.3.2 HIGH PERFORMANCE LIQUID CHROMATOGRAPHY

Problems associated with the microbiological assay of vitamin B-6 led to the early application of LC procedures for food and other biological matrices. Ubbink[8] and Gregory[28] provide in-depth reviews of LC procedures for vitamin B-6 analysis. We have summarized in Table 10.6 historically important method development publications and selected more recent methods of the application of LC to vitamin B-6 analysis. The most notable advantage of LC analysis compared with microbiological analysis is the high degree of specificity provided, allowing the quantitation of the six vitamers and various metabolites, such as 4-PA.

10.3.2.1 Extraction Procedures for Vitamin B-6 by HPLC

Extraction methods used prior to LC analysis can be categorized into the following approaches:

Approach 1—Hydrolysis of the phosphate esters with subsequent quantitation of PL, PM, and PN. Hydrolysis is usually enzymatically completed with a commercial phosphatase. Chromatography is simplified, but complete enzymatic conversion must be assured.[28] Treatment with H_2SO_4 has been used.[46]

Approach 2—Preservation of the phosphorylated vitamins with quantitation of the six biologically active forms, glycosylated forms (PN-glucoside), and metabolites such as 4-PA. Extraction is

Table 10.6
HPLC Methods for the Analysis of Vitamin B-6 in Foods, Feed, Pharmaceuticals and Biologicals

Sample Matrix	Sample Preparation			HPLC Parameters				References
	Analyte	Sample Extraction	Clean Up	Column	Mobile Phase	Detection	Quality Assurance Parameters	
Food								
1. Standards	PL, PM, PN, PLP, PMP, PNP, 4-PA	Centrifuge, 4°C Filter Evaporate under N^2 to 0.75 original volume Add equal volume Hex Vortex Draw off lower water layer Filter		Aminex A-25 55°C 24 cm × 6 mm	PH gradient Buffer 1 0.4 M NaCl—0.01 glycine, pH 10 Buffer 2 0.4 M NaCl —0.01 glycine, pH 2.5 Equilibrate column with Buffer 1 Inject Pump Buffer 1 for 80 min Pump Buffer 2 for 40 min 1.2 mL/min	Fluorescence Two filter fluorometers in series	—	J. Chromatogr., 176, 280, 1979[1]
2–5. Plasma, various foods	PL, PM, PN, PLP, PMP, PNP, 4-PA	Add 3-hydroxy-pyridine (IS) to 1 g sample Homogenize with 10 mL 5% SSA Centrifuge, 4°C Filter Evaporate under N_2 to 0.75 original value Add equal volume Hex Vortex Draw off lower water layer Filter	SSA removed by ion-exchange	Column 1 Aminex A-25 55°C 24 cm × 6 mm Column 2 Aminex A-25 18°C 24 cm × 3 mm Columns in series connected by a switching valve	Isocratic 0.4 M NaCl, 0.01 M glycine, 0.05 M semi-carbazide, pH 10 or Gradient See Reference 1.	Fluorescence PM, PMP, PN, PNP Ex λ = 310 Em λ = 380 PL, PLP Ex λ = 280 Em λ = 487	% Recovery 95–105 RSD = 3%	J. Chromatogr., 196, 176, 1980[2] 216, 338, 1981[3] J. Agric. Food Chem., 28, 1145, 1980[4] J. Food Sci., 46, 943, 1981[5]

Sample	Compounds	Sample preparation	Cleanup	Column	Mobile phase	Detection	Performance	Reference
6–7. Animal tissues, milk	PL, PM, PLP, PMP	Homogenize with 0.1 M KH$_2$PO$_4$, pH 7.0, with Polytron® (2 V) Add 4 mL 3 N perchloric acid Centrifuge Repeat extraction with 1 N perchloric acid	—	Ultrasphere IP, C$_{18}$ 5 μm 25 cm × 4.6 mm	Isocratic MeCN : 0.33 M KH$_2$PO$_4$, pH 2.2 (2.5 : 97.5) 2 mL/min	Fluorescence Treat extract with glyoxylic acid to deaminate PM and PMP Derivatize with semi-carbazide Ex λ = 365 Em λ = 400	% Recovery > 85 % CV 4.4–6.3	Anal. Biochem., 102, 374, 1980[6] J. Agric. Food Chem., 29, 921, 1981[7]
8. Biologicals, food, tissue	PL, PM, PN, PLP, PMP, PNP	Blend 3 g sample with 1 mL 20% SSA containing 4'-deoxypyridoxine (IS) Blend with 4 m CHCl$_3$ Centrifuge Inject aliquot of extract into preparative chromatographic system	Semi-Prep LC Bio-Rad AG2-8X 25 cm × 9 mm Monitor with fluorescence Ex λ = 295 Em λ = 405	C$_{18}$ 3 μm 3 cm × 4.6 mm	Gradient A$_1$—0.033 M KH$_2$PO$_4$ and 8 mM octane sulfonic acid, pH 2.2 A$_2$—0.033 M KH$_2$PO$_4$ and 8 mM octane sulfonic acid and 2.5% IPA, pH 2.2 B—0.033 M KH$_2$PO$_4$ and 6.5% IPA, pH 2.2 Linear 100% A$_1$ to 100% A$_2$ in 12 min with switch to 100% B in 15 min after injection 1.8 mL/min	Fluorescence Post-column derivatization by sodium bisulfate to hydroxy-sulfonates Ex λ = 330 Em λ = 440	RSD = 2% % Recovery 99–103 Except pork loin—lower for PL and PLP	J. Agric. Food Chem., 33, 359, 1985[8]
9. Human milk	PL, PM, PN	Add 4'-deoxypyridoxine (IS) Digest with potato acid phosphatase, 1 h, 37°C Add TCA Add CHCl$_3$ Centrifuge Adjust supernatant to pH 5.2 Filter	—	μBondapak C$_{18}$ 10 μm 30 cm × 3.9 mm	Gradient A—MeOH : water (85 : 15) B—0.005 M heptane sulfonic acid in 1% HAC 0–17 min 2% A to 40% A 17–20 min To 100% B	Fluorescence Ex λ = 300 Em λ = 375	DL (ng) On-column <1 (PM, PN) % Recovery PL—105 PN—83 QL (μg/L) 6	J. Chromatogr., 337, 249, 1985[9]

Table 10.6 Continued

Sample Matrix	Analyte	Sample Preparation		HPLC Parameters				
		Sample Extraction	Clean Up	Column	Mobile Phase	Detection	Quality Assurance Parameters	References
10. Chicken, raw, cooked	PL, PM, PLP, PMP	Extract with 1 M MPA and water, Polytron® Filter	—	Biosil ODS-55 25 cm × 4 mm	Isocratic 0.066 M KH$_2$PO$_4$ pH 3.0	Fluorescence Ex λ = 290 Em λ = 395	DL (ng) On-column PL—0.1 PLP—1.0 PM—0.5 PMP—0.1 % Recovery 90–108	*J. Food Sci.*, 53, 371, 1988[10]
11. Various foods	PL, PM, PN, PLP, PMP, PNP, 4-PA	Add 4-deoxy-pyridoxine (IS) Homogenize with 0.1–0.5 M cold perchloric acid Centrifuge Adjust supernatant to pH 7.5 and after filtration to pH 4.0 Digest with pH 7.5 filtrate with alkaline phosphatase, 30 min, 25°C Adjust to pH 4.0	—	Lichrosphere RP-18 5 μm 12.5 cm × 4 mm	Gradient A—MeOH B—0.03 M KH$_2$PO$_4$, pH 2.7 with 4 mM octane sulfonic acid 0–2 min 90% B 10%A 2–12 min To 60% B 12–17 min 60% B 40% A 17–19 min To 90% B 1.5 mL/min	Fluorescence Post-column derivatization sodium bisulfate Ex λ = 330 Em λ = 400	DL (pmol) On-column 0.4–0.7 % CV 1.1–5.0	*J. Chromatogr.*, 463, 207, 1989[11]
12-13. Various foods	PL, PM, PN, PLP, PMP, PNP, PN-glucoside	Extract with 1 M cold perchloric acid Centrifuge Adjust pH to 3.5 with 50% KOH Precipitate overnight	—	TSK Gel ODS-120A 25 cm × 4.6 mm	Isocratic 1% MeCN in 0.1 M sodium perchlorate and	Fluorescence Ex λ = 305 Em λ = 390 PLP determined as 4-PA-P or post-column	DL (ng) On-column PL—0.4 PM—0.2 PN—0.4 PLP—0.6	*J. Nutr. Sci. Vitaminol.*, 35, 171, 1989[19] *Agric. Biol. Chem.*,

Sample	Compounds	Sample preparation	Prep column	Column	Mobile phase	Detection	Results	Reference
		Divide into two parts Inject one and treat other with KCN to 5 mM to convert PLP to 4-PA-P	—		0.1 M KH$_2$PO$_4$, pH 3.5 0.5 mL/min	derivatization with sodium bisulfite	PMP—0.2 PNP—0.4 % CV 0.9–3.6	55, 563, 1991[13]
14–15. Various foods	Conversion of vitamins to PN	Add 25 mL 0.05 NaOAC pH 4.5, 2.5 mL 1 M glyoxylic acid, pH 4.5, 400 μL ferrous sulfate (2 g/L) and 20 mg acid phosphatase to 2.5 g sample. Incubate overnight, 37°C Dilute with water Filter To 5 mL aliquot, add 5 mL of 0.2 M NaOH and 0.1 M sodium borohydride Filter	—	Lichrosorb 60 RP Select B 5 μm 25 cm × 5 mm	Isocratic MeCN : 0.05 M KH$_2$PO$_4$ (4 : 96) containing 0.5 × 10^{-3} M Na heptane sulfonate, pH 2.5 1 mL/min	Fluorescence Ex λ = 290 Em λ = 395	RSD,% 3–18 % Recovery 90 QL (μg/g) 0.02 %CV <8	Food Chem., 48, 321, 1993[14] 52, 81, 1995[15]
16. Chicken, raw, fried	PL, PM, PN, PLP, PMP	2 g freeze-dried chicken was mixed with 10 mL 5% SSA containing 3-hydroxypyridine (IS) Mix 10 min, cold Add CH$_2$Cl$_2$ Centrifuge Filter	Prep LC Dowex AG 2-X8 34 cm × 1 cm Monitor by fluorescence Mobile phase 0.1 N HCl 1 mL/min	Diethyl amino ethyl G 500 power white Two columns in series 7.5 cm × 7.5 mm	Isocratic 0.12 M NaCl, 0.02 M glycine, pH 9.8 0.8 mL/min	Post-column derivatization with sodium bisulfite Fluorescence PM, PMP, PLP Ex λ = 330 Em λ = 400 PN, PL, IS Ex λ = 310 Em λ = 375	DL (ng) PL —1.24 PN—1.26 PM—0.79 PMP—0.78 PLP—2.68 % Recovery 96–102 PLP—83	J. Food Sci., 58, 505, 1993[15]
17. Food, feed	PL, PN, PM	Add 25 mL 5% TCA and 1 mL 4- deoxypyridoxine (IS) to 0.1–5.0 g sample Homogenize Dilute to 50 mL with 5% TCA	—	ODS Hypersil 3 μm 12.5 cm × 4.6 mm	Isocratic 3% MeOH, 1.25 mM 1-octane sulfonic acid in 0.1 M KH$_2$PO$_4$, pH 2.15 1.2 mL/min	Fluorescence Ex λ = 323 Em λ = 375	QL (μg/g) 0.02 % Recovery 96–104 %CV 2.5–9.3 PLP-19.2	J. Agric. Food Chem., 42, 1475, 1994[17]

Table 10.6 Continued

Sample Matrix	Analyte	Sample Preparation		HPLC Parameters				
		Sample Extraction	Clean Up	Column	Mobile Phase	Detection	Quality Assurance Parameters	References
		Centrifuge To 3 mL extract, add 0.4 mL 4 M NaOAC, pH 6.0 Digest with Takadiastase, 3 h, 45°C Filter						
18. Wheat	PL, PM, PN, PMP, PN-glucoside	Add 4′-deoxypyridoxine (IS) Homogenize in water Deproteinize with MPA Centrifuge Filter	—	Ultramex C$_{18}$ 3 μm 15 cm × 4.6 mm	Gradient A—0.033 KH$_2$PO$_4$ and 0.008 M l-octane sulfonic acid, pH 2.2 B—0.033 M phospheric acid and 10% MeCN, pH 2.2 0–10 min 100% A to 100% B 10–25 min 100% A Return to 100% A 1.2 mL/min	Fluorescence Ex λ = 311 Em λ = 360	% Recovery PN—101 PM—96 PL—57 PLP—34 PMP—79	*Cereal Chem.*, 72, 217, 1995[18]
Biologicals 1. Tissue	PLP	Homogenize in cold 0.1 M KH$_2$PO$_4$, pH 7.0 Deproteinize with 1 N perchloric acid Adjust pH to 6–7 with 3 N KOH Allow KClO$_4$ to precipitate	—	LiChrosorb RP-8 10 μm 25 cm × 4.6 mm	Isocratic 2.5% MeCN in 0.033 M KH$_2$PO$_4$, pH 2.2 1.3 mL/min	Pre-column derivatization with semi-carbazide Fluorescence Ex λ = 365 Em λ = 400	% Recovery 66–106 QL (μg/mL) 0.2	*Anal. Biochem.*, 102, 374, 1980

	Compounds	Sample preparation		Column	Mobile phase	Detection	Performance	Reference
2. Plasma	PL, PM, PN, PLP, PMP, PNP, 4-PA	Transfer aliquot of supernatant. Convert PLP to PLP-semi-carbazone with semi-carbazide HCl	—	Bio-Rad A-25 Two columns column-switching 24 cm × 6 mm 50°C 24 cm × 3 mm 18°C	Isocratic 0.4 M NaOH 0.01 M glycine 0.005 M semi-carbazide pH 10 1.25 mL/min	Fluorescence PM, PMP, PN and PNP are detected at Ex λ = 310 Em λ = 380 Flow directed through 2nd column PLP detected at Ex λ = 280 Em λ = 487 IS detected at Ex λ = 310 Em λ = 380	QL (ng/mL) <1 CV % 5 % Recovery 98	J. Chromatogr., 196, 176, 1980[2]
3. Blood	PLP	Add 5 mL 6% TCA to 1 mL blood Vortex Allow to stand 60 min at room temperature Mix, centrifuge	—	Hypersil-ODS 5 μm 25 cm × 4.6 mm	Isocratic 0.05 mM KH_2PO_4 pH 2.9 0.9 mL/min	Post-column derivatization with semi-carbazide Fluorescence Ex λ = 367 Em λ = 478	QL (mmol/L) 5 CV% 3.3–7.1 % Recovery 99–100	Int. J. Vit. Nutr. Res., 51, 216, 1981[3]
4. Tissue	PL, PM, PN, PLP, PMP, PNP, 4-PA	Add 3-hydroxyproline (IS) Extract with perchloric acid Adjust pH to 4.2 with 3 M KOH, stand overnight Centrifuge	Dowex H⁺, if required	μBondapak C_{18} 30 cm × 3.9 mm	Gradient A—10% IPA containing 0.09% HAC B—A containing 0.004 M sodium heptane sulfonate and 0.004 M sodium-l-octane sulfonate. Equilibrate with B. Pump for 5 min after injection, Switch to A.	313 nm	—	J. Chromatogr., 227, 181, 1982[4]

Table 10.6 Continued

Sample Matrix	Analyte	Sample Preparation — Sample Extraction	Sample Preparation — Clean Up	HPLC Parameters — Column	HPLC Parameters — Mobile Phase	HPLC Parameters — Detection	HPLC Parameters — Quality Assurance Parameters	References
5–6. Plasma, tissue, food	PL, PM, PN, PMP, PNP, 4-PA, other metabolites	Add TCA Mix Centrifuge Extract supernatant with EtO_2 Add 2-amino-5-chlorobenzoic acid (IS) prior to injection	—	Vydac 401 TP-B 10 μm 30 cm × 4.6 mm	Gradient A—0.02 N HCl B—0.1 M NaH_2PO_4, pH 3.3 C—0.05 M NaH_2PO_4, pH 5.9 0–13 min 100% A 13–17 min 100% B 17–25 min 88% B, 12% C 25–30 min To 100% C Maintain C until 40 min Reequilibrate with A	Post column addition of 1 M Na_2HPO_4 pH 7.5 containing sodium bisulfite (1 mg/mL) to increase fluorescence of PLP Fluorescence Ex λ = 330 Em λ = 400	—	Anal. Biochem., 129, 310, 1983[5] Meth. Enzymol., 280, 22, 1997[6] (chromatography parameters slightly modified)
7–8. Tissue, plasma	PL, PM, PN, PLP, PMP, PNP	Homogenize in water containing 4-deoxypyridoxine (IS) Deproteinize with 8% perchloric acid Centrifuge Adjust to alkaline pH with 6 M KOK Allow $KClO_4$ to settle Adjust pH to 5.2 with 1 M HCl Extract aliquot with equal	—	μBondapak ODS 10 μm 30 cm × 3.9 mm	Gradient A—MeOH : water (85 : 15) B—1% HAC containing 0.005 M heptane sulfonic acid 100% B to 40% A in 12 min Hold 5 min Back to 100% B in 15 min 1.5 mL/min	Fluorescence Ex λ = 300 Em λ = 375	% Recovery 82–96	J. Chromatogr., 306, 377, 1984[7] 374, 155, 1986[8]

Sample	Compounds	Sample preparation	Column	Mobile phase	Detection	Performance	Reference
		volume of CH$_2$Cl$_2$ Centrifuge Remove 2 mL aliquot of supernatant, add 2 mL 0.055 M HCl Autoclave, 5 h, 121°C Cool, adjust pH to 5.2					
9-13. Plasma, tissue, erythrocytes, lymphocytes	PL, PLP	Add 50 μL 6-methyl-2-pyridine carboxaldehyde semi-carbazone (IS) and 0.05 mL 10% TCA to 1 mL plasma Mix Centrifuge Add 50 μL 0.5 M semicarbazide to clear supernatnat Incubate, 40°C, 10 min Extract 2 × with 3 mL EtO$_2$	Partisil-10 ODS-3 25 cm ×4.6 mm Partisil-5 ODS 3 10 cm × 4.6 mm	—	Isocratic 0.05 M KH$_2$PO$_4$, pH 2.9, containing 7% MeCN 1.1 mL/min	Post-column alkalinization Fluorescence Ex λ = 367 Em λ = 478	QL (ng/mL) 0.25 %CV within day 5.9–8.1 % Recovery 92.3±8.6	J. Chromatogr., 342, 277, 1985[9] 375, 399, 1986[10] Am. J. Clin. Nutr. 46, 78, 1987[11] J. Lab. Clin. Med., 113, 15, 1989[12] Am. J. Clin. Nutr., 57, 47, 1993[13]
14. Plasma, tissue, urine	PL, PM, PN, PLP, PMP, PNP, 4-PA	Add 5% MPA and 4-deoxypyridoxine (IS) Homogenize Centrifuge Extract with CH$_2$Cl$_2$ Filter	Ultramex C$_{18}$ 3 μm 15 cm × 4.6 mm	—	Gradient A—0.033 M H$_3$PO$_4$ and 0.008 M l-octane sulfonic acid, pH 2.2 B—0.033 M H$_3$PO$_4$ and IPA (IS), pH 2.2 100% A 0–10 min To 100% B 10–25 min 100% B To 100% A at 30 min	Post-column addition of sodium bisulfite to enhance fluorescence of PLP Fluorescence Ex λ = 328 Em λ = 393	DL (ng) On-column 0.1–0.4 QL (pmol) 1.7–6.8 % Recovery 86.3–111 QL (pmol) 1.7–6.8	Nutr. Res., 9, 259, 1989[14]

Table 10.6 Continued

Sample Matrix	Analyte	Sample Preparation — Sample Extraction	Sample Preparation — Clean Up	HPLC Parameters — Column	HPLC Parameters — Mobile Phase	HPLC Parameters — Detection	HPLC Parameters — Quality Assurance Parameters	References
15. Serum	PLP as 4-PA phosphate	Mix 2 mL serum with 1 mL TCA Vortex Heat, 40°C, 30 min Centrifuge Mix 800 μL of supernatant with 300 mL 3.3 M K_2HPO_4 and 100 μL 40 mM KCN Heat, 50°C, 60 min Add 600 mL 0.2 M orthophosphoric acid to 1 mL extract prior to injection	—	μBondapak TMC$_{18}$ 10 μm 30 cm × 3.9 mm	Isocratic 3% MeCN in 0.033 M KH_2PO_4 and 0.05 M semi-carbazide HCl, pH 2.5 1.3 mL/min	Fluorescence Ex λ = 325 Em λ = 418	QL (ng/mL) 0.22 % Recovery 86–90 % CV 1.2–3.8	*Analyst,* 114, 1225, 1989[15]
16. Serum	PL, PM, PN, PLP, PMP	Deproteinize 2 mL serum with 100 μL perchloric acid Centrifuge Filter Use PMP as IS	—	Spherisorb C$_{18}$ ODS-2 12% C end-capped 5 μm 25 cm × 4.6 mm	Isocratic 0.067 M KH_2PO_4, pH 2.5, with 125 μM sodium hexane sulfonate	Post-column addition of sodium sulfite (1 mg/mL) in 0.067 M phosphate buffer, pH 7.5 Fluorescence Ex λ = 325 Em λ = 400	DL (pmol) On-column 0.3–2.5 % Recovery 100–110	*J. Liq. Chromatogr.,* 15, 897, 1992[16]
17. Plasma, various biologicals	PL, PM, PN, PLP, PMP, 4-PA	See Reference 13, Table 5—Biologicals.	—	Ultramex C$_{18}$ 3 μm 15 cm ×4.6 mm	Gradient A—0.033 M H_3PO_4 containing 0.1 M	Post-column addition of sodium sulfite (1 mg/mL) in	DL (pmol) On-column 0.3–1.5 QL (pmol)	*J. Chromatogr.,* 578, 45, 1992[17]

Sample	Compounds	Column	Sample preparation	Mobile phase	Detection	Performance	Reference
				1-octane sulfonic acid, pH 2.2 B—0.33 M H_3PO_4 in 10% IPA, pH 2.2 0 min 100% A Inject To 100% B in 10 min 10–25 min 100% B 25–29.5 min 100% A Equilibrate with 100% A from 29.5–35 min 1.2 mL/min	0.1 M phosphate buffer, pH 7.4 Fluorescence Ex λ = 328 Em λ = 393	2.5–10 % Recovery 88–104 CV% 0.83–8.33 levels near QL	
18–21. Plasma, erythrocytes	PL, PM, PN, PMP, PLP as 4-PA phosphate	TSK gel ODS 120A 25 cm × 4.6 mm	Add 1 mL 3 M cold perchloric acid to 2 mL plasma or erythrocyte lysate Vortex, centrifuge Adjust pH to 3.5 with 50% KOH Dilute to 5 mL with water Centrifuge Divide into two parts For PLP conversion to 4-PA-P, adjust pH to 7.5, add KCN to 5 mM Heat, 50°C, 3 h with shaking Readjust to pH 3.5 with HCl Allow to stand at ambient temperature for 24 h	Isocratic 1% MeCN, 0.1 M sodium perchlorate, 0.1 M KH_2PO_4, pH 3.5 30°C, 0.5 mL/min Mobile phase can be modified to improve resolution of trace metabolites.	Fluorescence Ex λ = 305 Em λ = 390 4-PA-P Ex λ = 320 Em λ = 420	—	Agric. Biol. Chem., 52, 1083, 1988[18] J. Nutr. Vitaminol., 36, 521, 1990[19] 40, 239, 1994[20] Meth. Enzymol., 280, 3, 1997[21]

completed with deproteinizing agents such as sulfosalicylic acid (SSA), trichloroacetic acid (TCA), metaphosphoric acid (MPA), and perchloric acid. Sample extraction at room temperature hydrolyzes Schiff bases, prevents enzymatic interconversions of the vitamers and increases water solubility by conversion of the pyridine bases to quaternary ammonium salts.[10] A major advantage is the ability to avoid hydrolysis of PN-glucoside. Acid hydrolysis procedures necessary for microbiological analysis hydrolyze PN-glucoside, therefore, biologically available vitamin B-6 is overestimated.

Approach 3—Conversion of all forms to PN, with quantitation of total vitamin B-6 as PN.[47]

Approach 4—Extraction of all non-bound vitamin B-6 with quantitation as free vitamin B-6. Such extractions can be used to determine relative amounts of free and bound vitamin B-6. Values obtained with required mild extractants such as 0.01 M sodium acetate[20] significantly underestimate nutritionally available vitamin B-6.

Various extractions for food and serum are summarized in Table 10.6.

10.3.2.2 Chromatography Parameters

10.3.2.2.1 Supports and Mobile Phases

Ion-exchange and reversed-phase chromatography resolve the multivitamin B-6 forms present in biological matrices. HPLC methods developed in the early 1970s largely relied upon ion-exchange resins while more recent methods have used C_{18} reversed-phase systems with ion-pairing agents. Vanderslice et al.[48] successfully resolved the six vitamers and 4-PA on Aminex A-25 anion-exchange resin. The procedure was based upon a complicated instrumentation set-up and laboratory packed columns, and was not extensively used by other researchers. However, the Vanderslice procedure and a series of subsequent papers adapting the procedure to food and serum analysis provided great insight into analysis of biological matrices by HPLC.[49–54] Two important developments resulted from the in-depth look at vitamin B-6 analysis. Vanderslice et al.[49] introduced and proved the worth of SSA for food extraction. SSA was subsequently used in many other studies as the extractant. Vanderslice and Maire[50] added 0.005 M semi-carbazide into the anion-exchange elution buffer to increase the fluorescence response of PL and PLP by conversion of the compounds to the oxime. This technique increased the fluorescence of the PL and PLP to levels comparable to the other vitamers. Application of the chromatography system developed by Vanderslice and colleagues was hampered by manufacturing changes in the Aminex A-25 resin that altered resolution of the vitamers.

Coburn and Mahuren[55] used cation-exchange chromatography on Vydac 401TP-B that resolved the vitamin B-6 vitamers and 4-PA. Important to the development of later procedures, the method introduced the post-column use of a potassium phosphate buffered (pH 7.5) bisulfite solution to enhance the fluorescence of PLP. The buffered solution allowed the detection of PNP which was not fluorescent in the acid mobile phase at the fluorescence wavelengths (Ex $\lambda = 330$, Em $\lambda = 400$) required for the other analytes. The post-column treatment permitted the detection of the six vitamers, 4-PA, and the internal standard (2-amino-5-chlorobenzoic acid) at the same wavelengths.

Since the methodology was introduced, chromatography parameters have been slightly modified for quantitation of other vitamin B-6 metabolites. These include 5-pyridoxic acid, 5-pyridoxic acid lactone, pyridoxo-4 : 5-lactone, and pyridoxo-5 : 4-lactone.[56] The authors state that cation exchange LC is better suited to resolution of the urinary metabolites than ion-pair, reversed-phase chromatography. The Vydac 401TP-B support is no longer available and was replaced with Nucleosil 5 SA.[56]

Reversed-phase chromatography on C_{18} has become the most common approach to vitamin B-6 analysis. As shown in Table 10.6, compositions of the mobile phases vary considerably, but most incorporate ion-pairing reagents to optimize resolution. Both gradient and isocratic systems successfully resolve the six vitamers and 4-PA as well as different internal standards used by the various investigators. One of the earliest applications of reversed-phase chromatography for vitamin B-6 was published by Gregory and Kirk.[57] Further method development by Gregory and colleagues was instrumental to development of current approaches for vitamin B-6 analysis. Important contributions included conversion of PLP to the semi-carbazone in tissue and plasma,[58] conversion of PMP and PM to PLP and PL by deamination with glyoxylate prior to derivatization with semi-carbazide,[59] and development of procedures to assay PN-glucoside.[22,60] The Gregory and Ink[22] procedure for identification and quantitation of PN-glucoside is summarized in Section 10.4. This method is highly significant to the accurate measurement of biologically active vitamin B-6 in plant foods.

Ubbink et al.[61,62] adapted Gregory's semi-carbazide enhancement of the fluorescent response of PLP to plasma and tissue analysis. Their studies showed that the semi-carbazones of PL and PLP were stable under conditions that rapidly decomposed free PL and PLP. The semi-carbazide derivatization agent was directly added to the extraction solution, simplifying previous pre-column and post-column derivatization procedures. Later studies proved the utility of TCA as a deproteinizing agent for plasma and tissue analysis. Because of the significance to plasma analysis of the Ubbink procedure, it is provided in Section 10.4.

Additional methods provided in Section 10.4 include serum analysis using PMP as the internal standard,[63] a pre-column derivatization method for conversion of all vitamers to PN,[47] and an LC procedure applicable to a wide range of sample matrices.[64]

10.3.2.2.2   Detection

UV detection is not usable for analysis of biological samples. $E_{1cm}^{1\%}$ values (Table 10.3) range from less than 10 to slightly above 400 depending upon the vitamer and solvent environment, indicating a relatively low UV detection sensitivity. For this reason, fluorescence is the universal detection mode unless highly fortified foods, medical foods, or pharmaceutical products are under study. Methods used to enhance the fluorescence of PL and PLP developed by the leading research groups on vitamin B-6 analysis include enhancement with bisulfite and the more accepted and simple enhancement with semi-carbazide. Method summaries (Table 10.6) show that semi-carbazide and sulfite enhancement are commonly used. Additionally, a more recent enhancement of PLP fluorescence has been developed by Tsuge et al.[65] that utilizes selective conversion of PLP to 4-pyridoxic acid 5'-phosphate. Methodology developed by Tsuge[66] permits resolution of 18 vitamin B-6 compounds. Supports were TSK-gel ODS 120A and TSK-gel ODS 80T. Resolution was achieved by an isocratic mobile phase of 1% acetonitrile—0.1 M perchloric acid—0.1 M phosphate buffer, pH 3.5. Small changes in acetonitrile concentration, mobile phase pH, or column temperature can be made to significantly alter retention times of the B-6 compounds. Potassium cyanide conversion of PLP to 4-pyridoxic acid 5'-phosphate increased fluorescence response ten times compared to native fluorescence of PLP.

10.3.2.2.3   Internal Standards

Due to the complexity of the chromatography, vitamin B-6 analysis of non-fortified foods and other biological samples should not be attempted without the use of a suitable internal standard. Gregory[28] reviewed the use of several compounds that have similar properties to the vitamin B-6 forms commonly found in biological samples. As shown in Table 10.6, these include 4-deoxypyridine, 3-hydroxypyridine, 6-methyl-2-pyridine carboxaldehyde, and 2-amino-5-chlorobenzoic acid. Of these, 4-deoxypyridine has been used most frequently. Addition of 4-deoxypyridine at levels required to provide sufficient fluorescence response can interfere with elution of low level metabolites in some systems.[66]

10.4   METHOD PROTOCOLS

Vitamin B-6 Analysis of Total Diet Samples, Food and Drug Administration Southeast Regional Laboratory Standard Operating Procedure, SOP N/AM/5/0/94, J.A. Martin and Marijane Lawson

Purpose

The purpose of this SOP is to set forth the operational parameters, methodology, and requirements for quality assurance and acceptability of data for the determination of vitamin B-6 in total diet samples.

Scope

Microbiological analysis for vitamin B-6 is applicable to most food matrices and vitamin supplements. The minimum detectable level on a wet weight basis is 2.5 μg/100 g for vitamin B-6. The minimum detection level assumes that the lowest practical sample dilution factor is 1 : 100.

Responsibility

The analysts assigned to the determination of folic acid and vitamin B-6, the program coordinator, the supervisory chemist, and Atlanta Center for Nutrient Analysis (ACNA) director will assure adherence to the following SOP. All revisions must be directed through and receive concurrence of the appropriate coordinator, the supervisory chemist, and the ACNA director. Major methodology revisions will require headquarters approval.

References

1. *Official Methods of Analysis,* (1990), 15th ed., AOAC, Arlington, VA, 960.46, 961.15, and 985.32.
2. Hazardous Waste Management Program, FDA Southeastern Regional Laboratory, Atlanta District, July 23, 1990.

Basic Principles

Vitamin B-6 is assayed by a modification of AOAC Method 961.15 "Vitamin B-6 (Pyridoxine, Pyridoxal, Pyridoxamine) in Food Extracts, Microbiological Method" and AOAC Method 985.32 "Vitamin B-6 (Pyridoxine, Pyridoxal, Pyridoxamine) in Ready-To-Feed Milk-Based Infant Formula, Microbiologial Method" (1). The assay organism is *Saccharomyces uvarum* ATCC 9080. Since *S. uvarum* does not respond equally to the vitamin B-6 vitamers, Method 961.15 uses open-column chromatography to separate the vitamers which are then quantitated individually by microbiological assay. Method 985.32 eliminates the chromatographic resolution step, since the primary form of vitamin B-6 in infant formula is pyridoxine. *Saccharomyces uvarum* is sensitized to the different vitamin B-6 vitamers by growing the cells in liquid culture broth containing added pyridoxine, pyridoxamine, and pyridoxal (Method 961.15). Assay of Total Diet samples follows Method 985.32. Elimination of the chromatographic step does not greatly affect quantification of vitamin B-6 vitamers from most foods. Pilot studies completed at ACNA prior to initiation of the Total Diet analysis program substantiated this fact (unpublished data, Dr. A. M. Soliman). Elimination of the chromatographic separation step allows rapid sample throughput which is not possible with the highly tedious nature of Method 961.15. Foods are extracted according to Method 961.15 which specifies 0.44 *N* HCl with autoclaving for 2 h at 121°C for plant products and 0.055 *N* HCl with autoclaving for 5 h at 121°C for animal products.

Apparatus

1. Autoturb® turbidimetric reader—160 tube capacity (Elan Co., Division of Eli Lilly & Co., Indianapolis, IN 46285) or equivalent.

2. Disposable Pyrex test tubes—18 × 150 mm, No. 9187—F83 (Thomas Scientific, Swedesboro, NJ 08085) or equivalent. Heat at 250°C to remove residual material.
3. Stainless steel test tube caps to fit 18 × 150 mm test tubes.
4. Environmental control orbital shaker incubator—capable of handling 3 autoturb racks at one time.
5. Balance accurate to 0.01 g.
6. Glass beads, 4 mm in diameter, add two per assay tube.

Reagents

1. Pyridoxine, pyridoxal, and pyridoxamine standard solutions—prepare separate solutions for each as follows:
   a. Stock solution—10.0 μg/mL. Dissolve 12.16 mg pyridoxine HCl, 12, 18 mg pyridoxal HC1, and 14.34 mg pyridoxamine HC1, respectively, in 1 *N* HCl and dilute to 1 L with 1 *N* HC1. Store in g-s bottles in refrigerator. *Note:* Use USP R.S. Pyridoxine HC1 for pyridoxine standard.
   Dilute 10.0 mL stock solution to 100.0 mL with H_2O.
   c. Working solution—1.0 ng/ml. Dilute 10.0 mL intermediate solution to 100.0 mL with H_2O. Mix, dilute 5.0 mL to 500.0 mL with H_2O. Prepare before each assay.
2. Mixed pyridoxine, pyridoxal, and pyridoxamine solution (for vitamin B-6 liquid culture broth). Pipet 2 mL of each intermediate solution (1.0 μg/mL) into a 1 L volumetric flask. Dilute to volume with H_2O.
3. Agar culture medium—Lactobacilli Agar AOAC, No. 0900—15 (Difco Laboratories, Detroit, MI 48232). Pipet hot agar in 10 mL portions into 18 × 150 mm screw cap tubes. Loosely cap and autoclave 15 min at 121°C. Tilt hot agar tubes to form slants and cool in the slant position.
4. Vitamin B-6 assay medium—Single strength Pyridoxine Y Medium, No. 0951-15-27 (Difco Laboratories, Detroit, MI 48232).
5. Inoculum rinse—vitamin B-6 assay medium diluted 1 : 1 with H_2O. Pipet 5 mL H_2O into test tubes containing 5 mL vitamin B-6 assay medium, loosely cap, autoclave 10 min to 121°C and cool.
6. Vitamin B-6 liquid culture broth—pipet 5 mL mixed solution (2) into 18 × 150 mm test tubes containing 5 mL inoculum rinse (5). Add two 4 mm glass beads, loosely cap and autoclave 10 min at 121°C. Store tubes in refrigerator.

Test Organism—Saccharomytes uvarum ATCC No. 9080. Maintain by weekly transfers on agar slants (3). Incubate agar slants 24 h at 30°C, refrigerate.

Safety precautions

The assays will be carried out with strict adherence to the District safety policies and waste management procedures (2).

Procedures

Series Definition

A series will consist of a maximum of ten assays.
1. A maximum of nine samples.
2. One QA control sample.
3. A recovery consisting of a sample with a known vitamin concentration is assayed periodically.

Sample Preparation and Extraction

Perform all sample preparations under subdued light with minimal contact with air.

Sample Preparation

All Total Diet samples are composited at the Kansas City Total Diet Research Center. The homogenous samples are shipped frozen to ACNA for analysis. Each sample consists of three subsamples packaged with double plastic bags. Subsamples are identified as subsamples 1, 2, and 3 with product name and an identifying code number. Prior to analysis a subsample is thawed, mixed well and the required portion (1.5 to 20 g) is removed for analysis.

Extraction

Weigh sample representing approximately 1 to 2 g dry solids into a 500 mL erlenmeyer. Add 200 mL 0.44 N HC1 to plant products and 200 mL 0.055 N HC1 to animal products. Autoclave plant product suspensions for 2 h at 121°C and animal product suspensions for 5 h at 121°C. Cool to room temperature, adjust to pH 4.5 with 6 N or saturated KOH. Dilute to 250.0 ml with H_2O in volumetric flask. Filter through Whatman No. 40 paper. Dilute to make a final concentration of approximately 1.0 μg/ml.

Inoculum Preparation

1. Incubate cells for inoculum in Latobacillus Agar slant for 24 h at 30°C before use.
2. Inoculate vitamin B-6 culture broth and incubate with shaking for 22 h at 30°C.
3. Centrifuge broth at 2500 rpm and resuspend cells with 10 ml of B-6 culture rinse. Repeat washing procedure and resuspend cells in a third 10 ml aliquot of the inoculum rinse. Prepare inoculum by adding 0.1 to 0.3 mL to 10 mL of inoculum rinse. The prepared inoculum suspension should have a %T of 65 to 75 as measured against the inoculum rinse.

Standard Curve Preparation

Construct an 8 point standard curve using the pyridoxine working solution. Add 0.0, 0.0, 0.5, 1.0, 1.5, 2.0, 2.5, 3.0, 4.0, and 5.0 ml of the working standard into triplicate 18 × 150 mm Pyrex test tubes. Add distilled water to adjust volume to 6.0 ml. Add 5.0 mL of Pyridoxine Y Assay Medium to each tube.

Blank Tubes

The first set of tubes containing 0.0 mL of standard represents the uninoculated blank used to set the Autoturb or specrophotometer to 100% T. The second set of tubes containing 0.0 mL standard is inoculated and represents the inoculated blank and is used to reset the spectrophotometer to 100% T.

Assay

Vitamin B-6 is assayed by the official AOAC turbidimetric method 960.46. Four sample extract levels (1, 2, 3, and 4 ml) are assayed in triplicate. Volume in each tube is adjusted to 5 ml with H_2O. Five mL of prepared assay media (Pyridoxine Y Assay Medium) is added to each tube. Pyridoxine assay tubes are steamed at 100°C for 10 min. The tubes are cooled to room temperature and inoculated with one drop of prepared inoculum per tube. Pyridoxine assay tubes are incubated at 30°C with orbital shaking for 22 h in a temperature controlled room. Growth response is measured as % T at 550 nm.

Calculations

Results are calculated from the regression line of the standard curve responses using fourth degree polynomial plots and a computer program written to conform to AOAC microbiological analysis protocol. Results are reported as μg vitamin per 100 g or per serving.

Stability of Pyridoxal-5-Phosphate Semicarbazone: Applications in Plasma Vitamin B-6 Analysis and Population Surveys of Vitamin B-6 Nutritional Status

Principle

- PL and PLP are converted pre-column to their respective semicarbazones. Vitamers are resolved isocratically on Partisil 10 ODS-3 and detected by fluorescence. Internal standard is 6-methyl-2-pyridine carboxaldehyde semi-carbazone.

Chemicals

- PL, PLP
- 6-methyl-2-pyridine carboxaldehyde (IS)
- CH_2Cl_2
- Acetonitrile
- Methanol
- Glacial acetic acid
- Semi-carbazide

Apparatus

- Liquid chromatograph
- Fluorescence detector

Procedure

Extraction

- Add 50 μL reconstituted 6-methyl-2-pyridine carboxaldehyde semi-carbazone (IS) to 1 mL plasma
- Add 0.5 mL 10% TCA
- Mix, centrifuge
- Add 50 mL of 0.5 M semi-carbazide to clear supernatant
- Incubate, 40°C, 10 min
- Extract, 2 × with 3 mL ethyl ether
- Aspirate ethyl ether, extract water phase with 3 mL CH_2Cl_2

Chromatography

See Figure 10.5.

Column	25 cm × 4.6 mm
Stationary phase	Patisil 10 ODS-3
Column temperature	Ambient
Mobile phase	0.05 KH_2PO_4 with 7% acetonitrile, pH 2.9
Flow	1.1 mL/min
Post-column reagent	4% NaOH, 0.1 mL/min
Detection	Fluorescence
	Ex λ = 367, Em λ = 478
Calculation	Internal standard 6-methyl-2-pyridine carboxaldehyde semi-carbazone

J. Chromatogr., 342, 277, 1985

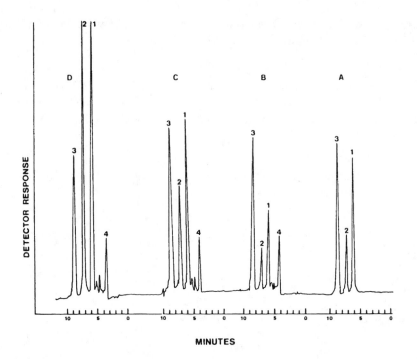

FIGURE 10.5   PL and PLP in plasma: A—standard; B—normal plasma; C—plasma spiked with PLP and PL; D—plasma, subject on oral supplements. Peak 1—PLPSC; Peak 2—PLSC; Peak 3—MPCSC (IS); Peak 4, unknown. Reproduced with permission from Reference 9, Table 6, Biologicals.

Identification and Quantification of Pyridoxine-β-Glucoside as a Major Form of Vitamin B-6 in Plant-Derived Foods

Principle

- Extract product with sulfosalicylic acid (SSA). Sample extracts are treated by anion-exchange chromatography to remove SSA. Vitamin B-6 vitamers and pyridoxine-β-glucoside are quantitated by reversed-phase chromatography and fluorescence detection following post-column enhancement of PL and PLP by buffered bisulfite.

Chemicals

- Hydrochloride salts of PN, PL, PM, and 4-deoxypyridoxine
- Pyridoxal-5′-phosphate
- 4-pyridoxic acid
- Pyridoxamine-5′-phosphate
- Isopropanol
- Sulfosalicylic acid
- l-octane sulfonic acid (sodium)

Apparatus

- Liquid chromatograph
- Fluorescence detector
- Gradient controller
- Anion-exchange column, AG2-x8 resin

Procedure

Extraction
- Mix 2 g sample with 9 mL 5% SSA
- Homogenize with Polytron, 45 s, setting 7
- Add 10 mL CH_2Cl_2
- Blend
- Centrifuge
- Remove aliquot of aqueous layer

Preparative Anion-Exchange Clean Up
- Inject 0.3 to 0.4 mL extract onto preparative LC column of AG2-x8 resin by injecting into flowing stream of 0.1M HCl
- SSA is bound to resin
- Monitor vitamin B-6 elution by fluorescence
- Collect effluent (6 to 10 mL)
- Neutralize with 1 M NaOH

β-Glucoside Treatment
- Dilute 0.9 mL of eluate with 0.1 mL 1 M sodium phosphate, pH 5
- Add 0.05 mL of β-glucoside (2 mg in water)
- Incubate, 37°C, 5 h
- Deproteinate with 0.07 mL 100% TCA

Chromatography
See Figure 10.6.

Stationary phase	Perkin-Elmer 3 × 3, ODS
Column temperature	Ambient

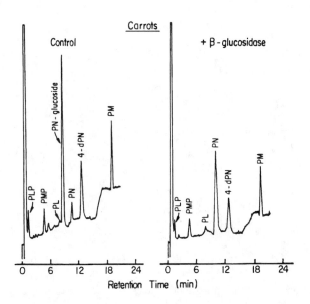

FIGURE 10.6   PN-glucoside chromography before and after β-glucosidase treatment. Reproduced with permission from Reference 22.

Mobile phase	A1—0.033 M KH$_2$PO$_4$ and 8 mM octanesulfonic acid, pH 2.2
	A2—0.033 M KH$_2$PO$_4$, 8 mM octanesulfonic acid, and 2.5% isopropanol, pH 2.2
	B—0.033 M KH$_2$PO$_4$, 6.5% isopropanol, pH 2.2
Gradient	100% A1 to 100% A2 in 12 min
	To 100% B in 15 min after injection
	Equilibration requires 10 mm after elution of PM
Flow	1.8 mL/min
Detection	Fluorescence : Ex λ = 330, Em λ = 400
Calculation	Internal standard, 4 deoxypyridoxine

J. Agric. Food Chem., 35, 76, 1987

A Simple Internally-Standardized Isocratic HPLC Assay for Vitamin B-6 in Human Serum

Principle

- Serum is deproteinized with perchloric acid. Vitamin B-6 (PL, PM, PN, PLP, and PMP) is determined by reversed-phase chromatography. Fluorescence is increased by post-column derivatization with sodium sulfite. PMP is a suitable internal standard.

Reagents

- PN, PL, PM, PMP, and PLP
- Sodium hexane sulfonic acid
- Sodium sulfite
- KH$_3$PO$_4$
- Na$_2$HP$_4$
- Orthophosphoric acid
- Trichloroacetic acid
- Perchloric acid

Apparatus

- Liquid chromatograph
- Fluorescence detector

Procedure

Extraction

- Add 100 μL 4 M perchloric acid and 100 μL 1000 mmol/L PMP (IS) to 2 mL serum
- Centrifuge
- Filter (0.45 μm)

Chromatography

Column	25 cm × 4.6 mm
Stationary phase	Spherisorb ODS2, 5 μm
Column temperature	Ambient
Mobile phase	0.067 M KH$_2$PO$_4$—125 μM sodium hexane sulfonate, pH 2.5
Flow	1 mL/min
Post-column reagent	0.067 phosphate buffer, pH 7.5, containing 1 g/L sodium sulfite at 0.5 mL/min
Injection volume	20 μL

Detection	Fluorescence
	Ex λ = 325,
	Em λ = 400
Calculation	Internal Standard —PMP

J. Liq. Chromatogr., 15, 897, 1992

Reliable and Sensitive HPLC Method with Fluorometric Detection for the Analysis of Vitamin B-6 in Foods and Feeds

Principle
- Vitamin B-6 is extracted with 5% TCA followed by enzymatic hydrolysis of PLP, PMP, and PNP. Non-phosphorylated vitamers are quantitated by paired-ion reversed-phase LC. Post-column addition of 1 M K_2PO_4 increased native fluorescence of the vitamers.

Chemicals
- PL, PM, PN, PLP, and PMP
- 4-deoxypyridoxine
- Takadiastase
- l-Octane sulfonic acid
- Phosphoric acid
- Trichloroacetic acid (TCA)
- Sodium acetate
- Methanol

Apparatus
- Liquid chromatograph
- Fluorescence detector

Procedure

Extraction
- Add 25 mL 5% TCA to 0.1 to 5.0 g sample
- Add 1 mL 4-deoxypyridine (IS) (100 μg/mL)
- Homogenize
- Dilute to 50 mL with TCA (5%)
- Shake, 30 min
- Centrifuge, filter

Dephosphorylation
- Transfer 3 mL filtrate to test tube
- Add 0.4 mL 4 M sodium acetate buffer, pH 6.0, and 0.1 mL Takadiastase (200 mg/mL)
- Incubate, 3 h, 45°C
- Vortex at 30 min intervals
- Cool
- Add 1.5 mL TCA (16.7%)
- Centrifuge, filter (0.45 μm)
- Inject

Chromatography
Column	12.5 cm × 4.6 mm

Stationary phase	Hypersil ODS, 3 μm
Column temperature	Ambient
Mobile phase	3% methanol and 1.25 mM l-octane-sulfonic acid (Pic B8) in 0.1 M KH$_4$, pH 2.15
Flow	1.2 mL/min
Post-column	Mix effluent with 1 M K$_2$HPO$_4$ (0.3 mL/min)
Detection	Fluorescence Ex λ = 333, Em λ = 375
Calculation	Internal standard, 4-deoxypyridoxine

J. Agric. Food Chem., 42, 1475, 1994

HPLC Determination of Vitamin B-6 in Foods After Pre-Column Derivatization of Free and Phosphorylated Vitamers into Pyridoxol

Principle
- Assay includes pre-column transformation of phosphorylated and free vitamers into pyridoxol with quantitation by ion-pair HPLC and fluorescence detection.

Chemicals
- Pyridoxamine — 2HCl standard
- Pyridoxal — HCl standard
- Pyridoxol — HCl standard
- Acid phosphatase
- Sodium acetate
- Glacial acetic acid
- Glyoxylic acid
- Ferrous sulfate
- Sodium hydroxide
- Sodium borohydride
- 1-Heptane sulfonic acid sodium salt
- 1-Octane sulfonic acid sodium salt
- Acetonitrile
- Potassium dihydrogen phosphate
- Orthophosphoric acid

Apparatus
- Liquid chromatograph
- Fluorescence detector

Procedure

Extraction
Assay applicable to baby food, biscuit, cereals, powdered milk, chocolate powder, tube-feeding solution, and yeast
- Weigh finely ground sample (2.5 g) into a conical flask
- Add 25 mL 0.05 M sodium acetate (pH 4.5)
- Add 2.5 mL 1 M glyoxylic acid (pH 4.5)
- Add 400 μL ferrous sulfate — 7H$_2$O (2 g/L)

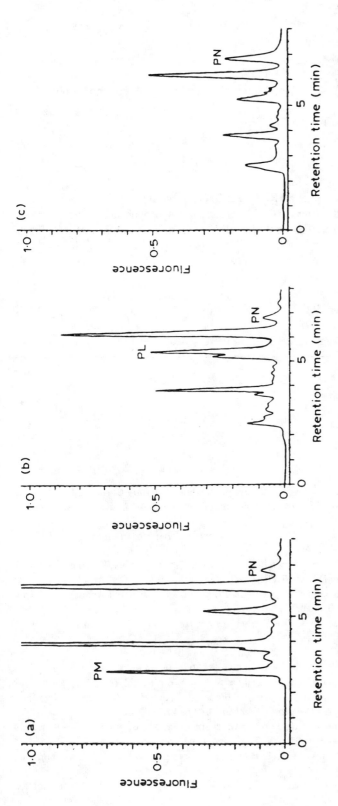

FIGURE 10.7 Chromatographic resolution of vitamin B-6 in yeast: a—without deamination and reduction; b—without reduction; c—complete method. Reproduced wth permission from Reference 14, Table 6, Food.

- Add 20 mg acid phosphatase
- Mix by continuous shaking
- Incubate in oven at 37°C overnight
- Dilute to 50 mL with H_2O
- Shake and filter
- Add 5 mL of reducing solution (0.2 M sodium hydroxide and 0.1 M sodium borohydride) to 5.0 mL aliquot
- Mix, filter (paper then 0.2 μm)

Chromatography
See Figure 10.7.

Column	25 cm × 5 mm
Stationary phase	Lichrospher 60 RP Select B, octysilyl, 5 μm
Mobile phase	Acetonitrile : 0.05 M potassium dihydrogen phosphate (4 : 96, V/V) containing 0.5×10^3 M sodium heptane sulfonate (pH 2.5)
Column temperature	Ambient
Flow	1 mL/min
Injection volume	20 μL
Detection	Fluorescence
	Ex λ = 290,
	Em λ = 395
Calculation	External standard, linear regression, 0.1 to 1.0 μg pyridoxol/mL

Food Chem., 48, 321, 1993; 52, 81, 1995

10.5   REFERENCES

Text

1. Snell, E. E., The vitamin activities of "pyridoxal" and pyridoxamine, *J. Biol. Chem.,* 154, 313, 1944.
2. Mueller, J. F. and Vilter, R. W., Pyridoxine deficiency in human beings induced with desoxypyridoxine, *J. Clin. Invest.,* 29, 193, 1950.
3. Combs, G. F., Jr., Vitamin B-6 in *The Vitamins: Fundamental Aspects in Nutrition and Health,* Academic Press, New York, 1992, chap. 13.
4. Leklem, J. E., Vitamin B-6, in *Present Knowledge in Nutrition,* 7th ed., Ziegler, E. E. and Filer, L. J., Jr., Eds., ILSI Press, Washington, DC, 1996, chap. 18.
5. Gibson, R. S., Assessment of vitamin B-6 status in *Principles of Nutritional Assessment,* Oxford University Press, New York, 1990, chap. 21.
6. National Research Council, *Recommended Dietary Allowances,* 10th ed., National Academy of Sciences, Washington, D.C., 1989, chap. 8.
7. *Nutritional Labeling and Education Act of 1990,* Fed. Reg., 58, 2070, 1993.
8. Ubbink, J. B., Vitamin B-6, in *Modern Chromatographic Analysis of Vitamins,* 2nd ed., De Leenheer, A. P., Lambert, W. E., and Nelis, H. J., Eds., Marcel Dekker, New York, 1992, chap. 10.
9. Bridges, J. W., Davies, D. S., and Williams, R. T., Fluorescence studies on some hydroxypyridines including compounds of the vitamin B-6 group, *Biochem. J.,,* 98, 451, 1966.
10. Ball, G. F. M., Chemical and biological nature of the water soluble vitamins, in *Water Soluble Vitamin Assays in Human Nutrition,* Chapman and Hall, New York, 1994, chap. 2.
11. Ang, C. Y. W., Stability of three forms of vitamin B-6 to laboratory light conditions, *J. Assoc. Off. Anal. Chem.,* 62, 1170, 1979.
12. Saidi, B. and Warthensen, J. J., Influence of pH and light on the kinetics of vitamin B-6 degradation, *J. Agric. Food Chem.,* 31, 876, 1983.

13. Vanderslice, J. T., Brownlee, S. G., Cortissoz, M. E., and Maire, C. E., Vitamin B-6 analysis: sample preparation, extraction procedures, and chromatographic separations, in *Modern Chromatographic Analysis of Vitamins,* De Leenheer, A. P., Lambert, W. E., and DeRuyter, M. G. M., Eds., Marcel Dekker, New York, 1985, chap. 10.

14. Gregory, J. F. III and Kirk, J. R., Interaction of pyridoxal and pyridoxal phosphate with peptides in a model food system during thermal processing, *J. Food Sci.,* 42, 1554, 1977.

15. Gregory, J. F. III, Ink, S. L., and Sartain, D. B., Degradation and binding to food proteins of vitamin B-6 compounds during thermal processing, *J. Food Sci.,* 51, 1345, 1986.

16. Yasumoto, K., Iwami, K., Tsuji, H., Okada, J., and Mitsuda, H., Bound forms of vitamin B-6 in cereals and seeds, *Vitamins,* 50, 327, 1976.

17. Yasumoto, K., Tsuji, H., Iwami, K., and Mitsuda, H., Isolation from rice bran of a bound form of vitamin B-6 and its identification as 5′-0-(β-D-glucopyranosyl) pyridoxine, *Agric. Biol. Chem.,* 41, 1061, 1977.

18. Kabir, H., Leklem, J. E., and Miller, L. T., Relationship of the glycosylated vitamin B-6 content of foods to vitamin B-6 bioavailability in humans, *Nutr. Rep. Int.,* 28, 709, 1983.

19. Kabir, H., Leklem, J., and Miller, L. T., Measurement of glycosylated vitamin B-6 in foods, *J. Food Sci.,* 48, 1422, 1983.

20. Addo, C. and Augustin, J., Changes in vitamin B-6 content in potatoes during storage, *J. Food Sci.,* 53, 749, 1988.

21. Tadera, K. and Orite, K., Isolation and structure of a new vitamin B-6 conjugate in rice bran, *J. Food Sci.,* 56, 268, 1991.

22. Gregory, J. F., III and Ink, S. L., Identification and quantification of pyridoxine-β-glucoside as a major form of vitamin B-6 in plant derived foods, *J. Agric. Food Chem.,* 35, 76, 1987.

23. Ink, S.L., Gregory, J. F. III, and Sartain, D. B., Determination of pyridoxine-β-glucoside bioavailability using intrinsic and extrinsic labeling in rats, *J. Agric. Food Chem.,* 34, 857, 1986.

24. Trumbo, P. R., Gregory, J. F., III, and Sartain, D. B., Incomplete utilization of pyridoxine-β-glucoside as vitamin B-6 in the rat, *J. Nutr.,* 118, 170, 1988.

25. Nakano, H. and Gregory, J. F., III, Pyridoxine and pyridoxine-5′-β-D-glucoside exert different effects on tissue B-6 vitamers but similar effects on β-glucosidase activity in rats, *J. Nutr.,* 125, 2751, 1995.

26. Polansky, M. M., Reynolds, R. D., and Vanderslice, J. T., Vitamin B-6 in *Methods of Vitamin Assay,* 4th ed., Augustin, J., Klein, B. P., Becker, D. A., and Venugopal, P. B., Eds., John Wiley & Sons, New York, 1985, chap. 17.

27. Lumley, I. D., Vitamin analysis in foods, in *The Technology of Vitamins in Food,* Ottaway, P. B., Ed., Chapman and Hall, London, 1993, chap. 8.

28. Gregory, J. F., III, Methods for determination of vitamin B-6 in foods and other biological materials: a critical review, *J. Food Comp. Anal.,* 1, 105, 1988.

29. Eitenmiller, R. and Landen, W. O., Jr., Vitamins, in *Analyzing Food for Nutrition Labeling and Hazardous Contaminants,* Jeon, I. G. and Ikins, W. G., Eds., Marcel Dekker, New York, 1995, chap. 8.

30. Strohecker, R. and Henning, H. M., *Vitamin Assay Tested Methods,* Verlag Chemie, Limburg, 1965, 143.

31. Atkin, L., Schultz, A. S., Williams, W. L., and Frey, C. N., Yeast microbiological methods for determination of vitamins—pyridoxine, *Ind. Eng. Chem. Anal. Ed.,* 15, 141, 1943.

32. Parrish, W. P., Loy, H. W., and Kline, O. L., A study of the yeast method for vitamin B-6, *J. Assoc. Off. Agric. Chem.,* 38, 506, 1955.

33. Parrish, W. P., Loy, H. W., and Kline, O. L., Further studies on the yeast method for vitamin B-6, *J. Assoc. Off. Agric. Chem.,* 39, 157, 1956.

34. MacArthur, M. J. and Lehmann, J., Chromatographic separation and fluorometric measurement of vitamin B-6 components in aqueous solutions, *J. Assoc. Off. Agric. Chem.,* 42, 619, 1959.

35. Toepfer, E. W. and Lehmann, J., Procedure for chromatographic separation and microbiological assay of pyridoxine, pyridoxal, and pyridoxamine in food extracts, *J. Assoc. Off. Agric. Chem.,* 44, 426, 1961.

36. Toepfer, E. W. and Polansky, M. M., Microbiological assay of vitamin B-6 and its components, *J. Assoc. Off. Agric. Chem.,* 53, 546, 1970.

37. Polansky, M., Microbiological assay of vitamin B-6 in foods, in *Methods in Vitamin B-6 Nutrition,* Leklem, J. E. and Reynolds, R. E., Eds., Plenum Press, New York, 1981, 21.

38. Barton-Wright, E. C., The microbiological assay of the vitamin B-6 complex (pyridoxine, pyridoxal, and pyridoxamine) with *Kloeckera brevis, Analyst,* 96, 314, 1971.

39. Guilarte, T. R., McIntyre, P. A., and Tsan, M., Growth response of the yeasts *Saccharomyces uvarum* and *Kloeckera brevis* to the free biologically active forms of vitamin B-6, *J. Nutr.*, 110, 954, 1980.

40. Gregory, J. F. III, Relative activity of the nonphosphorylated B-6 vitamers for *Saccharomyces uvarum* and *Kloeckera brevis* in vitamin B-6 microbiological assay, *J. Nutr.*, 112, 1643, 1982.

41. Guilarte, T. R., Shane, B., and McIntyre, P. A., Radiometric-microbiologic assay of vitamin B-6: application to food analysis, *J. Nutr.*, 111, 1869, 1981.

42. AOAC International, Official Methods of Analysis, 16th ed., AOAC International, Arlington, VA, 1995.

43. Rabinowitz, J. C. and Snell, E. E., The vitamin B-6 group. Extraction procedures for the microbiological determination of vitamin B-6, *Ind. Eng. Chem. Anal. Ed.*, 19, 277, 1947.

44. Rubin, S. H., Schener, J., and Hirschberg, E., The availability of vitamin B-6 in yeast and liver for growth of *Saccharomyces carlsbergensis*, *J. Biol. Chem.*, 167, 599, 1947.

45. Tanner, J. T. and Barnett, S. A., Methods of analysis for infant formula: Food and Drug Administration and Infant Formula Council collaborative study, *J. Assoc. Off. Anal. Chem.*, 68, 514, 1985.

46. Brubacher, G., Müller-Mulot, W., and Southgate, D. A. T., *Methods for the Determination of Vitamins in Foods Recommended by COST 91*, Elsevier Applied Science Publishers, New York, 1985, chap. 11.

47. Reitzer-Bergaentzle, M., Marchioni, E., and Hasselmann, C., HPLC determination of vitamin B-6 in foods after pre-column derivatization of free and phosphorylated vitamers into pyridoxol, *Food Chem.*, 48, 321, 1993.

48. Vanderslice, J. T., Stewart, K. K., and Yarmas, M. M., Liquid chromatographic separation and quantification of B-6 vitamers and their metabolite, pyridoxic acid, *J. Chromatogr.*, 176, 280, 1979.

49. Vanderslice, J. T., Maire, C. E., Doherty, R. F., and Beecher, G.R., Sulfosalicylic acid as an extraction agent for vitamin B-6 in food, *J. Agric. Food Chem.*, 28, 1145, 1980.

50. Vanderslice, J. T. and Maire, C. E., Liquid chromatographic separation and quantification of B-6 vitamers at plasma concentration levels, *J. Chromatogr.*, 196, 176, 1980.

51. Vanderslice, J. T., Maire, C.E., and Beecher, G. R., B-6 vitamer analysis in human plasma by high performance liquid chromatography: a preliminary report, *Amer. J. Clin. Nutr.*, 34, 947, 1981.

52. Vanderslice, J. T., Maire, C. E., and Yakupkovic, J. E., Vitamin B-6 in ready-to-eat cereals: analysis by high performance liquid chromatography, *J. Food Sci.*, 46, 943, 1981.

53. Vanderslice, J. T., Brown, J. F., Beecher, G. R., Maire, C. E., and Brownlee, S. G., Automation of a complex high performance liquid chromatography system. Procedures and hardware for a vitamin B-6 model system, *J. Chromatogr.*, 216, 338, 1981.

54. Vanderslice, J. T., Brownlee, S. G., Maire, C. E., Reynolds, R. D., and Polansky, M., Forms of vitamin B-6 in human milk, *Amer. J. Clin. Nutr.*, 37, 867, 1983.

55. Coburn, S. P. and Mahuren, J. D., A versatile cation-exchange procedure for measuring the seven major forms of vitamin B-6 in biological samples, *Anal. Biochem.*, 129, 310, 1983.

56. Mahuren, J. D. and Coburn, S. P., Determination of 5-pyridoxic acid, 5-pyridoxic acid lactone, and other vitamin B-6 compounds by cation-exchange high-performance liquid chromatography, *Meth. Enzymol.*, 280, 22, 1997.

57. Gregory, J. F. III and Kirk, J. R., Improved chromatographic separation and fluorometric determination of vitamin B-6 compounds in foods, *J. Food Sci.*, 42, 1073, 1977.

58. Gregory, J. F., III, Determination of pyridoxal 5'-phosphate as the semicarbazone derivative using high-performance liquid chromatography, *Anal. Biochem.*, 102, 374, 1980.

59. Gregory, J. F., III, Manley, D. B., and Kirk, J. R., Determination of vitamin B-6 in animal tissues by reverse-phase high-performance liquid chromatography, *J. Agric. Food Chem.*, 29, 921, 1981.

60. Gregory, J. F., III and Feldstein, D., Determination of vitamin B-6 in foods and other biological materials by paired-ion high performance liquid chromatography, *J. Agric. Food Chem.*, 33, 359, 1985.

61. Ubbink, J. B., Serfontein, W. J., and DeVilliers, L. S., Stability of pyridoxal 5'-phosphate semicarbazone: applications in plasma vitamin B-6 analysis and population surveys of vitamin B-6 nutritional status, *J. Chromatogr.*, 342, 277, 1985.

62. Ubbink, J. B., Serfontein, W. J., and DeVilliers, L. S., Analytical recovery of protein-bound pyridoxal 5'-phosphate in plasma analysis, *J. Chromatogr.*, 375, 399, 1986.

63. Reynolds, T. M. and Brain, A., A simple internally standardized isocratic HPLC assay for vitamin B-6 in human serum, *J. Liq. Chromatogr.*, 15, 897, 1992.

64. van Schoonhoven, J., Schrijver, J., Van den Berg, H., and Haenen, G., Reliable and sensitive high-performance liquid chromatographic method with fluorometric detection for the analysis of vitamin B-6 in foods and feeds, *J. Agric. Food Chem.,* 42, 1475, 1994.

65. Tsuge, H., Toukairin-Oda, T., Shoji, T., Sakamoto, E., Mori, M., and Suda, H., Fluorescence enhancement of PLP for application to HPLC, *Agric. Biol. Chem.,* 52, 1083, 1988.

66. Tsuge, H., Determination of vitamin B-6 vitamers and metabolites in a biological sample, *Meth. Enzymol.,* 280, 3, 1997.

Table 10.3   Physical Properties of Vitamin B-6

1. Budavari, S., *The Merck Index,* 12th ed., Merck and Company, Whitehouse Station, NJ, 1996, 1371, 1372.

2. Friedrich, W., Vitamin B-6, in *Vitamins,* Walter de Gruyter, Hawthorne, New York, 1988, chap. 9.

3. Ubbink, J. B., Vitamin B-6, in *Modern Chromatographic Analysis of Vitamins,* 2nd ed., De Leenheer, A. P., Lambert, W. E., and Nelis, H. J., Eds., Marcel Dekker, New York, 1992, chap. 10.

4. Ball, G. F. M., Chemical and biological nature of the water-soluble vitamins, in *Water-Soluble Vitamin Assays in Human Nutrition,* Chapman and Hall, New York, 1994, chap. 2.

Table 10.5   Compendium, Regulatory, and Handbook Methods for Analysis of Vitamin B-6

1. United States Pharmacopeial Convention, *U.S. Pharmacopoeia National Formulary,* USP23/NF18, Nutritional Supplements, Official Monographs, United States Pharmacopeial Convention, Rockville, MD, 1995.

2. Scottish Home and Health Department, *British Pharmacopoeia,* 15th ed., British Pharmacopoeic Commission, United Kingdom, 1993.

3. AOAC International, Official Methods of Analysis, 16th ed., AOAC International, Arlington, VA, 1995.

4. Toepfer, E. W. and Lehmann, J., Procedure for chromatographic separation and microbiological assay of pyridoxine, pyridoxal, and pyridoxamine in food extracts, *J. Assoc. Off. Anal. Chem.,* 44, 426, 1961.

5. Polansky, M. M., Murphy, E. W., and Toepfer, G. W., Components of vitamin B-6 in grains and cereal products, *J. Assoc. Off. Anal. Chem.,* 47, 750, 1964.

6. Toepfer, E. W. and Polansky, M. M., Microbiological assay of vitamin B-6 and its components, *J. Assoc. Off. Anal. Chem.,* 53, 546, 1970.

7. Tanner, J. T. and Barnett, S. A., Methods of analysis for infant formula: Food and Drug Administration and Infant Formula Council collaborative study, *J. Assoc. Off. Anal. Chem.,* 68, 514, 1985.

8. American Feed Ingredients Association, *Laboratory Methods Compendium,* Volume One: *Vitamins and Minerals,* American Feed Ingredients Association, West Des Moines, IA, 1991, 157.

9. Wills, R. B. H., Shaw, C. G., and Day, W. R., Analysis of water-soluble vitamins by high pressure liquid chromatography, *J. Chromatogr. Sci.,* 15, 262, 1977.

10. Polansky, M., Microbiological assay of vitamin B-6 in foods, in *Methods in Vitamin B-6 Nutrition,* Leklem, J. E. and Reynolds, R. D., Plenum Press, New York, 1981, 21.

11. Keller, H. E., *Analytical Methods for Vitamins and Carotenoids,* Hoffmann-LaRoche, Basel, 1988, 23.

12. American Association of Cereal Chemists, *AACC Approved Methods,* 9th ed., vol. 2, American Association of Cereal Chemists, St. Paul, MN, 1996.

13. Committee on Food Chemicals Codex, *Food Chemicals Codex,* 4th ed., National Academy of Sciences, Washington, DC, 1996, 334.

14. Brubacher, G., Müller-Mulot, W., and Southgate, D. A. T., *Methods for the Determination of Vitamins in Food, Recommended by COST 91,* Elsevier Applied Science Publishers, London, 1985, 129.

Table 10.6   HPLC Methods for the Analysis of Vitamin B-6 in Food, Feed, Pharmaceuticals, and Biologicals

Food

1. Vanderslice, J. T., Stewart, K. K., and Yarmas, M. M., Liquid chromatographic separation and quantification of B-6 vitamers and their metaoblite, pyridoxic acid, *J. Chromatogr.,* 176, 280, 1979.
2. Vanderslice, J. T. and Maire, C. E., Liquid chromatographic separation and quantification of B-6 vitamers at plasma concentration levels, *J. Chromatogr.,* 196, 176, 1980.
3. Vanderslice, J. T., Brown, J. F., Beecher, G. R., Maire, C. E., and Brownlee, S. G., Automation of a complex high-performance liquid chromatography system. Procedures and hardware for a Vitamin B-6 model system, *J. Chromatogr.,* 216, 338, 1981.
4. Vanderslice, J. T., Maire, C. E., Doherty, R. F., and Beecher, G. R., Sulfosalicylic acid as an extraction agent for vitamin B-6 in food, *J. Agric. Food Chem.,* 28, 1145, 1980.
5. Vanderslice, J. T., Maire, C. E., and Yakupkovic, J. E., Vitamin B-6 in ready-to-eat cereals: analysis by high performance liquid chromatography, *J. Food Sci.,* 46, 943, 1981.
6. Gregory, J. F., III, Determination of pyridoxal 5′-phosphate as the semicarbazone derivative using high-performance liquid chromatography, *Anal. Biochem.,* 102, 374, 1980.
7. Gregory, J. F., III, Manley, D. B., and Kirk, J. R., Determination of vitamin B-6 in animal tissues by reverse-phase high-performance liquid chromatography, *J. Agric. Food Chem.,* 29, 921, 1981.
8. Gregory, J. F., III and Feldstein, D., Determination of vitamin B-6 in foods and other biological materials by paired-ion high-performance liquid chromatography, J. Agric. *Food Chem.,* 33,359, 1985.
9. Morrison, L. A. and Driskell, J. A., Quantities of B-6 vitamers in human milk by high performance liquid chromatography, *J. Chromatogr.,* 337, 249, 1985.
10. Ang, C. Y. W., Cenciarelli, M., and Eitenmiller, R. R., A simple liquid chromatographic method for determination of B-6 vitamers in raw and cooked chicken, *J. Food Sci.,* 53, 371, 1988.
11. Bitsch, R. and Möller, J., Analysis of B-6 vitamers in foods using a modified high-performance liquid chromatographic method, *J. Chromatogr.,* 463, 207, 1989.
12. Toukairin-Oda, T., Sakamoto, E., Hirose, N., Mori, M., Itoh, T., and Tsuge, H., Determination of vitamin B-6 derivatives in foods and biological materials by reversed-phase HPLC, *J. Nutr. Sci. Vitaminol.,* 35, 171, 1989.
13. Tadera, K. and Naka, Y., Isocratic paired-ion high-performance liquid chromatographic method to determine B-6 vitamers and pyridoxine glucoside in foods, *Agric. Biol. Chem.,* 55, 563, 1991.
14. Reitzer-Bergaentzlé, M., Marchioni, E., and Hasselmann, C., HPLC determination of vitamin B-6 in foods after pre-column derivatization of free and phosphorylated vitamers into pyridoxol, *Food Chem.,* 48, 321, 1993.
15. Bergaentzle, M., Arella, F., Bourguignon, J. B., and Hasselmann, C., Determination of vitamin B-6 in foods by HPLC—a collaborative study, *Food Chem.,* 52, 81, 1995.
16. Olds, S. J., Vanderslice, J. T., and Brochetti, D., Vitamin B-6 in raw and fried chicken by HPLC, *J. Food Sci.,* 58, 505, 1993.
17. van Schoonhoven, J., Schrijver, J., van den Berg, H.,and Haenen, G. R. M. M., Reliable and sensitive high-performance liquid chromatographic method with fluorometric detection for the analysis of vitamin B-6 in foods and feeds, *J. Agric. Food Chem.,* 42, 1475, 1994.
18. Sampson, D. A., Eoff, L. A., Yan, X. L., and Lorenz, K., Analysis of free and glycosylated vitamin B-6 in wheat by high-performance liquid chromatography, *Cereal Chem.,* 72, 217, 1995.

Biologicals

1. Gregory, J. F. III, Determination of pyridoxal 5′-phosphate as the semicarbazone derivative using high-performance liquid chromatography, *Anal. Biochem.,* 102, 374, 1980.
2. Vanderslice, J. T. and Maire, C. E., Liquid chromatographic separation and quantification of B-6 vitamers at plasma concentration levels, *J. Chromatogr.,* 196, 176, 1980.
3. Schrijver, J., Speek, A. J., and Schreurs, W. H. P., Semiautomated fluorometric determination of pyridoxal 5′-phosphate (vitamin B-6) in whole blood by high-performance liquid chromatography, *Int. J. Vit. Nutr. Res.,* 51, 216, 1981.

4. Tryfiates, G. P. and Sattsangi, S., Separation of vitamin B-6 compounds by paired-ion high-performance liquid chromatography, *J. Chromatogr.,* 227, 181, 1982.

5. Coburn, S. P. and Mahuren, J. D., A versatile cation-exchange procedure for measuring the seven major forms of vitamin B-6 in biological samples, *Anal. Biochem.,* 129, 310, 1983.

6. Mahuren, J. D. and Coburn, S. P., Determination of 5-pyridoxic acid, 5-pyridoxic acid lactone, and other vitamin B-6 compounds by cation-exchange high-performance liquid chromatography, *Meth. Enzymol.,* 280, 22, 1997.

7. Pierotti, J. A., Dickinson, A. G., Palmer, J. K., and Driskell, J. A., Liquid chromatographic separation and quantitation of B-6 vitamers in selected rat tissues, *J. Chromatogr.,* 306, 377, 1984.

8. Hefferan, T. E., Chrisley, B. M., and Driskell, J. A., Quantitation of B-6 vitamers in rat plasma by high-performance liquid chromatography, *J. Chromatogr.,* 374, 155, 1986.

9. Ubbink, J. B., Serfontein, W. J., and DeVilliers, L. S., Stability of pyridoxal 5'-phosphate semicarbazone: applications in plasma vitamin B-6 analysis and population surveys of vitamin B-6 nutritional status, *J. Chromatogr.,* 342, 277, 1985.

10. Ubbink, J. B., Serfontein, W. J., and DeVilliers, L. S., Analytical recovery of protein-bound pyridoxal 5'-phosphate in plasma analysis, *J. Chromatogr.,* 375, 399, 1986.

11. Ubbink, J. B., Serfontein, W. J., Becker, P. J., and DeVilliers, L. S., Effect of different levels of oral pyridoxine supplementation on plasma levels of pyridoxal 5'-phosphate and pyridoxal levels and urinary vitamin B-6 excretion, *Am. J. Clin. Nutr.,* 46, 78, 1987.

12. Ubbink, J. B., Delport, R., Becker, P. J., and Bissbort, S., Evidence of a theophylline-induced vitamin B-6 deficiency caused by a non-competitive inhibition of pyridoxal kinase, *J. Lab Clin. Med.,* 113, 15, 1989.

13. Ubbink, J. B., Vermaak, W. J. H., van der Merwe, A., and Becker, P. J., Vitamin B-12, vitamin B-6 and folate nutritional status in men with hyperhomocysteinemia, *Am. J. Clin. Nutr.,* 57, 47, 1993.

14. Sampson, D. A. and O'Connor, D. K., Analysis of B-6 vitamers and pyridoxic acid in plasma, tissues and urine using high performance liquid chromatography, *Nutr. Res.,* 9, 259, 1989.

15. Millart, H. and Lamiable, D., Determination of pyridoxal 5'-phosphate in human serum by reversed-phase high-performance liquid chromatography combined with spectrofluorometric detection of 4-pyridoxic acid 5'-phosphate as a derivative, *Analyst,* 114, 1225, 1989.

16. Reynolds, T. M. and Brain, A., A simple internally-standardised isocratic HPLC assay for vitamin B-6 in human serum, *J. Liq. Chromatogr.,* 15, 897, 1992.

17. Sharma, S. K. and Dakshinamurti, K., Determination of vitamin B-6 vitamers and pyridoxic acid in biological samples, *J. Chromatogr.,* 578, 45, 1992.

18. Tsuge, H., Toukairin-Oda, T., Shoji, T., Sakamoto, E., Mori, M., and Suda, H., Fluorescence enhancement of PLP for application to HPLC, *Agric. Biol. Chem.,* 52, 1083, 1988.

19. Hirose, N., Kubo, N., and Tsuge, H., Highly sensitive determination of PLP in human plasma with HPLC method, *J. Nutr. Sci. Vitaminol.,* 36, 521, 1990.

20. Tsuge, H., Maeno, M., Nagae, K., Nohisa, C., and Hayakawa, T., Change in blood levels of vitamin B-6 derivatives in pregnant and lactating rats, *J. Nutr. Sci. Vitaminol.,* 40, 239, 1994.

21. Tsuge, H., Determination of vitamin B-6 vitamers and metabolites in a biological sample, *Meth. Enzymol.,* 280, 3, 1997.

11 Folate

11.1 REVIEW

Folate deficiency was recognized by Wills in 1931 through identification of a pernicious anemia prevalent in Indian women. The deficiency was inducible in monkeys fed the same diet and could be alleviated by feeding yeast or liver extracts. The antianemia factor was designated "vitamin M" in 1938.[1] In the following year, a similar anemia curable by liver extract was reported in chicks.[2] The name, folic acid, was first used by Snell's group in studies on the growth factors for *Lactobacillus casei* and *Streptococcus lactis*. Folic acid was isolated in quantity from spinach, and the name was derived from the Latin word "folium" for leaf.[3] The *L. casei* growth factor was purified and synthesized through the efforts of several biochemists (1941–1948). An excellent review of the history of folic acid research is provided by Friedrich.[4]

Identification of folic acid as a cure for megaloblastic anemia occurred in 1945.[5] Since then, folate deficiency is recognized as one of the most prevalent vitamin deficiencies common in all areas of the world. Deficiency results from inadequate intake, defective absorption, abnormal metabolism, or conditions such as drug therapy, leading to increased requirements.[5] Marginal deficiency produces general symptoms including tiredness, irritability, and decreased appetite. Severe deficiency produces megaloblastic anemia or the production of large immature red blood cells. Other symptoms include abdominal pain, diarrhea, ulcers in the mouth and pharynx, skin changes, and hair loss. Deficiency before or during pregnancy may result in premature birth or birth defects. Deficiency prior to conception is a causative factor in neural tube defect. Fortification of enriched cereal grain products was initiated in January 1988 to counteract this aspect of the deficiency. Other deficiency symptoms include various neurological disorders such as dementia and depression.[5] Close relationships between folate and vitamin B-12 deficiencies result owing to the involvement of the vitamins in DNA synthesis. Similarities in the megaloblastic anemias produced by deficiencies of the vitamins requires biochemical assessment for accurate diagnosis. Plasma folate levels (5-CH_3-H_4 folate) rapidly fluctuate with recent intake, therefore, erythrocyte folate levels are considered a more reliable status index.[6] An indirect clinical measure is the urinary excretion of formiminoglutamic acid (FIGLU). FIGLU is an intermediate in the conversion of histidine to glutamic acid by a folate-requiring enzyme—formimino transferase. Folate deficiency results in lowered enzyme activity and increased FIGLU excretion.[6] Unfortunately, increased excretion of FIGLU occurs under other metabolic disturbances and is not considered specific enough for completely accurate clinical diagnosis of folate deficiency. The test is, therefore, used infrequently.

Folates are present in most foods with legumes (peanuts, cowpeas, peas, etc.), leafy greens, citrus (orange juice), some fruits, vegetables (broccoli, cauliflower), and liver considered to be good sources. Enriched cereal products are fortified at 140 µg/100 g. The addition level is estimated to increase the intake of 19–50 year-old women to levels slightly below The Reference Daily Intake (RDI) of 400 µg.[7] Daly et al.[8] calculated the statistically expected reduction in risk of neural tube defects if women of child-bearing age with low red cell folate levels consumed the RDI. At the RDI, an approximate 50% reduction in neural tube defect was expected. For this reason, the current addition level required by FDA regulations is controversial. Higher levels of addition would further decrease the incidence of neural tube defect. However, the conservative FDA approach was dictated by the possibility that higher folate intake by the general population would mask vitamin B-12 deficiency.

The current folate RDA is 200 μg for adult males and 180 μg for adult women.[10] RDAs were decreased from 400 μg in the previous (1980) recommendations. RDA values increase to 400 μg during pregnancy, 280 μg during the first 6 months of lactation, and 260 μg during the second 6 months of lactation.

Folate is the general term inclusive of folic acid (pteroylglutamate) and poly-γ-glutamyl conjugates that exhibit the biological activity of folic acid. Structural characteristics are discussed in Section 11.2. Folates function in single-C metabolism as acceptors or donors of single C-units (methyl, methylene, methenyl, formyl, and formimino groups). Metabolically significant forms include 7,8-dihydrofolate (H_2 folate), 5,6,7,8-tetrahydrofolate (H_4 folate), 5-methyltetrahydrofolate (5-CH_3-H_4 folate), 5-formyltetrahydrofolate (5-CHO-H_4 folate), 10-formyltetrahydrofolate (10-CHO-H_4 folate), 5,10-methenyltetrahydrofolate (5,10-CH^+ = H_4 folate), 5,10-methylenetetrahydrofolate (5,10-CH_2-H_4 folate), 5-formiminotetrahydrofolate (5-CHNH-H_4 folate) and their respective γ-glutamyl conjugates. Metabolic interrelationships of the biologically significant forms are provided in Figure 11-1.[11,12] Enzymes indicated by numerals in Figure 11.1 are defined in Table 11.1.

11.2   PROPERTIES

11.2.1   CHEMISTRY

11.2.1.1   General Properties

The structure of folic acid is given in Figure 11.2. Pteroic acid, 4-[(pteridin-6-ylmethyl)amino] benzoic acid, is the parent compound.[13] Folate refers to the large group of heterocyclic compounds

---

TABLE 11.1
Enzymes of Folate Metabolism

[a]1. γ-Glutamyl hydrolase	EC 3.4.22.12 (Brush border)
2. Dihydrofolate reductase	EC 1.5.1.3
3. Folypoly-glutamate synthetase	EC 6.3.2.17
4. Serine hydroxymethyl transferase	EC 2.1.2.1
5. Methylenetetrahydrofolate reductase	EC 1.7.99.5
6. γ-Glutamyl hydrolase	EC 3.4.22.12 (lysosomal)
7. Cobalamin-dependent methionine synthase	EC 2.1.1.13
8. Glycine cleavage enzyme system	EC 1.4.4.2
	EC 2.1.2.10
9. Glutamate formiminotransferase	EC 2.1.2.5
10. Formiminotetrahydrofolate cyclodeaminase	EC 4.3.1.4
11. Methylenetetrahydrofolate dehydrogenase	EC 1.5.1.5
12. Methenyltetrahydrofolate cyclohydrolase	EC 3.5.4.9
13. Formyltetrahydrofolate synthetase	EC 6.3.4.3
14. Thymidylate synthase	EC 2.1.1.45
15. Formyltetrahydrofolate dehydrogenase	EC 1.5.1.6
16. Phosphoribosyl glycinamide (GAR) formyl transferase	EC 2.1.2.2
17. Phosphoribosyl aminoimidazole carboxamide (AICAR) formyl transferase	EC 2.1.2.3
18. 5-Formyltetrahydrofolate cycloligase	EC 6.3.3.2
19. Folate/MTX transport mechanism	
20. Glycine methyl transferase	EC 2.1.1.20

[a]Numbers refer to enzymes in Figure 11.1.

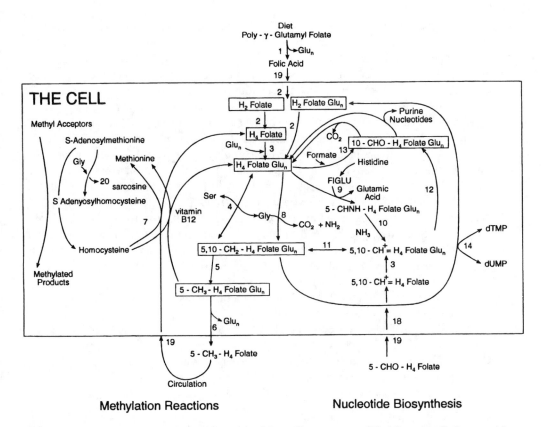

FIGURE 11.1   Metabolic interrelationships of the folates (figure was modified from text References 11 and 12).

based on the pteroic acid structure conjugated with one or more L-glutamates linked through the γ-carboxyl of the amino acid. Folic acid contains one glutamic acid residue with the accepted name "pteroylglutamic acid." Folic acid is not found in nature; however, it is the common, more stable, synthetic form used for food fortification and for formulation of pharmaceuticals. The USP Reference Standard is folic acid. Folic acid must be reduced to dihydrofolate (H_2 folate) or tetrahydrofolate (H_4 folate). Tetrahydrofolate is the active co-enzyme form of the vitamin. Folate structures and nomenclature are quite complicated owing to the number and diversity of biologically active forms. In general, structural variations encompass changes in the oxidation state of the pteridine ring structure, the one-carbon moiety carried by the specific folate, and the number of conjugated glutamate residues on the specific folate. For clarification, the IUPAC-IUB nomenclature rules are briefly summarized as follows.[13]

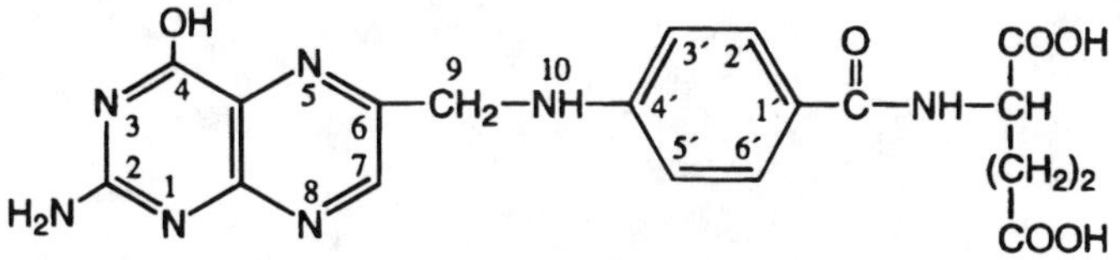

Folic Acid
2-amino-4-hydroxy-6-methyleneaminobenzoyl-
L-glutamic acid pteridine

FIGURE 11.2   The structure of folic acid.

1. Pteroic acid conjugated with one or more L-glutamate units are named pteroylglutamate, pteroyldiglutamate, etc. The name "pteroylmonoglutamate" should not be used (IUPAC-IUB Recommendation 2.3).
2. Folate and folic acid are the preferred synonyms for pteroylglutamate and pteroylglutamic acid, respectively (IUPAC-IUB Recommendation 2.4).
3. "Folate" may be used to designate any members of the family of pteroylglutamates or mixtures with various levels of reduction of the pteridine ring, single-C substitutions, and numbers of conjugated glutamate residues (IUPAC-IUB Recommendation 2.5).
4. Reduced compounds are indicated by the prefixes dihydro-, tetrahydro-, etc., with numerals indicating the positions of the additional hydrogens. Tetrahydrofolate is assumed to be substituted in the 5, 6, 7, and 8 positions, and dihydrofolate is assumed to be substituted in the 7 and 8 position unless otherwise indicated (IUPAC-IUB Recommendation 2.6).
5. Substituent groups are indicated by prefixes together with the locations of the positions substituted. Substituent prefixes indicate that the substituent replaces one hydrogen atom in the parent structure in the case of formyl, methyl, or formimino, or two hydrogens in the case of methylene and methenyl (IUPAC-IUB Recommendation 2.7).
6. Rules for use of symbols and abbreviations include the following:
   a. Folate is preferred to folic acid and should not be abbreviated.
   b. Pteroate, pteroyl, or pteroic acid is indicated by the symbol "Pte."
   c. Pteroylglutamates and the corresponding acids are indicated by the symbols PteGlu, $PteGlu_2$, $PteGlu_3$, etc. The subscript indicates the number of glutamate units.
   d. Reduced states are indicated by H_2 or H_4 in front of the main symbol. H_4 folate and H_2 folate are preferred abbreviations. TH and DH should not be used.
   e. Substituents are indicated as follows:

Substituent	Symbol	Formula
Formimino	NHCH-	$HN = CH-$
Formyl	HCO-	$O = CH-$
Methyl	CH_3-	CH_3-
Methylene	$-CH_2-$	$-CH_2-$
Methenyl	$-CH^+$	$-CH =$ as a component of $[> N-CH = N^+ <\leftrightarrow> >N^+ = CH-N<]$

The above rules regarding symbols and abbreviations are found in IUPAC-IUB Recommendation 2.8. Names of substituted folates, abbreviations, and substituent positions are provided in Table 11.2. Structural relationships are shown in Figure 11.3.

TABLE 11.2
Substituent Groups and Their Positions in Folic Acid Coenzymes

Name	Abbreviation	Position	
		N-5	N-10
Pteroylglutamic Acid	Folic acid	—	-H
7,8-Dihydrofolate	H_2 folate	-H	-H
5-Methyl-5,6-dihydrofolate		$-CH_3$	-H
5,6,7,8-Tetrahydrofolate	H_4 folate	-H	-H
5-Methyltetrahydrofolate	$5-CH_3-H_4$ folate	$-CH_3$	-H
5-Formyltetrahydrofolic acid	$5-CHO-H_4$ folate	-CHO	-H
10-Formyltetrahydrofolate	$10-CHO-H_4$ folate	-H	-CHO
5-Methyltetrahydrofolate	$5-CH_3-H_4$ folate	$=CH_3$	-H
5,10-Methenyltetrahydrofolate	$5,10-CH^+=H_4$ folate	$=CH-^\pm$ bridge	—
5,10-Methylenetetrahydrofolate	$5,10-CH_2H_4$ folate	$-CH_2-$ bridge	—
5-Formiminotetrahydrofolate	$5-CHNH-H_4$ folate	-CHNH	-H

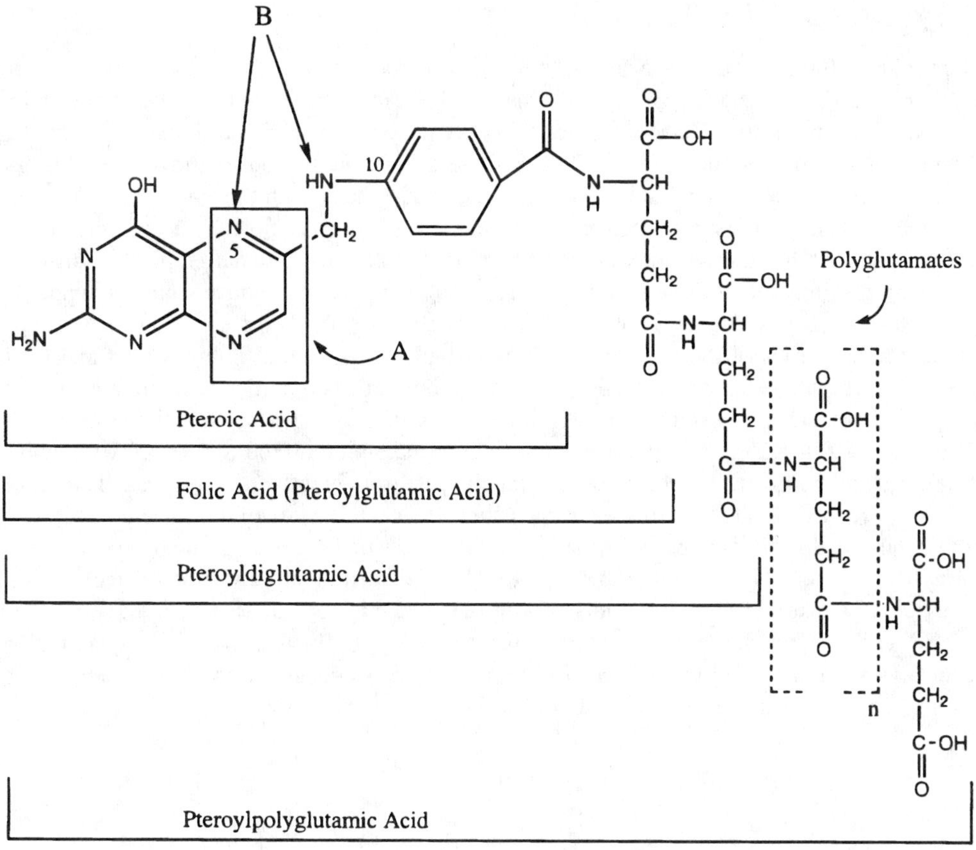

A - Pterin ring oxidation - reduction
B - One carbon fragment attachment
n - Number of glutamates

FIGURE 11.3   Structural relationships of the folates.

Physical and chemical properties of folic acid and reduced folates were reviewed in detail by Temple and Montgomery[14] and Gregory.[15] Solubility characteristics summarized by Gregory[15] include the following:

1. Folates exhibit minimum solubility in mildly acidic solvents (pH 2 to 4) where mono-cationic and neutral forms predominate.
2. Solubility increases in proportion to the pH above this range as anionic species increase in concentration.
3. Solubility increases at very low pH in strong acid solutions. At such low pH levels, highly cationic species exist.
4. Pteroic acid is less soluble than folic acid over most of the pH scale. The solubility of folic acid is influenced by the polar hydrophilic character of the α-carboxyl group of glutamic acid.
5. At neutral to alkaline pH levels, polyglutamyl folates are more anionic than folic acid due to the presence of additional ionizable α-carboxyl groups.
6. Long-chain polyglutamyl folates are more hydrophobic than short-chain polyglutamyl folates at low pH levels where the α-carboxyl groups are predominantly protonated.

11.2.1.2   Spectral Properties

Absorption and fluorescence properties of folic acid and commonly occurring derivatives are given in Table 11.3. For more detailed spectral information, the reader is referred to extensive tabular information provided by Temple and Montgomery.[14] Descriptive UV spectra and fluorescence excitation and emission spectra were provided by Ball.[16] These spectra are reproduced in Figures 11.4.I and 11.4.II. Folates show characteristic UV absorption spectra usually with three absorbance maxima. A maxima attributable to the p-aminobenzoyl-glutamic acid (PABG) moiety exists from 270 to 280 nm.[17] H_4 folate exhibits a single maximum at 286 nm in 0.1 M phosphate buffer, pH 7.1.[16] Likewise, PABG strongly influences fluorescence properties of the folates. Reduced pterins without the p-aminobenzoyl moiety do not exhibit native fluorescence.[16] The most comprehensive study on fluorescence properties of the pteridines was published by Uyeda and Rabinowitz[18] and is often referenced as the single most significant source on fluorescence properties of the folates. H_2 folate and H_4 folates other than 5,10-methenyl-H_4 folate fluoresce maximally at excitation 300 to 320 nm and emission 360 to 425 nm. Folate has an excitation maximum at 360 to 380 nm with emission maximum at 450 to 460 nm.[17,18] Fluorescence intensity is strongly influenced by pH and buffer composition. For reduced folates, fluorescence intensity increases as acidity of the solvent increases. For HPLC determination by fluorescence, native fluorescence of H_4-folate, 5-methyl-H_4 folate, and 5-formyl-H_4 folate is sufficient at pH 2.3 to allow detection at low pmol detection limits. Fluorescence intensity of H_2-folate and 10-formyl-H_4 folate is not sufficient to allow quantitation, and folic acid does not fluoresce.[18,19] Procedures used to apply fluorescence to LC quantitation of these analytes are discussed in Section 11.4. Fluorescence is considered the most specific and, in most cases, most sensitive detection mode for LC detection.[15,19,20]

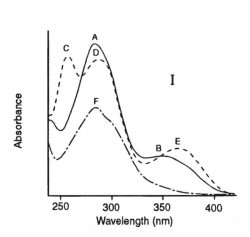

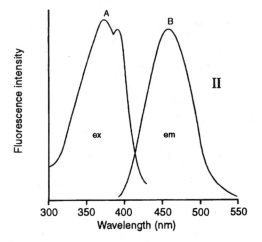

FIGURE 11.4.I   Absorption spectra of folic acid, A, 282 nm; B, 347 nm (0.1 M phosphate buffer, pH 7.1, solid line). Folic acid, C, 255 nm; D, 283 nm; E, 364 nm (0.1 M NaOH, pH 13.0, dashed line). Tetrahydrofolate, F, 286 nm (0.1 M phosphate buffer, pH 7.1, broken line). Spectra reproduced with permission from text Reference 16.

FIGURE 11.4.II   Fluorescence excitation and emission spectra of folic acid in 0.1 M phosphate buffer, pH 9.0. A =360 nm; B = 450 nm. Spectra reproduced with permission from text Reference 16.

TABLE 11.3
Physical Properties of Folates

Substance[a]	Molar Mass	Formula	Absorbance[b]				Fluorescence[c]		
			λ max	$E_{1cm}^{1\%}$	$\varepsilon \times 10^{-3}$	Solvent	Ex (nm)	Em (nm)	pH
Folic Acid CAS No. 59-20-3 **4253**	441.40	$C_{19}H_{19}N_7O_6$	282	[611.7]	27.0	Phosphate buffer, pH 7.0	363	450–460	9
			350	[158.6]	7.0	Phosphate buffer, pH 7.0			
			254	[566.4]	25.0	0.1 M NaOH, pH 13			
			282	[532.2]	23.8	0.1 M NaOH, pH 13			
			363	[197.1]	8.7	0.1 M NaOH, pH 13			
H_4 folate	445.44	$C_{19}H_{23}N_7O_6$	297	[606.1]	27.0	Phosphate buffer, pH 7.0	305–310	360	3
10-CHO-H_4 folate	473.45	$C_{20}H_{23}N_7O_7$	288	[384.4]	18.2	Phosphate buffer, pH 7.0	313	360	7
5-CHO-H_4 folate CAS No. 58-05-9	473.45	$C_{20}H_{23}N_7O_7$	287	[665.3]	31.5	Phosphate buffer, pH 7.0	314	365	7
			282	[688.5]	32.6	0.1 M NaOH, pH 13			
4254 5-CH$_3$-H_4 folate	459.46	$C_{20}H_{25}N_7O_6$	290	[696.5]	32.0	Phosphate buffer, pH 7.0	—	—	—
5-CHNH-H_4 folate	472.46	$C_{20}H_{24}N_8O_6$	285	[749.3]	35.4	Phosphate buffer, pH 7.0	308	360	7
5,10-CH=H_4 folate	456.44	$C_{20}H_{22}N_7O_6$	352	[547.1]	25.0	Phosphate buffer, pH 7.0	370	470	4
5,10-CH$_2$-H_4 folate	457.45	$C_{20}H_{23}N_7O_6$	294	[699.5]	32.0	Phosphate buffer, pH 7.2	—	—	—

[a] Common or generic name; CAS No. - Chemical Abstract Service number, bold print designates the Merck Index monograph number.
[b] Values in brackets are calculated from corresponding ε values.
[c] pH of optimum fluorescence.

Ball, G.F.M., *Water-Soluble Vitamin Assays in Human Nutrition.*[1]
Budavari, S. *The Merck Index.*[2]
Freidrich, W., *Vitamins.*[3]
Temple, C., Jr., Montgomery, J.A., *Folates and Pterins.*[4]

11.2.1.3   Stability

Several excellent reviews exist that comprehensively cover the extensive information available on folate stability.[15,16,17,21,22] To call attention to specific stability properties of importance to the analyst, the following summary is provided along with primary and secondary literature references. The summary of stability characteristics is not meant to be all inclusive, but to provide a guide to analysts to be aware of the many factors that affect folate stability in biological systems and during analysis.

1. Loss of biological activity occurs through oxidative cleavage of the C-9-N-10 bond.
    a. p-Aminobenzoylglutamate is the major oxidation product at pH 4, 7, and 10. Pterin fragments include predominantly pterin at pH 4 and 6, and formylpterin at pH 7 and 10.[17,21,23]
    b. H_4 Folate is more susceptible to oxidation than folic acid.[15,21,24]
    c. Substitution at the N-5 and N-10 positions increases oxidative stability of reduced folates.[15,16,20,23]
    d. Reducing agents including ascorbic acid, 2-mercaptoethanol and dithiothrietol stabilize folates.[15,16,21,22,24,25,26,27,28]
    e. Folic acid is more stable than naturally occurring folates at both ambient and elevated temperatures.[15,16,22]
    f. Folic acid is stable to 100°C when protected from light at pH 5.0 to 12.0.
    g. 5-Formyl-H_4 folate is stable at neutral pH. Under acid conditions with heating, it is converted to 5,10-methenyl-H_4 folate.
2. The number of glutamate residues attached to the folate does not influence stability.[16,21]
3. Folates are cleaved through photochemical and reductive mechanisms.[15,16,29,30]
4. Folate is subject to food processing and storage losses; however, the losses are variable owing to the variations in food matrices, oxygen availability, chemical environment, extent of heating, and forms of folate in the food.
    a. Folates, being water soluble, are subject to large leaching losses. Canning liquid can contain a significant proportion of the folate originally present in the raw product.[31]
    b. Presence of reducing agents (ascorbic acid) in the food can increase folate retention during thermal processing.[21,32,33]
    c. Presence of metals (Fe^{++}) can increase folate loss.[21,34]
    d. Common food additives including sodium nitrite used in some cured products cause folate destruction.[15,35]
    e. Kinetics of thermal loss generally follow first-order rates and depend on oxygen concentration (pseudo-first-order rate).[21,22,36]
    f. As dissolved or headspace oxygen levels decrease, folate stability increases.[15,16,21,37]
    g. Folate is quite stable in dry products in the absence of light and oxygen. Of significance to the addition of folic acid to cereal products, the vitamin is stable in flour during storage and subject to only small losses during baking.[38]
    h. Folic acid is used for fortification. Its stability is greater than naturally occurring folates in most foods.

Considerable data are available on the stability of 5-methyl-H_4 folate in fluid milk. Milk provides an ideal product for thermal processing studies because 90 to 95% of the folate in milk is 5-methyl-H_4 folate.[39] Its stability in milk has been well defined.[32,33,40,41,42] Loss during UHT pasteurization is usually less than 20%. Recent UHT thermal processing studies in model systems showed 5-methyl-H_4 folate degradation as second order in the presence of oxygen.[42] Degassing of liquid foods before thermal processing to reduce dissolved oxygen levels greatly improves folate retention.

11.2.1.4   Bioavailability

In-depth discussion of the bioavailability of folate to the human is much beyond the scope of this text. An excellent summary of factors influencing vitamin bioavailability is given in Table 11.4.[43] Most, if not all, of these factors apply to folate. Significant to absorption, polyglutamylfolates are hydrolyzed to monoglutamylfolates in the brush border (Figure 11.1).[44,45,46] The enzyme(s), γ-glutamyl hydrolase or human conjugase, can be inhibited by food substances.[47] Processing and cooking effects on conjugase inhibitors are largely unknown. Conversely, folate-binding protein from milk may increase folate absorption by protecting dietary folates from uptake by bacteria in the gut, thus increasing absorption in the small intestine.[48] Other studies, however, have contradicted early suggestions regarding the role that dietary binding proteins might play in human or animal absorption of folates.[49]

Food component interactions with dietary folates may act to either increase or decrease efficiency of folate absorption. Excellent studies on fiber effects on folate bioavailability indicate lack of binding, but potential for physical interferences with absorption mechanisms at the surface of the intestinal mucosa.[15,50,51,52] Other dietary interactions include effects of foods on intestinal pH with potential modification of conjugase activity, presence of folate antagonists, intestinal changes influenced by dietary factors (alcoholism), chelation, and factors that influence the rate of gastric

---

TABLE 11.4
Factors Influencing Bioavailabity of Vitamins[a]

Factor	Biological or Physical Variable
Extrinsic	
Chemical form of vitamin	Solubility or dispersibility
	Difference in rates of absorption, transport, and metabolism
	Potential variation in tissue uptake, renal, and biliary excretion
Concentration of vitamin	Concentration dependence of intestinal absorption
	Solubility of vitamin
Physical form of vitamin	Formulation variables (coatings, counter-ions, emulsifiers, etc.)
	Physical interactions with other food components
Composition of diet/food	Digestibility (protein, fat, fiber)
	Influence on intestinal digestion processes
	Influence on intestinal emulsification and absorption of lipids and fat-soluble vitamins
	Influence on intestinal absorption processes
	Intestinal transit time
	Influence of diet on intestinal microflora
Non-food antagonists	Impaired absorption or metabolism caused by pharmaceuticals or alcohol
Intrinsic	
Age of individual	Developmental changes in digestive function
	Age-induced changes in gastrointestinal function
Species	Human versus animal model
	Is animal model appropriate?
Health	Digestive function (e.g., secretion of gastric HCl and pepsin, pancreatic enzymes, and bile acids)
	Nutritional status

[a] Table reproduced with permission from Reference 43.

emptying. In spite of the large amount of information available on folate bioavailability, knowledge of this important part of folate nutrition has been recently described as fragmentary.[12] Informative reviews include those by Gregory,[15,46,53] Bailey,[45] and Hawkes and Villota.[22]

11.3   METHODS

Methods for folate analysis include bioassays, microbiological, LC, ligand-binding, and radioimmunoassay. LC methods are becoming highly refined and offer the best approach to precisely define specific folate profiles in biological samples. Notable, more recent reviews on methods include Gregory,[15] Ball,[16] Mullin and Duch,[20] and Eitenmiller and Landen.[54] Keagy[55] reviewed chick and rat bioassays. Folate analysis is complicated by the multiple metabolic forms present in biological samples, variable γ-glutamyl polymer lengths of 2 to 12, and instability, which must be of primary concern to all analysts involved with folate assay. Many older, established procedures are available in published compendiums and handbooks. These methods are summarized in Table 11.5; however, folate analysis is rapidly advancing and newer methods offer many advantages.

11.3.1   MICROBIOLOGICAL

11.3.1.1   Folate Assay Organisms

Three bacteria and the protozoan *Tetrahymena pyriformis* have been used for folate assay. The bacteria, *Lactobacillus rhamnosus* ATCC No. 7469 (formerly *L. casei*), *Enterococcus hirae* ATCC No. 8043 (formerly *Streptococcus faecalis*), and *Pediococcus acidilactici,* ATCC No. 8081 (formerly *P. cerevisiae*) have different responses to the folates available in biological matrices. Their responses and the limited information available on the response of *T. pyriformis* are shown in Table 11.6. *L. rhamnosus* is the most commonly used and most accepted organism for folate analysis of natural products. It responds to natural folate forms present in biologicals, and does not respond to pteroic acid—a common folate degradation product. *E. hirae* lacks specificity in that it does not respond to 5-methyl-H_4 folate, the most common folate present in milk, other foods, tissue, and serum, and does respond to pteroic acid.[56] None of the organisms efficiently responds to γ-glutamyl folate with greater than three glutamic acid residues. *L. rhamnosus* has greater capacity for response to the γ-glutamyl folate polymers compared to the other assay organisms; however, its response is limited to no greater than three glutamates with much lower response to higher polymeric folates. The response of *L. rhamnosus* to pteGlu$_3$ has been shown to be less than to folic acid and pteGlu$_2$.[57] Lack of response to the higher γ-glutamyl folate polymers requires γ-glutamyl hydrolase (conjugase) treatment during the extraction phase of the assay (Section 11.3.1.2.1) for each of the bacteria. *P. acidilactici* has the most limited response and can grow on only mono-, di-, and triglutamates of 5- or 10-HCO-H_4 folate. It does not respond to methyl-substituted folates.[16]

Even though *L. rhamnosus* is considered to be the best available bacteria for folate assay of food and other biologicals, its ability to respond equally on a molar basis to metabolically active folates has been questioned.[57] Goli and Vanderslice[57] reported significant growth response differences to various folates. Under the conditions of their study, the relative growth response to H_2 folate and H_4 folate were only 29% and 15% at higher vitamin concentration levels compared to folic acid. Response to 5-CH_3-H_4 folate, 5-CHO-H_4 folate, and 10-HCO-H_4 folate were 83%, 115%, and 95%, respectively, compared to folic acid. Reports of growth variations by *L. rhamnosus* are not common. Newman and Tsai[58] reported small differences between folic acid, 5-CH_3-H_4 folate, and 5-HCO-H_4 folate using a microtiter plate technique. Since standard curves are, in most circumstances, established with folic acid when the assay organism is *L. rhamnosus,* unequal growth response to the naturally occurring forms in a biological sample could significantly affect accuracy. Therefore, all analysts using the *L. rhamnosus* assay should determine growth response under their laboratory con-

TABLE 11.5
Compendium, Regulatory and Handbook Methods for Analysis of Folate

Source	Form	Methods and Application	Approach	Most Current Cross-Reference
U.S. Pharmacopeia National Formulary, 1995, USP23/NF18[1]				
1. pages 2142, 2146, 2148, 2152	Pteroylglutamic acid	Folic acid in oil- and water-soluble vitamin capsules/tables w/wo minerals	HPLC 280 nm	None
2. pages 2160, 2166, 2169, 2172	Pteroylglutamic acid	Folic acid in water-soluble vitamin capsules/tables w/wo minerals	HPLC 280 nm	None
3. pages 691–692	Pteroylglutamic acid	Folic Acid (NLT 95.0%, NMT 102.0%)	HPLC 254 nm	None
4. page 692	Pteroylglutamic acid	Folic acid Injection/tablets	HPLC 254 nm	None
British Pharmacopoeia, 15th ed., 1993[2]				
1. vol. II, pages 293–294	Pteroylglutamic acid	Folic acid	Spectrophotometric 550 nm	None
2. vol. II, pages 922–923	Pteroylglutamic acid	Folic acid tablets	HPLC 283 nm	None
3. addend., 1996, pages 1725–1726	Calcium folinate	Calcium folinate 280 nm	HPLC	None
AOAC Official Methods of Analysis, 16th ed., 1995[3]				
1. 45.2.03	Pteroylglutamic acid	AOAC Official Method 944.12, Folic Acid (Pteroylglutamic acid) in Vitamin Preparations	Microbiological	
2. 50.1.21	Pteroylglutamic acid and naturally occurring forms	AOAC Official Method 992.05 Folic Acid (Pteroylglutamic acid) in Infant Formula	Microbiological	*J. AOAC Int.*, 76, 399, 1993[4]

TABLE 11.5 Continued

Source	Form	Methods and Application	Approach	Most Current Cross-Reference
American Feed Ingredients Association, *Laboratory Methods Compendium*, vol. 1, 1991[5]				
1. pages 83–86	Pteroylglutamic acid and naturally occurring forms	Folic acid in complete feeds and premixes (70.2 µg/kg)	Microbiological	Hoffmann-LaRoche, *Analytical Methods for Vitamins and Carotenoids in Feed*, 1988, 30[6]
Food Chemicals Codex, 4th ed., 1996[7]				
1. page 157	Folic acid	Folic acid (NLT 95.0%, NMT 102.0%)	HPLC 254 nm	None
Hoffmann-LaRoche, *Analytical Methods for Vitamins and Carotenoids in Feed*, 1988[6]				
1. pages 50–52	Folic acid	Microbiological assay of folic acid in complete feeds and premixes	Microbiological	None

TABLE 11.6
Responses Induced by Folate Derivatives Relative to Folic Acid[a]

Folate	L. rhamnosus	E. hirae	P. acidilactici	T. pyriformis
Folic acid	+	+	—	+
H_2 folate	+	+	—	*[b]
H_4 folate	+	+	+	+
5-HCO-H_4 folate	+	+	+	+
10-HCO-H_2 folate	+	+	—	*
10-HCO-H_4 folate	+	+	+	*
5-CH_3-H_4 folate	+	—	—	—
5,10-CH^+ = H_4 folate	+	+	—	*
5-CHNH-H_4 folate	+	+	+	*
PteGlu$_2$	+ (100%)	+	—	+
PteGlu$_3$	+ (100%)	—	—	+
PteGlu$_4$	+ (65%)	—	—	*
PteGlu$_5$	+ (20%)	—	—	*
PteGlu$_6$	+ (3.6%)	—	—	*
PteGlu$_7$	+ (2.4%)	—	—	*
Pteroic acid	—	+	—	—

[a]Table adapted from Reference 56. [b]Asterisk indicates that data is unavailable.

ditions to folic acid and major metabolic forms. Unequal response adds uncertainty to quantitative studies unless response factors are unequivocally proven.[54]

11.3.1.2 Extraction Procedures

11.3.1.2.1 General Requirements

Many procedures exist in the literature for extraction of folates for microbiological analysis, and procedures are still being refined. Some procedures are summarized in Table 11.7. Traditional procedures include homogenization of the sample in buffers containing reducing agents such as ascorbic acid, 2-mercaptoethanol, and dithiothreitol to prevent oxidation. Protection from light and air help to maintain natural folates in their native states. Following homogenization, the sample homogenate is usually heated briefly at 100°C. The initial steps are designed to free the folate from the sample matrix, deproteinate the extract, and protect the native state folates. Additionally, higher fat samples should be defatted to prevent fatty acid stimulation of the growth response of *L. rhamnosus*.[59] Plasma analysis follows similar protocols used for food and other biologicals. Simple dissolution in buffer containing reducing agents is sufficient for pharmaceuticals containing only folic acid.

Biological samples must be hydrolyzed with γ-glutamyl hydrolase, (conjugase) to cleave poly-γ-glutamyl folates to the triglutamate level or lower for growth of *L. rhamnosus* and to lower degrees of polymerization for *E. hirae*. Conjugases from several sources are usable. Chicken pancreas conjugase is specified in AOAC International[60] Methods. Crude, dried chicken pancreas is available commercially and provides a convenient source for the enzyme. Other common sources are hog kidney, rat, and human plasma. Hog kidney, rat, and human plasma conjugase produce monoglutamyl folates and, therefore, serve as the hydrolases for LC methods requiring complete deconjugation. Keagy[55] provides properties of several conjugases used by various investigators (Table 11.8). Unless organisms other than *L. rhamnosus* are used as the assay organism or LC analysis is to be completed that requires only monoglutamates in the digest, chicken pancreas provides a suitable and reliable conjugase source. Properly handled, residual folate from the chicken pancreas preparations will be

TABLE 11.7
Microbiological Assay of Folate in Food and Biologicals

| Matrix | Analyte | Extraction | | | Microorganism | Detection | Reference |
		Buffer	Conjugase	Conditions			
1. Standards	PteGlu$_{1-7}$	0.05 M phosphate, pH 6.1, 0.1% AA	Hog kidney	*Digestion* Digest with HK conjugase Homogenize fresh hog kidney with 3 vol of 0.32% cysteine-HCl adjusted to pH 5.4 Digest 2 h at 37°C Centrifuge, treat with Dowex (5 g/100 mL) at pH 4.5 for 1 h	*L. rhamnosus*	Turbidimetric	*Anal. Biochem.*, 49, 517, 1972[1]
2. Bread, flour	Folate	0.1 M phosphate, pH 6.1 5 mg/mL AA	Hog kidney	Homogenize in buffer Digest with HK conjugase Homogenize fresh hog kidney with 3 vol of 0.32% cysteine-HCl adjusted to pH 5.4 Digest 2 h at 37°C Centrifuge, treat with Dowex (5 g/100 ml) at pH 4.5 for 1 h	*L. rhamnosus*	Turbidimetric	*Cereal Chem.*, 52, 348, 1975[2]
3. Plasma, erythrocytes	5-CH$_3$-H^4 folate	0.05 M phosphate, pH 6.1, 200 mg/100 mL AA	—	Dilute 1 : 10 with water Dilute 1 : 1 with buffer Incubate, 37°C, 20 min	*L. rhamnosus*	Radiometric	*J. Nucl. Med.*, 19, 906, 1978[3]

No. Food	Analyte	Buffer	Enzyme	Procedure	Organism	Method	Reference
4. Spinach	Folate	0.1 M phosphate, pH 7.0, 1% AA	Chicken pancreas	Blend 50–100 g in 50 mL buffer Add 30 mL buffer to 15–20 g homogenate Heat at 100°C, 10 min Cool Digest with CP conjugase 37°C, 24 h	L. rhamnosus	Turbidimetric Radiometric	J. Food Sci., 46, 552, 1981[4]
5. Various foods	Folate	0.05 M phosphate, pH 6.1, 0.5 g/100 mL AA	Chicken pancreas	Homogenize 50–100 g in 200–400 mL buffer Dilute with buffer to 500–1000 mL Boiling water bath, 10 min Dilute with buffer Digest with CP conjugase 37°C, 2 h	L. rhamnosus	Radiometric	J. Nutr., 113, 2192, 1983[5]
6. Various foods	Folate	57 mM AA, pH 6.0	Hog kidney Chicken pancreas	Add diced food to boiling 57 mM AA, pH 6.0, 5 min Homogenize Dilute with 57 mM AA Centrifuge Digest at 37°C, 6 h	L. rhamnosus Growth at pH 6.2 and 6.8	Turbidimetric	Br. J. Nutr., 49, 181, 1983[6]
7–8. Spinach	Folate	0.1 M phosphate, pH 7.0, 0.15% AA	Hog kidney Chicken pancreas	Microwave blanch Homogenize in buffer Autoclave, 121°C, 10 min Centrifuge with HK or CP conjugase, 37°C, 2 h Various conditions were studied	L. rhamnosus	Turbidimetric	Nutr. Rep. Int., 28, 317, 1983[7] J. Food Sci., 49, 94, 1984[8]

TABLE 11.7 Continued

Matrix	Analyte	Extraction Buffer	Conjugase	Conditions	Microorganism	Detection	Reference
9. Plasma	5-HCO-H$_4$ folate	0.1 M K$_2$HPO$_4$, pH 6.1, 0.1% AA	—	Add AA to plasma to 0.5% Dilute to 2 × volume with buffer Incubate, 37°C, 90 min Heat, 100°C, 30 min Centrifuge	L. rhamnosus P. acidilactici	Turbidimetric Microtiter plate assay	Anal. Biochem., 154, 509, 1986[9]
10. Various	Folate foods	0.1 M NaOAC, pH 4.7, 5 g/L AA	Endogenous	Blend 10 g with buffer Incubate, 37°C, 4 h Heat at 100°C Dilute with 0.05 M phosphate buffer, pH 6.1 1.5 g/L AA	L. rhamnosus	Turbidimetric	J. Assoc. Off. Anal. Chem., 69, 773, 1986[10]
11. Spinach, broccoli	Folate	0.1 M phosphate, pH 6.8, 1% AA	Chicken pancreas	Homogenize in buffer Digest with CP conjugase, 37°C, overnight Digest with Pronase® 37°C, 4 h Steam, 5 min Centrifuge	L. rhamnosus	Turbidimetric	J. Food Sci., 51, 626, 1986[11]
12. Food, plasma, diets, tissue	Folate	Food—100 mM phosphate, pH 6.1, 0.5% AA Blood—50 mM phosphate	Hog kidney	Dilute and homogenize in buffer, dilute to final volume of 20 mL Autoclave 10 min, 121°C	L. rhamnosus	Turbidimetric	J. Micronutr. Anal., 3, 55, 1987[12]

	Sample/Analyte	Extraction buffer	Enzyme	Procedure	Organism	Method	Reference
13. Various foods	Folate	pH 6.1, 1% AA *Orange juice*— 100 mM phosphate, pH 6.1, 0.2% AA 0.2 M phosphate, pH 6.1, 5 g AA	Chicken pancreas Hog kidney	Autoclave samples in 100 mL buffer, 5 min, 121°C Homogenize, if necessary Filter, dilute with buffer Keep frozen at −20°C Digest with CP conjugase, incubate 37°C, overnight Digest with HK conjugase, incubate 37°C, 6 h Make up to 10 mL with buffer (pH 4.6 for HK, pH 6.1 for CP) Incubate for 2h or 20 h, 37°C, overnight Steam, dilute Add amylase and amyloglucosidase Centrifuge both digest and non-digest (37°C, 4 h) with HK conjugase	*L. rhamnosus*	Turbidimetric	*Br. J. Nutr.*, 59, 261, 1988[13]
14. Standards	PteGlu.H$_4$ folate H$_2$ folate 5-CH$_3$-H$_4$ folate 5-CHO-H$_2$ folate 10-CHO-H$_2$ folate	pH 6.1, 0.05 M phosphate buffer, 0.15% AA	—	*PteGlu*— Dissolve in 0.1 M NaOH in 20% ethanol *Others*— Dissolve in 0.05 M Tris buffer, pH 7.5 with 0.05 M 2-MCE	*L. rhamnosus*	CO$_2$ analyzer Turbidimetric	*J. Micronutr. Anal.*, 6, 19, 1989[14]

TABLE 11.7 Continued

Matrix	Analyte	Extraction			Microorganism	Detection	Reference
		Buffer	Conjugase	Conditions			
15–20. Infant formula Baby foods Cowpea flour Various foods Feeds	Folate	(A)—0.1 M sodium phosphate (dibasic), 1% AA, pH 6.8 16.—1.42% sodium phosphate 1% AA, pH 6.8	Chicken pancreas Pronase®	Blend composited food Homogenize in buffer Digest with CP conjugase, incubate overnight, 37°C Add 0.2% Pronase®, incubate, 37°C, 4 h	L. rhamnosus	Turbidimetric	J. Micronutr. Anal., 7, 37, 1990[15] J. Assoc. Off. Anal. Chem., 73, 805, 1990[16] J. Sci. Food Agri., 64, 389, 1994[17] Poultry Sci., 74, 1447, 1995[18] Poultry Sci., 74, 1456, 1995[19] J. Food Sci., 61, 1039, 1996[20]
21. Standards	PteGlu$_{1-7}$	(A)—0.05 M tris buffer, pH 7.5 (B)—0.10 M phosphate buffer, 0.10% AA, pH 4.5 (C)—0.1 M phosphate buffer, 0.17% AA, pH 6.0, 6.5, 7.2 (D)—0.1 M phosphate buffer, 0.1% AA, pH 7.2	Human blood plasma Chicken pancreas	Stock solution— PteGlu$_{1-7}$ in buffer (A) Conjugase treatment Dilute stock solution in buffer (B) Incubate 3 h or 20 h with 100 mM 2-MCE 0.2 M sodium acetate buffer, pH 4.5, plasma and toluene Digest with plasma conjugase with buffer (C) Digest with CP conjugase with buffer (D)	L. rhamnosus	CO$_2$ analyzer	Food Chem., 143, 57, 1992[21]

No.	Sample	Analyte	Buffer	Enzyme	Procedure	Organism	Method	Reference
22.	Serum and red cells	Folate	0.5% sodium ascorbate	—	Dilute serum and red cell lysate in sodium ascorbate Mix and add to plate wells	L. rhamnosus	Microtiter plate technique Turbidimetric	J. Clin. Pathol., 45, 344, 1992[22]
23.	Infant formula	Folate	0.05 M phosphate buffer 0.05 M phosphate buffer + 0.05% AA	Chicken pancreas	Reconstitute powders and adjust to volume 100 mL with water or Dilute liquids and adjust to 100 mL with water Pipet 1 mL dilute sample and 1 mL CP conjugase Add buffer (A) Add 18 mL buffer (B) and 1 mL toluene Incubate 16 h, 37°C	L. rhamnosus	Tritimetric Turbidimetric	J. AOAC Int., 76, 399, 1993[23]
24.	Multivitamin formulations	PetGlu	A—0.1 M phosphate buffer, pH 8.0 B—0.05 M phosphate buffer, 0.05% AA, pH 6.1	—	Shake samples with 50 mL buffer (A), 15 min Autoclave 5 min, 121°C Centrifuge Prepare different dilutions of sample with buffer (B)	S. faecalis	Microplate	J. AOAC Int., 78, 1173, 1995[24]
25.	Freeze dried space shuttle foods Frozen vegetables	Folate	50 mm Hepes/Ches buffer, pH 7.85	Chicken pancreas	Heat 10 g aliquot of sample 100°C, 10 min, with buffer Homogenize Digest (modified trienzyme Martin et al., 1990)	L. rhamnosus	Microplate	J. Food Sci., 60, 538, 1995[25]

TABLE 11.7 Continued

| Matrix | Analyte | Extraction | | | Microorganism | Detection | Reference |
		Buffer	Conjugase	Conditions			
26. Mixed foods	Folate	A—0.1 M potassium phosphate buffer, 57 mM AA, pH 6.3 B—As (A), pH 4.1	Chicken pancreas	Homogenize dietary composites in buffer (A) Mix homogenate with 2 vol of buffer (B)	L. rhamnosus	Microplate Turbidimetric	J. Agri. Food Chem., 45, 135, 1997[26]
27. Cereal-grain products	Folate 5-CH₃-H₂ folate 10-CHO-H₂ folate 10-CHO-folate 5-CHO-H₂ folate PteGlu	50 mM Hepes/Ches buffer, pH 7.85 containing 2% (W/V) AA and 10 mM 2-MCE	Rat plasma conjugase	Add 2 g dry sample to buffer, mix Boil 10 min Homogenize Digest with rat plasma or trienzyme treatment (Martin et al., 1990)	L. rhamnosus	PDA, HPLC Turbidimetric	J. Agri. Food Chem., 45, 407, 1997[27]

TABLE 11.8
Properties of γ-Glutamyl Hydrolases Used for Folate Assay

Source	pH Optimum	Glutamate Residues in Product
Chicken pancreas	7.8	2
Hog kidney	4.5	1
Rat pancreas	5.5–6.0	1
Human jejunum	4.5	1
Human plasma	6.5	1
Liver	4.5	1
Cabbage	5.0	1 or 2
Cabbage	8.0	2

Table adapted from Reference 55.

low and will not interfere with the assay. A method provided by Keagy[55] can be used to produce a low folate chicken pancreas preparation. Steps in the clean up are the following:

1. Suspend 10 g of dessicated chicken pancreas (Difco) in 300 mL 0.1 M phosphate buffer, pH 7.0. Stir 1 h at room temperature.
2. Incubate overnight at 30°C under toluene, centrifuge.
3. Mix the supernatant with an equal volume of 0.1 M tricalcium phosphate gel suspension (Sigma) for 30 min. Cool in an ice bath. Centrifuge cold.
4. Cool the upper layer below 5°C and slowly add an equal volume of ice cold ethanol with vigorous stirring. Refrigerate overnight.
5. Centrifuge. Dissolve precipitate in 100 mL of 0.1 M phosphate buffer, pH 7.0, by stirring. Container should be kept cold in an ice bath.
6. Centrifuge. Mix supernatant with 10% by weight of Dowex 1 × 8 (chloride) for 1 h at 0°C.
7. Remove Dowex by centrifugation and filter the supernatant through gauze.
8. Store frozen in volumes required for batch usage depending on laboratory requirements.

Goli and Vanderslice[61] reported that *L. rhamnosus* response to di- and triglutamates was 90% and 60%, respectively, compared to the response to folic acid. Use of plasma conjugase at pH 4.5 produces monoglutamates, but significant folate degradation. The authors recommend pH 6.0 for use of plasma conjugase. Chicken pancreas conjugase yields a mixture of mono- and diglutamate folates at pH 6.0 and pH 7.0. The authors cautioned that a commonly used hog kidney conjugase digestion at pH 4.9 might lead to substantial folate degradation. Conversely, use of 0.05 M sodium acetate buffer, with 1% ascorbate was reported to give greater stability during extraction than at pH 7.0.[15,19] Gregory[15] concluded that mildly acidic buffers containing ascorbate are generally useful for folate extraction from most matrices.

11.3.1.2.2 Buffers and Antioxidants

Many different buffer systems and stabilizing antioxidants have been used to extract folate from biological samples. Recent work is beginning to give a clearer picture of required parameters for optimal extraction. Buffer systems provide optimal pH conditions for enzymatic deconjugation in later extraction steps.[15] Examination of the methods for microbiological assay given in Table 11.7 shows that phosphate buffers are used for pHs between pH 6.1 and 7.0 for use with chicken pancreas and hog kidney conjugase. Although the pH optimum of hog kidney conjugase is 4.5, use of buffers near pH 6.0 gives sufficient deconjugation, and avoids reported loss of folate at lower pH levels.[27] At pH

4.9, folate is stable at 100°C for 60 min if 1.0% ascorbate is present.[15] Acetate buffer has been used in conjunction with plasma conjugase for both blood and food analysis; however, acetate inhibits this conjugase.[27,61]

Phosphate buffer, pH 6.0, containing 52 mM (1%) ascorbic acid/ascorbate and 0.1% 2-mercaptoethanol is an excellent extractant for foods prior to HPLC analysis. This buffer system could be easily incorporated into microbiological assay protocols. The addition of the 2-mercaptoethanol produced better folate stability than use of only ascorbic acid. As discussed in Section 11.3.1.2.1, use of 0.05 M sodium acetate buffer, pH 4.9, with 1% ascorbate stabilizes folates during extraction. Acidic systems increase the stability of ascorbic acid, and are thought to eliminate degradation products from the extraction solution that can interact with the folate.[25]

Studies by Wilson and Horne[25,62] led to the use of 50 mM N-2-hydroxyethylpiperazine-N'-ethanesulfonic acid (Hepes), 50 mM 2-(N-cyclohexylamino) ethanesulfonic acid (Ches) containing 100 mM sodium ascorbate and 200 mM 2-mercaptoethanol, pH 7.85, for folate extraction from biological samples. The buffer is now commonly referred to as the Wilson and Horne buffer. The buffer system avoids folate interconversions attributed to ascorbate degradation products. Gregory et al.[63] evaluated the Wilson and Horne buffer (Hepes/Ches), pH 7.85; acetate buffer with 1% ascorbate, pH 4.9, and phosphate buffer with 1% ascorbate, pH 7.0, and found that the Wilson and Horne buffer was superior for folate extraction. Since this work, the Wilson and Horne buffer has been used by several investigators with good success.[27,64,65]

11.3.1.2.3 Trienzyme Extractions

Folate extraction is often optimized from foods by the addition of α-amylase and/or protease digestion to the conjugase digestion protocol. Yamada[66] in 1979 reported that total measurable folate could be significantly increased by addition of protease digestion during extraction to the traditional thermal extraction and conjugase digestion. The effect was demonstrated with human milk, hog liver, and cod muscle. Other researchers showed that addition of α-amylase digestion increased folate extraction from high starch and glycogen products.[67,68] Polysaccharide binding was demonstrated.[67] DeSouza and Eitenmiller[69] incorporated previous studies in development of a trienzyme approach to folate extraction applicable to most foods. The method substantially increased measurable folate from many food samples and was particularly effective on cereal-based and dairy products. The broad specificity protease from *Streptomyces griseus,* Pronase®, and α-amylase together with chicken pancreas conjugase constituted the trienzyme treatment. The DeSouza and Eitenmiller procedure was adapted into analysis protocols at the Atlanta Center for Nutrient Analysis for folate analysis of FDA Total Diet Market Basket Samples.[70] The standard operating procedure for the FDA Total Diet method is given in Section 11.4.

Further application of the trienzyme method did not occur until recently. Tamura et al.[64] in 1997 used the trienzyme method with modified buffers and order of enzyme addition, and showed significant increase in measurable folates in many food mixtures compared to traditional conjugase digestion. The suggestion was made that food composition databases should be revised using the trienzyme extraction. Such observations dramatically substantiate recommendations made by DeSouza and Eitenmiller[69] and Martin et al.[70] that traditional conjugase digestions may significantly underestimate the true folate value of the food supply. Another recent study has shown the applicability and worth of the trienzyme methodology for analysis of cereal-based foods. Pfeiffer et al.[65] modified the original methodology[69,70] by using Hepes/Ches buffer, pH 7.85, and rat plasma conjugase and quantitated the folate by HPLC. The trienzyme treatment led to variable increases of measured total folates in the products studied. Overall, significant increases as high as 34% were obtained. Additionally, close agreement to microbiological results were obtained by the HPLC method when the trienzyme digests were assayed by both methods. The authors concluded that the trienzyme extraction is applicable to both HPLC and microbiological assays, and that traditional methods of extraction are not appropriate for folate assay of cereal-grain products. The Pfeiffer et al.[65] method is provided in Section 11.4.

11.3.1.3 Modification of Traditional Microbiological Assays for Folate

Traditional microbiological assays have been modified to increase speed and decrease labor intensiveness. Microtiter 96-well plates and autoplate readers have been successfully used in several laboratories.[68,71,72,73,74,75,76] Additionally, rapid microbiological procedures based upon release of $^{14}CO_2$[77] and the use of CO_2[57] analyzers have been developed which offer significant time savings. Such methods generally provide good agreement with traditional microassay techniques. Use of the microtiter plate assay should be seriously considered by all laboratories involved in microbiological vitamin analysis. Significant savings in labor and materials are obtainable. Detection limits are comparable to traditional methods as well as precision. Readers are encouraged to read Tamura's excellent review on use of the 96-well microplate assay.[71] This laboratory has been a pioneer in use of such assays. Techniques for the microplate assay are provided by Tamura.[71]

11.3.1.4 Recommendations for the Microbiological Assay of Folate

1. Traditional extraction procedures for foods should be modified in light of recent research findings.[64,65,67,68,69]
2. Modified trienzyme extractions as published by Tamura et al.[64] and Pfeiffer et al.[65] offer viable approaches for improved folate extraction from foods.
3. Extraction buffers based on the Wilson and Horne buffer, pH 7.85, or the phosphate buffer, pH 6.0, of Vahteristo et al.[27] are excellent stabilization systems. Both extractants contain ascorbic acid and 2-mercaptoethanol.
4. *L. rhamnosus* should be the assay organism for natural products. *E. hirae* is suitable for products containing only folic acid.
5. Microplate methods offer significant savings in time and materials.

Traditional microbiological techniques can be modified to the microplate procedures.

11.3.1.5 AOAC International Official Methods

AOAC International[60] does not provide HPLC methods for folate assay. Methods currently available use either *E. hirae* ATCC No. 8043 or *L. rhamnosus* ATCC No. 7469 for microbiological assay.

AOAC Official Method 944.12, Folic Acid (Pteroylglutamic Acid) in
Vitamin Preparations, Microbiological Method, AOAC Official Methods
of Analysis, 45.2.03

Method 944.12 uses the response of *E. hirae* for measurement of folic acid in pharmaceutical products formulated with folic acid. The method is not designed for assay of naturally occurring forms because *E. hirae* does not respond to $5\text{-}CH_3\text{-}H_4$ folates. Additionally, the method does not provide extraction conditions necessary for extraction and deconjugation of poly-γ-glutamyl folates. The extraction procedure for vitamin preparations has the following steps:

1. Add water equal in mL to greater than or equal to ten times the dry weight of sample. Folic acid concentration must be less than or equal to 1.0 mg folic acid/mL.
2. Add equivalent of 2 mL NH_4OH (2 + 3) /100 mL liquid.
3. Disperse, wash down sides of flask with 0.1 N NH_4OH.
4. Autoclave, 121 to 123°C, 15 min.

5. Cool and filter or centrifuge.
6. Dilute, adjust to pH 6.8.

AOAC Official Method 992.05, Folic Acid (Pteroylglutamic Acid) in
Infant Formula, Microbiological Method, AOAC Official Methods
of Analysis, *50.1.21*

Method 992.05 is applicable only to the assay of folic acid in infant formula. *L. rhamnosus* is the
assay organism. While the method is not intended for measurement of total folate, a conjugase digestion step is included in the extraction, so the method undoubtedly measures folate originating from
natural ingredients.[54] Extraction steps include the following:

1. Reconstitute or dilute formula with water to a concentration of ca 5 μg folic acid per
   100 mL.
2. Pipet 1 mL diluted sample and 1 mL chicken pancreas preparation into 18 × 150 mm
   screw top culture tubes, mix. Add 18 mL 0.05 *M* phosphate-ascorbate buffer (50 mg
   ascorbic acid/100 mL).
3. Add 1 mL toluene.
4. Incubate for 16 h at 37°C.
5. Autoclave, 121°C, 10 min.
6. Centrifuge.
7. Dilute with 0.05 *M* phosphate-ascorbate buffer to required folic acid concentration.

AOAC International does not provide a collaborated method for total folates in natural products.
However, the trienzyme extraction has been used to measure folates in FDA Total Diet samples at
the Atlanta Center for Nutrient Analysis.[70] The procedure essentially uses methodology developed
by DeSouza and Eitenmiller[69] at the University of Georgia (Section 11.3.1.2.3). The FDA standard
operating procedure (SOP N/AM/4/0/94) is provided in Section 11.4. The trienzyme extraction
increases folate values in many foods compared with the traditional conjugase digestion; however,
as previously discussed in Section 11.3.1.2.3, the effects can not be predicted by food matrix type.
The FDA approach has been to apply the trienzyme procedure to all total diet samples to ensure maximal assay results.

11.3.2   LIGAND BINDING ASSAYS

Various biospecific methods using ligand binding have been developed for folate analysis of clinical and food samples. Biospecific methods for water-soluble vitamins were classified into two
groups by Finglas and Morgan.[78] Methods based upon the specific interaction of antibody with its
antigen include radioimmunoassay (RIA) and enzyme-linked immunoabsorbent assay (ELISA).
Assays using naturally occurring vitamin binding proteins with isotope labels or enzyme labels
include radio-labeled protein binding assays (RPBA) based on isotope dilution procedures and
enzyme protein binding assays (EPBA).

Folate assay methods have been developed using each of these ligand binding approaches.
RPBA procedures and to a limited extent EPBA methods are used for folate assay of clinical samples. Such methods have largely replaced use of microbiological methods for the assay of folate in
blood and serum.[74] Because of the significance to clinical laboratory operations, the performance of
the most widely-used techniques have been extensively evaluated and compared to microbiological
and LC methods for the analysis of serum, blood, and erythrocyte folate levels. Two such extensive
studies of commercial RPBA kits were conducted by the Center for Food Safety and Applied
Nutrition (CFSAN), FDA, and Centers for Disease Control (CDC) in the United States, and by the
Food-Linked Agro-Industrial Research Program (FLAIR) in the European Community. These stud-

ies have been widely discussed in the scientific literature. Reports that analysts should read before attempting to initiate blood analysis using RPBA techniques include conclusive papers on both the U.S. and EC studies.[80,81] Both reports discussed problems with standards used for calibration of available kits up to 1994. Overestimation of serum and red blood cell folate values occurred over several years and produced questionable data regarding folate status. Since the commercial kits were used in the U.S. National Health and Nutrition Surveys (II and III), the calibration problems led to the extensive study. FLAIR comparative studies showed that commercial diagnostic kits were subject to between-kit and between-laboratory variability. Also, RPBA results often did not compare with LC or microbiological analyses. FLAIR recommendations include the need for further standardization and optimization of assay and extraction procedures, the need for appropriate, clinically, and nutritionally relevant reference materials, and more extensive information on kit calibrants from manufacturers. Further, laboratories using the kits should verify reference standards, before use, by use of pure, calibrated standards, and in-house quality control samples. All can learn from the European and U.S. experiences earlier in this decade. Quality assurance programs are now demanding proper control of problems associated with the extensive use of RPBA kits in clinical situations.

Wigertz and Jägerstad[79] compared LC folate analysis of milk and blood to data obtained by a commercial RPBA assay. Their data showed that the RPBA method overestimated H_4 folate. Plasma folate values were higher as measured by RPBA and compared to LC values. LC profiles showed only 5-methyltetrahydrofolate in the plasma. Overestimation by RPBA was thought to be owing to the use of folic acid rather than 5-methyltetrahydrofolate as the calibrating standard. It has been known for many years that milk folate binding protein has greater affinity for folic acid than for 5-methyl-tetrahydrofolate between pH 7.2 and 8.0. At pH 9.3, binding affinity was equal.[15]

Use of competitive binding assays for food analysis have been hampered by problems arising from variation of ligand binding affinity for the multiple folate forms present in many foods.[15,54] Gregory[15] stated the following, "On the basis of the known specificity of the bovine milk folate-binding protein, it is difficult to rationalize studies reporting good correlation between the results of competitive binding and microbiological assays." Even if the RPBA is completed at pH 9.3, RPBA results frequently do not compare to microbiological assay results. DeSouza and Eitenmiller[69] found good agreement between RPBA and microbiological assay of infant formula which contains predominantly folic acid added during manufacture, but poor agreement for assay of baby foods containing natural folates. Such differences in results by microbiological and radioassay procedures are common throughout the literature on application of RPBA to food analysis. Recent comparison of HPLC, microbiological, and RPBA assays of milk show close agreement.[41,79] This is expected since up to 95% of the folate in milk is 5-methyltetrahydrofolate.

Another approach to FBPA for food analysis has been developed by Finglas et al.[82,83] The method utilized a folate binding protein-peroxidase conjugate and did not use isotopes. The EPBA assay showed similar responses for 5-formyltetrahydrofolate and 5-methyltetrahydrofolate. The authors stressed that folic acid must be used for calibration if fortified foods are assayed. The method was used to assay raw and cooked vegetables with good comparative results to microbiological assay by *L. rhamnosus*. Analysis time was four hours by EPBA compared to two to three days for the microbiological assay. The method was included in a Community Bureau of Reference of the Commission of the European Communities (BRC) comparative study.[84] Results between laboratories varied from 378 to 1051 μg/100 g when human plasma conjugase was used in the analysis with EPBA assay of a reference brussels sprout sample. Similar large variations occurred with use of chicken pancreas conjugase. The conclusion was that EPBA and RPBA methods for food analysis are limited by the response of the binding protein to natural folate forms, and that application of the ligand binding methods "may yield tenuous results." Failure to obtain acceptable ligand binding assays for folate analysis of foods leads to the need for good LC methods. As discussed in the next section, LC methods have been significantly improved and can be routinely applied in food analysis programs for folate.

11.3.3 HIGH PERFORMANCE LIQUID CHROMATOGRAPHY

HPLC methods for folate analysis have been refined to the point that most analytical laboratories equipped with modern LC systems and detectors, specifically a fluorescent or photodiode array detector, can successfully assay naturally occurring folates. The primary advantage of LC analysis is the ability to quantify the specific folate forms and, if so desired, the γ-glutamylfolate polymers. Such specificity is not obtainable by other methods. Several excellent reviews of HPLC methods are available.[15,16,20] Our attention will be given to a few recently published methods that have advanced the LC analysis of folate. Additionally, method summaries provided in Table 11.9 give details of extraction methods and LC chromatography and detection parameters. The papers included in Table 11.9 were chosen from the standpoint to provide an historical perspective of method development for the LC analysis of folate in food and clinical samples. The methods were carefully chosen from a quite large pool of LC method development papers on folate analysis.

11.3.3.1 Folate Extraction for LC Analysis

Procedures for extraction of folate have their basis in studies completed for microbiological assay in earlier decades. Such information discussed in Section 11.3.1.2 has been refined for preparatory methods useful for LC analysis. Procedural steps include the following:

1. *Dispersion or Homogenization in a Stabilizing Buffer*—Buffer systems were discussed in Section 11.3.1.2 for microbiological assays. Buffers must contain a stabilizing agent to protect labile folates from oxidative degradation. For food analysis, recent papers recommend the addition of ascorbic acid and 2-mercaptoethanol.[27,65] The Wilson and Horne buffer contains 2% ascorbate and 0.2 M 2-mercaptoethanol. Other researchers use only ascorbic acid with good results.[79,85] Ascorbic acid can not be used with electrochemical (EC) detection owing to high background current.[86] Lucock et al.[26,86] recommended dithiothreitol for stabilization of plasma in conjunction with EC detection. In a recent paper, Lucock et al.[87] indicated that ascorbic acid and dithiothreitol are suitable antioxidants for most biological samples depending on detection systems and pH conditions. Thus, these antioxidants should be used selectively. Ascorbic acid is most effective under acid conditions, and dithiothreitol is most effective at neutral pH. Antioxidants convert 5-methyldihydrofolates to reduced forms. 5-Methyltetrahydrofolic acid is stabilized at pH 7.3 and pH 9.0 by dithiothreitol, but not at pH 3.5.[26] For quantitation of 10-formyltetrahydrofolate, the Wilson and Horne buffer at pH 7.85 is useful, preventing thermal conversion of the 10-formyl form to 5-formyltetrahydrofolate.[15] Additionally, 5-formyltetrahydrofolate is unstable under acidic conditions.[20]

2. *Destruction of Sample Matrix and Release of Folates*—In order to facilitate later determinative steps and ensure complete folate extraction, biological samples are usually heated at 100°C or autoclaved to precipitate proteins and inactive enzymes that catalyze folate oxidation or interconversion. Additionally, enzyme digestion by α-amylase and protease is now becoming accepted as necessary to completely free non-specifically bound folates (Section 11.3.1.2.3). Thermal treatment has been considered sufficient to free folate from specific folate binding proteins. Extraction of serum includes protein removal by perchloric acid, heating, or addition of organic solvents (acetonitrile, acetone).[20] Various extraction approaches for serum are provided in procedures summarized in Table 11.9. Solid phase extraction (SPE) is finding increased use as an integral step in serum extractions. Urine can be diluted, treated by SPE, and directly injected.[88] Extensive studies in Finland by Vahteristo and colleagues[27,85,89,90,91] on the LC quantitation of folates in food use SPE clean up by strong anion exchange following deconjugation by hog kidney conjugase. The extracts are relatively free of chromatographic interference. Affinity chromatography, discussed below,

TABLE 11.9
HPLC Methods for the Analysis of Folates in Food, Feeds, Pharmaceuticals and Biologicals

| | Sample Preparation | | | | HPLC Parameters | | | | |
Sample Matrix	Analyte	Sample Extraction	Clean Up	Column	Mobile Phase	Detection	Quality Assurance Parameters	References
Food								
1–2. Fortified cereal, beef liver	Folic acid 5-CH$_3$-H$_4$ folate H$_2$-folate 5-CHO-H$_4$ folate and/or 10-CHO-H$_4$ folate	*Infant formula—* Dilute with 0.1 M KH$_2$PO$_4$, 0.25% AA, pH 7.0 Adjust pH to 4.5 Centrifuge, filter (0.45 µm) *Cereal—* Homogenize in 0.1 M KH$_2$PO$_4$, 0.25% AA, pH 7.0 Centrifuge; filter *Liver—* Homogenize in 0.1 M KOAC, 0.25% AA, pH 4.0 Incubate, 37 °C, 2 h Heat, 100 °C, 10 min Centrifuge	Liver Biobeads SM-2	Ultrasphere IP 25 cm × 4.6 mm in series with µBondapak phenyl 30 cm × 3.9 mm Pre-column silica 25 cm × 4.6 mm	Isocratic 0.033 M KH$_2$PO$_4$: MeCN : pH 2.3 (91.5 : 9.5) 0.7 mL/min	Post-column oxidation by Ca hypochlorite to form highly fluorescent pterin fragments Fluorescence Ex λ = 365 Em λ = 415 or UV 280 nm	DL (ng) On-column 2–40 (UV) 0.2–0.9 (Fluorescence) % Recovery 65–82	*J. Agric. Food Chem.* 29, 374, 1981[1] *J. Food Sci.,* 47, 1568, 1982[2]
3. Pharmaceuticals, infant formula, meal replacer, egg replacer	Folic acid	*Pharmaceuticals—* Extract with 0.05 M phosphate/citrate buffer, pH 8.0, containing 0.5 mg/mL	Infant formula DEAE cellulose	Spherisorb ODS 10 µm 25 cm × 4.6 mm	Gradient A— 0.1 M NaOAC, pH 4.0 : MeCN (98 : 2) B— 0.1 M NaOAC, pH 4.0 : MeCN (70 : 30)	280 nm	DL (ng) On-column 4.6 % CV 5.9–6.8	*J. Liq. Chromatogr.,* 5, 953, 1982[3]

TABLE 11.9 Continued

Sample Matrix	Analyte	Sample Preparation		HPLC Parameters				References
		Sample Extraction	Clean Up	Column	Mobile Phase	Detection	Quality Assurance Parameters	
		AA			100% A to 100% B in 30 min 1 mL/min		% Recovery 96–98	
		Infant formula— Disperse in water Dilute with phosphate/citrate/AA buffer Digest with papain, 40 °C, < 4 h or overnight Centrifuge Filter						
4. Various foods	Folic acid H_2 folate H_4 folate 5-CH_3-H_4 folate 5-CHO-H_4 folate	Add 0.05 *M* NaOAC, pH 4.9, containing 1% AA Add 50 μL 2-octanol Homogenize with Polytron Bubble N_2 through sample Seal Incubate, 100°C, 60 min Centrifuge Remove supernatant Digest with HK conjugase, 37°, 60 min Adjust to pH 7.0	DEAE- Sephadex	A-25 Guard column C_{18}, 10μm 30 cm × 4.6 mm Analytical μBondapak Phenyl 10 μm 30 cm × 3.9 mm	Gradient 7.2 to 11.3% MeCN in 0.033 *M* Phosphate, pH 2.3 over 15 min 1 mL/min	Post-column oxidation by Ca hypochlorite to form highly fluorescent pterin fragments Fluorescence Ex λ = 365 Em λ = 415	DL (pmol/mL) On-column 0.03–2.3 QL (nmol/g) 0.01-1.1 % Recovery 68.3–107	*J. Nutr.*, 114, 341, 1984[4]

Sample	Analytes	Sample preparation	SPE / column prep	Column	Mobile phase	Detection	Performance	Reference
5. Commercial diets	Folic acid	Disperse in 0.01 M phosphate, pH 7.4 Filter	SPE Bond elute Quaternary amino anion-exchange	μBondapak C	Isocratic 0.01 M NaOAC, pH 5.7 : MeCN (94 : 6) 2 mL/min	365 nm or PDA	% Recovery 100–102	*J. Liq. Chromatogr.*, 7, 2659, 1984[5]
6. Diets, plasma	Folic acid H$_2$ folate H$_4$ folate 5-CH$_3$-H$_4$ folate 5-CHO-H$_4$ folate 10-CHO-H$_4$ folate	Diet samples Disperse in MeCN : 25 mM Phosphate, pH 7.0 (50 : 50) Sonicate, 5 min	Pre-column automatic switching Nucleosil C$_{18}$ 5 μm Two in series	Spherisorb ODS-2 5 μm 25 cm × 4.6 mm	Isocratic Column switching A—25 mM phosphate buffer, pH 7.0 : MeOH (95 : 5) B—50 mM phosphate buffer, pH 7.0 Precolumn 1—100% B Precolumn 2—100% A Analytical—100% A 1 mL/min	280 nm	DL (pmol) 1-10 % Recovery 90-95	*J. Chromatogr.*, 378, 55, 1986[6]
7. Milk, dairy products	Folic acid H$_2$ folate H$_4$ folate 5-CHO-H$_4$ folate 10-CHO-H$_4$ folate	Adjust pH to 4.5 with HAC Homogenize, Waring blender Centrifuge Decant supernatant Add phosphate buffer, pH 4.5, containing 10% AA and 1 M 2-MCE to concentration of 0.1% AA and 0.1 M 2-MCE Digest with HK conjugase, 37°C, 2 h Centrifuge, filter (0.45 μ8/m)	—	C$_{18}$, Microsorb 3 μm 10 cm × 4.6 mm	Isocratic Phosphate buffer, pH 6.8 : MeOH (50 : 50) containing 50 mL/L of 1.0 M TBAP 1 mL/min	EC + 900 mV vs Ag/AgCl or Fluorescence Ex λ = 238 Em λ = 340 Post-column pH adjustment with 4.25% phosphoric acid or enhancement with hypochlorite oxidation	QL (ng/g) 0.3 - 7.3	*J. Chromatogr.*, 449, 271, 1988[7]
8-9. Various foods	Polyglutamyl folates 1–7 Folic acid 1–7 H$_2$ folate 1–7	Suspend or dilute in solution of 2% AA, 10 mM 2-MCE and 100 mM Bis-Tris, pH 7.8 in autoclave,	Folate binding protein—Sepharose 4B affinity column	Econosphere 5 μm 10 cm × 4.6 mm	Gradient A- 5 mM TBAP, 0.5 mM DET in 25 mM phosphate/ Tris buffer, pH 7.4 or	PDA 350 nm 10-CHO-H$_4$ folate 258 nm	%CV 5–19	*Anal. Biochem.*, 182, 94, 1989[8] *J. Nutr. Biochem.*, 4, 488, 1993[9]

TABLE 11.9 Continued

Sample Matrix	Sample Preparation			HPLC Parameters				References
	Analyte	Sample Extraction	Clean Up	Column	Mobile Phase	Detection	Quality Assurance Parameters	
	H_4 folate 1–7 5-CH_3-H_4 folate 1–7 5-CHO-H_4 folate 1–7 10-CHO-H_4 folate 1–7	30 min Cool Homogenize, Waring blender Centrifuge Mix with [^{3}H] folic acid			25 mM NaCl in water B—5 mM TBAP, 0.5 mM DET in 25 mM phosphate/ Tris buffer, pH 7.4 in MeCN : EtOH : water (64 : 9 : 27) Equilibrate with 90% A, 10% B Increase B to 60% over 40 min 1 mL/min			
10. Various foods	Folic acid PteGlu$_{1-3}$	Homogenize in 50 mM NaOAC, pH 4.9, containing 50.5 mM AA Transfer aliquot to screw cap tube Flush with N_2 Seal Boil, 60 min Cool Centrifuge Adjust pH to 4.9 Filter Digest with HK conjugase	—	Perkin Elmer 3×3 C$_{18}$	Isocratic 0.1 M KOAC, pH 5.0, containing 1.2% MeCN 1.5 mL/min	Post-column oxidation with hypochlorite Fluorescence Ex λ = 365 Em λ = 415	—	*J. Agric. Food Chem.,* 38, 154, 1990[10]

	Analyte	Sample preparation	Cleanup	Column	Mobile phase	Detection	Performance	Reference
11–12. Citrus juice	5-CH3-H4 folate	Centrifuge diluted juice. Adjust pH to 5.0 (1.0 M NaOH). Digest with HK conjugase, 37°, 90 min. Cool. Centrifuge, filter (0.45 μM)	SPE Bond Elut Phenyl. Pre-column backflushed to analytical column	Zorbax ODS C18 5 μm 25 cm × 4.6 mm	Gradient A—MeOH : phosphate/acetate buffer, pH 5.0 (10 : 90) containing 0.005 TBAP B—(30 : 90). Inject into A. B backflushes from pre-column onto analytical column and through detector	EC +200 mV vs Ag/AgCl	% CV 2.8	J. Agric. Food Chem., 38, 1515, 1990[11] 39, 714, 1991[12]
13. Elemental diets	Folic acid	Dissolve in water containing NaCl (10 g/60 mL), 50°C. Allow to stand 30 min at ambient temperature. Dilute to 100 mL with water. Extract with Hex. Inject aqueous layer	—	Capcellpak C18 5 μcm 25 cm × 4.6 mm	MeCN : water (9 : 91) containing 1 mM Na₂EDTA 1 mL/min	360 nm	% Recovery 95	J. Chromatogr., 609, 399, 1992[13]
14. Infant formula Medical foods	Folic acid	Dilute to 15 mL with water. Heat, 100°C, 5 min. Do not heat sterilized samples. Digest with mixture of papain and bacterial protease, 40°C, 1 h. Filter	In-line Strong anion-exchange Bio-Series SAX	Zorbax RX C8 25 cm × 4.6 mm	Gradient A—NaOAC/NaSO₄, pH 5.3 B—640 mL + 360 mL MeCN 0–20 min 100% A 20–33 min 84.5% A—15.5% B 33–40 min To 100% B 40–44 min To 100% B	345 nm	DL (μg/kg) 10 QL (μg/kg) 28 % Recovery 95.9 % CV 3.6	J. AOAC Int., 75, 891, 1992[14]

TABLE 11.9 Continued

Sample Matrix	Analyte	Sample Preparation		HPLC Parameters				References
		Sample Extraction	Clean Up	Column	Mobile Phase	Detection	Quality Assurance Parameters	
15–19. Milk, whole blood, plasma, various foods	Folic acid H_4 folate $5\text{-}CH_3\text{-}H_4$ folate $5\text{-}CHO\text{-}H_4$ folate $10\text{-}CHO$ folic acid	Milk—Add AA to 1% concentration boiling water bath, 15 min Cool Digest with human plasma conjugase (Conjugase in 100 mM 2-MCE, 37°C, 2 h) Discontinued due to low activity of commercial sources, replace with HK conjugase Solid foods, milk powder, whole meal flour—Extract with 5–6 vol 75 mM KH_2PO_4 containing 52 mM AA and 0.1% 2-MCE, pH 6.0 Homogenize under N_2 Add 2-octanol to reduce foaming Microwave 1 min Boiling water bath, 10 min Cool	SPE Baker quaternary amine (N^+) strong anion-exchange	Hypersil ODS 3 μm 15 cm × 4.6 mm	Gradient MeCN : 30 mM KH_2PO_4, pH 2.0 0–4 min 10% MeCN—90% 30 mM KH_2PO_4 To 24% MeCN in 8 min Back to 10% MeCN in 3 min 0.8 mL/min Change gradient to optimize resolution or verify peaks	Fluorescence Ex λ = 290 Em λ = 356 $10\text{-}CHO\text{-}H_4$ folate Ex λ = 360 Em λ = 460	DL (ng) On-column 0.03–0.1 % CV 2.4–11.6 % Recovery 50–90	*Food Chem.,* 57, 109, 1996[15] *J. Agric. Chem.,* 44, 477, 1996[16] *J. Food Sci.,* 61, 524, 1996[17] *J. AOAC Int.,* 80, 373, 1997[18]

					% Recovery	J. Agric. Food Chem., 45, 407, 1997[20]
					87–107	

| | | Folate binding protein-Affigel | Ultremex C$_{18}$ 5 μm 25 cm × 4.6 mm | Gradient A—MeCN B—0.033 M phosphoric acid, pH 2.3 0–8 min Isocratic 5% A, 95% B 8–33 min Linear gradient to 17.5% A 1 mL/min | PDA UV Monitor at 280 nm | |

| 20. Cereal foods | Folic acid 10-CHO-folate 5-CHO-H$_4$ folate 10-CHO-H$_2$ folate 5-CH$_3$-H$_4$ folate | Add 10 volumes Hepes/Ches buffer, pH 7.85 (50 mM Hepes, 50 mM Ches) containing 2% AA and 10 mM 2-MCE Vortex; Boiling water bath, 10 min Cool; Homogenize (Polytron) Digest rat plasma conjugase and ∝-amylase (37°C, 4 h) followed by protease (37°C, 1 h) Boiling water bath, 5 min Cool Centrifuge Resuspend residue in extraction buffer Centrifuge Filter (Whatman #1) Flush, N$_2$) | | | | |

Centrifuge
Redissolve residue with extraction buffer
Centrifuge
Combine extract
Adjust aliquot to pH 4.9
Digest with HK conjugase, 37°C, 2 h
Boiling water bath, 5 min

TABLE 11.9 Continued

Sample Matrix	Analyte	Sample Preparation — Sample Extraction	Clean Up	HPLC Parameters — Column	Mobile Phase	Detection	Quality Assurance Parameters	References
Biologicals								
1–3. Liver	Folic acid	Extract with 100°C buffer containing	—	Ultrasphere I.P. 15 cm × 4.6 mm	Gradient	Microbiological *L. rhamnosus*	—	*Anal. Chem.*, 116, 393, 1981[1]
	H_4 folate	2% AA, 0.2 M 2-MCE,		A—Water				*Anal. Biochem.*, 142, 529, 1984[3]
	5-CH_2-H_4 folate	50 mM Chess, pH 7.5		B—Water:95% EtOH				
	5-CHO-H_4 folate	Heat at 100°C, 10 min		(1 : 1) A and B contain 5 mM				*Proc. Natl. Acad. Sci., USA*, 80, 6500, 1983[2]
	10-CHO-H_4 folate	Homogenize			TBAP and 5 mM			
		Centrifuge, 40,000 g			2-MCE			
		Remove supernatant			15% B to 30% B in			
		Recentrifuge			60 min			
		Aspirate lipid layer			1 mL/min			
		Digest with rat plasma conjugase						
		Filter						
4. Serum	Folic acid	Add 2-MCE to 0.1 M	—	Cosmosil 5 pH	Isocratic	EC	DL (pg)	*J. Chromatogr.*, 382, 303, 1986[4]
	H_4 folate	Store serum at −30°C		Phenyl bonded	50 mM KH_2PO_4,	+350 mV vs	On-column	
	5-CH_3-H_4 folate	Mix with 2 vol of		5 μm	pH 3.5 containing	Ag/AgCl	1–150	
	5-CHO-H_4 folate	acetone		15 cm × 4.6 mm	0.1 mM EDTA and		% Recovery	
	10-CHO-H_4 folate	Centrifuge			15% MeOH		5-CH_3-H_4 folate	
		Filter (0.45 μm)			0.5 mL/min		92.9	
5–10. Tissue	Polyglutamyl folates, 1–7	Liver	Folate binding protein—	Econosphere C_{18}	Gradient	PDA	—	*Anal. Biochem.*, 168, 247, 1988[5]; 182, 89, 1989[6]
		Add 5–10 vol of	Sepharose	5 μm	See References 8, and 9	350 nm		
	H_2 folate 1–7	boiling extraction	4B affinity column	10 cm × 4.6 mm	(Table 9, Foods)	10-CHO-H_4		*Cancer Res.*, 51, 16, 1991[7]
	H_4 folate 1–7	solution				folate		
	5-CH_3-H_4	2% AA, 10 mM 2-MCE				258 nm		
		in 0.1 M Bis-Tris,						

	Compound	Sample preparation	Cleanup	Column	Mobile phase	Detection	Recovery / DL	Reference
	folate 1–7 5-CHO-H$_4$ folate 1–7 folate 1–7 10-CHO-H$_4$ folate 1–7	pH 7.85 Boil 10–15 min Homogenize Centrifuge Store, evacuated, –70°C						J. Nutr. Biochem., 2, 44, 1991[8]; 3, 519, 1992[9] J. Nutr., 122, 986, 1992[10] J. Chromatogr., 487, 456, 1989[11]
11. Tissue	H$_4$ folate 5-CH$_3$-H$_4$ folate 5-CHO-H$_4$ folate	Add 4 volumes 0.1 M NaOAC, pH 4.9, containing 20 mM 2-MCE Homogenize under N$_2$ Boiling water bath, 60 min Cool Centrifuge	DEAE - Sephadex	μBondapak phenyl 10 × 10 Radial-Pak	Isocratic Gradient A—5% MeCN in 0.033 NaH$_2$PO$_4$, pH 2.3 B—15% MeCN in 0.033 NaH$_2$PO$_4$, pH 2.3 Isocratic A for 6 min over 2 min To 25% A, 75% B Continue for 4 min Return to A over 2 min	Fluorescence Ex λ = 300 Em λ = 356	% Recovery 79.8–92	
12. Liver	H$_4$ folate 5-CH$_3$-H$_4$ folate 5-CHO-H$_4$ folate	Homogenize in ice-cold 1% AA solution Flush with N$_2$ Incubate overnight, 37°C Centrifuge Adjust pH to 4.9 Boiling water bath, 60 min Centrifuge Add 3 vol acetone to supernatant Centrifuge Rotovap Adjust volume to 50 mL	SPE (Baker-10) Quaternary amine (N$^+$) Strong anion-exchange	Spherisorb-ODS 30 cm × 3.9 mm	Isocratic MeCN : water containing 30 mM NaH$_2$PO$_4$ (10.5 : 89.5) 1 mL/min	Fluorescence Ex λ = 300 Em λ = 360	DL (pmol) On-column 0.4–2.0 % Recovery 95–123	Anal. Biochem., 176, 406, 1989[12]

TABLE 11.9 Continued

Sample Matrix	Analyte	Sample Preparation		HPLC Parameters				References
		Sample Extraction	Clean Up	Column	Mobile Phase	Detection	Quality Assurance Parameters	
13. Plasma	5-CH$_3$-H$_4$ folate	To 1.5 mL plasma, add 150 µL of β-hydroxy ethyltheophylline (2 mg/mL) (IS) Bond Elut Phenyl SPE Elute with MeOH Evaporate Reconstitute with mobile phase	—	Nova-Pak Phenyl cartridge 4 µm 10 cm × 8 mm	Isocratic MeOH : 0.05 M KH$_2$PO$_4$, pH 3.5 (15 : 85) 2 mL/min	Internal Standard 254 nm 5-CH$_3$-H$_4$ folate EC +350 mV vs Ag/AgCl	% Recovery 81–89	*Biomed. Chromatogr.,* 3, 58, 1989[13]
14. Serum, whole blood	5-CH$_3$-H$_4$ folate	*Whole blood*— To 0.4 mL, add 1.8 mL AA, 10 g/L Incubate 1 h, ambient Add 0.2 mL 60% perchloric acid Centrifuge Mix 0.2 mL supernatant with 0.5 mL AA (30 g/L) *Serum*—To 1 mL, add 40 mg AA and 0.1 mL perchloric acid Centrifuge	—	Spherisorb S5 ODS 5 µm 25 cm x 4.6 mm	Isocratic MeCN:0.033 M orthophosphoric acid, pH 2.3 1.5 mL/min	Fluorescence Ex λ = 295 Em λ = 365	DL (pg) On-column 10 % Recovery Serum–84.7 Blood–86.3	*Metabolism,* 3 39, 902, 1990[14]
15. Plasma	H$_4$ folate 5-CH$_3$-H$_4$ folate	Store, frozen with addition of 1 mg/mL AA	—	IRICA phenyl 15 cm × 4.6 mm	Isocratic MeCNC : 20 mM NaOAC, pH 3.6,	EC + 300 mV vs Ag/AgCl	QL (ng/mL) 0.13–0.15 % Recovery	*J. Vet. Med. Sci.,* 54, 249, 1992[15]

No. / Sample	Compounds	Sample preparation	Column	Mobile phase	Detection	DL (ng)	Reference
16. Standards	Folic acid, H_2 folate, H_4 folate, 5-CH_3-H_4 folate, 5-CHO-H_4 folate, Methotrexate, P-amino-benzoyl-glutamic acid, Dichlorofolic aid, Pterin, Pterin-6-carboxylic acid	Thaw, add equal volume 0.5 M perchloric acid, Centrifuge, Filter (0.45 μm), Dilute standards in 1% AA; —	Hypersil ODS, 3 μm, 25 cm × 4.6 mm	Gradient, A—5 mM KH_2PO_4 containing 0.1 M EDTA (3.5 : 96.5), B—MeCN, 0 min 93% A, 7% B; 0–15 min 87% A, 13% B; 15–18 min 81% A, 19% B; 18–21 min 79% A, 21% B	UV 295 nm, Fluorescence, Post-column oxidation with potassium peroxidisulfate	DL (ng), On-column UV—295 nm 1.1–2.4, Fluorescence Ex λ = 295 Em λ = 356; 77.6–83.0	J. Chromatogr., 540, 207, 1991[16]
17–20. Tissues, blood, erythrocytes, serum cerebrospinal fluid, foods	Folic acid, H_2 folate, H_4 folate, 5-CH_3-H_2 folate, 5-CH_3-H_4 folate, 5-CHO-H_4 folate, 5,10-CH_2-H_4 folate, Amino-pterin	Erythrocytes, Add 400 mL AA (20 g/L) to 200 mL blood, Incubate 3 h, 25°C, Add 50 μL 11M perchloric acid, Vortex, Neutralize 11 M KOH, Centrifuge; —	Nova-Pak Phenyl, 4 μm, 7.5 cm × 3.9 mm	Isocratic, MeOH : 0.05 M KH_2PO_4, pH 3.5 (15 : 85), 25°C, 0.4 mL/min	EC +650 mV vs Ag/AgCl, Fluorescence Ex λ = 295 Em λ = 365 5,10-CH=H_4 folate Ex λ = 360 Em λ = 470 DAD Monitor at 200–400 nm	DL (ng), On-column Fluorescence 0.3–0.52	Food Chem., 47, 79, 1993[17]; 50, 307, 1994[18]; 53, 329, 1995[19]; Biochem. Mol Med., 58, 93, 1996[20]

TABLE 11.9 Continued

| | Sample Preparation | | | HPLC Parameters | | | | |
| | | | | | | Quality Assurance Parameters | | |
Sample Matrix	Analyte	Sample Extraction	Clean Up	Column	Mobile Phase	Detection		References
	Teropterin P-amino-benzoyl-glutamic acid					280 nm		
21. Standard	Folic acid	Dissolve in 0.1 M NaOAC	—	Shim-Pack CLC ODS 15 cm × 6 mm	Isocratic MeOH : water (30 : 70) 50°C 1 mL/min	Fluorescence Ex λ = 295 Em λ = 365 Oxidation with potassium permanganate to 2-amino-4-hydroxy-pteridine-6-carboxylic	DL (ng) 1.5 %CV 6.6	*Fres. J. Anal. Chem.,* 346, 841, 1993[21]
22. Serum, urine	5-CH$_3$-H$_4$ folate 5-CHO-H$_4$ folate	*Serum—* Stabilize samples with addition of AA (0.5 mg/mL) Add MeCN—1.5 mL to 1 mL sample Vortex Centrifuge Extract MeCN supernatant with 7 mL CHCl$_3$ Centrifuge Remove aqueous phase	Column switching to direct analytes to analytical column from enrichment column	Nova-Pak Phenyl 4 μm 7.5 cm × 3.9 mm *In-Line Enrich-ment—* C$_{18}$-Macherez + Nagel Centrifuge 5 μm 3 cm × 4 mm *Analytical* C$_{18}$-Macherez +	*Eluent A—* 0.005 M TBAP adjusted to pH 6.5 with phosphoric acid *Eluent B—* 0.0015 Na$_2$PO$_4$, 0.00075 M TBAP containing 7.5% IPA 1.5 mL/min *Eluent C—* 0.028 M phosphate	Fluorescence Ex λ = 308 Em λ = 365	—	*J. Chromatogr. B,* 669, 319, 1995[22]

			Column	Mobile phase	Detection/Quantitation	Performance	Reference
		Dilute with 0.005 TBAP adjusted to pH 6.5 with phosphoric acid (Eluent A)	Nagel 25 cm × 2 mm 3 μm	containing 0.006 M sodium azide			
				Eluent D— Phosphoric acid			
		Urine— Dilute with Eluent A SPE-Supelco C$_{18}$ Elute with 2 mL 50% MeCN Extract MeCN with CHCl$_3$ Centrifuge, collect aqueous phase Dilute with Eluent A	*Chiral—* Resolvosil B5A7 7 μm 15 cm × 4.6mm				
23. Serum	Folic acid H$_4$ folate 5-CH$_3$-H$_4$ folate 5-CHO-H$_4$ folate	Add [3',5',7,9-^{3}H] folic acid (IS) to 1 mL serum Deproteinize with 100 mL perchloric acid (60%) Vortex; Centrifuge Adjust pH to 7.0 with 100 mL 6 M KOH	— μBondapak C$_{18}$ Radial Pak 10 cm × 8 mm	Isocratic Citrate/phosphate, 0.1 M, pH 4 : 1% HAC : MeOH (43 : 42 : 15) 3 mL/min Collect 3 mL fractions Dilute 1 : 1 with 0.5% sodium ascorbate	Radiolabel Quantitation by *L. rhamnosus* microplate assay	QL (ng/mL) 0.1 DL (pg/mL) 1 CV % 10.3–20.7 % Recovery 104–105	*Anal. Biochem.,* 238, 179, 1996

is an excellent concentration and clean-up approach prior to LC analysis of folate; however, the Finnish procedure is simpler to implement and useful for many matrices. Table 11.9 gives details of the method (food references 15 to 19).

3. *Deconjugation*—Depending on the objectives of the study, the analyst has the choice of determining folates as the monoglutamylfolates or quantifying the folates as the γ-glutamyl polymers. If the polymeric forms are to be chromatographed, all indigenous conjugase enzymes must be quickly inactivated by heating. Older literature states that rapid heating to 70°C inactivates conjugases.[15,89] Although most LC methods are based on resolution of monoglutamylfolates, excellent LC methods are available to resolve the γ-glutamyl polymeric folates. Inclusion of a conjugase digestion is necessary to convert the γ-glutamyl polymeric folates to the monoglutamate form. Differing from conjugase treatments for microbiological assay, an enzyme must be used that converts the polymeric forms only to the monoglutamate level. Hog kidney conjugase treatment is common[27,89,90,91,92]; however, rat plasma conjugase is used in recent reports.[65,93] Chicken pancreas is not suitable for methods requiring only monoglutamylfolates in the extract because it yields a mixture of mono- and diglutamate.[61]

4. *Affinity Chromatography*—Over the past decade, affinity chromatography developed into an integral part of sample preparation procedures for food, serum, and other biologicals. The methodology was developed by Selhub and colleagues and applied to various matrices.[94,95,96,97] The procedure for isolation of the bovine milk folate binding protein was detailed by Selhub et al.[94,98] Selhub's work, since the early 1980's, has provided a significant tool that allows folates in biological extracts to be purified and concentrated extensively before chromatography. Further, the extract is clean enough to allow use of PDA detectors. Affinity chromatography was recently integrated into the LC analysis of cereal-grain products by Pfeiffer et al.[65] Pfeiffer's procedure incorporates several procedural steps developed by various researchers over the last decade. The method is provided in Section 11.4. Anyone considering the use of LC for folate analysis should become familiar with the application of affinity chromatography to the sample preparation protocol. Bagley and Selhub[99] provide a recent, in-depth, procedural guide to the combined use of affinity chromatography and LC for folate assay from biologicals.

11.3.3.2   Chromatography Parameters

11.3.3.2.1   Supports and Mobile Phases

Monoglutamylfolates can be resolved by ion-exchange or reversed-phase chromatography. Ion exchange on several supports using open-column chromatography provided the first chromatographic resolution of folates. Quantification during this time period (1960 to 1970s) relied upon microbiological assay of the column eluates. Mullin and Duch,[20] in their 1992 review, showed that most LC methods to that time relied upon C_{18} reversed-phase supports and, more infrequently, use of phenyl supports. Procedures published since 1992 (Table 11.9) have in most cases used reversed-phase chromatography with C_{18}. When ion pairing is used, the reagent has been predominantly tetrabutylammonium phosphate (TBAP). Most systems require gradient elution. Mobile phase systems are given in Table 11.9 for recently published procedures. Figure 11.5 is an example of chromatography suitable for resolution of polyglutamylfolates and monoglutamyl forms. Descriptions in Table 11.9 (food references 8 and 9) give parameters for the ion-pair system used by Selhub's group in conjunction with affinity chromatography clean up and PDA detection.

11.3.3.2.2   Detection

UV absorbance, fluorescence, and electrochemical (EC) detection can be used effectively for folate quantitation. Microbiological assay of column eluents were used in earlier studies prior to the avail-

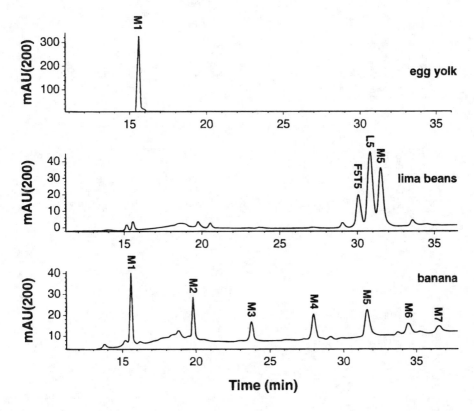

FIGURE 11.5 Ion-pair LC of purified food folates chromatography: see References 8 and 9 (Foods, Table 11.9). F = 10-CHO-H$_4$ folate, T = O unsubstituted tetrahydrofolates, L = 5-CHO-H$_4$ folates, M = 5-CH$_3$-H$_4$ folates. Numbers following letters indicate number of glutamate residues. Reproduced with permission.

ability of more effective LC detectors. Quite recently, Lucock et al.[87] optimized detection parameters for UV, fluorescence, and EC detection of 11 monoglutamylfolates. UV spectra were obtained by PDA. Data provided by Lucock et al.[87] is highly useful for anyone initiating LC analysis of folates (Tables 11.10 and 11.11).

11.3.3.2.3 Internal Standards

Owing to the complexity and varying responses of folates to different detection modes, internal standards have not been routinely applied in LC methods. Recently, [^{3}H] folic acid was effectively used as an internal standard (IS) for folate analysis.[100] The IS was used in conjunction with a *L. rhamnosus* assay of LC resolved 5-methyl-H$_4$ folate. Use of a microplate assay allowed effective quantitation of the 5-methyl-H$_4$ folate. The tritiated IS was quantified by scintillation counting. A detection limit of 1 ng/mL was obtained and recoveries approximated 100%.

TABLE 11.10
Physico-Chemical Data Useful for the LC Analysis of Monogutamylfolates.[a]

Folymono-gluamate	Chromatographic Retention Time (min) at 0.4 mL/min[c]	λ_{max} (nm) for UV detection between 240 and 400nm [Relative Absorptivity (%) Is Given in Parentheses]	Optimum Voltage for Electrochemical Detection Using a Glassy Carbon Electrode (mV)	Optimum Emission Wavelength (nm) at an Excitation Wavelength of 295 nm[b]	Purity angle Purity Threshold Value <1.0 Peak Implies Peak Homogeneity
P-ABG	2.82	272 (100)	900	(1)358 (2) 609	0.23
$5CH_3$-H_3PteGlu	4.32	276 (100)	No signal below 1000	607	0.10
H_4PteGlu	4.06	267 (100) 290 (7)	400	358	0.58
$5CH_3$-H_4PteGlu	6.16	267 (100) 290 (99)	400	(1) 358 (2) 607	0.18
5CHO-H_4PteGlu	9.75	285 (100)	600	(1) 372 (2) 607	0.86
$5,10CHH_4$PteGlu	11.43	(1) 355 (100) (2)255 (36) (3) 280 (26)	900	607[b]	0.08
H_2PteGlu	12.79	(1) 280 (100) (2) 300 (82) (3) 325–350 (27–46)	400	607	0.04
PteGlu	14.31	(1) 280 (100)[d] (2) 300 (82) (3) 350 (25)	850	No emission in the 350–365 region	0.06
$5,10CH_2H_4$PteGlu	21–26	300 (100)	500	(1) 363 (2) 607	0.01

[a] Reproduced with permission from Reference 87.
[b] Excitation λ is not optimum.
[c] Mobile phase—15% (v/v) methanol in 0.05 M KH_2PO_4, pH 3.5.
[d] Spectral characteristics of $PteGlu_3$ are almost identical to PteGlu.

TABLE 11.11
Comparison of UV, Fluorescence, and Electrochemical Detection Sensitivity for Monoglutamylfolates and Related compounds[a]

Congener	Minimum UV Detection Limit Equivalent to 0.0003 au	Minimum Electrochemical Detection Limit[e] 450 mV	800 mV	Minimum Fluorescence Detection Limit at 295 nm Excitation/ 365 nm Emission	Common Reason for Measurement
p-ABG	530 pg	b	b	3.12 ng	Stability studies on C9–N10 cleavage
$5CH_3H_2PteGlu$	1.2 ng	b	b	c	Stability studies, $5CH_3$-$H_4PteGlu$ purity analysis
$H_4PteGlu$	790 pg	1.1ng	440 pg	4.9 ng	Biochemical studies
$5CH_3$-$H_4PteGlu$	1.7 ng	300 pg	240 pg	300 pg	Food, plasma, whole blood, and pharmaceutical analysis; can be used for methotrexate rescue
$PteGlu_3$	2.3 ng	d	—	—	Synthetic substrate useful in biochemical studies
$5CHOH_4PteGlu$	3.8 ng	No signal	800 pg	18.8 ng	Plasma and pharmaceutical analysis in relation to methotrexate rescue; is a precursor for $10CHOH_4PteGlu$
$5,10CHH_4PteGlu$	7.4 ng (280 nm) / 2.4 ng (355 nm)	b	b	c	Precursor for synthesis of $10CHOH_4PteGlu$
$H_2PteGlu$	2.7 ng	1.7 ng	180 pg	c	Biochemical studies
PteGlu	3.3 ng	b	b	c	Found in food and plasma following supplementation; pharmaceutical analysis
Aminopterin	2.64 ng	—	—	—	Antifolate
$5,10CH_2H_4PeGlu$	9.6 ng	2 ng	—	52.4 ng	Biochemical studies

[a]Table reproduced with permission from Reference 87.
[b]Oxidation state or occurence makes this form of detection inappropriate.
[c]Inappropriate form of detection or excitation wavelength.
[d]Not studied.
[e]Mobile phase—15% (v/v) methanol in 0.05 M KH_2PO_4, pH 3.5.

11.4   METHOD PROTOCOLS
Microbiological Assay of Total Diet Samples, Food and Drug Administration, Southeast Regional Laboratory, Standard Operating Procedure, N/AM/4/0/94, Marijane Lawson and James I. Martin.

Purpose:

The purpose of this SOP is to set forth the operational parameters, methodology and requirements for quality assurance and acceptability of data for determination of total folate in Total Diet Samples.

Scope:

Microbiological analysis for folic acid is applicable to most food matrices and vitamin supplements. The minimum detectable level on a wet basis is 0.25 μg/100 g for folic acid. The minimum detection level assumes that the lowest practical sample dilution factor is 1:100.

Responsibility:

The analysts assigned to the determination of folic acid, the program coordinator, the supervisory chemist, and Atlanta Center for Nutrient Analysis (ACNA) director will assure adherence to the following SOP. All revisions must be directed through and receive concurrence of the appropriate coordinator, the supervisory chemist, and the ACNA director. Major methodology revisions will require concurrence with headquarters and ACNA.

References:

1. *Official Methods of Analysis,* 15th ed., AOAC International, Arlington, VA, 960.46, 961.15, and 985.32, 1990.
2. DeSouza, S. and Eitenmiller, R.R., *J. Micronutr. Anal.* 7, 37, 1990.
3. Martin, J.I., Landen, W.O., Jr., Soliman, A.G., and Eitenmiller, R.R., *J. Assoc. Off. Anal. Chem.* 73, 805, 1990.
4. Hazardous Waste Management Program, FDA Southeastern Regional Laboratory, Atlanta District, 1990.

Basic Principles:

Folic acid is assayed microbiologically with *Lactobacillus rhamnosus* ATCC 7469. Samples are digested by a trienzyme procedure using Pronase®, α-amylase, and conjugase (2). The trienzyme procedure is used routinely for total folate analysis at the ACNA (3). Current AOAC procedures are not suitable for measurement of total folate.

Apparatus:

1. Autoturb® turbidimetric reader—160 tube capacity (Elan Co., Division of Eli Lilly & Co., Indianapolis, IN 46285) or equivalent.
2. Stainless steel centrifuge tubes—50 mL capacity, No. 00579 (DuPont Instruments).
3. Constant-temperature water bath—Model No. MW-1140A-1 (Blue M Co., Blue Island, IL 60406), set at 37 $\pm$ 0.5°.
4. Thick-walled screw cap glass digestion test tubes—40 $\times$ 20 mm, No. 9212-C90 (Thomas Scientific, Swedesboro, NJ 08085) or equivalent.
5. Disposable Pyrex test tubes—18 $\times$ 150 mm, No. 9187-F83 (Thomas Scientific, Swedesboro, NJ 08085) or equivalent. Heat 2 h at 250°C to remove residue material.
6. Stainless steel test tube caps. To fit 18 $\times$ 150 mm test tubes.
7. Presterilized filtering system—Type TC, No. 150-0020, 150 mL/0.2 μm (Nalgene Co., Rochester, NY 14602) or equivalent.
8. Polytron® homogenizer— Basic assembly Model PT 10-35 with Model PT 20 ST sawtooth generator (Brinkmann Instruments, Inc., Westbury, NY 11590).
9. Analytical balance accurate to 0.01 g.

Reagents:

1. Agar culture medium—LactobacilliAgar AOAC, No. 0900-15 (Difco Laboratories, Detroit, MI 48232).
2. Culture suspension medium—Lactobacilli Broth AOAC, No. 0901-15 (Difco Laboratories).
3. Folic acid *Lactobacillus casei* assay medium—No. 0822-15, prepare as per label instructions and add designated amount of ascorbic acid (Difco Laboratories).
4. Culture—*Lactobacillus rhamnosus,* ATCC No. 7469 (American Type Culture Collection, Rockville, MD 20852). (formerly *L. casei*).
5. Distilled water—Do not use deionized water.
6. Extraction buffer—Dissolve 1 g ascorbic acid (reagent grade) in 100 mL 1.42% Na_2HPO_4. Adjust pH to 6.8 $\pm$ 0.1 with 2 *N* NaOH. (Stable overnight if kept cold and in the dark.)
7. Inoculum resuspension medium—Prepare 5 test tubes (18 $\times$ 150 mm, each containing 10 mL single-strength folic acid assay medium [5 mL reagent(3) plus 5 mL water]. Cap, autoclave 5 min at 121°C, cool and incubate overnight in 37 $\pm$ 0.5° water bath. This resuspension medium will be used to prepare the folate-depleted assay inoculum.
8. Folic acid standard solutions—(1) Stock solutions—100 μg/mL pteroylglutamic acid prepared as per AOAC, 15th ed., 944.12 B(a). (2) Working standard solution—0.200 ng/mL. Dilute stock solution with water to obtain desired concentration. The final volume must contain 2 mL buffer [Reagent(6)]/100 mL.
9. Enzymes—(1) Conjugase (chicken pancreas)—5 mg/mL. Extract 0.2 g acetone-washed dry conjugase powder, No. 0459-12 (Difco Laboratories) in 40 mL buffer as follows: Transfer powder to cold mortar, add 1 to 2 mL buffer, and mix until fine suspension is formed. Transfer suspension to stainless steel 50 mL centrifuge tube with 35 to 40 mL buffer and centrifuge 10 min at 5000 rpm, preferably in a refrigerated system and keep cold until ready to use. (2) α-Amylase—20 mg/mL. Dissolve 0.25 g α-amylase No. AO273 (Sigma Chemical Co., St. Louis, MO 63178) in 25 mL water. Keep cold until ready to use. (3) Protease—2 mg/mL. Dissolve 0.05 g Pronase.® No. P-5147 (Sigma Chemical Co.) or equivalent in 50 mL water. Pass conjugase and Pronase® solutions through separate sterile filters and keep cold until ready to use. Do not filter α-amylase solution.

Test Organism—*Lactobacillus rhamnosus* ATCC 7469 (formerly *L. casei.*). Maintain by weekly stab transfers into agar culture medium (1). Incubate at 37°, 18 to 24 h. Store refrigerated.

Safety Precautions:

The assays will be carried out with strict adherence to the District safety policies and waste management procedures (4).

Procedure

Series Definition

A series will consist of a maximum of 10 assays.

1. A maximum of 8 samples.
2. One enzyme blank.
3. One QA control sample.
4. A recovery consisting of a sample with a known vitamin concentration is assayed periodically.

Sample Preparation and Digestion

1. *Sample Preparation*—Perform all sample preparations under subdued light with minimal contact with air. Use nitrogen gas to blanket product whenever possible.

   All Total Diet samples are composited at the Kansas City Total Diet Research Center. The homogenous samples are shipped frozen to ACNA for analysis. Each sample consists of three subsamples packaged in double plastic bags. Subsamples are identified as subsamples 1, 2, and 3 with product name and an identifying code number. Prior to analysis a subsample is thawed, mixed well and the required portion (1.5 to 20 g) is removed for analysis. Add 50 mL buffer [Reagent 6] to the weighed sample and homogenize using Polytron®. for 1 min (medium setting). Avoid excess foaming. Rinse Polytron® tip and dilute sample to 100.0 mL with buffer. Transfer 25.0 mL to digestion tube, add 10 mL buffer, and proceed to digestion procedure. Weights and volumes may be adjusted to obtain desired folate levels in final extract solutions.

NOTE: For samples containing high levels of fat and/or oils, which become gummy when added to the buffer, omit the homogenization step and add the sample directly into the digestion tube and defat by adding 20 to 25 mL hexane to the weighed sample, mix well, centrifuge and decant off the hexane/fat supernate. Evaporate to dryness gently using nitrogen gas and continue by adding 35 mL of buffer to the sample making sure it is completely mixed. (This will not get rid of all of the fat, but will remove most and reduce or eliminate the problem.)

2. *Digestion Procedure*—Place loosely capped digestion tubes containing sample/buffer suspension and enzyme blank in vigorously boiling water bath for 5 min (begin counting time when water in bath begins to boil). Cool to room temperature (water or ice bath). For all sample and blank tubes, add 1 mL conjugase solution/1 g solid sample material. Add 1 mL α-amylase solution, gently swirl, tighten caps, and incubate at 37° 4 h. After 4 h incubation, add 1 mL protease solution/1 g solid material, gently swirl, add 2 drops toluene, cap tightly, and incubate overnight at 37° in water bath. The reason for this order and the time for addition of enzymes to samples is to allow conjugase and α-amylase to act on respective substrates before possible enzyme deactivation by Pronase® which has very broad, non-specific protease activity.

To deactivate enzymes after incubation period, add 2 mL buffer/tube and heat for 5 min in boiling water bath. Cool tubes, transfer contents of each tube to 100 mL volumetric flask, and bring to volume with water. Mix and filter through Whatman No. 40 paper. Dilute an appropriate aliquot of the filtrate, with water containing 2% buffer to give a final concentration of about 0.15 ng/mL.

Inoculum Preparation

1. Transfer *L. rhamnosus* cells from stab to test tube containing 10 mL Lactobacilli Broth AOAC.
2. Incubate at 37° for 16 to 20 h.
3. Centrifuge broth at 2500 rpm and resuspend cells in 10 ml sterile saline. Repeat washing procedure three times.
4. After final centrifugation, resuspend cells in 10 mL of inoculum resuspension medium.
5. Incubate 5 to 6 h at 37°. (Significant cell growth should be observed.)
6. Vortex test tube, transfer 4 to 8 drops of the culture suspension to 10 mL of the resuspension medium. Percent transmission of the cell preparation should be 65 to 75% as measured against the resuspension medium.

Standard Curve Preparation

Construct an eight point standard curve by adding 0.0, 0.0, 0.5, 1.0, 1.5, 2.0, 2.5, 3.0, 4.0 and 5.0 ml of the working standard into triplicate 18 × 150 mm Pyrex test tubes. Add distilled water to adjust volume to 5.0 mL. Add 5.0 mL of *Lactobacillus casei* assay medium to each tube.

Blank Tubes

The first set of tubes containing 0.0 mL of standard represents the uninoculated blank used to set the Autoturb or spectrophotometer to 100% T. The second set of tubes containing 0.0 ml standard is inoculated and represents the inoculated blank and is used to reset the instrument to 100%T.

Enzyme Blank

An enzyme blank is carried through the sample digestion procedure. The blank is prepared by adding 1 mL conjugase and 1 mL α-amylase to 25 mL extraction buffer. After 4 h at 37°, add 1 mL of Pronase® and two drops of toluene and incubate overnight at 37°. Enzyme blanks are diluted to levels comparable to the final sample dilutions and assayed to determine contribution of the enzyme to the *L. rhamnosus* growth response. Usually, at dilutions used for most foods, blank corrections are not required.

Assay

Folic acid is assayed by the official AOAC turbidimetric method (1). Four sample extract levels (1, 2, 3, and 4 mL) are assayed in triplicate. Volume in each tube is adjusted to 5 ml with H_2O. Five mL of single-strength assay media (folic acid *Lactobacillus casei* media) is added to each tube. Prepared assay tubes, standard curve tubes, blank and enzyme blank tubes are autoclaved at 121° for 5 min. The tubes are cooled to room temperature and inoculated with one drop of prepared inoculum per tube. Assay tubes are incubated at 37° for 20 to 24 h. Growth response is measured as % T at 550 nm. The tubes are removed when the growth response of an extra 5.0 ml standard (1 ng/tube) is 2% T or less per hour.

Calculations:

Results are calculated from the regression line of the standard curve responses using fourth degree polynomial plots and a computer program written to conform to AOAC microbiological analysis protocol. Results are reported as μg vitamin per 100 g or per serving.

Determination of Folate in Cereal-Grain Food Products Using Trienzyme Extraction and Combined Affinity and Reversed-Phase Liquid Chromatography

Principle

• Extract folates by digestion with rat plasma conjugase, α-amylase, and protease in Hepes/Ches buffer, pH 7.85. The extract is purified by affinity chromatography with immobilized folate binding protein. Folates are resolved by reversed-phase gradient LC and quantitated with UV diode array detection.

Chemicals and Materials

• Hepes/Ches buffer
• Affigel 10
• Isolated folate binding protein (FBP)
• 5-Methyltetrahydrofolate
• 5-Formyltetrahydrofolate
• Folic Acid
• 10-Formylfolic acid
• 5, 10-methenyltetrahydrofolate HCl
• Pteroyltriglutamate
• Sodium ascorbate
• Dithiothreitol
• 2-Mercaptoethanol
• Trifluoroacetic acid

Enzymes

- Rat plasma conjugase
- α-Amylase
- Protease

Apparatus

- Polytron® homogenizer
- Liquid chromatograph
- Diode array detector
- Glass columns (0.7 cm × 20 cm)

Procedure

Trienzyme Extraction

- Add 10 volumes Hepes/Ches buffer, pH 7.85 containing 2% sodium ascorbate and 10 mM 2-mercaptoethanol to 2 g dry sample
- Boiling water bath, 10 min
- Cool
- Homogenize, Polytron®
- Digest with rat plasma conjugase and α-amylase, 4 h, 37°C
- Digest with protease, 1h, 37°C
- Boiling water bath, 5 min
- Cool
- Centrifuge
- Resuspend residue in extraction buffer
- Centrifuge and combine supernatants
- Filter, Whatman #1
- Flush with N_2, store at 4°C

Extract Purification

- Prepare affinity chromatography sorbent : FBP coupled to Affigel 10 in 0.7 cm × 20 cm glass columns
- Apply sample extract to affinity column equilibrated with 0.1 M potassium phosphate buffer, pH 7.0
- Wash with 5 mL 0.25 M potassium phosphate, pH 7.0, containing 1.0 M NaCl
- Follow with 5 mL 0.025 M potassium phosphate, pH 7.0
- Elute folate with 2 mL 0.02 M trifluoroacetic acid/0.01 M dithiothreitol (discard) followed by 5.0 mL of 0.02 M trifluoroacetic acid/0.01 M dithiothreitol (contains all folates)
- Add 30 mL 1 M piperazine
- Add sodium ascorbate to 0.02 % v/v
- Add 2-mercaptoethanol to 10 mM
- Flush with N_2
- Store frozen

Chromatography

Column	25 cm × 4.6 mm
Stationary phase	Ultramex C_{18}, 5 μm
Mobile phase	Gradient
	A—MeCN
	B—0.033 M phosphoric acid, pH 2.3
	0 to 8 min, 5% A, 95% B
	8 to 33 min, linear to 17.5% A

Column temperature	Ambient
Detection	Diode array, 280 nm
Calculation	Peak area
	External standard, peak area, least squares regression

J. Agric. Food Chem., 45, 407, 1997

11.5   REFERENCES

Text

1. Day, P. L., Langston, W. C., and Shukers, C. F., Failure of nicotinic acid to prevent nutritional cytopenia in monkeys, *Proc. Exp. Biol. Med.,* 38, 860, 1938.
2. Hogan, A. G. and Parrott, E. M., Anemia in chicks due to vitamin deficiency, *J. Biol. Chem.,* 128, 46, 1939.
3. Mitchell, H. K., Snell, E. E., and Williams, R. J., The concentration of folic acid, *J. Am. Chem. Soc.,* 63, 2284, 1941.
4. Friedrich, W., Folic acid and unconjugated pteridines, in *Vitamins,* Walter de Gruyter, Berlin, 1988, chap. 10.
5. Machlin, L. J. and Hüni, J. E. S., in *Vitamin Basics,* Hoffmann-LaRoche, Basel, 1994, 49.
6. Gibson, R. S., *Principles of Nutritional Assessment,* Oxford University Press, New York, 1990, chap. 22.
7. *Nutritional Labeling and Education Act of 1990,* Fed. Reg., 58, 2070, 1993.
8. Daly, L. E., Kirke, P. N., Molloy, A., Weir, D. G., and Scott, J. M., Folate levels and neural tube defects, *JAMA,* 274, 1698, 1995.
9. Czeizel, A. E., Folic acid in the prevention of neural tube defects, *J. Ped. Gastroenterol. Nutr.,* 20, 4, 1995.
10. National Research Council, *Recommended Dietary Allowances,* 10th ed., National Academy of Sciences, Washington, D. C., 1989, chap. 8.
11. Munson, P. L., Mueller, R. A., and Breese, G. R., in, *Principles of Pharmacology,* Chapman and Hall, New York, 1995, chap. 59.
12. Selhub, J. and Rosenberg, I. H., Folic acid, in *Present Knowledge in Nutrition,* Ziegler, E. E. and Filer, L. J., Jr., Eds., ILSI Press, Washington, D. C., 1996, chap. 21.
13. Blakley, R. L., IUPAC-IUB Joint Commission on Biochemical Nomenclature (JCBN). Nomenclature and symbols for folic acid and related compounds. Recommendations 1986, *Eur. J. Biochem.,* 168, 251, 1987.
14. Temple, C., Jr. and Montgomery, J. A., Chemical and physical properties of folic acid and reduced derivatives, in *Folates and Pterins,* vol. 1, Blakley, R. L. and Benkovic, S. J., Eds., John Wiley & Sons, New York, 1984, chap. 2.
15. Gregory, J. F., III, Chemical and nutritional aspects of folate research: analytical procedures, methods of folate synthesis, stability, and bioavailability of dietary folates, in *Advances in Food and Nutrition Research,* vol. 33, Kinsella, J. E., Ed., Academic Press, New York, 1989, 1.
16. Ball, G. F. M., Chemical and biological nature of the water-soluble vitamins, in *Water-Soluble Vitamin Assays in Human Nutrition,* Chapman and Hall, London, 1994, chap. 2.
17. Blakley, R. L., The biochemistry of folic acid and related pteridines, in *Frontiers of Biology,* vol. 13, Neuberger, A. and Tatum, E. L., Eds., North-Holland, Amsterdam, 1969, chap. 3.
18. Uyeda, K. and Rabinowitz, J. C., Fluorescence properties of tetrahydrofolate and related compounds, *Anal. Biochem.,* 6, 100, 1963.
19. Gregory, J. F., III, Sartain, D. B., and Day, B. P. F., Fluorometric determination of folacin in biological materials using high performance liquid chromatography, *J. Nutr.,* 114, 341, 1984.
20. Mullin, R. J. and Duch, D. S., Folic acid, in *Modern Chromatographic Analysis of Vitamins,* De Leenheer, A. P., Lambert, W. E., and Nelis, H. J., Eds., Marcel Dekker, New York, 1992, chap. 6.
21. Gregory, J. F., III, Chemical changes of vitamins during food processing, in *Chemical Changes in Food During Processing,* Richardson, T. and Finley, J. W., Eds., AVI Publishing Company, Westport, CN, 1985, chap. 17.

22. Hawkes, J. G. and Villota, R., Folates in foods: reactivity, stability during processing, and nutritional implications, *Crit. Rev. Food Sci. Nutr.,* 28, 439, 1989.

23. Reed, L. S. and Archer, M.C., Oxidation of tetrahydrofolic acid by air, *J. Agric. Food Chem.,* 28, 801, 1980.

24. O'Broin, J. D., Temperley, I. J., Brown, J. P., and Scott, J. M., Nutritional stability of various naturally occurring monoglutamate derivatives of folic acid, *Am. J. Clin. Nutr.,* 28, 438, 1975.

25. Wilson, S. D. and Horne, D. W., Evaluation of ascorbic acid in protecting labile folic acid derivatives, *Proc. Natl. Acad. Sci. USA,* 80, 6500, 1983.

26. Lucock, M. D., Green, M., Hartley, R., and Levene, M. I., Physiochemical and biological factors influencing methylfolate stability: use of dithiothreitol for HPLC analysis with electrochemical detection, *Food Chem.,* 47, 79, 1993.

27. Vahteristo, L. T., Ollilainen, V., Koivistoinen, P. E., and Vara, P., Improvements in the analysis of reduced folate monoglutamates and folic acid in food by high-performance liquid chromatography, *J. Agric. Food Chem.,* 44, 477, 1996.

28. Paine-Wilson, B. and Chen, T. S., Thermal destruction of folacin: effect of pH and buffer ions, *J. Food Sci.,* 44, 717, 1979.

29. Stokstad, E. L. R., Fordham, D., and Degronigen, A., Inactivation of pteroylglutamic acid (Liver *Lactobacillus casei* factor) by light, *J. Biol. Chem.,* 167, 877, 1947.

30. Hutchings, B. L., Stokstad, E. L. R., Mowat, J. H., Boothe, J. H., Waller, C. W., Angier, R. B., Senb, J., and Subbarow, Y., The degradation of the fermentation *Lactobacillus casei* factor, II., *J. Am. Chem. Soc.,* 70, 10, 1948.

31. DeSouza, S. C. and Eitenmiller, R. R., Effects of processing and storage on the folate content of spinach and broccoli, *J. Food Sci.,* 51, 626, 1986.

32. Ford, J. E., The influence of the dissolved oxygen in milk on the stability of some vitamins towards heating and during subsequent exposure to sunlight, *J. Dairy Res.,* 34, 239, 1967.

33. Chen, T. S. and Cooper, R. G., Thermal destruction of folacin: effect of ascorbic acid, oxygen, and temperature, *J. Food Sci.,* 44, 713, 1979.

34. Day, B. P. F. and Gregory, J. F. III, Thermal stability of folic acid and 5-methyltetrahydrofolic acid in liquid model food systems, *J. Food Sci.,* 48, 581, 1983.

35. Wogan, G. N., Paglialunga, S., Archer, M. C., and Tannenbaum, S. R., Carcinogenicity of nitrosation products of ephedrine, sarcosine, folic acid and creatinine, *Cancer Res.,* 35, 1981, 1975.

36. Ruddick, J. E., Vanderstoep, J., and Richards, J. F., Kinetics of thermal degradation of methyltetrahydrofolic acid, *J. Food Sci.,* 45, 1019, 1980.

37. Mnkeni, A. P. and Beveridge, T., Thermal destruction of 5-methyltetrahydrofolic acid in buffer and model food systems, *J. Food Sci.,* 48, 595, 1983.

38. Keagy, P. M., Stokstad, E. L. R., and Fellers, D. A., Folacin stability during bread processing and family flour storage, *Cereal Chem.,* 52, 348, 1975.

39. Shin, Y. S., Kim, E. S., Watson, J. E., and Stokstad, E. L. R., Studies on folic acid compounds in nature, IV. Folic acid compounds in soybeans and cow milk, *Can. J. Biochem.,* 53, 338, 1975.

40. Andersson, I. and Öste, R., Loss of ascorbic acid, folacin and vitamin B_{12}, and changes in oxygen content of UHT milk. I. Introduction and methods, *Milchwissenschaft,* 47, 223, 1992.

41. Andersson, I. and Öste, R., Loss of ascorbic acid, folacin and vitamin B_{12}, and changes in oxygen content of UHT milk. II. Results and discussion, *Milchwissenschaft,* 47, 299, 1992.

42. Viberg, U., Jägerstad, M., Öste, R., and Sjoholm, I., Thermal processing of 5-methyltetrahydrofolic acid in the UHT region in the presence of oxygen, *Food Chem.,* 59, 381, 1997.

43. Gregory, J. F., III, Recent developments in methods for the assessment of vitamin bioavailability, *Food Technol.,* 42, 230, 1988.

44. Reisenaurer, A. M., Krumdieck, C. L., and Halsted, C. H., Folate conjugase: two separate activities in human jejunum, *Science,* 198, 196, 1977.

45. Bailey, L. B., Factors affecting folate bioavailability, *Food Technol.,* 42, 206, 1988.

46. Gregory, J. F., III, The bioavailability of folate, in *Folate in Health and Disease,* Bailey, L. B., Ed., Marcel Dekker, New York, 1995, chap. 8.

47. Krumdieck, C. L., Newman, A. J., and Butterworth, C. E., Jr., A naturally occurring inhibitor of folic acid conjugase (pteroylpolyglutamyl hydrolase) in beans and other pulses, *Am. J. Clin. Nutr.,* 26, 460, 1973.

48. Ford, J. E., Salter, D. N., and Scott, K. J., The folate-binding protein in milk, *J. Dairy Res.*, 36, 435, 1969.

49. Swiatlo, N. L. and Picciano, M. F., Relative folate bioavailability from human, bovine and goat milk containing diets, *Fed. Proc.*, 2, Abstract 4600, 1988.

50. Ristow, K. A., Gregory, J. F. III., and Damron, B. L., Effects of dietary fiber on the bioavailability of folic acid monoglutamate, *J. Nutr.*, 112, 750, 1982.

51. Keagy, P. M. and Oace, S. M., Folic acid utilization from high fiber diets in rats, *J. Nutr.*, 114, 1252, 1984.

52. Keagy, P. M., Stokstad, B., and Oace, S. M., Folate bioavailability in humans: effects of wheat bran and beans, *Am. J. Clin. Nutr.*, 47, 80, 1988.

53. Gregory, J. F., III, Bioavailability of folate, Eur. J. Clin. Nutr., 51, 554, 1997.

54. Eitenmiller, R. R. and Landen, W. O., Jr., Vitamins, in *Analyzing Food for Nutrition Labeling and Hazardous Contaminants,* Jeon, I. J. and Ikins, W. G., Eds., Marcel Dekker, New York, 1995, chap. 9.

55. Keagy, P. M., Folacin. Microbiological and animal assays, in *Methods of Vitamin Assay,* Augustin, J., Klein, B. P., Becker, D. A., and Venugopal, P. B., Eds., John Wiley & Sons, New York, 1985, chap. 18I.

56. Voigt, M. N. and Eitenmiller, R. R., Comparative review of the thiochrome microbial and protozoan analyses of B-vitamins, *J. Food Prot.*, 41, 730, 1978.

57. Goli, D. M. and Vanderslice, J. T., Microbiological assays of folacin using a CO_2 analyzer, *J. Micronutr. Anal.*, 6, 19, 1989.

58. Newman, E. M. and Tsai, J. F., Microbiological analysis of 5-formyltetrahydrofolic acid and other folates using an automatic 96-well plate reader, *Anal. Biochem.*, 154, 509, 1986.

59. Snell, E. E. and Strong, F. M., A microbiological assay for riboflavin, *Ind. Eng. Chem., Anal. Ed.*, 11, 346, 1939.

60. AOAC International, *Official Methods of Analysis,* 16th ed., AOAC International, Arlington, VA, 1995.

61. Goli, D. M. and Vanderslice, J. T., Investigation of the conjugase treatment procedure in the microbiological assay of folate, *Food Chem.*, 43, 57, 1992.

62. Wilson, S. D. and Horne, D. W., High-performance liquid chromatographic determination of the distribution of naturally occurring folic acid derivatives in rat liver, *Anal. Biochem.*, 142, 529, 1984.

63. Gregory, J. F., III, Engelhardt, R., Bhandari, S. D., Sartain, D. B., and Gustafson, S. K., Adequacy of extraction techniques for determination of folate in foods and other biological materials, *J. Food Comp. Anal.*, 3, 134, 1990.

64. Tamura, T., Mizuno, Y., Johnston, K. E., and Jacob, R. A., Food folate assay with protease, α-amylase, and folate conjugase treatments, *J. Agric. Food Chem.*, 45, 135, 1997.

65. Pfeiffer, C. M., Rogers, L. M., and Gregory, J. F., III, Determination of folate in cereal-grain food products using trienzyme extraction and combined affinity and reversed-phase liquid chromatography, *J. Agric. Food Chem.*, 45, 407, 1997.

66. Yamada, M., Folate contents of milk, *Vitamins* (in Japanese), 53, 221, 1979.

67. Cerna, L. and Kas, J., New conception of folacin assay in starch or glycogen containing food samples, *Nahrungs*, 27, 957, 1983.

68. Pedersen, J. C., Comparison of γ-glutamyl hydrolase (conjugase; EC 3.4.22.12) and amylase treatment procedures in microbiological assay for food folates, *Br. J. Nutr.*, 59, 261, 1988.

69. DeSouza, S. and Eitenmiller, R. R., Effects of different enzyme treatments on extraction of total folate from various foods prior to microbiological and radioassay, *J. Micronutr. Anal.*, 7, 37, 1990.

70. Martin, J., Landen, W. O., Jr., Soliman, A. M., and Eitenmiller, R. R., Application of a tri-enzyme extraction for total folate determination in foods, *J. Assoc. Off. Anal. Chem.*, 73, 805, 1990.

71. Tamura, T., Microbiological assay of folates, in *Folic Acid Metabolism in Health and Disease. Contemporary Issues in Clinical Nutrition,* vol. 13, Picciano, M. F., Stokstad, E. L., and Gregory, J.F., III, Eds., Wiley-Liss, New York, 1990, 121.

72. O'Broin, S. and Kelleher, B., Microbiological assay on microtiter plates of folate in serum and red cells, *J. Clin. Pathol.*, 45, 344, 1992.

73. Das Sarma, J., Duttagupta, C., Ali, E., and Dhar, T. K., Improved microbiological assay for folic acid based on microtiter plating with *Streptococcus faecalis*, *J. AOAC Int.*, 78, 1173, 1995.

74. Newman, E. M. and Tsai, J. F., Microbiological analysis of 5-formyltetrahydrofolic acid and other folates using an automatic 96-well plate reader, *Anal. Biochem.*, 154, 509, 1986.

75. Horne, D. W. and Patterson, D., *Lactobacillus casei* microbiological assay of folic acid derivatives in 96-well microtiter plates, *Clin. Chem.,* 34, 2357, 1988.
76. Horne, D. W., Microbiological assay of folates in 96-well microtiter plates, *Meth. Enzymol.,* 281, 38, 1997.
77. Chen, M. F., Hill, J. W., and McIntyre, P. A., The folacin contents of food as measured by a radiometric microbiologic method, *J. Nutr.,* 113, 2192, 1983.
78. Finglas, P. M., and Morgan, M. R. A., Application of biospecific methods to the determination of B-group vitamins in food—a review, *Food Chem.,* 49, 191, 1994.
79. Wigertz, K. and Jägerstad, M., Comparison of a HPLC and radioprotein-binding assay for the determination of folates in milk and blood samples, *Food Chem.,* 54, 429, 1995.
80. van den Berg, H., Finglas, P. M., and Bates, C., FLAIR intercomparisons on serum and red cell folate, *Int. J. Vit. Nutr. Res.,* 64, 288, 1994.
81. Raiten, D. J. and Fisher, K. ., Assessment of folate methodology used in the Third National Health and Nutrition Examination Survey (NHANES III, 1988–1994), Life Sciences Research Office, FASEB, Report to the Center for Food Safety and Applied Nutrition, Food and Drug Administration, November 1994.
82. Finglas, P. M., Faulks, R. M., and Morgan, M. R. A., The development and characterization of a protein binding assay for the determination of folate-potential use in food analysis, *J. Micronutr. Anal.,* 4, 295, 1988.
83. Finglas, P. M., Kwiatkowska, C., Faulks, R. M., and Morgan, M. R. A., Comparison of a non-isotopic, microtitration plate folate-binding protein assay and a microbiological method for the determination of folate in raw and cooked vegetables, *J. Micronutr. Anal.,* 4, 309, 1988.
84. Finglas, P. M., Faure, U., and Southgate, D. A. T., First BCR-intercomparison on the determination of folates in food, *Food Chem.,* 46, 199, 1993.
85. Vahteristo, L., Finglas, P. M., Witthöft, C., Wigertz, K., Seale, R., and de Froidmont-Görtz, I., Third EU MAT intercomparison study on food folate analysis using HPLC procedures, *Food Chem.,* 57, 109, 1996.
86. Lucock, M. D., Hartley, R., and Smithells, R. W., A rapid and specific HPLC-electrochemical method for the determination of endogenous 5-methyltetrahydrofolic acid in plasma using solid phase sample preparation with internal standardization, *Biomed. Chromatogr.,* 3, 58, 1989.
87. Lucock, M. D., Green, M., Priestnall, M., Daskalakis, I., Levene, M. I., and Hartley, R., Optimisation of chromatographic conditions for the determination of folates in foods and biological tissues for nutritional and clinical work, *Food Chem.,* 53, 329, 1995.
88. Schleyer, E., Reinhardt, J., Unterhalt, M., and Hiddemann, W., Highly sensitive coupled-column high-performance liquid chromatographic method for the separation and quantitation of the diastereomers of leucovorin and 5-methyltetrahydrofolate in serum and urine, *J. Chromatogr. B.,* 669, 319, 1995.
89. Vahteristo, L. T., Ollilainen, V., and Vara, P., HPLC determination of folate in liver and liver products, *J. Food Sci.,* 61, 524, 1966.
90. Vahteristo, L. T., Ollilainen, V., and Vara, P., Liquid chromatographic determination of folate monoglutamates in fish, meat, eggs, and dairy products consumed in Finland, *J. AOAC Int.,* 80, 373, 1997.
91. Vahteristo, L. T., Lehikoinen, K., Ollilainen, V., and Vara, P., Application of an HPLC assay for the determination of folate derivatives in some vegetables, fruits, and berries consumed in Finland, *Food Chem.,* 59, 589, 1997.
92. Wittenberg, J. B., Noronha, J. M., and Silverman, M., Folic acid derivatives of the gas gland of *Physalia physalis* L, *Biochem. J.,* 85, 9, 1962.
93. Engelhardt, R. and Gregory, J. F., III, Adequacy of enzymatic deconjugation in quantification of folate in foods, *J. Agric. Food Chem.,* 38, 154, 1990.
94. Selhub, J., Darcy-Vrillon, B., and Fell, D., Affinity chromatography of naturally occurring folate derivatives, *Anal. Biochem.,* 168, 247, 1988.
95. Selhub, J., Determination of tissue folate composition by affinity chromatography followed by high-pressure ion pair liquid chromatography, *Anal. Biochem.,* 182, 84, 1989.
96. Varela-Moreiras, G., Seyoum, E., and Selhub, J., Combined affinity and ion-pair liquid chromatographies for the analysis of folate distribution in tissues, *J. Nutr. Biochem.,* 2, 44, 1991.
97. Seyoum, E. and Selhub, J., Combined affinity and ion pair column chromatographies for the analysis of food folate, *J. Nutr. Biochem.,* 4, 488, 1993.

98. Selhub, J., Osman, A., and Rosenberg, I.H., Preparation and use of affinity columns with bovine milk folate binding protein (FBP) covalently linked to Sepharose 4B. *Meth. Enzymol.,* 66, 686, 1980.

99. Bagley, P. J. and Selhub, J., Analysis of folates using combined affinity and ion-pair chromatography, *Meth. Enzymol.,* 281, 16, 1997.

100. Kelly, P., McPartlin, J., and Scott, J., A combined high-performance liquid chromatographic-microbiological assay for serum folic acid, *Anal. Biochem.,* 238, 179, 1996.

Table 11.3 Physical Properties of Folates

1. Ball, G. F. M., Folate, in *Water-Soluble Vitamin Assays in Human Nutrition,* Chapman and Hall, New York, 1994, chap. 2.

2. Budavari, S., *The Merck Index,* 12th ed., Merck and Company, Whitehouse Station, NJ, 1996, 715–716.

3. Freidrich, W., Folic acid and unconjugated pteridines in *Vitamins,* Walter de Gruyter, Berlin, 1988, chap. 10.

4. Temple, C., Jr. and Montgomery, J. A., Chemical and physical properties of folic acid and reduced derivatives, in *Folates and Pterins,* vol. 1, Blakely, R. L., and Benkovic, S. J., Eds., John Wiley & Sons, New York, 1984, chap. 2.

Table 11.5 Compendium, Regulatory, and Handbook Methods for Analysis of Folate

1. The United States Pharmacopeial Convention, in *U. S. Pharmacopeia National Formulary,* USP23/NF18, Nutritional Supplements, Official Monographs, United States Pharmacopeial Convention, Rockville, MD, 1995.

2. Scottish Home and Health Department, *British Pharmacopoeia,* 15th ed., British Pharmacopoeia Commission, United Kingdom, 1993.

3. AOAC International, *Official Methods of Analysis,* 16th ed., AOAC International, Arlington, VA, 1995.

4. Tanner, J. T., Barnett, S. A., and Mountford, M. K., Analysis of milk-based infant formula. Phase V. Vitamin A, and E, folic acid, and pantothenic acid: Food and Drug Administration Infant Formula Council collaborative study, *J. AOAC Int.,* 76, 399, 1993.

5. American Feed Ingredients Association, *Laboratory Methods Compendium,* vol. 1. *Vitamins and Minerals,* American Feed Ingredients Association, West Des Moines, IA, 1991, 153.

6. Keller, H. E., *Analytical Methods for Vitamins and Carotenoids in Feeds,* Hoffmann-LaRoche, Basel, 1988, 30, 50.

7. Committee on Food Chemical Codex, *Food Chemicals Codex,* 4th ed., National Academy of Sciences, Washington, D. C., 1996, 157.

Table 11.7 Microbiological Assay of Folate in Foods and Biologicals

1. Tamura, T., Shin, Y. S., Williams, M. A., and Stokstad, E. L. R., *Lactobacillus casei* response to pteroylpolyglutamates, *Anal. Biochem.,* 49, 517, 1972.

2. Keagy, P. M., Stokstad, E. L. R., and Fellers, D. A., Folacin stability during bread processing and family flour storage, *Cereal Chem.,* 52, 348, 1975.

3. Chen, M. F., McIntyre, P. A., and Kertcher, J. A., Measurement of folates in human plasma and erythrocytes by a radiometric microbiologic method, *J. Nuc. Med.,* 19, 906, 1978.

4. Klein, B. P. and Kuo, C. H. Y., Comparison of microbiological and radiometric assays for determining total folacin in spinach, *J. Food Sci.,* 46, 552, 1981.

5. Chen, M. F., Hill, J. W., and McIntyre, P. A., The folacin contents of foods as measured by a radiometric microbiologic method, *J. Nutr.,* 113, 2192, 1983.

6. Phillips, D. R. and Wright, A. J. A., Studies on the response of *Lactobacillus casei* to folate vitamin in foods, *Br. J. Nutr.,* 49, 181, 1983.

7. Chen, T. S., Song, Y. O., and Kirsch, A. J., Effects of blanching, freezing and storage on folacin contents of spinach, *Nutr. Rep. Int.,* 28, 317, 1983.

8. Kirsch, A. J. and Chen, T. S., Comparison of conjugase treatment procedures in the microbiological assay for food folacin, *J. Food Sci.,* 49, 94, 1984.

9. Newman, E. M. and Tsai, J. F., Microbiological analysis of 5-formyltetrahydrofolic acid and other folates using an automatic 96-well plate reader, *Anal. Biochem.*, 154, 509, 1986.

10. Keagy, P. M., Computerized semiautomated microbiological assay of folacin, *J. Assoc. Off. Anal. Chem.*, 69, 773, 1986.

11. DeSouza, S. C. and Eitenmiller, R. R., Effects of processing and storage on the folate content of spinach and broccoli, *J. Food Sci.*, 51, 626, 1986.

12. Wilson, D. S., Clifford, C. K., and Clifford, A. J., Microbiological assay for folic acid-effects of growth medium modification, *J. Micronutr. Anal.*, 3, 55, 1987.

13. Pedersen, J. C., Comparison of γ-glutamyl hydrolase (conjugase; EC 3.4.22.12) and amylase treatment procedures in the microbiological assay for food folates, *Br. J. Nutr.*, 59, 261, 1988.

14. Goli, D. M. and Vanderslice, J. T., Microbiological assays of folacin using a CO_2 analyzer system, *J. Micronutr. Anal.*, 6, 19, 1989.

15. DeSouza, S. and Eitenmiller, R. R., Effects of different enzyme treatments on extraction of total folate from various foods prior to microbiological assay and radioassay, *J. Micronutr. Anal.*, 7, 37, 1990.

16. Martin, J. I., Landen, W. O., Jr., Soliman, A. G. M., and Eitenmiller, R. R., Application of a tri-enzyme extraction for total folate determination in foods, *J. Assoc. Off. Anal. Chem.*, 73, 805, 1990.

17. Ryu, K. S., Eitenmiller, R. R., and Pesti, G. M., A comparison of enzyme preparations to liberate folic acid for the microbiological assay of feed ingredients, *J. Sci. Food Agric.*, 64, 389, 1994.

18. Ryu, K. S., Roberson, K. D., Pesti, G. M., and Eitenmiller, R. R., The folic acid requirements of starting broiler chicks fed diets based on practical ingredients. 1. Interrelationships with dietary choline, *Poultry Sci.*, 74, 1447, 1995.

19. Ryu, K. S., Pesti, G. M., Robertson, K. D., Edwards, H. J., Jr., and Eitenmiller, R. R., The folic acid requirements of starting broiler chicks fed diets based on practical ingredients, 2. Interrelationships with dietary methionine, *Poultry Sci.*, 74, 1456, 1995.

20. Prinyawiwatkul, W., Eitenmiller, R. R., Beuchat, L. R., McWatters, K. H., and Phillips, R. D., Cowpea flour vitamins and trypsin inhibitor affected by treatment and fermentation with *Rhizopus microsporus*, *J. Food Sci.*, 61, 1039, 1996.

21. Goli, D. M. and Vanderslice, J. T., Investigation of the conjugase treatment procedure in the microbiological assay of folate, *Food Chem.*, 43, 57, 1992.

22. O'Broin, S. and Kelleher, B., Microbiological assay on microtiter plates of folate in serum and red cells, *J. Clin. Pathol.*, 45, 344, 1992.

23. Tanner, J. T., Barnett, S. A., and Mountford, M. K., Analysis of milk-based infant formula. Phase V. Vitamins A and E, folic acid, and pantothenic acid: Food and Drug Administration-Infant Formula Council collaborative study, *J. AOAC Int.*, 76, 399, 1993.

24. Das Sarma, J. D., Duttagupta, C., Ali, E., and Dher, T. K., Improved microbiological assay for folic acid based on microtiter plating with *Streptococcus faecalis*, *J. AOAC Int.*, 78, 1173, 1995.

25. Lane, H. W., Nillen, J. L., and Kloeris, V. L., Folic acid content in thermostabilized and freeze-dried space shuttle foods, *J. Food Sci.*, 60, 538, 1995.

26. Tamura, T., Mizuro, Y., Johnston, K. E., and Jacob, R. A., Food folate assay with protease, α-amylase, and folate conjugase treatments, *J. Agric. Food Chem.*, 45, 135, 1997.

27. Pfeiffer, C. M., Rogers, L. M., and Gregory, J. F., III, Determination of folate in cereal-grain food products using trienzyme extraction and combined affinity and reversed-phase liquid chromatography, *J. Agric. Food Chem.*, 45, 407, 1997.

Table 11.9   HPLC Methods for the Analysis of Folates in Food, Feeds, Pharmaceuticals, and Biologicals

Food

1. Day, B. P. and Gregory, J. F., III, Determination of folacin derivatives in selected foods by high-performance liquid chromatography, *J. Agric. Food Chem.*, 29, 374, 1981.

2. Gregory, J. F., III, Day, B. P. F., and Ristow, K. A., Comparison of high performance liquid chromatographic, radiometric, and *Lactobacillus casei* methods for the determination of folacin in selected foods, *J. Food Sci.*, 47, 1568, 1982.

3. Hoppner, K. and Lampi, B., The determination of folic acid (pteroylmonoglutamic acid) in fortified products by reversed phase high pressure liquid chromatography, *J. Liq. Chromatogr.*, 5, 953, 1982.

4. Gregory, J. F., III, Sartain, D. B., and Day, B. P. F., Fluorometric determination of folacin in biological materials using high performance liquid chromatography, *J. Nutr.,* 114, 341, 1984.

5. Schieffer, G. W., Wheeler, G. P., and Cimino, C. O., Determination of folic acid in commercial diets by anion-exchange solid-phase extraction and subsequent reversed-phase HPLC, *J. Liq. Chromatogr.,* 7, 2659, 1984.

6. Wegner, C., Trotz, M., and Nau, H., Direct determination of folate monoglutamates in plasma by high-performance liquid chromatography using an automatic precolumn-switching system as sample clean-up procedure, *J. Chromatogr.,* 378, 55, 1986.

7. Holt, D. L., Wehling, R. L., and Zeece, M. G., Determination of native folates in milk and other dairy products by high-performance liquid chromatography, *J. Liq. Chromatogr.,* 449, 271, 1988.

8. Selhub, J., Determination of tissue folate composition by affinity chromatography followed by high-pressure ion pair liquid chromatography, *Anal. Biochem.,* 182, 84, 1989.

9. Seyoum, E. and Selhub, J., Combined affinity and ion pair column chromatographies for the analysis of food folate, *J. Nutr. Biochem.,* 4, 488, 1993.

10. Engelhardt, R. and Gregory, J. F., III, Adequacy of enzymatic deconjugation in quantification of folate in foods, *J. Agric. Food Chem.,* 38, 154, 1990.

11. White, D. R., Jr., Determination of 5-methyltetrahydrofolate in citrus juice by reversed-phase high-performance liquid chromatography with electrochemical detection, *J. Agric. Food Chem.,* 38, 1515, 1990.

12. White, D. R., Jr., Lee, H. S., and Krüger, R. E., Reversed-phase HPLC/EC determination of folate in citrus juice by direct injection with column switching, *J. Agric. Food Chem.,* 39, 714, 1991.

13. Iwase, H., Determination of folic acid in an elemental diet by high-performance liquid chromatography with UV detection, *J. Chromatogr.,* 609, 399, 1992.

14. Jacoby, B. T. and Henry, F. T., Liquid chromatographic determination of folic acid in infant formula and adult medical nutritionals, *J. AOAC Int.,* 75, 891, 1992.

15. Vahteristo, L., Finglas, P. M., Witthöft, C., Wigertz, K., Seale, R., and de Froidmont-Görtz, I., Third EU MAT intercomparison study on food folate analysis using HPLC procedures, *Food Chem.,* 57, 109, 1996.

16. Vahteristo, L. T., Ollilainen, V., Koivistoinen, P. E., and Vara, P., Improvements in the analysis of reduced folate monoglutamates and folic acid in food by high-performance liquid chromatography, *J. Agric. Food Chem.,* 44, 477, 1996.

17. Vahteristo, L., Ollilainen, V., and Varo, P., HPLC determination of folate in liver and liver products, *J. Food Sci.,* 61, 524, 1996.

18. Vahteristo, L. T., Ollilainen, V., and Varo, P., Liquid chromatographic determination of folate monoglutamates in fish, meat, egg, and dairy products consumed in Finland, *J. AOAC Int.,* 80, 373, 1997.

19. Vahteristo, L., Lehikoinen, K., Ollilainen, V., and Varo, P., Application of an HPLC assay for the determination of folate derivatives in some vegetables, fruits and berries consumed in Finland, *Food Chem.,* 59, 589, 1997.

20. Pfeiffer, C. M., Rogers, L. M., and Gregory, J. F., III, Determination of folate in cereal-grain food products using trienzyme extraction and combined affinity and reversed-phase liquid chromatography, *J. Agric. Food Chem.,* 45, 407, 1997.

Biologicals

1. Horne, D. W., Briggs, W. T., and Wagner, C., High pressure liquid chromatographic separation of the naturally occurring folic acid monoglutamate derivatives, *Anal. Biochem.,* 116, 393, 1981.

2. Wilson, S. D. and Horne, D. W., Evaluation of ascorbic-acid in protecting labile folic acid derivatives, *Proc. Natl. Acad. Sci. USA,* 80, 6500, 1983.

3. Wilson, S. D. and Horne, D. W., High-performance liquid chromatographic determination of the distribution of naturally occurring folic acid derivatives in rat liver, *Anal. Biochem.,* 142, 529, 1984.

4. Kohashi, M., Inoue, K., and Sotobayashi, H., Microdetermination of folate monoglutamates in serum by liquid chromatography with electrochemical detection, *J. Chromatogr.,* 382, 303, 1986.

5. Selhub, J., Darcy-Vrillon, B., and Fell, D., Affinity chromatography of naturally occurring folate derivatives, *Anal. Biochem.,* 168, 247, 1988.

6. Selhub, J., Determination of tissue folate composition by affinity chromatography followed by high-pressure ion pair liquid chromatography, *Anal. Biochem.,* 182, 89, 1989.

7. Selhub, J., Seyoum, E., Pomfret, E. A., and Zeisel, S. H., Effects of choline deficiency and methotrexate treatment upon liver folate content and distribution, *Cancer Res.,* 51, 16, 1991.

8. Varela-Moreiras, G., Seyoum, E., and Selhub, J., Combined affinity and ion pair liquid chromatographies for the analysis of folate distribution in tissues, *J. Nutr. Biochem.,* 2, 44, 1991.

9. Varela-Moreiras, G., Selhub, J., da Costa, K. A., and Zeisel, S. H., Effect of chronic choline deficiency in rats on liver folate content and distribution, *J. Nutr. Biochem.,* 3, 519, 1992.

10. Varela-Moreiras, G. and Selhub, J., Long-term folate deficiency alters folate content and distribution differentially in rat tissues, *J. Nutr.,* 122, 986, 1992.

11. Case, G. L. and Steele, R. D., Determination of reduced folate derivatives in tissue samples by high-performance liquid chromatography with fluorometric detection, *J. Chromatogr.,* 487, 456, 1989.

12. Gounelle, J. C., Ladjimi, H., and Prognon, P., A rapid and specific extraction procedure for folates determination in rat liver and analysis by high-performance liquid chromatography with fluorometric detection, *Anal. Biochem.,* 176, 406, 1989.

13. Lucock, M.D., Hartley, R., and Smithells, R.W., A rapid and specific HPLC-electrochemical method for the determination of endogenous 5-methyltetrahydrofolic acid in plasma using solid phase sample preparation with internal standardization, *Biomed. Chromatogr.,* 3, 58, 1989.

14. Leeming, R. J., Pollock, A., Melville, L. J., and Hamon, C. G. B., Measurement of 5-methyltetrahydrofolic acid in man by high-performance liquid chromatography, *Metabolism,* 39, 902, 1990.

15. Shimoda, M., Simultaneous determination of tetrahydrofolate and N^5-methyltetrahydrofolate in pig plasma by high-performance liquid chromatography with electrochemical detection, *J. Vet. Med. Sci.,* 54, 249, 1992.

16. Hahn, A., Stein, J., Rump, U., and Rehner, G., Optimized high-performance liquid chromatographic procedure for the separation and quantification of the main folacins and some derivatives, *J. Chromatogr.,* 540, 207, 1991.

17. Lucock, M. D., Green, M., Hartley, R., and Levene, M. I., Physico-chemical and biological factors influencing methylfolate stability: use of dithiothreitol for HPLC analysis with electrochemical detection, *Food Chem.,* 47, 79, 1993.

18. Lucock, M. D., Nayeemuddin, F. A., Habibzadeh, N., Schorah, C. J., Hartley, R., and Levene, M. I., Methylfolate exhibits a negative *in vitro* interaction with important dietary metal cations, *Food Chem.,* 50, 307, 1994.

19. Lucock, M. D., Green, M., Priestnall, M., Daskalakis, I., Levene, M. I., and Hartley, R., Optimisation of chromatographic conditions for the determination of folates in foods and biological tissues for nutritional and clinical work, *Food Chem.,* 53, 329, 1995.

20. Lucock, M. D., Daskalakis, I., Schorah, C. J., Levene, M. I., and Hartley, R., Analysis and biochemistry of blood folate, *Biochem. Mol. Med.,* 58, 93, 1996.

21. Ichinose, N., Tsuneyoshi, T., Kato, M., Suzuki, T., and Ikeda, S., Fluorescent high-performance liquid chromatography of folic acid and its derivatives using permanganate as a fluorogenic reagent, *Fres. J. Anal. Chem.,* 346, 841, 1993.

22. Schleyer, E., Reinhardt, J., Unterhalt, M., and Hiddemann, W., Highly sensitive coupled-column high-performance liquid chromatographic method for the separation and quantitation of the diastereomers of leucovorin and 5-methyltetrahydrofolate in serum and urine, *J. Chromatogr. B.,* 669, 319, 1995.

23. Kelly, P., McPartlin, J., and Scott, J., A combined high-performance liquid chromatographic-microbiological assay for serum folic acid, *Anal. Biochem.,* 238, 179, 1996.

12 Vitamin B-12, Biotin, and Pantothenic Acid

12.1 VITAMIN B-12

12.1.1 REVIEW

Vitamin B-12 deficiency, or pernicious anemia, was identified in 1824 with clinical symptoms being described in 1855.[1] It was not until 1925 that treatment protocols became apparent through the discovery by Whipple and Robscheit-Robbins that raw liver had curative effects for anemic dogs.[2] In 1926, Minot and Murphy reported that raw liver cured pernicious anemia in humans. That same decade (1927), Castle suggested the presence of the extrinsic factor in food and the intrinsic factor in the gastrointestinal system as the preventative factors for pernicious anemia.[1] In 1934, Whipple, Minot, and Murphy were awarded the Nobel Prize for Medicine for advances made in the treatment of pernicious anemia. Significant events in the more recent history of vitamin B-12 include the isolation and naming of vitamin B-12 and the first use of injections of the vitamin to cure deficiency (1948), the isolation of crystalline forms and identification of cyanocobalamin (CNCbl) and hydroxocobalamin (OHCbl) (1949), establishment of the structure of vitamin B-12 and its microbial synthesis (1955), and chemical synthesis (1973).[1] Dorothy Hodgkin was awarded the Nobel Prize in 1964 for her work with X-ray crystallography to determine the structure.

Absorption of vitamin B-12 requires enzyme and acid hydrolysis in the stomach to liberate Cbl from macromolecules, primarily protein. After digestive release, Cbl binds to salivary proteins (R-binders), and subsequently is bound by the intrinsic factor secreted by gastric parietal cells.[3] Absorption occurs in the ileum through binding of Cbl with cell surface receptors and release of the intrinsic factor. After absorption, vitamin B-12 is complexed with the B-12 delivery protein (TCII) to form holoTCII or with the B-12 storage protein (haptocorrin) to form holohaptocorrin. TCII and haptocorrin complexes contain 20% and 80%, respectively, of serum total vitamin B-12.[3]

Pernicious anemia evolves through abnormal absorption of vitamin B-12 resulting from inadequate digestion, lack of necessary binding factors including Ca^{++}, lack of intrinsic factor due to lack of synthesis or autoimmune inactivation, absence of the delivery or storage proteins, and various other pathological states. Lack of sufficient dietary intake is usually not the cause of deficiency.[4]

Signs of pernicious anemia include macrocytic, megaloblastic anemia, and neurologic involvement resulting from demyelination of the spinal cord, brain, optic, and peripheral nerves.[4] General symptoms include glossitis, weakness, loss of appetite, loss of weight, loss of taste and smell, impotence, irritability, memory impairment, mild depression, and hallucinations.[1] Hebert[3] summarized sequential stages of vitamin B-12 status and the use of various indicators to assess human status. Low serum holoTCII is the earliest indicator of negative vitamin B-12 balance which indicates inadequate delivery of vitamin B-12 to DNA synthesizing cells. Serum holoTCII falls to low levels before total serum vitamin B-12 lowers or deficiency occurs. Measurement of serum and erythrocyte concentrations remain common biochemical tests for status assessment; however, such measurements are often difficult to interpret.

All vitamin B-12 found in the diet is derived from microbial synthesis. Food sources include fermented foods and animal products. Low, but measurable, levels of vitamin B-12 can sometimes be found in plant products owing to the presence of bacteria. In the animal kingdom, vitamin B-12 is derived from the animal's diet or from synthesis by the gut microflora. The richest food sources include meats, seafoods, eggs, and dairy products. Vegetarian diets can produce deficiency; however, most "true" vegetarians are aware of their need to supplement the vegetarian diet with vitamin B-12.[5] For vegetarians, 1 to 5 μg, orally, is sufficient. Therapeutic treatment of pernicious anemia requires 100 μg of vitamin B-12 parenterally per month.[6] OHCbl is retained at higher levels than CNCbl.[1] Recommended Dietary Allowances (RDA) are 2 μg for adults, increasing to 2.2 μg during pregnancy, and 2.6 μg during lactation.[4] The Reference Daily Intake (RDI) specified by the Nutritional Labeling and Education Act of 1990 is 6 μg.[7]

Metabolically active co-enzyme forms of Cbl are 5′-deoxyadenosyl cobalamin (adoCbl) and methylcobalamin (MeCbl). AdoCbl dependent reactions include conversion of methylmalonyl CoA to succinyl CoA by methylmalonyl CoA mutase in the degradation of propionate and the conversion of leucine to 3-aminoisocapronate by leucine mutase. MeCbl functions with methionine synthetase in the methylation of homocysteine in methionine synthesis. Vitamin B-12 is required for the enzymatic removal of the methyl group from methylfolate which regenerates tetrahydrofolate required for formation of 5,10-methylene tetrahydrofolate. 5,10-Methylene tetrahydrofolate is the source of thymidylate (dTMP) synthesis. Therefore, vitamin B-12 deficiency causes folate to be trapped as methylfolate. Adequate amounts of 5,10-methylene tetrahydrofolate become unavailable for DNA synthesis. The folate-trap mechanism and its biochemistry are explained in detail by Hebert.[3] In both folate and vitamin B-12 deficiency, megaloblastic changes in red blood cells are similar owing to defective synthesis of DNA.

12.1.2 PROPERTIES

12.1.2.1 Chemistry

12.1.2.1.1 General Properties

Vitamin B-12 is the collective name for cobalt-containing corrinoids with the biological activity of CNCbl. The corrin structure includes four reduced pyrrole rings joined by three methene bridges with two pyrroles linked directly. The central cobalt atom is bound by coordinate linkages to the nitrogen atoms of the four pyrrole rings. The corrin ring is structurally similar to heme except it has one less α-methene bridge and has cobalt in place of iron.[3] The structural formula of cobalamin given by Hebert[3] is shown in Figure 12.1. Cyanocobalamin (CNCbl) is the permissive name for vitamin B-12. Nutritionally vitamin B-12 includes all cobalamins biologically active in the human. In CNCbl, the β-position of the cobalt atom is occupied by a cyano-ligand (CN⁻). In addition to CN⁻, the β-position may be occupied by OH⁻ to form hydroxocobalamin (OHCbl), water to form aquocobalamin (H_2OCbl), NO_2 to form nitrocobalamin (NO_2Cbl), deoxyadenosyl to form co-enzyme B-12 (adoBCbl), methyl to form methylcobalamin (MeCbl), and SO_3 to form sulfitocobalamin (SO_3Cbl). Use of the terms vitamin B-12$_a$ (OHCbl), vitamin B-12$_b$ (H_2OCbl), and vitamin B-12$_c$ (NO_2Cbl) are not recommended by IUPAC-IUB.[8]

General properties of the various cobalamins important in metabolism are given in Table 12.1. CNCbl is a tasteless, odorless, red crystalline substance with good water solubility (1 g/80 mL at 25°C). In the amorphous form, the vitamin is hygroscopic and absorbs about 12% by weight of water.[9] The vitamin is soluble in alcohols, phenols, and other polar solvents with hydroxy groups. CNCbl is not soluble in other organic solvents including acetone, ether, and benzene. Crystals do not melt, but decompose above 200°C. The USP standard is CNCbl.

CNCbl and OHCbl are the forms of vitamin B-12 available for medical use and fortification by the food industry. CNCbl is predominantly used in vitamin preparations, supplements, medical foods, and fortified foods because of its better stability compared to OHCbl. OHCbl is used to treat specific disease states including tobacco amblyopia and optic neuropathy.[3,10]

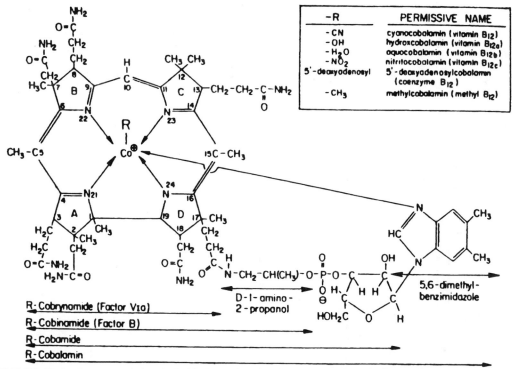

FIGURE 12.1 Structure of vitamin B-12. Reproduced with permission from Reference 3.

12.1.2.1.2 Spectral Properties

Aqueous solutions of CNCbl have absorption maxima at 278, 361, and 551 nm.[11,12] The spectra of CNCbl, H_2OCbl, and OHCbl are similar. Maximal absorbance is in the region of 350 to 368 nm.[11] AdoCbl and MeCbl show less intense absorption around 360 nm and change color from red to yellow in weakly acidic solutions.[11] Absorption spectra of CNCbl and H_2OCbl are shown in Figure 12.2.[12]

12.1.2.2 Stability

Crystalline forms of vitamin B-12 are stable when protected from light.[11] The vitamin is generally considered to be stable under most food processing operations, but, like all water-soluble vitamins, it is subject to large losses through leaching into the cooking water. CNCbl is the most stable form of vitamin B-12.[13] Light exposure cleaves the cyanide with the production of OHCbl.[14] Other ions or groups can attach to the cobalt with production of other cobalamins. In excess cyanide, cyanide can replace other moieties bound to the β-position of the cobalt. CNCbl has optimum stability at pH 4.0 to 4.5.[15] It is stable to autoclaving between pH 4.0 and 7.0.[14] Severe alkaline and acid conditions, UV, or strong visible light, and oxidizing agents inactivate the vitamin.[15] There is some indication in the literature that stability can be decreased in multinutrient preparations in the presence of thiamin, niacin, and ascorbic acid. However, the literature is not definitive.[10,13]

12.1.3 METHODS

Available methods for assay of vitamin B-12 include polarographic, spectrophotometric, various chromatographic procedures including paper, thin-layer, open-column, GC and LC procedures, microbiologic, and radio-ligand binding procedures. Almost all available data of vitamin B-12 in

TABLE 12.1
Physical Properties of Vitamin B-12

Substance[a]	Molar Mass	Formula	Solubility	Crystal Form	λ max nm	Absorbance[b] E$_1^{1\%}$cm	ε × 10^{-3}	Solvent
Cyanocobalamin B$_{12}$ CAS No. 68-19-9 10152	1355.38	C$_{63}$H$_{88}$CoN$_{14}$O$_{14}$P	Soluble in water (1g/80ml)	Dark red hygroscopic Darkens at 210–220°C	278 361 551	115 204 64	[15.6] [27.6] [8.7]	Water Water Water
Hydroxocobalamin B12a CAS No. 13422-51-0 4854	1346.37	C$_{62}$H$_{89}$CoN$_{13}$O$_{15}$P	Moderately soluble in water Insoluble in acetone, ether, petroleum ether, benzene	Dark red orthorhombic Darkens at 200°C	279 325 359 516 537	[141] [85] [153] [66] [71]	19.0 11.4 20.6 8.9 9.5	Water Water Water Water Water
Aquacobalamin B12b CAS No. 13422-52-1	1347.0	C$_{62}$H$_{90}$CoN$_{13}$O$_{15}$POH	—	—	274 317 351 499 527	[153] [45] [197] [60] [63]	20.6 6.1 26.5 8.1 8.5	Water Water Water Water Water
Nitrocobalamin B12c CAS No. 20623-13-6 4854	1374.6	C$_{62}$H$_{88}$CoN$_{14}$O$_{16}$P	—	Red crystalline solids	352 528 357 535	153 60 139 63	[21.0] [8.4] [19.1] [8.7]	Water Water 0.01 N NaOH 0.01 N NaOH
Sulfitocobalamin CAS No 15671-27-9 4854	1409.5	C$_{62}$H$_{89}$CoN$_{13}$O$_{17}$PS	—	—	275 365 418 516	328 130 49 61	[46.2] [18.3] [6.9] [8.6]	Water Water Water Water

Common name / CAS No. / Merck[a]	MW	Formula	Solubility	Appearance	λ_{max}	$E_{1\,cm}^{1\%}$[b]	$\epsilon \times 10^{-3}$	Solvent
Adenosylcobalamin	1579.6	$C_{72}H_{100}CoN_{1815}O_{17}P$	Soluble in ethanol, phenol	yellow-orange	288	[115]	18.1	Water, pH 7.0
Cobamamide			Insoluble in acetone, ether	6-faced crystal	340	[78]	12.3	Water, pH 7.0
CAS No. 13870-90-1			dioxane		375	[60]	10.9	Water, pH 7.0
2513					522	[51]	8.0	Water, pH 7.0
Methylcobalamin	1344.4	$C_{63}H_{91}CoN_{13}O_{14}P$	—	Bright red	266	[148]	19.9	Water, pH 7.0
CAS No. 13422-55-4					342	[107]	14.4	Water, pH 7.0
6125					522	[70]	9.4	Water, pH 7.0
					264	[184]	24.7	0.1 N HCl
					304	[170]	22.9	0.1 N HCl
					462	[71]	9.6	0.1 N HCl

[a] Common or generic name; CAS No.—Chemical Abstract Service number, bold print designates the Merck Index monograph number.

[b] Values in brackets are calculated from corresponding ϵ value or $E_{1\,cm}^{1\%}$ value.

Budavari, S., *The Merck Index*. 12th ed., 1996[1]

Friedrich, W., *Vitamins.*, 1988[2]

Food Chemicals Codex.[3]

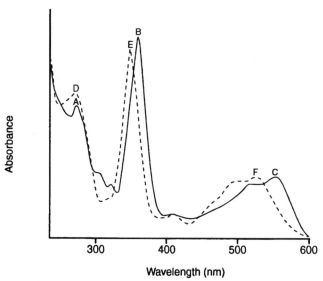

FIGURE 12.2   Absorption spectra of cyanocobalamin (solid line) and aquocobalamin (broken line), aqueous solution, pH 5.8. λ max, A = 278 nm; B = 361 nm; C = 550 nm; D = 274 nm; E = 351 nm; F = 525 nm. Reproduced with permission from Reference 12.

food has been obtained by microbiological assay.[5] Assay of naturally occurring vitamin B-12 in most biological matrices is difficult owing to the low concentrations normally present. Except for organ meats, vitamin B-12 levels usually are less than 10 μg/100 g and often below 1.0 μg/g.[5] Detection after LC resolution requires 10 ng on-column when monitored at 350 nm.[14] The relatively high detection limit combined with low, natural levels in animal products makes vitamin B-12 assay by LC difficult even if preconcentration steps are used.[14] For clinical tissue and serum samples, radio-ligand binding assays with [57]Co-labeled CNCbl are routine and dependable. However, radioassay kits for clinical assay are not reliable for assay of food (Section 12.1.3.2). Normal vitamin B-12 content of serum ranges from 150 to 750 pg/mL.[1]

LC can effectively resolve natural cobalamins. However, owing to low levels of the analytes, radio-ligand binding assays are necessary to quantitate eluted cobalamins. Excellent discussions of LC methods useful for vitamin B-12 assay were presented by Lindemans[14] and Lindemans and Abels.[16] Summaries of available LC methodologies are given in these reviews.

LC can be conveniently applied to the assay of vitamin B-12 in high concentration supplements and pharmaceutical preparations.[17,18,19] Regulatory, compendium, and handbook procedures are summarized in Table 12.2. These methods use spectrophotometric, microbiological, and LC approaches for the assay of CNCbl in pharmaceuticals and microbiological assay for foods.

12.1.3.1   AOAC International Methods (*Lactobacillus delbrueckii*)

AOAC International[20] methods use microbiological assay with *Lactobacillus delbrueckii* (*leichmannii*) ATCC 7830. The methodology was originally collaborated for use on vitamin preparations, but the AOAC Task Force on Methods for Nutrition Labeling[21] recommended the procedure for use on all food matrices.

**TABLE 12.2
Compendium, Regulatory and Handbook Methods for Analysis of Vitamin B-12**

Source	Form	Methods and Application	Approach	Most Current Cross-Reference
U.S. Pharmacopeia, National Formulary, USP 23/NF 18, Nutritional Supplements, Official Monographs[1]				
1. pages 2142, 2145, 2148, 2152	Cyanocobalamin	Cyanocobalamin in oil- and water-soluble vitamin capsules/tablets w/wo minerals	Method 1— HPLC 550 nm Method 2— Microbiological	None
2. pages 2160, 2164, 2169, 2171	Cyanocobalamin	Cyanocobalamin in water-soluble capsules/tablets w/wo minerals	Method 1— HPLC 550 nm Method 2— Microbiological	None
3. pages 413–414, 1719–1721	Cyanocobalamin	Cyanocobalamin Co[57] capsule/oral solution	Microbiological	None
4. page 435	Cyanocobalamin	Cyanocobalamin injection	Spectrophotometric 361 nm	None
5. page 435	Cyanocobalamin	Cyanocobalamin (NLT 96.0%, NMT 100.5%)	Spectrophotometric 361 nm	None
British Pharmacopoeia, 15th ed., 1993[2]				
1. vol. I, page 189	Cyanocobalamin	Cyanocobalamin	Spectrophotometric 361 nm	None
2. vol. II, page 860	Cyanocobalamin	Cyanocobalamin injection	Spectrophotometric 361 nm	None
3. vol. II, page 861	Cyanocobalamin	Cyanocobalamin tablets	HPLC 361 nm	None
4. vol. II, pages 1222–1223	Cyanocobalamin	Cyanocobalamin Co[57] capsules	HPLC 361 nm and Gamma detector for Co[57]	None

TABLE 12.2   continued

Source	Form	Methods and Application	Approach	Most Current Cross-Reference
5. vol. II, page 1223	Cyanocobalamin	Cyanocobalamin Co^{57} solution	HPLC 361 nm and Gamma detector for Co^{57}	None
6. vol. II, page 1224	Cyanocobalamin	Cyanocobalamin Co^{58} solution	HPLC 361 nm and Gamma detector for Co^{58}	None
7. addend. 1995, page 1556	Hydroxocobalamin acetate	Hydroxocobalamin acetate	Spectrophotometric 351 nm / HPLC 351 nm	None
8. addend. 1995, page 1557	Hydroxocobalamin chloride	Hydroxocobalamin chloride	Spectrophotometric 351 nm / HPLC 351 nm	None
9. addend. 1995, page 1557	Hydroxocobalamin sulphate	Hydroxocobalamin sulphate	Spectrophotometric 351 nm / HPLC 351 nm	None
AOAC Official Methods of Analysis, 16th ed. 1995[3]				
1. 45.2.02	Cyanocobalamin	AOAC Official Method 952.20, Cobalamin (Vitamin B_{12} Activity) in Vitamin Preparations	Microbiological	*J. Assoc. Off. Anal. Chem.*, 42, 529, 1959[4]
2. 50.1.20	Cyanocobalamin	AOAC Official Method 986.23, Cobalamin (Vitamin B_{12} Activity) in Milk-Based Infant Formula	Microbiological	*J. Assoc. Off. Anal. Chem.*, 69, 777, 1986[5]
American Feed Ingredients Association, *Laboratory Methods Compendium*, vol. 1, 1991[6]				
1. pages 163–164	Cyanocobalamin	Vitamin B_{12} in concentrates	HPLC 550 nm	

Source	Compound	Description	Method	Reference
2. pages 165–168	Cyanocobalamin	Microbiological assay of vitamin B_{12} in complete feeds and premixes	Microbiological	Hoffman-LaRoche, *Analytical Methods for Vitamins and Carotenoids in Feeds*, 36–38[7] *The Vitamins*, Vol. VIII, 1967, 282[8]
American Association of Cereal Chemists, *Approved Methods*, vol. 2, 1996[9] 1. AACC 86–40	Cyanocobalamin	Vitamin B_{12} in cereal products	Microbiological	AOAC 16th ed. 45.2.01, 45.2.02, 1995[3]
Food Chemicals Codex, 4th ed. 1996[10] 1. pages 431–432	Cyanocobalamin	Vitamin B_{12} (NLT 96.0%, NMT 100.5%)	Spectrophotometric 361 nm	None
Hoffmann-LaRoche, *Analytical Methods for Vitamins and Carotenoids*, 1988[7] 1. pages 36–38	Cyanocobalamin	Microbiological assay of vitamin B_{12} complete feeds and premixes	Microbiological	*The Vitamins*, vol. VIII, 1967, 282[8]

AOAC Official Method 952.20, Cobalamin (Vitamin B-12 Activity) in Vitamin
Preparations, Microbiological Method, *Official Methods of Analysis of AOAC
International, 45.2.02*

Lactobacillus delbrueckii growth response is sensitive enough to quantitate CNCbl at concentrations
approaching 1.0 pg/mL of assay growth media. This sensitivity is sufficient to quantitate vitamin
B-12 in foods containing less than 0.5 μg/100 g.[5]

Vitamin B-12 active compounds are extracted in phosphate buffer containing 1.3 g Na_2HPO_4,
1.2 g citric acid, and 1.0 g anhydrous sodium metabisulfite per 100 mL. Extracting solutions must
contain a reducing agent such as metabisulfite or ascorbic acid to protect the cobalamins throughout
the extraction.[22,23] Many methods incorporate sodium cyanide to ensure the conversion of the more
labile OHCbl to the more stable dicyanocobalamin $(CN)_2Cbl$.[15] Method 952.20 does not use sodium
cyanide. Of importance, sodium metabisulfite must be at a concentration less than 0.03 mg/mL in
the final assay solution to avoid inhibition of *L. delbrueckii* growth. The extraction is completed by
homogenizing the sample in the extraction solution, autoclaving the mixture at 121°C for 10 min,
adjusting the cooled mixture to pH 4.5, diluting with water to a vitamin B-12 concentration of
approximately 0.2 ng/mL, and filtering. Standard microbiological assay techniques are used to quantitate the vitamin (AOAC Method 960.46).

AOAC Official Method 986.23 (50.1.20) "Cobalamin (Vitamin B-12 Activity) in Milk-Based
Infant Formula" is basically the same as Method 952.20. At this point in time, AOAC International
has not collaborated the method for use on other types of infant formula; however, the AOAC Task
Force on Methods for Nutrient Labeling listed Method 986.23 as acceptable for all infant formulas.[21]

Lactobacillus delbrueckii has variable response to various cobalamins. Muhammad et al.[22]
determined the growth response of *L. delbrueckii* to CNCbl, OHCbl, SO_3Cbl, $(CN)_2Cbl$, NO_2Cbl,
MeCbl, and adoCbl since the potential exists for these cobalamins to be present in extracts of biological samples prepared with the addition of sodium cyanide, potassium cyanide, sodium
metabisulfite, or sodium nitrite. Similar growth response was found for CNCbl, OHCbl, SO_3Cbl,
$(CN)_2Cbl$, and NO_2Cbl. However, adoCbl produced a greater response and MeCbl a lesser growth
response (Figure 12.3). When CNCbl is used as the calibration standard in the *L. delbrueckii* assay,
accurate determinations can be obtained for OHCbl, SO_3Cbl, CNCbl, and adoCbl when the extracting solution contains excess cyanide; however, MeCbl will be underestimated. In the presence of
sodium metabisulfite or sodium nitrite only OHCbl, SO_3Cbl, and CNCbl can be assayed with confidence. AdoCbl will be overestimated if extracted in the presence of sodium metabisulfite or sodium
nitrite because these compounds do not modify adoCbl. Conversely, MeCbl, which is also stable in
the presence of metabisulfite and nitrite, will be underestimated. Excess cyanide converts OHCbl,
SO_3Cbl, and adoCbl to the $(CN)_2Cbl$ form, and MeCbl remains unchanged.[22] Because adoCbl and
OHCbl are the predominant cobalamins in food,[22,24] the AOAC International assay potentially can
overestimate naturally occurring vitamin B-12 activity as cyanide is omitted from the extracting solution.

Muhammad et al.[22] concluded that vitamin B-12 activity can not be accurately measured by *L.
delbrueckii* using CNCbl as the calibration standard if adoCbl and/or MeCbl are present in the sample extract. To circumvent the inability of commonly used extractants to convert adoCbl and MeCbl
to cobalamins with equal response to CNCbl in the *L. delbrueckii* assay, photoconversion of these
forms to OHCbl was suggested prior to assay. Complete conversion occurs under exposure to fluorescent light within 1 h.[22] This approach has not been incorporated into published work or analysis
of vitamin B-12 activity in food. However, improvement in the reliability of data obtained by assay
with *L. delbrueckii* might be possible through addition of this simple extraction step.

Lactobacillus delbrueckii can utilize vitamin B-12 analogs, deoxyribonucleotides, and deoxyribonu-
cleosides in addition to biologically active cobalamins. Older literature suggests that dilution of deoxyri-
boside levels (e.g., thymidine) to less than 1 μg/mL of the assay medium will eliminate the effect.[25]
Comparative studies on animal products assayed by *L. delbrueckii* and *Ochromonas malhamensis*, a

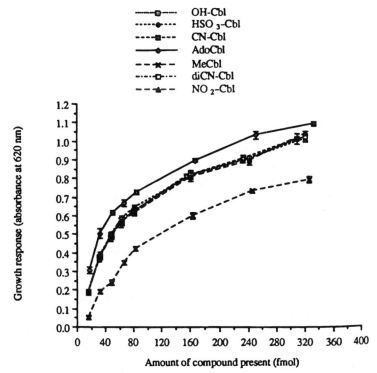

FIGURE 12.3 Growth responses of *Lactobacillus delbrueckii* (ATCC 7830) to OHCbl, HSO₃Cbl, CNCbl, AdoCbl, MeCbl, DiCNCbl, and NO₂Cbl. Reproduced with permission from Reference 22.

protozoan considered to be the most specific assay organism for measurement of vitamin B-12 activity, indicated little difference in the values obtained by the two organisms.[26] The ease of using *L. delbrueckii*, compared to the protozoan, makes it a clear choice for vitamin B-12 analysis in most laboratories.

12.1.3.2 Radio-Ligand Binding Assays

Radio-ligand binding assays have been routinely used for blood and tissue analysis since early work by Rothenberg,[27] Barakat and Elkins,[28] and Lau et al.[29] established the use of intrinsic factor as the binding protein and [⁵⁷Co]CNCbl as the radiolabeled ligand for a competitive binding assay for vitamin B-12 in serum. Other binding proteins in addition to intrinsic factor have been used, including transcobalamin I (TC-I), transcobalamin II (TC-II), and haptocorrin or R-binder from saliva. Early studies established that such binding proteins were not specific for Cbl and bound non-biologically active cobalamins. Porcine intrinsic factor is routinely used as the binding protein in most clinical applications.

Specific radioimmunoassays (RIA) are available for CNCbl[30] and adoCbl.[31] The RIA methods are based on monospecific antisera and eliminate cross-reaction with other cobalamins. Such assays are not in routine use in most clinical laboratories.

Studies by several research groups indicated that radio-ligand binding assays with intrinsic factor could be used for food analysis.[23,32–39] The early research established extraction procedures necessary to liberate bound cobalamins from food matrices. When optimized extraction procedures were used, radio-ligand and microbiological procedures showed agreement for most foods; however,

TABLE 12.3
Conversion[a] of Cobalamins by Excess Potassium Cyanide, Sodium Metabisulfite, and Sodium Nitrite

Before Conversion	+KCN	After Conversion $+Na_2S_2O_5$	$+NaNO_2$
OHCbl	diCNCbl	HSO_3Cbl	NO_2Cbl
HSO_3Cbl	diCNCbl	HSO_3Cbl	HSO_3Cbl
CNCbl	diCNCbl	HSO_3Cbl	CNCbl
AdoCbl	diCNCbl	AdoCbl	AdoCbl
MeCbl	MeCbl	MeCbl	MeCbl

[a] Based on absorption spectrophotometry of aqueous solutions. Spectra were determined 30 min after addition of the compound and incubation in the dark. The ratio, in terms of number of moles of KCN, Na_2S_2O5, and $NaNO_2$ to each cobalamin was 50 : 1, 1.5 : 1, and 15 : 1, respectively. Reproduced with permission from Reference 41.

differences were noted often enough to conclude that the two methods are not universally interchangeable for the assay of all foods. Differences in results between the two methods indicated that radio-ligand assay gave lower values than microbiological assay in situations when variation existed.[40] This trend was postulated to be due to inefficient extraction of vitamin B-12 in chemical forms bindable to the intrinsic factor and to the lower specificity of *L. delbrueckii*.[40]

Muhammad et al.[41] studied the relative binding affinities of CNCbl, CN_2Cbl, OHCbl, SO_3Cbl, NO_2Cbl, adoCbl, and MeCbl with porcine intrinsic factor. Equivalent binding was noted for CNCbl, CN_2Cbl, NO_2Cbl, and MeCbl (P > 0.2) (Figure 12.4). Significantly different binding affinities were found for OHCbl, SO_3Cbl, and adoCbl. Therefore, porcine intrinsic factor can not be used as the binding protein with CNCbl as the calibration standard unless equal cyanide is used in the extraction procedure to convert OHCbl, SO_3Cbl, and adoCbl to CN_2Cbl.[41] Effects of excess potassium cyanide, sodium metabisulfite, and sodium nitrite on the conversion of cobalamins are given in Table 12.3.

A protein binding assay developed by Alcock et al.[42] appears to be useful for fortified foods in which CHCbl is the predominant cobalamin. The procedure uses a R-protein-enzyme conjugate and microtitration plate techniques for quantitation of CNCbl. Since R-proteins bind Cbl and Cbl analogs, the assay has not been applied to non-fortified foods. Applications to fortified breakfast cereals gave a limit of detection of 9 pg per well and a quantitation limit of 0.09 μg per 100 g.

Currently, protein ligand binding assays are not routinely used for food analysis. Although the Alcock et al.[42] procedure could be a time and labor-saving method for analysis of vitamin B-12 in fortified foods, the lack of a commercial source of the R-protein enzyme conjugate is a hindrance to use of the assay by most laboratories involved with analysis of vitamin B-12 in foods. It appears that the microbiological assay by *L. delbrueckii* will continue to be the method of choice for food analysis for the foreseeable future.

12.2 BIOTIN

12.2.1 REVIEW

Wildiers (1901) reported the presence of a growth factor in yeast and meat extracts referred to as "bios" which was required for yeast growth.[1] Bios was fractionated over the next decades into bios I (meso-inositol), bios II (an impure preparation of pantothenic acid), and bios II B (later identified as biotin). Recognition of the toxic effects of raw egg white in the animal diet occurred before the

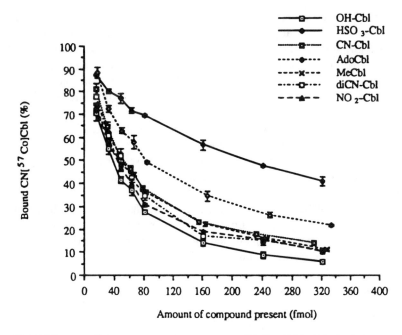

FIGURE 12.4 The relative binding affinity of OHCbl, HSO$_3$Cbl, CNCbl, AdoCbl, McCbl, DiCNCbl and NO$_2$Cbl with porcine intrinsic factor. Reproduced with permission from Reference 41.

turn of the century and was further defined in 1916 by Bateman. Boas[43] (1927) confirmed earlier descriptions of egg white injury in rats fed raw egg white and showed the curative effects of raw liver. In 1936, Kögl and Tonnis[44] isolated and crystallized a growth factor from egg yolk which they named biotin. Snell, in 1941, reported that the glycoprotein, avidin, was the biotin antagonist responsible for the toxicity of raw egg white.[45] The structure was determined in 1942 with synthesis in 1943.

Biotin deficiency is characterized by anorexia, nausea, vomiting, glossitis, pallor, mental depression, hair loss (alopecia), dry scaly dermatitis, and an increase in serum cholesterol and bile pigments.[4] Human deficiency is rare but can occur through prolonged consumption of raw egg and parenteral feeding without biotin supplementation in patients with short-gut syndrome.[46] Biotin deficiency occurs in infants through an inborn error of metabolism that leads to lack of biotinidase, the enzyme necessary to cleave biotinyl-lysine bonds in biocytin (biotinyllisine). Mock[46] indicates that the lack of biotinidase produces biotin deficiency by leading to inefficient release of protein-bound biotin in the gastrointestinal tract, less salvage of biotin at the cellular level, and through increased renal loss. Biotin deficiency has been linked to sudden infant death syndrome; however, firm conclusions have not been made in this significant area. Biotin deficiency is diagnosed by reduced urinary excretion of biotin, increased urinary excretion of 3-hydroxy-isovaleric acid, and curative effects of supplementation.[46] Blood levels do not adequately reflect deficiency.[46]

Biotin occurs in relatively low concentrations in most foods. Liver and yeast, which contain in excess of 100 µg/100 g, are high in biotin content compared to other foods. Substantial sources are egg yolk, dairy products, soy products, cereals, and vegetables. Meat and fruit are low in biotin.[4] Hoppner et al.[47] published one of the latest studies on biotin content in foods. The study quantitated biotin in 45 vegetables and 16 nuts. In vegetables, biotin content ranged from 0.3 µg/100 g (iceberg lettuce and green peppers) to 8.4 µg/100 g (mushrooms). Other, higher contents in vegetables were 7.5 µg/100 g (cauliflower), 7.0 µg /100 g (snow peas), and 5.9 µg/100 g (yams). Biotin content in nuts ranged from 0.7 µg/100 g (coconut) to 91.1 µg/100 g (oil roasted peanuts). Most nuts contained greater than 10 µg/100 g. The Hoppner et al.[47] data was obtained by microbiological assay with *Lactobacillus plantarum* ATCC 8014. Microbial synthesis in the gut is a source of biotin; however, the significance of microbial synthesis to total biotin available to the human is unknown. The role of avidin as a biotin antagonist is understood. Nutritionally, the binding phenomenon has little impact since cooking destroys the avidin-biotin complex and denatures avidin, preventing additional complex formation. Raw egg white, if added to foods without further cooking or ingested with cooked foods, provides avidin that binds the low amounts of biotin in the food. The avidin-biotin complex resists digestive proteases and prevents absorption.

A Recommended Dietary Allowance (RDA) has not been set. The Estimated Safe and Adequate Daily Dietary Intake is 30 to 100 µg.[4] The Reference Daily Intake (RDI) for use in calculation of nutrition label information is 300 µg.[7]

Metabolically, biotin is the co-enzyme for carboxylases that incorporate bicarbonate into various substrates. Mammalian carboxylases are acetyl-CoA carboxylase (fatty acid synthesis), pyruvate carboxylase (oxaloacetate formation), methylcrotonyl-CoA carboxylase (leucine degradation), and propionyl-CoA carboxylase (methylmalonyl-CoA formation).

12.2.2 PROPERTIES

12.2.2.1 Chemistry

12.2.2.1.1 General Properties

Biotin is cis-hexahydro-2-oxo-1H-thieno [3,4-d] imidazole-4-pentanoic acid.[8] Eight stereoisomers exist. d(+) Biotin is the only biologically active form and other isomers are not found in nature.[48] The biotin structure is shown in Figure 12.5. The bicyclic ring structure contains an ureido ring which is fused to a tetrahydrothiophene ring with a valeric acid side chain. Binding with carboxylase enzymes is through an amide linkage between the carboxyl group of biotin and an ε-amino group of the enzyme protein. Biocytin (Figure 12.6) is formed by proteolysis of the biotin-enzyme complex. Biotin is released from biocytin by biotinidase to conserve biotin in the cellular pool.

In nature, biotin occurs free or bound through ε-amino linkages with lysine as biocytin or to carrier proteins and peptides. It exists in the free state in plants to a greater extent than in animal tissues.[49] Mock et al.[50] reported that greater than 95% of the biotin in human milk was present as free biotin. Scheiner[51] showed that various animal-based feed ingredients contained from 11 to 29% free biotin; whereas, cereal and plant ingredients contained from 23 to 80% free biotin. Because of the bound nature, extraction procedures to measure total biotin must liberate the vitamin. Complexity of the bind-

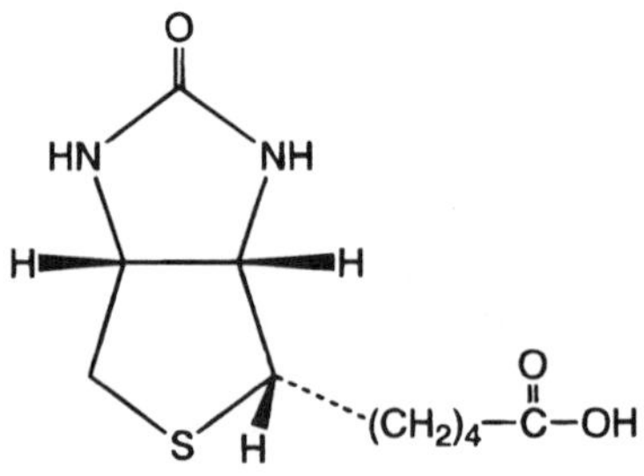

d-Biotin
Hexahydro-2-oxo-lH-thieno[3,4-d]
imidazole-4-pentanoic acid

FIGURE 12.5 Structure of biotin.

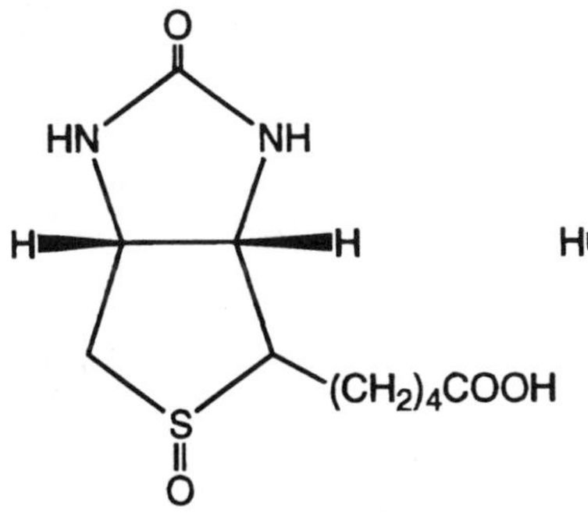

Biotin sulfoxide

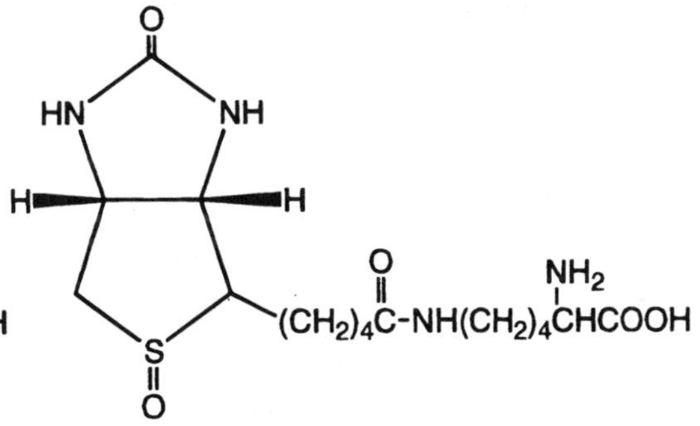

Biocytin

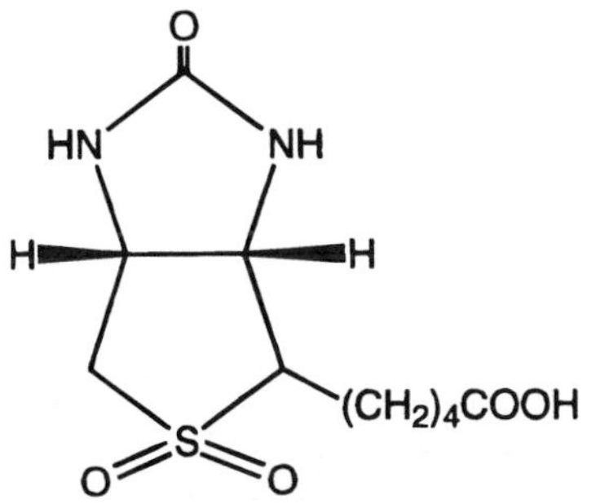

Biotin sulfone

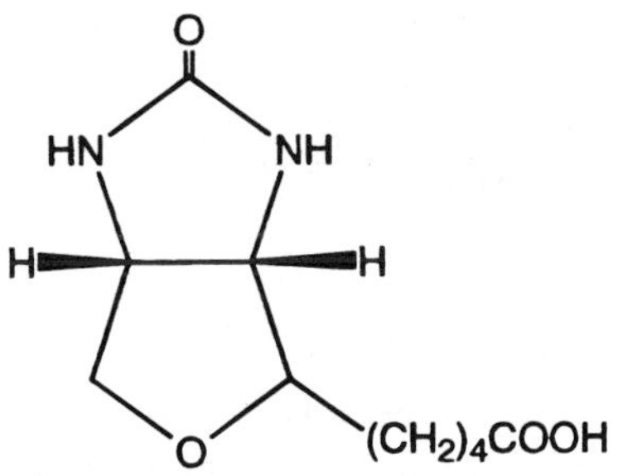

Oxybiotin

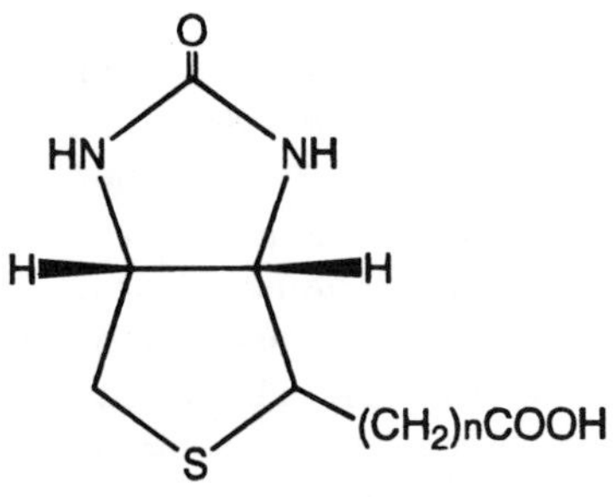

Bisnorbiotin, n = 2
Tetranobiotin, n = 0

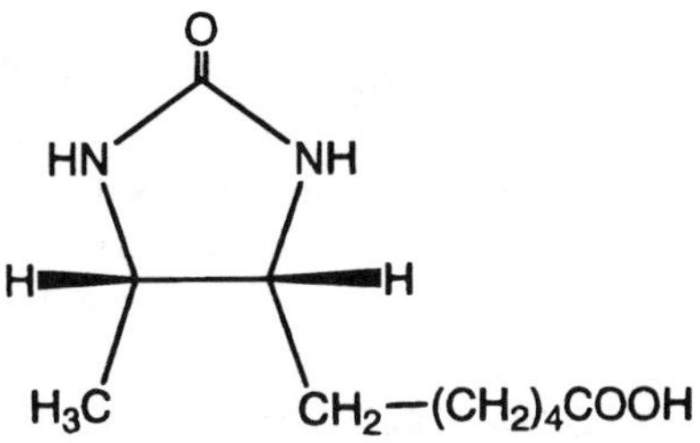

Dethiobiotin

FIGURE 12.6 Structures of biotin metabolites and analogs.

ing systems in foods promotes variability in biological availability due to differential susceptibilities of the biotin-protein linkages to digestion.[52] Biotin availability in cereals ranges from 0% in wheat to 100% in corn. In most grains, bioavailability of biotin is 20 to 30%. Availability from meat is low.[52] Extraction by strong acid hydrolysis yields total biotin and does not indicate bioavailability.

Physical properties of biotin are given in Table 12.4. The USP standard is d-biotin. Formulations for use by the pharmaceutical and food industry and for the animal feed industry include crystalline biotin, combination premixes, and with diluents such as dicalcium phosphate to aid in dispersibility and ease of blending. It is soluble in alkali solutions but sparingly soluble in water (20 mg/100 mL at 25°C) and 95% ethanol. It is insoluble in organic solvents.

TABLE 12.4
Physical Properties of Biotin

Substance[a]	Molar Mass	Formula	Solubility	Melting Point °C	Crystal Form	Absorbance λ max nm
Biotin CAS No. 58-85-5 **1272**	244.31	$C_{10}H_{16}N_2O_3S$	Soluble in dilute alkali Sparingly soluble in water, alcohol Insoluble in most organic solvents	232–233	Colorless, fine, long needles	204 very weak

[a] Common or generic name; CAS No.—Chemical Abstract Service number, bold print designates the *Merck Index* monograph number.

Ball, G. F. M., *Water-Soluble Vitamin Assays in Human Nutrition,* 1988[1]

Budavari, S. *The Merck Index,* 12th ed. 1996[2]

12.2.2.1.2 Spectral Properties

Biotin has weak absorbance at 200 to 220 nm with an absorption maxima at 204 nm from the carbonyl group.[12] LC methods are only useful for assay of highly concentrated pharmaceuticals or vitamin premixes unless UV absorbance or fluorescence is enhanced through derivatization. Such approaches are discussed in Section 12.2.3.3.

12.2.2.2 Stability

The sulfur atom in biotin is subject to oxidation with the sequential formation of biotin sulfoxide and biotin sulfone (Figure 12.6). The susceptibility of sulfur to oxidation provides a primary route for loss of biotin activity in processed foods. Oxidation produces a mixture of l- and d-biotin sulfoxides. Further oxidation to the sulfone leads to complete loss of biological activity. Humans have limited capability to reduce d-biotin sulfoxide back to d-biotin. β-Oxidation of the valeric acid side chain yields bisnorbiotin and tetranorbiotin (Figure 12.6). Susceptibility to sulfur oxidation and β-oxidation can produce degradation; however, losses in foods have not been well defined under specific processing and storage conditions. This is owing, in part, to the fact that deficiencies have not been commonly diagnosed, and dietary supplies have been considered sufficient. As biochemists and nutritionists learn more about biotin metabolism and various disease state relationships, a better understanding of processing effects might be required.

Biotin in solution is quite stable at pH 4.0 to 9.0.[12] Biotin is commonly extracted by autoclaving biological samples in 2 *N* or 6 *N* sulfuric acid for two h (Section 12.2.3.1). UV light exposure leads to loss of biological activity.[53]

12.2.3 METHODS

Biotin was assayed by microbiological methods for many decades. Avidin-binding assays developed in the 1970s were substantially based on the work of Hood.[54,55,56] Initial methods were based upon isotope dilution assays; however, many modifications adapting the strong and specific binding of avidin with biotin incorporate immunological and enzyme protein binding assay (EPBA) approaches. Most clinical studies and research on biological tissues and fluids have relied heavily on the avidin-binding assays. Conversely, such specific and highly sensitive methods have not been adapted to food studies. Almost all available data on the biotin content of the food supply has been obtained by assay with *Lactobacillus plantarum* ATCC 8014. LC methods can efficiently separate biotin, the sulfoxides, sulfones, and other biotin analogs. Commonly available LC detectors can not be used for direct quantitation for biotin owing to its low, non-specific absorbance and lack of fluorescence. LC methods coupled with avidin-binding detection, formation of fluorescent derivatives, and other approaches have been developed and used effectively to dramatically improve quantitation of biotin and its metabolites in serum and urine. These methods are discussed in Section 12.2.3.3. This methodology has not been extensively used for food assay, but there is no reason that LC coupled with newer detection approaches would not add a new dimension to biotin determination in foods.

Useful reviews on biotin analysis include Scheiner,[49] Bowers-Komro et al.,[57] Stein et al.,[58] Eitenmiller and Landen,[5] Mock,[59] Hentz and Bachas,[60] Rehner and Stein,[61] Lizano et al.,[62] Huang and Rogers,[63] and Shiuan et al.[64] These reviews, particularly with the availability of the 1997 articles in *Methods of Enzymology*, vol. 279, provide extensive and current sources for procedures for biotin assay. Table 12.5 provides a summary of compendium, regulatory, and handbook methods for biotin assay. HPLC methods of the USP are only applicable to highly concentrated pharmaceuticals or pure biotin. Other methods are microbiological procedures for feeds and premixes. AOAC

TABLE 12.5
Compendium, Regulatory, and Handbook Methods for the Analysis of Biotin

Source	Form	Methods and Application	Approach	Most Current Cross-Reference
U.S. Pharmacopeia, National Formulary, USP 23/NF 18, Nutritional Supplements, Official Monographs, 1995[1]				
1. pages 2142, 2145, 2148, 2152	Biotin	Biotin in in oil- and water-soluble vitamin capsules/tablets w/wo minerals	HPLC 200 nm or Microbiological	None
2. pages 2159, 2162, 2169, 2171	Biotin	Biotin in water-soluble capsule/ tablets w/wo minerals	HPLC 200 nm or Microbiological	None
3. page 206	Biotin	Biotin (NLT 97.5%, NMT 100.5%)	Titration, Sodium hydroxide	None
American Feed Ingredients Association, *Laboratory Methods Compendium,* vol. 1, 1991[2]				
1. pages 67–71	Biotin	Biotin in complete feeds and premixes ($> 10 \, \mu g/kg$)	Microbiological	Int. *J. Vit. Nutr. Res.*, 46, 314, 1976[3]
Food Chemicals Codex, 4th ed., 1996[4]				
1. page 46	Biotin	Biotin (NLT 97.5%, NMT 100.5%)	Titration, Sodium hydroxide	None
Hoffman, La-Roche, *Analytical Methods for Vitamins and Carotenoids,* 1988[5]				
1. pages 45–49	Biotin	Microbiological assay of biotin in complete feeds and premixes	Microbiological	*Clinical Vitaminology*[6] Int. *Vit. Nutr. Res.*, 46, 314, 1996[3]

International[20] does not provide a method for biotin. The AOAC International Task Force on Methods for Nutrition Labeling recommended that a microbiological assay by *L. plantarum* ATCC 8014 be considered for collaborative study.[21] At present, collaborative studies are not underway.

12.2.3.1 Microbiological Assay of Biotin

Traditionally, biotin in foods and other biological samples was quantitated by microbiological assay with *L. plantarum* ATCC 8014. The *L. plantarum* assay was originally introduced by Wright and Skeggs in 1944.[65] Less frequently used microorganisms include *Lactobacillus rhamnosus*, *Saccharomyces cerevisiae*, *Neurospora crassa*, *Ochramonas danica*,[15] *Escherichia coli* KS302bio,[66] and *Kloeckera apiculata (brevis)*.[67,68] *L. plantarum* is more specific for biologically active forms of biotin than other biotin requiring microorganisms.[49] It does, however, respond to dethiobiotin which spares biotin and can cause significant overestimation of the biotin content, if present in sample extracts.[69] Langer and Gÿorgy[70] reviewed early work on microbial responses to biotin and related compounds. Growth response characteristics of *L. plantarum* include:

1. Lack of response to bound forms of biotin. Biocytin must be cleaved by extraction conditions, usually by autoclaving in 2 *N* or 6 *N* sulfuric acid.
2. Equal growth response to biotin sulfoxide, but no response to biotin sulfone.
3. Fatty acids can stimulate growth. Lipids should be extracted prior to acid hydrolysis to avoid fatty acid effects.[51]

Details of the *L. plantarum* assay were provided by Scheiner.[49,51] Extraction procedures by product matrix include the following:

- **Tablets and capsules**—Homogenize in 0.1 *N* sodium hydroxide. Dilute and centrifuge to clarify. Dilute and adjust the final dilution to pH 6.8. The assay solution should approximate 0.2 ng/mL in concentration.
- **Granulations and premixes**—Mix with 0.1 *N* sodium hydroxide. Swirl for 10 min, dilute and centrifuge. Make final dilution (0.2 ng/mL), adjust to pH 6.8.
- **Pure biotin**—Add 1 mL of 0.1 *N* sodium hydroxide for each 10 mg. Dissolve by swirling. Transfer to 1 L volumetric flask and bring to volume. Dilute an aliquot to proper assay range (0.2 ng/mL).
- **Solutions and suspensions**—Pipet an aliquot into volumetric flask, bring to volume. Dilute aliquot to the proper assay range (0.2 ng/mL). For suspensions, it may be necessary to add a few drops of 1 *N* sodium hydroxide to the first dilution to ensure complete solubilization of biotin.
- **Foods and feeds**—To 5 g of sample, add 2 *N* sulfuric acid to plant products and 6 *N* sulfuric acid to animal products. The ratio of acid to sample should be 20 : 1. Autoclave at 121°C for 2 h. Cool, dilute with water, filter or centrifuge an aliquot, adjust pH to 6.8 with 20% sodium hydroxide, and dilute to the proper assay range (0.2 ng/mL).

Note: High fat samples should be extracted with hexane or ethyl ether to avoid fatty acid stimulation of the growth response.

The standard curve range is 0.025 to 2.5 ng biotin per 10 mL volume in the assay tube.

Few modifications have been made to the standard biotin assay by *L. plantarum*. However, an innovative radiometric assay by *Kloeckera apiculata* (brevis, ATCC 9774) was introduced by Guilarte[67,68] for analysis of plasma and foods. [14]CO$_2$ produced by the metabolism of L-1-[^{14}C]-methionine in the presence of biotin was measured. CO$_2$ production was proportional to the amount of biotin present in the growth medium. *K. apiculata* did not respond to dethiobiotin, dehydrobiotin, and biotin sulfone. Biotin-d-sulfoxide was as active as biotin, but biotin-L-sulfoxide was only 10 to

15% as active. Unlike *L. plantarum*, *K. apiculata* responds to intact biocytin. *K. apiculata* response was not affected by fatty acids and aspartic acid which can stimulate growth of *L. plantarum*. For plasma analysis, *K. apiculata* values were lower than those obtained by *L. plantarum*. Guilarte[67] attributed the higher values obtained by the *L. plantarum* assay to plasma fatty acids that spared the organism's biotin requirement. For food products,[68] the radiometric assay gave comparable data to the *L. plantarum* assay except for cereals. For all cereal samples, the radiometric assay indicated higher content of biotin compared to the *L. plantarum* assay. The research showed that biotin was removed from the sample extract by filtering, after acid hydrolysis. Filtration is commonly used to clarify sample extracts prior to microbiological assay and is not necessary for the radiometric assay. Although the *K. apiculata* radiometric procedure was shown to have advantages of better specificity, easier sample preparation, and other time saving attributes, it has not been routinely used for food analysis. Use of radioisotopes has been mentioned by several authors as undesirable in food analysis laboratories. Stricter regulations and higher disposal costs make their use more difficult today, compared to the time the methods were originally developed.

12.2.3.2   Avidin-Binding Assays

The ability of avidin to bind stoichometrically to biotin in a stable complex is the basis of current methods to quantitate biotin and certain metabolites from biological materials. Radio-ligand binding assays were initially developed by Dakshinamurti et al.[71] and Hood[54,55,56] using ${}^{14}C$-biotin. During the same time period, an avidin-binding assay with [${}^{3}H$]-biotin was reported.[72] Later modifications include the introduction of ${}^{125}I$-biotin[73] and ${}^{125}I$-biotin derivatives combined with double antibody techniques to separate free from bound ligand.[74] Later changes introduced biotinylated enzymes in place of the radio-ligand; thus, replacing γ-counting as the detection method with a measurement of enzyme activity.[75,76] One of the more recent modifications of radioligand binding procedures was the introduction of solid-phase sequential assays.[77,78] The assay as described by Mock[78] has the following sequence:

1. A constant amount of ${}^{125}I$-avidin is incubated with known amounts of biotin and with dilutions of sample to produce the standard curve and unknown response.
2. An aliquot of the first incubation is transferred to microtiter plates coated with biotin covalently linked to bovine serum albumin.
3. The assay solutions are incubated in the coated wells for at least 4 h at room temperature.
4. The wells are washed with buffer and the bound ${}^{125}I$ is counted in a scintillation counter.

As biotin increases in the standard additions or unknown samples, more biotin-binding sites on the ${}^{125}I$-avidin are occupied during the initial incubation. Thus, fewer radiolabels are bound to the well in the second incubation. Mock[78] fully describes the traditional methodology, and the reader is directed to his detailed procedural guide.

Use of radio-ligands are now unnecessary for biotin quantitation through the application of conventional enzyme protein binding (EPBA) procedures. As early as 1988, Finglas et al.[79] reported a procedure based on avidin-horseradish peroxidase conjugates and microtiter plate techniques for the assay of biotin in liver. This early use of EPBA was sensitive with a limit of detection of 10 pg biotin per well. Since avidin binds with biotin analogs, the EPBA was thought to compare closely with the *L. plantarum* assay.[80] The assay, however, has not been widely applied to foods.

More recently, avidin-horseradish peroxidase linked protein binding assays have been advantageously applied to clinical chemistry.[81,82,83] Specificity is dramatically increased by coupling the spectrophotometric assay to LC resolution.[59,82,83] Methodology for this significant modification in biotin assay capability is provided by Mock.[59] Zempleni et al.[82] proved that many substances known to compete with biotin or biotinylated protein for binding to avidin do not interfere with the LC/avidin-binding assay. Development of LC procedures are discussed in the following section.

12.2.3.3 Quantitation of Biotin and Biotin Metabolites by LC

Quantitation of biotin in food and other biological samples was hampered by the lack of sensitive and specific detection systems for underivatized biotin. Röder et al.[84] derivatized biotin with 9-anthryldiazomethane to produce fluorescent biotin-9-anthryl-methylester. The fluorescent derivative was resolved on Nucleosil C_{18}, mobile phase of acetonitrile : water (6 : 4) with fluorescence detection at Ex $\lambda = 365$, Em $\lambda = 425$. The on-column detection limit was 1 ng. The method was applied with good success to various pharmaceuticals. Desbene et al.[85] produced p-bromophenacyl bromide esters and 4-bromomethylmethoxycoumarin derivatives for the UV and fluorescence detection, respectively, of biotin. The derivatives were formed pre-column and chromatographed on C_{18}. Chastain et al.[86] showed that reversed-phase chromatography on C_{18} was superior to anion-exchange LC for the resolution of biotin and 13 metabolites and analogs. Chastain's procedure forms the basis of more recent LC applications for biotin research. In the method, a 35 min linear gradient from 0.05% trifluoroacetic acid, pH 2.5 to 0.05% trifluoroacetic acid : acetonitrile (70 : 30) successfully resolved the standards. Detection was at 220 nm which limited the application of the method directly to biological samples.

Only recently has the power of LC resolution been put into a practical and more routine working situation. Mock's research group has successfully coupled the LC method of Chastain et al.[86] with avidin-binding detection using avidin-horseradish peroxidase as the reporter. Research applications of the method include papers by Zempleni et al.[82,83] that demonstrate the excellent specificity and sensitivity of the method. Mock[59] conclusively states that without LC resolution as an integral part of the methodology, a direct assay of total avidin-binding substances in serum or urine overestimates biotin and underestimates the total biotin plus biotin metabolites. Application of this procedure needs to be investigated for food analysis. It appears to have the necessary attributes to remove the ambiguity from available food compositional data. Procedural details of the avidin-horseradish peroxidase/LC approach to biotin analysis have been recently published.[59] Chastain's LC method[86] was modified by equilibrating the C_{18} column with 0.05% trifluoroacetic acid buffered ammonium acetate to pH 2.5 (A) and forming a linear gradient with 0.05% trifluoroacetic acid : acetonitrile (1 : 1) (B). The gradient runs for 35 min, reaching 40% B. After the analytical run, the mobile phase is increased to 100% B over 5 min and held for 5 min to elute non-polar substances. The limit of detection is low at 5 fmol.[59]

Stein et al.[58] developed an LC method useful for complex matrices based upon the formation of fluorescent esters of biotin with panacyl bromide in the presence of crown ether. The esters are formed pre-column and resolved either by normal- or reversed-phase chromatography (Figure 12.7). A disadvantage of the method compared to avidin-horseradish peroxidase/LC method is the extensive clean up required of biological sample extracts prior to derivatization. Nevertheless, the method shows the rapid advances being made in analytical method development for biotin, its metabolites, and analogs.

A post-column reaction with avidin labeled with fluorescein isothiocyanate (FITC) was developed by Przyjazny et al.[87] for the quantitation of biotin and biocytin. The procedural details of the avidin-FITC method and a method using the fluorescent probe 2-amilinonaphthalene-6-sulfonic acid for post-column reaction with biotin and biocytin were given by Hentz and Bachas[60] in *Methods of Enzymology*, vol. 279. In-depth discussions on the above procedures and other approaches for biotin assay are provided in this source.

Undoubtedly, the success of coupling HPLC with detection systems using avidin binding principles will have significant impact on all areas of biotin research. We now have sensitive and specific LC procedures which were not available until quite recently. Most likely, such methods can be adapted to food analysis to provide the same impact in compositional studies as they have in clinical research and biochemistry.

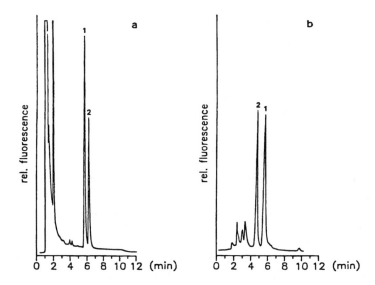

FIGURE 12.7   Resolution of the panacyl esters of dethiobiotin (1) and biotin (2). (A) Normal-phase, (B) Reversed-phase. Reproduced with permission from Reference 58.

12.3   PANTOTHENIC ACID

12.3.1   REVIEW

Pantothenic acid was fractionated from bios (Section 12.2) as an acid component in 1931. It was identified and named by R. J. Williams in 1933. The name was derived from the Greek word "panthos," meaning everywhere which indicates its widespread occurrence in nature. Williams et al.[88] determined the structure in 1939. Other significant historical events include relating the chick anti-dermatitis factor to pantothenic acid (1939),[89,90] synthesis (1940),[91] and identification of the structural role in co-enzyme A (CoA).[92] A Nobel Prize was awarded to Lipmann and Krebs in 1953 for their research on the function of CoA in metabolism. Recognition of the acyl-carrier protein (ACP) and its role in acyl group transfer (fatty acid synthesis) occurred in 1965.[93]

Because of the availability of pantothenic acid in the food supply, human deficiency has been diagnosed only in severely malnourished patients.[94, 95] Various animal species have been studied under conditions to induce pantothenic acid deficiency. Deficiency arising from reduced lipid synthesis and energy production include retarded growth rates, infertility, abortion, neonatal death, skin and hair, pigmentation, feather abnormalities, neuromuscular disorders, gastrointestinal malfunction, adrenal failure, and sudden death.[4,95] Inducement of the deficiency in humans produced many symptoms including headache, fatigue, insomnia, intestinal disturbances, and paresthesia (abnormal sensations) in the hands and feet.[94,95] Because of the variability in symptoms and the possible inter-relationships with other vitamin and nutritional deficiencies, human status indicators are difficult to interpret. Total pantothenic acid levels in blood that fall below 100 µg/100 mL may indicate low dietary intake.[96] Total pantothenic acid in urine, serum, and blood have been used to indicate status; however, their sensitivity and interpretation remain problematic.[97]

Most foods contain measurable pantothenic acid levels because of its diverse metabolic functions. Richest food sources are yeast, organ meats, egg yolk, whole grains, and yeast. Relatively low amounts are present in fresh and cooked vegetables, nuts, fruits, meat, milk, and processed cereals.[98]

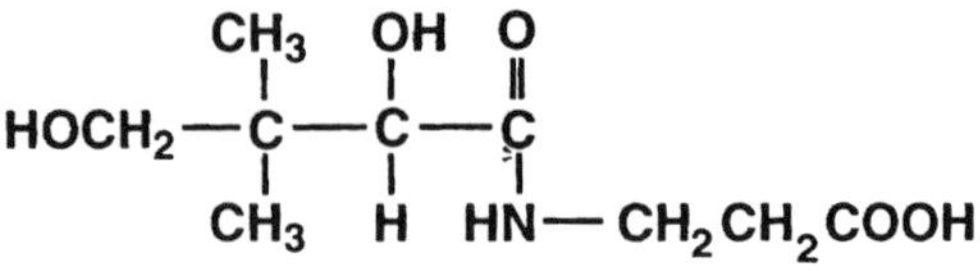

$$CH_3 \quad OH \quad O$$
$$HOCH_2 - \underset{\underset{CH_3}{|}}{\overset{\overset{CH_3}{|}}{C}} - \underset{\underset{H}{|}}{\overset{\overset{OH}{|}}{C}} - \underset{\underset{HN - CH_2 CH_2 COOH}{|}}{\overset{O}{\underset{\|}{C}}}$$

Pantothenic Acid
N-(2,4-dihydroxy-3,3-dimethyl-1-
oxobutyl) β-alanine

FIGURE 12.8   Structure of pantothenic acid.

However, these foods are consumed in quantity in most diets and represent significant dietary sources. A Recommended Dietary Allowance (RDA) has not been set, but the Estimated Safe and Adequate Daily Dietary Intake has been recommended at 4 to 7 mg for the adult.[4] The Reference Daily Intake (RDI) is 10 mg.[7]

Pantothenic acid occurs in the free state, as pantethine, bound to proteins, or in CoA. In ACP, 4′-phosphopantotheine is the prosthetic group that provides the binding site for two-carbon fragments. CoA is the acyl carrier for oxidative removal of acyl groups, and ACP is the carrier of acyl groups for synthesis of fatty acids. Characteristic reactions requiring CoA are regulation of alcohols, amines, and amino acids, and the oxidation of pyruvate by the pyruvate dehydrogenase complex to form acetyl-CoA. β-oxidation of fatty acids results in the removal of two-carbon fragments transferred as acetyl-CoA. CoA participates in condensation reactions to form a variety of intermediary metabolites including formation of citric acid from oxaloacetic acid in the TCA cycle.

12.3.2   PROPERTIES

12.3.2.1   Chemistry

12.3.2.1.1   General Properties

The structure of pantothenic acid is given in Figure 12.8. The compound is systematically named d(+)-N-(2,4-dihydroxy-3,3-dimethyl-1-oxobutyl)-β-alanine.[8] The trivial name is d(+)-α,γ-dihydroxy-β,β-dimethylbutyrl-β-alanine. It consists of pantoic acid linked through an amide linkage to β-alanine. Due to the chirality at the hydroxylated carbon atom of the pantoic acid moiety, the vitamin is optically active and racemic mixture results from synthesis. Only the d(+)-enantiomers are biologically active and present in nature. The structure of CoA is provided in Figure 12.9.

The USP standard is d(+)-pantothenic acid. Commercial forms include the sodium and calcium salts and the alcohol, pantothenol. Pantothenic acid is highly hygroscopic and more unstable than the salts. Therefore, the salts, predominantly calcium pantothenate, are the usual forms chosen for food fortification and dry pharmaceutical products. Pantothenol is a hygroscopic viscous oil. It is commonly used in liquid pharmaceuticals. The alcohol is slightly soluble in water and very soluble in alcohol.[99] Pantothenol is equivalent to pantothenic acid in biological activity. The alcohol has better stability at pH 3 to 5 compared to the salts.[98] Equivalent to 1 g of calcium pantothenate is 0.92 grams of pantothenic acid, and 1 g of pantothenol is equivalent to 1.16 g of calcium pantothenate.[100] Physical properties are summarized in Table 12.6.

12.3.2.1.2   Spectral Properties

Pantothenic acid does not contain a chromophore. The carbonyl group weakly absorbs below 210 nm.

12.3.2.2   Stability

Pantothenic acid is most stable to thermal processing at pH 5 to 7.[101] Large losses can occur through leaching into the cooking water during preparation of vegetables. In milk, pantothenic acid is stable

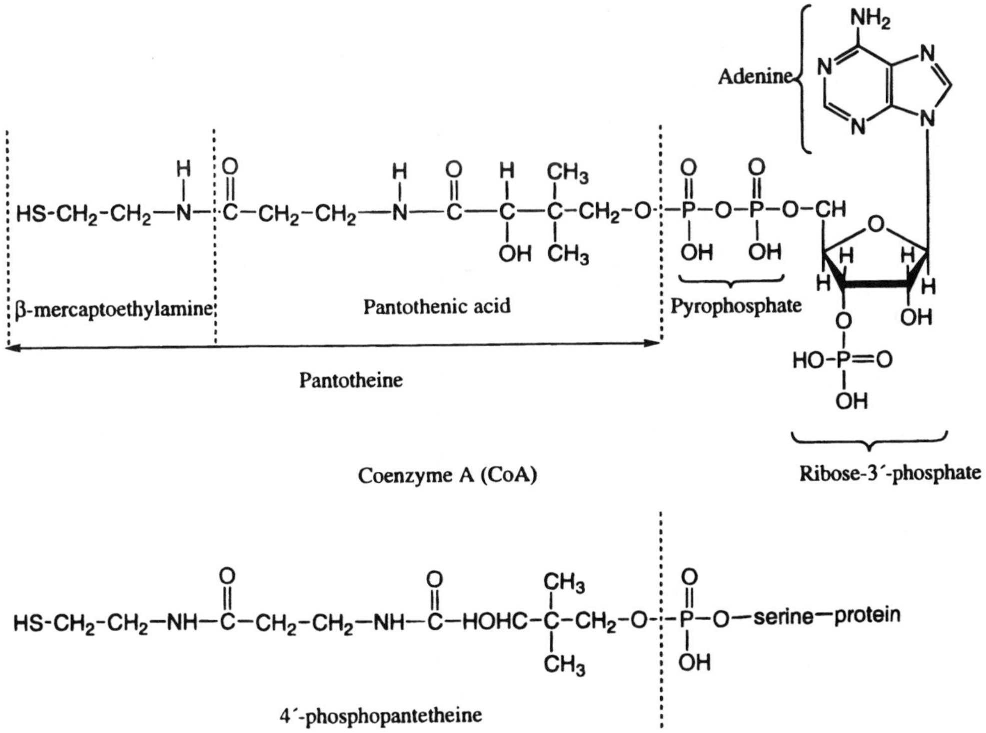

FIGURE 12.9   Structure of coenzyme A.

to pasteurization, since the normal pH of milk is in the optimal pH stability range.[101] Goldsmith et al.[102] showed that pantothenic acid in human milk withstood a wide range of pasteurization conditions including low temperature long time (LTLT) at 62.5°C for 30 min, high temperature short time (HTST) at 72°C for 15 s and 88°C for 5 s, and sterilization at 100°C for 5 min. Only biotin, niacin, and riboflavin were as stable as pantothenic acid among the nine water-soluble vitamins studied. Further, pantothenic acid was not affected by frozen storage at −20°C for one month.

Pantothenase, a bacterial amidase, cleaves pantothenic acid into a β-alanine and pantoic acid.[103] Action of this enzyme provides an enzymatic route for pantothenic acid destruction. Unlike many vitamins, pantothenic acid is stable to oxidative environments and light exposure.

12.3.3   METHODS

Methods for assay of pantothenic acid vary widely in approach. However, LC methods have not been used to analyze biological samples because of the lack of sensitive and specific detection modes. Thus, applications of LC have been limited to the analysis of pharmaceuticals, vitamin premixes, and foods such as infant formula, in which the vitamin is present in higher concentration compared to non-formulated foods. Historically, methodology for pantothenic acid assay relied on various chemical and physical methods, animal bioassays, microbiological methods, and, more recently, gas chromatographic, and immunological methods. Older literature sources discuss the animal assays, microbiological, and chemical and physical methods in detail. These sources include Strohecker and Henning,[104] Baker and Frank,[105] and Freed.[106] Chemical and physical methods are available for the determination of pantothenic acid and its salts in dry or liquid vitamin preparations. Such procedures use hydrolysis under acidic or basic conditions, or reductive splitting of the

TABLE 12.6
Physical Properties of Pantothenic Acid, Salts, and Pantothenol

Substance[a]	Molar Mass	Formula	Solubility	Crystal Form	Melting Point °C	λ max nm
Pantothenic Acid CAS No. 79-83-4 **7147**	219.24	$C_9H_{17}NO_5$	Freely soluble in water, ethylacetate, dioxane Moderately soluble in ether, amyl alcohol Insoluble in $CHCl_3$	None, oil		204 very weak
Sodium Pantothenate CAS No. 867-81-2 **7147**	241.20	$C_9H_{16}NNaO_5$	Soluble in water Sparingly soluble in ether, amyl alcohol Insoluble in $CHCl_3$	Crystals	122–124	No chromophore
Calcium Pantothenate CAS No. 137-08-6 **7147**	476.53	$C_{18}H_{32}CaN_2O_{10}$	Soluble in water Slightly soluble in alcohol and acetone	Minute needles	195-196 (Dec.)	No chromophore
D(+) Pantothenol CAS No. 81-13-0 **2988**	205.25	$C_9H_{19}NO_4$	Freely soluble in alcohol, methanol Slightly soluble in water, ether	None, viscous liquid		No chromophore

[a]Common or generic name; CAS No.—Chemical Abstract Service number, bold print designates the *Merck Index* monograph number.
Ball, G. F. M., *Water-Soluble Vitamin Assays in Human Nutrition*, 1988[1]
Budavari, S. *The Merck Index*, 12th ed., 1996[2]

vitamin into end-products (β-alanine, pantoic acid, pentoyl lactone) that can be measured by spectrophotometry, fluorometry, or gas chromatography. More recent literature that provides methodology discussions include reviews written by Wyse et al.,[107] El-Habashy and Eitenmiller,[98] Eitenmiller and Landen,[5] Ball,[12] and Velisek et al.[99]

Compendium and handbook methods provided in Table 12.7 are mostly limited to microbiological and titration procedures for assay of vitamin tablets and pantothenol preparations. The USP/NSF[108] methods include an LC procedure for pharmaceutical preparations with detection at 210 nm. AOAC International[20] methods are microbiological assays by *Lactobacillus plantarum* ATCC 8014. Method 945.74 (45.2.05) "Pantothenic Acid in Vitamin Preparations" does not include an enzymatic hydrolysis treatment and is limited to assay of free pantothenic acid and its salts. Method 992.07 (50.1.22) "Pantothenic Acid in Milk-Based Infant Formula" includes the traditional enzyme treatments (Section 12.3.3.1) for natural products, but has not been collaborated for other food matrices. AOAC International[20] does not provide LC based methods.

12.3.3.1 Microbiological Assay of Pantothenic Acid

L. plantarum ATCC 8014 has been the preferred microorganism for pantothenic acid assay for decades. Other organisms, both bacteria and protozoa, are suitable for the assay (*Saccharomyces cerevisiae, Saccharomyces uvarum, Lactobacillus delbrueckii,* and *Tetrahymena pyriformis.*[98]) *L. plantarum* responds on an equimolar basis to free pantothenic acid and pantetheine. It does not respond to phosphopantetheine or intact forms of CoA.[15] Voigt et al.[109,110] completed in-depth studies of factors that interfere with microbiological assays and reported that *L. plantarum* was affected to a lesser degree than other commonly used organisms by sample matrix effects.

Because of the requirement of *L. plantarum* for free pantothenic acid and pantetheine, biological samples must be treated enzymatically by a "double-enzyme" treatment with alkaline phosphatase and pantetheinase that cleaves pantothenic acid from CoA and dephosphorylates pantetheine. Pantetheinase preparations from hog kidney, chicken liver, or pigeon liver are normally used. Endogenous pantothenic acid must be removed from tissue preparations prior to the addition of sample digests. These procedures are provided in detail by Wyse et al.[107] Sample preparation procedures for the microbiological and radioimmunoassays (Section 12.3.3.2) are also provided in this excellent, highly descriptive reference.

12.3.3.2 Radioimmunoassay and Enzyme-Linked Immunosorbent Assay

A radioimmunoassay (RIA) for pantothenic acid was developed by Wyse et al.[111] for analysis of biological samples. Pantothenic acid was extracated by the "double-enzyme" digestion used for the *L. plantarum* assay. Results were shown to compare closely to the microbial assay.[112,113] The RIA was used to assay 75 processed and cooked foods.[113] Findings indicated relatively low amounts of pantothenic acid in some highly processed foods. Non-fortified cereals and fruit products were low in pantothenic acid compared to most other foods. All fruit products contained less than 0.2 mg per serving. Boiled or baked potatoes and canned tomato products contained higher levels of the vitamin. This study, to date, is one of the most comprehensive investigations completed on the pantothenic acid content of the U.S. food supply.

The RIA procedure developed by Wyse et al.[111] remains a viable alternative to the *L. plantarum* assay. This assay, like RIA methods for other water-soluble vitamins, has not been used extensively by other research groups.

Smith et al.[114] developed the first direct enzyme-linked immunosorbent assay (ELISA) for pantothenic acid. Antibodies specific for pantothenic acid were covalently linked to alkaline phosphatase with glutarylaldehyde. Immobilized pantothenate substrate was formed by attaching human serum albumin-pantothenate conjugate to the surface of polystyrene tubes by passive absorption. The binding of the enzyme-linked antibody to immobilized substrate is inhibited by free pantothenic

TABLE 12.7
Compendium, Regulatory, and Handbook Methods for the Analysis of Pantothenic Acid

Source	Form	Methods and Application	Approach	Most Current Cross-Reference
U.S. Pharmacopeia, National Formulary, USP23/NF 18, Nutritional Supplements, Official Monographs, 1995[1]				
1. pages 2142, 2146, 2148, 2153	Pantothenic acid as calcium pantothenate	Pantothenic acid in oil- and water-soluble vitamin capsules/tablets w/wo minerals	Method 1—HPLC 210 nm Method 2—Microbiological	None
2. pages 2161, 2166, 2169, 2172	Pantothenic acid as calcium pantothenate	Pantothenic acid in water-soluble vitamin capsules/tablets w/wo minerals	Method 1—HPLC 210 nm Method 2—Microbiological	None
3. page 258	Calcium pantothenate	Calcium pantothenate tablets (NLT 95.0%, NMT 115.0%)	Microbiological	None
4. page 1154	Panthenol	Panthenol (NLT 99.0%, NMT 102.0%)	Titration, perchloric acid	None
5. pages 2160, 2169	Panthenol Dexpanthenol	Assay for dexpanthenol or panthenol	Microbiological	None
AOAC Official Methods of Analysis, 16th ed., 1995[2]				
1. 45.2.05	Pantothenic acid	AOAC Official Method, 945.74, Pantothenic Acid in Vitamin Preparations	Microbiological	*J. Assoc. Off. Anal. Chem.,* 42, 529, 1959[3]; *J. Biol. Chem.* 192, 181, 1951[4]
2. 50.1.22	Calcium pantothenate	AOAC Official Method, 992.07 Pantothenic Acid in Milk-Based Infant Formula	Microbiological	*J. AOAC Int.,* 76, 398, 1993[5]

Source	Substance	Description	Method	Reference
American Feed Ingredients Association, *Laboratory Methods Compendium*, vol. 1, 1991[6] 1. pages 73–76	Calcium pantothenate	Calcium D-pantothenate in complete feeds and premixes (> 1 mg/kg)	Microbiological	Hoffmann-LaRoche, *Analytical Methods for Vitamins and Carotenoids*, 1988, 42[7]
Food Chemicals Codex, 4th ed., 1996[8] 1. page 116	Dex-Panthenol	Dex-Panthenol (NLT 98.0%, NMT 102.0%)	Titration, perchloric acid	None
Hoffmann-LaRoche, *Analytical Methods for Vitamins and Carotenoids*, 1988[7] 1. pages 42–44	Calcium D-pantothenate	Microbiological assay of calcium D-pantothenate (calpan) in complete feeds and premixes	Microbiological	None

acid in the standards or samples. Binding ratios were determined by the extent of hydrolysis of p-nitrophenyl phosphate by alkaline phosphatase. In 1988, Morris et al.[115] reported an indirect double-antibody ELISA that was highly specific for pantothenic acid. The assay was specifically applied to food analysis.[116] Results compared closely to microbiological assay of *L. plantarum*. Song et al.[117] developed an indirect ELISA for plasma analysis with good results. The method requires no preparation of the plasma and was reported to be easier to use, less expensive, and more sensitive than other RIA or ELISA procedures for assay of free pantothenic acid. Finglas and Morgan[118] reviewed existing biospecific methods for water-soluble vitamins. This review provides excellent background material for the overall area.

RIA and ELISA tests are sensitive, less labor intensive, and provide acceptable alternatives to the microbiological assay of pantothenic acid in biological samples. The method of choice depends on availability of equipment, budget, and expertise available.[98] RIA and ELISA tests require pantothenic acid to be in the free state, and enzyme digestion is necessary if total pantothenic acid is to be determined.

12.3.3.3 Chromatographic Approaches to the Quantitation of Pantothenic Acid

Chromatography, even though LC techniques have not played a central role in analytical approaches, remains an important part of pantothenic acid methodology. Earliest methods were based on paper and thin layer chromatographic (TLC) procedures. TLC coupled with scanning densitometers, provides a simple and rapid method for analysis of pharmaceutical preparations. Gas liquid chromatography (GLC) also is adaptable to analysis of higher concentration products. GLC, from a basic research approach, has not been amenable to food, blood, or tissue assay due to the necessity to use quite complex preparatory methods. Velisek et al.[99] provide recent information on chromatographic approaches to pantothenic acid assay. Recently published methods are discussed below.

Nag and Das[119] used TLC to quantitate pantothenol and pantothenic acid in pharmaceutical preparations. Tablets and capsules were powdered, extracted with water and ethanol, centrifuged, and diluted to volume. Liquid preparations were diluted with ethanol, precipitates removed by centrifugation, and the clean supernatants applied directly to TLC plates. Syrups were treated with ammonium sulfate and benzoyl alcohol, and the alcohol layer was used directly for TLC.

Chromatographic conditions included Silica 60 precoated, aluminum-backed sheets, and chloroform : isopropanol-water, 4+1, v/v (85 : 15) as the developing solvent. After chromatography, plates were heated in a hot-air oven at 160°C to degrade the pantothenic acid and panthenol into β-alanine or β-alanol, respectively. Plates were developed with ninhydrin and quantitated by scanning densitometry at 490 nm. The method was reported to be simple, specific, and highly accurate. Over 500 products were assayed by the procedure, and other ingredients in the products did not interfere with the analysis. Recoveries for pantothenic acid and pantothenol approached 100%.

Iwase[120] introduced a column-switching LC method for assay of pantothenic acid in commercial, elemental diets. Diet preparations were dissolved in water at 50°C. Sodium chloride was added, and the solution was diluted with water. After hexane extraction, aliquots of the aqueous phase were injected. Chromatography included pre-column fractionation on Capcellpak C_{18} (150 cm × 4.6 mm) with switching to a Capcellpak C_{18} (25 cm × 4.6 mm) analytical column. The pre-column was eluted with acetonitrile : water, pH 2.1, (5 : 95). After washing with the mobile phase, adsorbed compounds were introduced onto the analytical column with acetonitrile : water, pH 2.1, (9 : 91), containing 1.5 mM sodium l-heptane sulfonate. Detection was at 210 nm. Recovery was 95% and within-day RSD was low at 1.8%. While the procedure gives excellent results, the complexity of the LC set-up shows the problems inherently present in applying LC to the pantothenic acid analysis.

Recently, Romera and Gil[121] applied reversed-phase chromatography to analysis of pantothenic acid in infant formulas. Powdered formulas were homogenized in water at 40°C, cooled, and treated with acetic acid and sodium acetate in precipitate protein. After centrifugation, the supernatant was filtered and injected directly onto the LC column. Chromatography was completed on C_{18} with a mobile phase of 0.25 M sodium phosphate : acetonitrile, pH 2.5 (97 : 3) with detection at 197 nm. Recovery ranged from 89 to 98%. Coefficients of variation ranged from 1.3 to 3.2%. The procedure was stated to be an ideal replacement for the microbiological assay of pantothenic acid in infant formula. The simplicity of the procedure indicates that it could be widely applied to infant formula, medical foods, and other fortified foods.

12.4 REFERENCES

Text

1. Machlin, L. J. and Hüni, J. E. S., Vitamin B-12, in *Vitamins Basics*, Hoffmann-LaRoche, Basel, 1994, 40, 56.
2. Whipple, G. H. and Robscheit-Robbins, F. S., Blood regeneration in severe anemia: favorable influence of liver, heart and skeletal muscle in diet, *Am. J. Physiol.*, 72, 408, 1925.
3. Herbert, V., Vitamin B-12, in *Present Knowledge in Nutrition*, 7th ed., Ziegler, E. E. and Filer, L. J., Jr., Eds., ILSI Press, Washington, D.C., 1996, chap. 20.
4. National Research Council, *Recommended Dietary Allowances*, 10th ed., National Academy of Sciences, Washington, D.C., 1989, chap. 8.
5. Eitenmiller, R. R. and Landen, W. O., Jr., Vitamins, in *Analyzing Food for Nutrition Labeling and Hazardous Contaminants*, Jeon, I.J. and Ikins, W.G., Eds., Marcel Dekker, New York, 1995, chap. 9.
6. Olson, R. E., Water-soluble vitamins, in *Principles of Pharmacology*, Munson, P. L., Mueller, R. A. and Breese, G. R., Eds., Chapman and Hall, New York, 1995, Chap. 59.
7. *Nutritional Labeling and Education Act of 1990*, Fed. Reg., 58, 2070, 1993.
8. Anon., Nomenclature policy: generic descriptions and trivial names for vitamins and related compounds, *J. Nutr.*, 120, 12, 1990.
9. Committee on Food Chemicals Codex, *Food Chemicals Codex*, 4th ed., National Academy of Sciences, Washington, D.C., 1996, 431.
10. Ellenbogen, L. and Cooper, B. A., Vitamin B-12, in *Handbook of Vitamins*, 2nd ed., Machlin, L. J., Ed., Marcel Dekker, New York, 1991, chap. 13.
11. Friedrich, W., Vitamin B-12, in *Vitamins*, Walter de Gruyter, Berlin, 1988, chap. 13.
12. Ball, G.F.M., Chemical and biological nature of the water-soluble vitamins, in *Water-Soluble Vitamin Assays in Human Nutrition*, Chapman and Hall, New York, 1994, chaps. 2, 8.
13. Chin, H. B., Vitamin B-12, in *Methods of Vitamin Assay*, 4th ed., Augustin, J., Klein, B. P., Becker, D. A. and Venugopal, P. B., Eds., John Wiley & Sons, New York, 1985, chap. 19.
14. Lindemans, J., Cobalamins, in *Modern Chromatographic Analysis of Vitamins*, 2nd ed., De Leenheer, A. P., Lambert, W. E. and Nelis, H. J., Eds., Marcel Dekker, New York, 1992, chap. 12.
15. Voigt, M. N. and Eitenmiller, R. R., Comparative review of the thiochrome, microbial and protozoan analyses of B-vitamins, *J. Food Prot.*, 41, 730, 1978.
16. Lindemans, J. and Abels, J., Vitamin B-12 and related corrinoids, in *Modern Chromatographic Analysis of the Vitamins*, De Leenheer, A. P., Lambert, W. E. and De Ruyter, M. G. M., Eds., Marcel Dekker, New York, 1985, chap. 12.
17. Woollard, D. C., New ion-pair reagent for the high-performance liquid chromatographic separation of B-group vitamins in pharmaceuticals, *J. Chromatogr.*, 301, 470, 1984.
18. Amin, M. and Reusch, J., Simultaneous determination of vitamins B_1, B_2, B_6 and B_{12} and C, nicotinamide and folic acid in capsule preparations by ion-pair reversed-phase high-performance liquid chromatography, *Analyst*, 112, 989, 1987.
19. Amin, M. and Reusch, J., High performance liquid chromatography of water-soluble vitamins. II. Simultaneous determination of vitamins B_1, B_2, B_6 and B_{12} in pharmaceutical preparations, *J. Chromatogr.*, 390, 448, 1987.
20. AOAC International, *Official Methods of Analysis*, 16th ed., AOAC International, Arlington, VA, 1995.
21. AOAC International, Report of the AOAC International Task Force on Methods for Nutrient Labeling Analyses, *J. AOAC Int.*, 76, 180A, 1993.

22. Muhammad, K., Briggs, D. and Jones, G., The appropriateness of using cyanocobalamin as calibration standards in *Lactobacillus leichmanni* ATCC 7830 assay of vitamin B$_{12}$, *Food Chem.*, 48, 427, 1993.

23. Marcus, M., Prabhudesai, M. S. M. and Wassef, S., Stability of vitamin B-12 in the presence of ascorbic acid in food and serum: restoration by cyanide of apparent loss, *Am. J. Clin. Nutr.*, 33, 137, 1980.

24. Farquharson, J. and Adams, J. F., The forms of vitamin B-12 in foods, *Br. J. Nutr.*, 36, 127, 1976.

25. Freed, M., Vitamin B-12, in *Methods of Vitamin Assay*, 3rd ed., Interscience Publishers, New York, 1966, chap. 13.

26. Lichtenstein, H., Beloian, A. and Reynolds, H., Comparative vitamin B-12 assay of foods of animal origin by *Lactobacillus leichmannii* and *Ochromonas malhamensis*, *J. Agric. Food Chem.*, 7, 771, 1959.

27. Rothenberg, S. P., Radioassay of serum vitamin B-12 by quantitating the competition between CO^{57} B$_{12}$ and unlabeled B$_{12}$ for the binding sites of intrinsic factor, *J. Clin. Invest.*, 42, 1391, 1963.

28. Barakat, R. M. and Ekins, R. P., An isotopic method for the determination of vitamin B-12 levels in blood, *Blood*, 21, 70, 1963.

29. Lau, K. S., Gottlieb, C. W., Wasserman, L. R. and Herbert, V., Measurement of serum vitamin B-12 level using radioisotope dilution and coated charcoal, *Blood*, 26, 202, 1965.

30. Rothenberg, S. P., Marcoullis, G. P., Schwarz, S. and Lader, E., Measurement of cyanocobalamin in serum by a specific radio-immunoassay, *J. Lab. Clin. Med.*, 103, 959, 1984.

31. Quadros, E. V., Rothenberg, S. P. and Polu, S., A specific radioimmunoassay for 5'-deoxyadenosyl cobalamin in serum, *Br. J. Haema..*, 69, 551, 1988.

32. Richardson, P. J., Favell, D. J., Gidley, G. C. and Jones, G. H., Application of a commercial radioassay test kit to the determination of vitamin B-12 in food, *Analyst*, 103, 865, 1978.

33. Beck, R. A., Comparison of two radioassay methods for cyanocobalamin in seafoods, *J. Food Sci.*, 44, 1077, 1979.

34. Samson, R. R. and McClelland, D. B. L., Vitamin B$_{12}$ in human colostrum and milk: quantitation of the vitamin and its binder and the uptake of bound vitamin B$_{12}$ by intestinal bacteria, *Acta Paediatr. Scand.*, 69, 93, 1980.

35. Casey, P. J., Speckman, K. R., Ebert, F. J. and Hobbs, W. E., Radioisotope dilution technique for the determination of vitamin B-12 in foods, *J. Assoc. Off. Anal. Chem.*, 65, 85, 1982.

36. Kralova, B., Rauch, P. and Cerna, J., Use of vitamin B$_{12}$ radioassay in the analysis of biological materials, mainly of foods, *Die Nahr.*, 26, 803, 1982.

37. Osterdahl, B., Janne, K., Johansson, E. and Johnsson, H., Determination of vitamin B-12 in gruel by a radioisotope dilution assay, *Int. J. Vit. Nutr. Res.*, 56, 95, 1986.

38. Osterdahl, B. and Johansson, E., Comparison of two radioisotope dilution assay kits for measuring vitamin B-12 in gruel, *Int. J. Vit. Nutr. Res.*, 58, 303, 1988.

39. Andersson, I., Lundqvist, R., and Öste, R., Analysis of vitamin B-12 in milk by a radioisotope dilution assay, *Milchwissenschaft*, 45, 507, 1990.

40. Muhammad, K., Briggs, D. and Jones, G., Comparison of a competitive binding assay with *Lactobacillus leichmannii* A.T.C.C. 7830 assay for the determination of vitamin B$_{12}$ in foods, *Food Chem.*, 48, 431, 1993.

41. Muhammad, K., Briggs, D. and Jones, G., The appropriateness of using cyanocobalamin as calibration standards in competitive binding assays of vitamin B$_{12}$, *Food Chem.*, 48, 423, 1993.

42. Alcock, S. C., Finglas, P. M. and Morgan, M. R. A., Production and purification of an R-protein-enzyme conjugate for use in an microtitration plate protein-binding assay for vitamin B$_{12}$ in fortified food, *Food Chem.*, 45, 199, 1992.

43. Boas, M. A., Effect of desiccation upon the nutritional properties of egg white, *Biochem J.*, 21, 712, 1927.

44. Kogl, F. and Tonnis, B., Isolation of chrystalline biotin from egg yolk. *Z. Physiol. Chem.*, 242, 73, 1936.

45. Friedrich, W., Biotin, in *Vitamins*, Walter de Gruyter, Berlin, 1988, chap. 11.

46. Mock, D. M., Biotin, in *Present Knowledge in Nutrition*, 7th ed., Ziegler, E.E. and Filer, L. J., Eds., ILSI Press, Washington, D.C., 1996, chap. 22.

47. Hoppner, K., Lampi, B. and O'Grady, E., Biotin content in vegetables and nuts available on the Canadian market, *Food Res. Int.*, 27, 495, 1994.

48. Gaudry, M. and Ploux, O., Biotin, in *Modern Chromatographic Analysis of Vitamins*, 2nd ed., De Leenheer, A. P., Lambert, W. E. and Nelis, H. J., Eds., Marcel Dekker, New York, 1992, chap. 11.

49. Scheiner, J., Biotin, in *Methods of Vitamin Assay*, 4th ed., Augustin, J., Klein, B.P., Becker, D.A., and Venugopal, P.B., Eds., John Wiley & Sons, New York, 1985, chap. 21.

50. Mock, D. M., Mock, N. I. and Langbehn, S. E., Biotin in human milk: methods, location and chemical form, *J. Nutr.*, 122, 535, 1992.
51. Scheiner, J. M., Extraction of biotin from pharmaceuticals, premixes, food and feeds, *Ann. New York Acad. Sci.*, 477, 420, 1985.
52. Combs, G. F., Jr., Biotin, in *The Vitamins*, Academic Press, New York, 1992, chap. 14.
53. Bonjour, J.-P., Biotin, in *Handbook of Vitamins*, 2nd ed., Machlin, L. J., Ed., Marcel Dekker, New York, 1991, chap. 10.
54. Hood, R. L., A radiochemical assay for biotin in biological materials, *J. Sci. Food Agric.*, 26, 1847, 1975.
55. Hood, R. L., The use of linear regression in the isotope dilution assay of biotin, *Anal. Biochem.*, 79, 635, 1977.
56. Hood, R. L., Isotope dilution assay for biotin: use of [^{14}C]-biotin, *Meth. Enzymol.*, 62, 279, 1979.
57. Bowers-Kömro, D. M., Chastain, J. L. and McCormick, D. B., Separation of biotin and analogs by high-performance liquid chromatography, *Meth. Enzymol.*, 122, 63, 1986.
58. Stein, J., Hahn, A., Lembcke, B., and Rehner, G., High-performance liquid chromatographic determination of biotin in biological materials after crown ether-catalyzed fluorescence derivatization with panacyl bromide, *Anal. Biochem.*, 200, 89, 1992.
59. Mock, D. M., Determinations of biotin in biological fluids, *Meth. Enzymol.*, 279, 265, 1997.
60. Hentz, N. G. and Bachas, L. G., Fluoropore-linked assays for high-performance liquid chromatography postcolumn reaction detection of biotin and biocytin, *Meth. Enzymol.*, 279, 275, 1997.
61. Rehner, G. I. and Stein, J., High-performance liquid chromatographic determination of biotin in biological materials after crown-ether-catalyzed fluorescence derivatization with panacyl bromide, *Meth. Enzymol.*, 279, 286, 1997.
62. Lizano, S., Ramanathan, S., Feltus, A., Witkowski, A., and Daunert, S., Bioluminescence competitive binding assays for biotin based on photoprotein aequorin, *Meth. Enzymol.*, 279, 296, 1997.
63. Huang, E. Z. and Rogers, Y. H., Competitive enzymatic assay of biotin, *Meth. Enzymol.*, 279, 304, 1997.
64. Shiuan, D., Wu, C. H., Chang, Y. S., and Chang, R. J., Competitive enzyme linked immunosorbent assay for biotin, *Meth. Enzymol.*, 279, 321, 1997.
65. Wright, L. D. and Skeggs, H. R., Determination of biotin with *Lactobacillus arabinosus*, *Proc. Soc. Exp. Biol. Med.*, 56, 95, 1944.
66. Sanyal, I., Cohen, G., and Flint, D. H., Biotin synthase: purification, characterization as a [^{2}Fe-2S] cluster protein and *in vitro* activity of *Escherichia coli* bio B gene product, *Biochemistry*, 33, 3625, 1994.
67. Guilarte, T. R., Measurement of biotin levels in human plasma using a radiometric microbiological assay, *Nutr. Rep. Int.*, 31, 1155, 1985.
68. Guilarte, T. R., Analysis of biotin levels in selected foods using a radiometric-microbiological method, *Nutr. Rep. Int.*, 32, 837, 1985.
69. De Moll, E. and Shive, W., Assay for biotin in the presence of dethiobiotin with *Lactobacillus plantarum*, *Anal. Biochem.*, 158, 55, 1986.
70. Langer, B. W., Jr. and György, P., Biotin, VIII., active compounds and antagonists, in *The Vitamins*, 2nd ed., Sebrell, W. H. and Harris, R. S., Eds., Academic Press, New York, 1968, 294.
71. Dakshinamurti, K., Landman, A. D., Ramamurti, L., and Constable, R. J., Isotope dilution assay for biotin, *Anal. Biochem.*, 61, 225, 1974.
72. Landman, A. D., A sensitive assay for biotin analogs and biotin-proteins, *Int. J. Vit. Nutr. Res.*, 46, 310, 1976.
73. Horsburgh, T. and Gompertz, D., A protein-binding assay for measurement of biotin in physiological fluids, *Clin. Chim. Acta*, 82, 215, 1978.
74. Livaniou, E., Evangelatos, G. P., and Ithakissios, D. S., Biotin radioligand assay with an ^{125}I-labeled biotin derivative, avidin and avidin double-antibody reagents, *Clin. Chem.*, 33, 1983, 1987.
75. Niedbala, R. S., Gergits, F., and Schray, K. J., Spectrophotometric assay for nanogram quantities of biotin and avidin, *J. Biochem. Biophys. Meth.*, 13, 205, 1986.
76. Bayer, E. A., Ben-Hur, H., and Wilchek, M., A sensitive enzyme assay for biotin, avidin and streptavidin, *Anal. Biochem.*, 154, 367, 1986.
77. Mock, D. M. and DuBois, D. B., A sequential, solid-phase assay for biotin in physiologic fluids that correlates with expected biotin status, *Anal. Biochem.*, 153, 272, 1986.

78. Mock, D. B., Sequential solid-phase assay for biotin based on ^{125}I-labeled avidin, *Meth. Enzymol.*, 184, 224, 1990.

79. Finglas, P. M., Faulks, R. M. and Morgan, M. R. A., The analysis of biotin in liver using a protein-binding assay, *J. Micronutr. Anal.*, 2, 247, 1986.

80. Finglas, P. M. and Morgan, M. R. A., Application of biospecific methods to the determination of B-group vitamins in foods—a review, *Food Chem.*, 49, 191, 1994.

81. Rosebrough, S. F. and Hartley, D. F., Quantification and lowering of serum biotin, *Lab. Anim. Sci.*, 45, 554, 1995.

82. Zempleni, J., McCormick, D. B., Stratton, S. L., and Mock, D. M., Lipoic acid (thioctic acid) analogs, tryptophan analogs and urea do not interfere with the assay of biotin and biotin metabolites by high-performance liquid chromatography/avidin-binding assay, *Nutr. Biochem.*, 7, 518, 1996.

83. Zempleni, J., McCormick, D. B., and Mock, D. M., Identification of biotin sulfone, bisnorbiotin methyl ketone and tetranorbiotin-l-sulfoxide in human urine, *Am. J. Clin. Nutr.*, 65, 508, 1997.

84. Röder, E., Engelbert, U., and Troschütz, J., Hochdruckflüssig-chromatographesche bestimmung von biotin in arzneimitteln, *Fres. Z. Anal. Chem.*, 319, 426, 1984.

85. Desbene, P. L., Coustal, S., and Frappier, F., Separation of biotin and its analogs by high-performance liquid chromatography: convenient labeling for ultraviolet or fluorimetric detection, *Anal. Biochem.*, 128, 359, 1983.

86. Chastain, J. L., Bowers-Komro, D. M., and McCormick, D. B., High-performance liquid chromatography of biotin and analogs, *J. Chromatogr.*, 330, 153, 1985.

87. Przyjazny, A., Hentz, N. G., and Bachas, L. G., Sensitive and selective liquid chromatographic post-column reaction detection system for biotin and biocytin using a homogenous fluorophore-linked assay, *J. Chromatogr. A*, 654, 79, 1993.

88. Williams, R. J., Weinstock, H. H., Jr., Rohrmann, E., Truesdail, J. H., Mitchell H. K. and Meyer, C. E., Pantothenic acid: III. Analysis and determination of constituent groups, *J. Am. Chem. Soc.*, 61, 454, 1939.

89. Jukes, T. H., Pantothenic acid requirement of chicks, *J. Am. Chem. Soc.*, 61, 975, 1939.

90. Wooley, D. W., Waisman, H. A., and Elvejhem, C. A., Nature and partial synthesis of the chick anti-dermatitis factor, *J. Am. Chem. Soc.*, 61, 977, 1939.

91. Stiller, E. T., Harris, S. A., Finkelstein, J., Keresztesy, J. C., and Folkers, K., Pantothenic acid. VIII. The total synthesis of pure pantothenic acid, *J. Am. Chem. Soc.*, 62, 1785, 1940.

92. Ochoa, S., Mehler, A., and Kornberg, A., Coenzyme for acetylation, a pantothenic acid derivative, *J. Biol. Chem.*, 167, 869, 1947.

93. Pugh, E. L. and Wakil, S. J., Studies on the mechanism of fatty acid synthesis, *J. Biol. Chem.*, 240, 4727, 1965.

94. Plesofsky-Vig, N., Pantothenic acid, in *Present Knowledge in Nutrition,* 7th ed., Ziegler, E. E. and Filer, L. J., Jr., Eds., ILSI Press, Washington, D.C., 1996, chap. 23.

95. Smith, C. M. and Song, W. O., Comparative nutrition of pantothenic acid, *Nutr. Biochem.*, 7, 312, 1996.

96. Sauberlich, H. W. and Skala, J. H., in *Laboratory Tests for the Assessment of Nutritional Status*, CRC Press, Cleveland, OH, 1974, 88.

97. Annous, K. F. and Song, W. O., Pantothenic acid uptake and metabolism by red blood cells of rats, *J. Nutr.*, 125, 2586, 1995.

98. El-Habashy, M. and Eitenmiller, R. R., Pantothenic acid, in *Encyclopedia of Food Science,* Macrae, R., Robinson, R. K., and Sadler, M. J., Eds., Academic Press, San Diego, CA, 1993, 3399.

99. Velisek, J., Davidek, J. and Davidek, T., Pantothenic acid, in *Modern Chromatographic Analysis of Vitamins*, 2nd ed., De Leenheer, A. P., Lambert, W. E., and Nelis, H. J., Eds., Marcel Dekker, New York, 1992, chap. 13.

100. Ottaway, P. B., Appendix 1, in *The Technology of Vitamins in Food*, Chapman and Hall, Glasgow, 1993.

101. Fox, H. M., Pantothenic acid, in *Handbook of Vitamins*, 2nd ed., Machlin, L. J., Ed., Marcel Dekker, New York, 1991, chap. 11.

102. Goldsmith, S. J., Eitenmiller, R. R., Toledo, R. T., and Barnhart, H. M., Effects of processing and storage on the water-soluble vitamin content of human milk, *J. Food Sci.*, 48, 994, 1983.

103. Friedrich, W., Pantothenic acid, in *Vitamins*, Walter de Gruyter, New York, 1988, chap. 12.

104. Strohecker, R. and Henning, H. M., *Vitamin Assay, Tested Methods*, Verlag Chemie, Darmstadt, 1965.

105. Baker, H. and Frank, O., Pantothenic acid, in *Clinical Vitaminology*, Interscience Publishers, New York, 1968, chap. 6.

106. Freed, M., Pantothenic acid, in *Methods of Vitamin Assay*, 3rd ed., Interscience Publishers, 1966, chap. 9.

107. Wyse, B. V., Song, W. O., Walsh, J. H., and Hansen, R. G., Pantothenic acid, in *Methods of Vitamin Assay,* 4th ed., Augustin, J., Klein, B. P., Becker, D. A., and Venugopal, P.B., Eds., John Wiley & Sons, New York, 1985, chap. 16.

108. The United States Pharmacopeial Convention, *U.S. Pharmacopeia National Formulary*, USP/NF18, Nutritional Supplements, Official Monographs, United States Pharmacopeial Convention, Rockville, MD, 1995.

109. Voigt, M. N., Eitenmiller, R. R., and Ware, G. O., Vitamin assay by microbial and protozoan organisms: response to vitamin concentration, incubation time and assay vessel size, *J. Food Sci.,* 43, 1418, 1978.

110. Voigt, M. N., Eitenmiller, R. R., and Ware, G. O., Vitamin analysis by microbial and protozoan organisms: response to food preservatives and neutralization salts, *J. Food Sci.,* 44, 723, 1979.

111. Wyse, B. W., Wittwer, C., and Hansen, G., Radioimmunoassay for pantothenic acid in blood and other tissues, *Clin. Chem.,* 25, 108, 1979.

112. Walsh, J. H., Wyse, B. W., and Hansen, R. G., A comparison of microbiological and radioimmunoassay methods for the determination of pantothenic acid in foods, *J. Food Biochem.,* 3, 175, 1979.

113. Walsh, J. H., Wyse, B. W., and Hansen, R. G., Pantothenic acid content of 75 processed and cooked foods, *J. Am. Diet. Assoc.,* 78, 140, 1981.

114. Smith, A. H., Wyse, B. W., and Hansen, R. G., The development of an ELISA for pantothenate, *Fed. Proc.,* 40, 915, 1981.

115. Morris, H. C., Finglas, P. M., Faulks, R. M., and Morgan, M. R. A., The development of an enzyme-linked immunosorbent assay (ELISA) for the analysis of pantothenic acid and analogues, part I—production of antibodies and establishment of ELISA systems, *J. Micronutr. Anal.,* 4, 33, 1988.

116. Finglas, P. M., Faulks, R. M., Morris, H. C., Scott, K. J., and Morgan, M. R. A., The development of an enzyme-linked immunosorbent assay (ELISA) for the analysis of pantothenic acid analogues, part II—determination of pantothenic acid in foods, *J. Micronutr. Anal.,* 4, 47, 1988.

117. Song, W. O., Smith, A., Wittwer, C., Wyse, B., and Hansen, G., Determination of plasma pantothenic acid by indirect enzyme linked immunosorbent assay, *Nutr. Res.,* 10, 439, 1990.

118. Finglas, P. M. and Morgan, M. R. A., Application of biospecific methods to the determination of B-group vitamins in food—a review, *Food Chem.,* 49, 191, 1994.

119. Nag, S. S. and Das, S. K., Identification and quantitation of pantothenol and pantothenic acid in pharmaceutical preparations by thin-layer chromatography and densitometry, *J. AOAC Int.,* 75, 898, 1992.

120. Iwase, H., Determination of pantothenic acid in an elemental diet by column-switching high-performance liquid chromatography with ultraviolet detection, *Anal. Sci., 9 ,* 149, 1993.

121. Rômera, J. M., Ramirez, M., and Gil, A., Determination of pantothenic acid in infant milk formulas by high performance liquid chromatography, *J. Dairy Sci.,* 79, 523, 1996.

Table 12.1

Physical Properties of Vitamin B-12

1. Budavari, S., *The Merck Index*, 12th ed., Merck and Company, Whitehouse Station, NJ, 1996, 415, 825, 1033, 1710.

2. Friedrich, W., Vitamin B_{12}, in *Vitamins*, Walter de Gruyter, Berlin, 1988, chap. 13.

3. Committee on Food Chemicals Codex, *Food Chemicals Codex,* 4th ed., National Academy of Sciences, Washington, D.C., 1996, 431.

Table 12.2

Compendium, Regulatory and Handbook Methods for Analysis of Vitamin B-12

1. The United States Pharmacopeial Convention, *U.S. Pharmacopeia National Formulary*, USP23/NF18, Nutritional Supplements, Official Monograph, United States Pharmacopeial Convention, Rockville, MD, 1995, 2142.

2. Scottish Home and Health Department, *British Pharmacopoeia*, 15th ed., British Pharmacopoeia Commission, United Kingdom, 1993.

3. AOAC International, *Official Methods of Analysis*, 16th ed., AOAC International, Arlington, VA, 1995.

4. Loy, H. W., Report on revision of microbiological methods for the B vitamins, *J. Assoc. Off. Anal. Chem.,* 42, 529, 1959.
5. Tanner, J. T. and Barnett, S. A., Methods of analysis for infant formula: Food and Drug Administration and Infant Formula Council collaborative study, phase III, *J. Assoc. Off. Anal. Chem.,* 69, 777, 1986.
6. American Feed Ingredients Association, *Laboratory Methods Compendium. Vitamins and Minerals,* American Feed Ingredients Association, West Des Moines, IA, 1991, 163.
7. Keller, H. W., *Analyical Methods for Vitamins and Carotenoids*, Hoffmann-LaRoche, Basel, 1988, 36.
8. Skeggs, H. R., Vitamin B-12, in *The Vitamins,* vol, VIII, György, P. and Pearson, W.N., Eds., Academic Press, New York, 1967, chap. 9.
9. American Association of Cereal Chemists (AACC), *Approved Methods,* 9th ed., vol. 2, American Association of Cereal Chemists, St. Paul, MN, 1996.
10. Committee on Food Chemicals Codex, *Food Chemicals Codex,* 4th ed., National Academy of Sciences, Washington, D.C., 1996, 431.

Table 12.4

Physical Properties of Biotin

1. Ball, G. F. M., Chemical and biological nature of the water-soluble vitamins, in *Water-Soluble Vitamin Assays in Human Nutrition*, Chapman and Hall, New York, 1994, chap. 2.
2. Budavari, S., *The Merck Index*, 12th ed., Merck and Company, Whitehouse Station, NJ, 1996, 207.

Table 12.5

Compendium, Regulatory and Handbook Methods for the Analysis of Biotin

1. The United States Pharmacopeial Convention, *U.S. Pharmacopeia National Formulary,* USP23/NF18, Nutritional Supplements, Official Monographs, United States Pharmacopeial Convention, Rockville, MD, 1995, 2142.
2. American Feed Ingredients Association, *Laboratory Methods Compendium. Vitamins and Minerals,* American Feed Ingredients Association, West Des Moine, IA, 1991, 67.
3. Frigg, M. and Brubacher, G., Biotin deficiency in chicks fed a wheat-based diet, *Int. J. Vit. Nutr. Res.,* 46, 314, 1976.
4. Committee on Food Chemicals Codex, *Food Chemicals Codex*, 4th ed., National Academy of Sciences, Washington, D.C., 1996, 46.
5. Keller, H. E., *Analytical Methods for Vitamins and Carotenoids*, Hoffmann-LaRoche, Basel, 1988, 45.
6. Baker, H. and Frank, O., Biotin, in *Clinical Vitaminology*, Interscience Publishers, New York, 1968, chap. 3.

Table 12.6

Physical Properties of Pantothenic Acid, Salts and Pantothenol

1. Ball, G.F.M., Chemical and biological nature of the water-soluble vitamins, in *Water-Soluble Vitamin Assays in Human Nutrition*, Chapman and Hall, New York, 1994, chap. 2.
2. Budavari, S., *The Merck Index*, 12th ed., Merck and Company, Whitehouse Station, NJ, 1996, 499, 1205.

Table 12.7

Compendium, Regulatory, and Handbook Methods for the Analysis of Pantothenic Acid

1. The United States Pharmacopeial Convention, *U.S. Pharmacopeia National Formulary*, USP23/NF18, Nutritional Supplements, Official Monographs, United States Pharmacopeial Convention, Rockville, MD, 1995, 2142.
2. AOAC International, *Official Methods of Analysis*, 16th ed., AOAC International, Arlington, VA, 1995.

3. Loy, H.W., Report on revision of microbiological methods for the B vitamins, *J. Assoc. Off. Anal. Chem.*, *42,* 529, 1959.

4. Novelli, G.D. and Schmetz, F.J., An improved method for the determination of pantothenic acid in tissues, *J. Biol. Chem.*, 192, 181, 1951.

5. Tanner, J.T., Barnett, S.A. and Mountford, M. K., Analysis of milk-based infant formula, phase V. Vitamins A and E, folic acid and pantothenic acid. Food and Drug Administration—Infant Formula Council collaborative study, *J. AOAC Int.*, 76, 399, 1993.

6. American Feed Ingredients Association, *Laboratory Methods Compendium*, Vol. 1. *Vitamins and Minerals,* American Feed Ingredients Association, West Des Moines, IA, 1991, 73.

7. Keller, H.E., *Analytical Methods for Vitamins and Carotenoids*, Hoffmann-LaRoche Basel, 1988, 42.

8. Committee on Food Chemicals Codex, *Food Chemicals Codex*, 4th ed., National Academy of Sciences, Washington, D.C., 1996, 116.

Index

A